DEVELOPMENTS IN FOOD SCIENCE 29

FOOD SCIENCE AND HUMAN NUTRITION

DEVELOPMENTS IN FOOD SCIENCE 29

FOOD SCIENCE AND HUMAN NUTRITION

Edited by
GEORGE CHARALAMBOUS

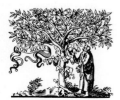

ELSEVIER
Amsterdam – London – New York – Tokyo 1992

ELSEVIER SCIENCE PUBLISHERS B.V.
Molenwerf 1
P.O. Box 211, 1000 AE Amsterdam, The Netherlands

Library of Congress Cataloging-in-Publication Data

Food science and human nutrition / edited by George Charalambous.
    p.   cm. -- (Developments in food science ; 29)
  ISBN 0-444-88834-9 (acid-free paper)
  1. Food--Composition. 2. Food--Analysis. 3. Nutrition.
I. Charalambous, George, 1922-   . II. Series.
TX531.F672 1992
664'.07--dc20   92-9175
                                                              CIP

ISBN 0-444-88834-9

© 1992 Elsevier Science Publishers B.V. All rights reserved.

No part of this publication may be reproduced, stored in a retrieval system or transmitted in any form or by any means, electronic, mechanical, photocopying, recording or otherwise, without the prior written permission of the publisher, Elsevier Science Publishers B.V., Permissions Department, P.O. Box 521, 1000 AM Amsterdam, The Netherlands.

Special regulations for readers in the USA – This publication has been registered with the Copyright Clearance Center Inc. (CCC), Salem, Massachusetts. Information can be obtained from the CCC about conditions under which photocopies of parts of this publication may be made in the USA. All other copyright questions, including photocopying outside of the USA, should be referred to the copyright owner, Elsevier Science Publishers B.V., unless otherwise specified.

No responsibility is assumed by the Publisher for any injury and/or damage to persons or property as a matter of products liability, negligence or otherwise, or from any use or operation of any methods, products, instructions or ideas contained in the material herein. Because of rapid advances in the medical sciences, the Publisher recommends that independent verification of diagnoses and drug dosages should be made.

pp. 183–210, 211–228, 437–450, 695–710, 711–722: copyright not transferred.

Printed on acid-free paper.

Printed in The Netherlands

DEVELOPMENTS IN FOOD SCIENCE

Volume 1   J.G. Heathcote and J.R. Hibbert
Aflatoxins: Chemical and Biological Aspects

Volume 2   H. Chiba, M. Fujimaki, K. Iwai, H. Mitsuda and Y. Morita (Editors)
Proceedings of the Fifth International Congress of Food Science and Technology

Volume 3   I.D. Morton and A.J. MacLeod (Editors)
Food Flavours
Part A. Introduction
Part B. The Flavour of Beverages
Part C. The Flavour of Fruits

Volume 4   Y. Ueno (Editor)
Trichothecenes: Chemical, Biological and Toxicological Aspects

Volume 5   J. Holas and J. Kratochvil (Editors)
Progress in Cereal Chemistry and Technology. Proceedings of the VIIth World Cereal and Bread Congress, Prague, 28 June-2 July 1982

Volume 6   I. Kiss
Testing Methods in Food Microbiology

Volume 7   H. Kurata and Y. Ueno (Editors)
Toxigenic Fungi: their Toxins and Health Hazard. Proceedings of the Mycotoxin Symposium, Tokyo, 30 August–3 September 1983

Volume 8   V. Betina (Editor)
Mycotoxins: Production, Isolation, Separation and Purification

Volume 9   J. Holló (Editor)
Food Industries and the Environment. Proceedings of the International Symposium, Budapest, Hungary, 9–11 September 1982

Volume 10   J. Adda (Editor)
Progress in Flavour Research 1984. Proceedings of the 4th Weurman Flavour Research Symposium, Dourdan, France, 9–11 May 1984

Volume 11   J. Holló (Editor)
Fat Science 1983. Proceedings of the 16th International Society for Fat Research Congress, Budapest, Hungary, 4–7 October 1983

Volume 12   G. Charalambous (Editor)
The Shelf Life of Foods and Beverages. Proceedings of the 4th International Flavor Conference, Rhodes, Greece, 23–26 July 1985

Volume 13   M. Fujimaki, M. Namiki and H. Kato (Editors)
Amino-Carbonyl Reactions in Food and Biological Systems. Proceedings of the 3rd International Symposium on the Maillard Reaction, Susuno, Shizuoka, Japan, 1–5 July 1985

Volume 14   J. Škoda and H. Škodova
Molecular Genetics. An Outline for Food Chemists and Biotechnologists

Volume 15   D.E. Kramer and J. Liston (Editors)
Seafood Quality Determination. Proceedings of the International Symposium, Anchorage, Alaska, U.S.A., 10–14 November 1986

Volume 16   R.C. Baker, P. Wong Hahn and K.R. Robbins
Fundamentals of New Food Product Development

Volume 17   G. Charalambous (Editor)
Frontiers of Flavor. Proceedings of the 5th International Flavor Conference, Porto Karras, Chalkidiki, Greece, 1–3 July 1987

Volume 18   B.M. Lawrence, B.D. Mookherjee and B.J. Willis (Editors)
Flavors and Fragrances: A World Perspective. Proceedings of the 10th International Congress of Essential Oils, Fragrances and Flavors, Washington, DC, U.S.A., 16–20 November 1986

Volume 19   G. Charalambous and G. Doxastakis (Editors)
Food Emulsifiers: Chemistry, Technology, Functional Properties and Applications

Volume 20   B.W. Berry and K.F. Leddy
Meat Freezing. A Source Book

Volume 21	J. Davídek, J. Velíšek and J. Pokorný (Editors)	
	Chemical Changes during Food Processing	
Volume 22	V. Kyzlink	
	Principles of Food Perservation	
Volume 23	H. Niewiadomski	
	Rapeseed. Chemistry and Technology	
Volume 24	G. Charalambous (Editor)	
	Flavors and Off-Flavors '89. Proceedings of the 6th International Flavor Conference, Rethymnon, Crete, Greece, 5–7 July 1989	
Volume 25	R. Rouseff (Editor)	
	Bitterness in Foods and Beverages	
Volume 26	J. Chełkowski (Editor)	
	Cereal Grain. Mycotoxins, Fungi and Quality in Drying and Storage	
Volume 27	M. Verzele and D. De Keukeleire	
	Chemistry and Analysis of Hop and Beer Bitter Acids	
Volume 28	G. Charalambous (Editor)	
	Off-Flavors in Foods and Beverages	
Volume 29	G. Charalambous (Editor)	
	Food Science and Human Nutrition	

PREFACE

As Burns phrased it, the best laid schemes, etc., and plans for the Seventh International Conference scheduled for June 1991 at Samos did gang agley because of the uncertainties of the then political situation.

Frustrated would-be participants dubbed the aborted Conference "notional", "mirage", "now-you-see-it, now-you-don't". They all lobbied the Organizers for publication of their current research reports at this point in time, pledging other up-to-date papers and chapters for a rescheduled Conference in 1992.

This series of meetings, going back to 1977, has always attempted to bring together active researchers from all parts of the world for a relaxed discussion of their research results and technological interests, resulting in a timely publication of a compilation of up-to-date working documents.

In view of this, the Conference Organizers and the Publishers decided to include in this volume the sixty-odd papers that would have been presented at Samos in 1991. Their authors include both some founding fathers (and mothers) of these fourteen-year-old meetings and some new blood. We would particularly like to welcome newcomers from Egypt, Turkey, Brazil, Singapore - all educated in Europe and/or North America and now successfully conducting research in their own countries.

We wish to thank the Publishers for their forbearance and all contributors to this "mirage" Conference for up-to-date reports on their current research in Food Science and Human Nutrition.

The Seventh International Conference on Recent Developments in Food Science and Human Nutrition has been rescheduled for June 24-26, 1992 at Pythagorion, Samos Island in Greece, and its Proceedings will again be published by Elsevier.

The Editor

CONTENTS

Preface vii

List of Contributors xv

Developments of a Microbially Catalyzed Oxidation System 1
    S.J.B. DUFF and W.D. MURRAY

Evaluation of *Urtica* Species as Potential Sources of Important Nutrients 15
    H. WETHERILT

Alternates to Synthetic Antioxidants 27
    R.J. EVANS and G.S. REYNHOUT

Utilization of Cottonseed Protein in Preparing New Edible Food Products 43
    Y.G. MOHARRAM and N.S. ABU-FOUL

Computer-Aided Organic Synthesis Applied to the Study of Formation of
Aroma Compounds. Thermal Degradation of Diallyl Disulfide 75
    G. VERNIN, J. METZGER, P. AZARIO, R. BARONE, M. ARBELOT
    and M. CHANON

Formation of Aroma by Hydrolysis of Glycosidically Bound Components 99
    V. REYNE, C. SALLES and J. CROUZET

The Effect of Carbon and Nitrogen Sources on the Growth and Aroma
Production of *Penicillium italicum* 115
    L.F.M. YONG

The Computer Simulation of the Chemical Kinetics of Flavor Compounds
in Heated Foods 123
    A.E. GROSSER

Flavor Compounds in Maple Syrup 131
    I. ALLI, E. AKOCHI-K and S. KERMASHA

A Rapid Method for Monitoring Food Volatiles 141
    J.R.J. PARE, J.M.R. BELANGER, A. BELANGER and N. RAMARATHNAM

Bramble Dried Leaf Volatiles 145
    J.A. MAGA, C.K. SQUIRE and H.G. HUGHES

Influence of Variety and Location of Growth on Resulting
Bramble Dried Leaf Volatiles 149
    J.A. MAGA, C.K. SQUIRE and H.G. HUGHES

Steam Volatile Constituents from Seeds of *Momordica charantia* L. 153
    M. KIKUCHI, T. ISHIKAWA, T. IIDA, S. SETO, T. TAMURA
    and T. MATSUMOTO

Comparison of Volatile Components in Two Naranjilla Fruit (*Solanum quitoense* Lam.) Pulp from Different Origins 163
    P. BRUNERIE and P. MAUGEAIS

Analysis of the Volatile Constituents of a Special Type of White Bread 175
    M.E. KOMAITIS, G. ANGELOUSIS and N. GIANNONITS-ARGYRIADIS

Defining Roasted Peanut Flavor Quality. Part I. Correlation of GC Volatiles with Roast Color as an Estimate of Quality 183
    J.R. VERCELLOTTI, K.L. CRIPPEN, N.V. LOVEGREN and T.H. SANDERS

Defining Roasted Peanut Flavor Quality. Part II. Correlation of GC Volatiles and Sensory Flavor Attributes 211
    K.L. CRIPPEN, J.R. VERCELLOTTI, N.V. LOVEGREN and T.H. SANDERS

Growth Response of the Mushroom *Agaricus campestris* to Nitrogen Sources when Cultivated in Submerged Fermentation 229
    A.M. MARTIN

Study of the Growth and Biomass Composition of the Edible Mushroom *Pleurotus ostreatus* 239
    A.M. MARTIN

Improved Retention of Mushroom Flavor in Microwave-Hot Air Drying 249
    L.F. DI CESARE, M. RIVA and A. SCHIRALDI

Study of the Interaction between Polyvinyl Chloride and Vinyl Chloride Monomer using Inverse Gas Chromatography - Thermodynamic and Structural Considerations 257
    D. APOSTOLOPOULOS

Inverse Gas Chromatographic Study of Moisture Sorption by Wheat and Soy Flour and the Effect of Specific Heat Treatment on their Sorption Behavior 277
    K.A. RIGANAKOS, P.G. DEMERTZIS and M.G. KONTOMINAS

Application of a Modified I.G.C. Method in the Study of the Water Sorptional Behavior of Selected Proteins. I. Lysozyme-Water Interactions 287
    P.G. DEMERTZIS, S.G. GILBERT and H. DAUN

Application of a Modified I.G.C. Method in the Study of the Water Sorptional Behavior of Selected Proteins. II. Gliadin-Water Interactions 303
    P.G. DEMERTZIS, S.G. GILBERT and H. DAUN

Water Sorption Hysteresis in Potato Starch and Egg Albumin 313
    M. LAGOUDAKI and P.G. DEMERTZIS

Study of Water Vapor Diffusion Through Plastic Packaging Materials Using Inverse Gas Chromatography 321
    P.J. KALAOUZIS and P.G. DEMERTZIS

Diffusion of Water in Starch Materials 329
    G.D. SARAVACOS, V.T. KARATHANOS and S.N. MAROUSIS

→Soluble Coffee's New Biotechnology 341
    R.L. COLTON

Aroma of Chinese Scented Green Tea with *Citrus aurantium* var. *arama* 347
    S.-J. LUO, W.-F. GUO and H.-J. FU

Design and Application of a Multifunctional Column Switching
GC-MSD System 351
    K. MacNAMARA, P. BRUNERIE, S. KECK and A. HOFFMANN

Sensory and Analytical Evaluation of Hop Oil Oxygenated Fractions 371
    N.B. SANCHEZ, C.L. LEDERER, G.B. NICKERSON, L.M. LIBBEY
    and M.R. McDANIEL

→Sensory and Analytical Evaluation of Beers Brewed with Three Varieties
of Hops and an Unhopped Beer 403
    N.B. SANCHEZ, C.L. LEDERER, G.B. NICKERSON, L.M. LIBBEY
    and M.R. McDANIEL

Nitrate Mass-Balance in the Brewing Industry 427
    M. MOLL, S. CHEVRIER, N. MOLL and J.P. JOLY

Extractability of Catechins and Proanthocyanidins of Grape Seeds 437
    E. REVILLA, E. ALONSO, M. BOURZEIX and V. KOVAC

→Low-Alcohol Content Wine-Like Beverages. Storage Stability of
those Obtained from Dealcoholized Wines 451
    M.D. SALVADOR, R. PEREZ, M.D. CABEZUDO, P.J. MARTIN-ALVAREZ
    and L. IZQUIERDO

Synthesis of Optically Active Whisky Lactone 469
    Y. NODA and M. KIKUCHI

Effect of Copper, Potassium, Sodium and Calcium on Alcoholic Fermentation
of Raisin Extract and Sucrose Solution 475
    K. AKRIDA-DEMERTZI and A.A. KOUTINAS

Microbiological Changes During the Ripening of Turkish White Pickled Cheese 491
    M. KARAKUS and I. ALPERDEN

Problems Associated with the Processing of Cucumber Pickles: Softening,
Bloater Formation and Environmental Pollution 499
    A.A. GUILLOU and J.D. FLOROS

Retention of Added Acids During the Extrusion of Corn Starch/Isolated Soy
Protein Blends 515
    J.A. MAGA and C.H. KIM

Binding During Extrusion of Added Flavorants as Influenced by
Starch and Protein Types 519
    J.A. MAGA and C.H. KIM

Capsaicinoids: Analogue Composition of Commercial Products 526
    J.A. MAGA and H. BEL-HAJ

Influence of Cultivar and Processing on Peach Drink
Acceptability and Yield 531
    J.A. MAGA and R.A. RENQUIST

Subjective and Objective Comparison of Baked Potato Aroma as Influenced
by Variety/Clone 537
    J.A. MAGA and D.G. HOLM

Investigation of the Properties Influencing Popcorn Popping Quality 543
    J.A. MAGA and B. BLACH

Spaghetti Products Containing Dried Distillers Grains 551
    K. VAN EVEREN, J.A. MAGA and K. LORENZ

Comparison of Preferences for Salty and Umami Flavours Between Two
Ethnic Groups of Different Dietary Habits 565
    M.L. LAW and J.R. PIGGOTT

Enzymatic Hydration of (4R)-(+)-Limonene to (4R)-(+)-alpha-Terpineol 571
    K.R. CADWALLADER and R.J. BRADDOCK

Interesterification of Palm Oil Mid Fraction by Immobilized Lipase in
n-Hexane: Effect of Lecithin Addition 585
    L. MOJOVIC and S. SHILER-MARINKOVIC

Potential Applications of Supercritical Carbon Dioxide
Separations in Soybean Processing 595
    Ž.L. NIKOLOV, P. MAHESHWARI, J.E. HARDWICK, P.A. MURPHY
    and L.A. JOHNSON

Effects of Glucose Oxidase-Catalase on the Flavor Stability
of Model Salad Dressings 617
    D.B. MIN and B.S. MISTRY

Fatty Acid Composition of the Total, Neutral and Phospholipids
of the Brazilian Freshwater Fish *Colossoma macropomum* 633
    E.L. MAIA and D.B. RODRIGUEZ-AMAYA

Carotenoid Composition of the Tropical Fruits *Eugenia uniflora* and
Malpighia glabra 643
    M.L. CAVALCANTE and D.B. RODRIGUEZ-AMAYA

Food Emulsions in Extruded Glassy Materials 651
    F.Z. SALEEB, J.L. CAVALLO and S. VIDAL

An Overview of Aseptic Processing of Particulate Foods 665
    N.G. STOFOROS

Diabetes: Food Nutrition, Diet and Weight Control 679
    A.A. KHAN

Current Approaches to the Study of Meat Flavor Quality 695
    A.M. SPANIER

Preparation and Use of Food Grade N-Carboxymethylchitosan to Prevent
Meat Flavor Deterioration 711
    A.J. St. ANGELO and J.R. VERCELLOTTI

Consumer Acceptability of Algin Restructured Beef 723
    J.A. MAGA, L. DWYER and G.R. SCHMIDT

Formation of Dialkylthiophenes in Maillard Reactions Involving Cysteine 731
    G.P. RIZZI, A.R. STEIMLE and D.R. PATTON

Listeria monocytogenes and its Fate in Meat Products 743
    J.N. SOFOS

Extrusion Cooking of Chicken Meat with Various Nonmeat Ingredients 761
    A.S. BA-JABER, J.N. SOFOS, G.R. SCHMIDT and J.A. MAGA

A Method for Determining Binding of Hexanal by Myosin and Actin Using
Equilibrium Headspace Sampling Gas Chromatography 783
    R.A. GUTHEIL and M.E. BAILEY

Subject Index 817

LIST OF CONTRIBUTORS

Numbers in parentheses indicate where contributions begin

N.S. ABU FOUL (43) Omar El-Mokhtar Street, El Remal, 54-163 Gaza Palestine

E. AKOCHI-K. (131) Food Science and Agricultural Chemistry Department,
McGill University, P.O. Box 187, Macdonald Campus, Ste-Anne de Bellevue,
Québec, Canada H9X 1CO

K. AKRIDA-DEMERTZI (475) Department of Chemistry, University of Ioannina,
P.O. Box 1186, GR-45 110 Ioannina, Greece

I. ALLI (131) Food Science and Agricultural Chemistry Department,
McGill University, P.O. Box 187, Macdonald Campus, Ste-Anne de Bellevue,
Québec, Canada H9X 1CO

E. ALONSO (437) Departamento de Química Agrícola, Geología y Geoquímica,
Universidad Autónoma de Madrid, E-28049 Madrid, Spain

I. ALPERDEN (491) Department of Nutrition and Food Technology, TÜBITAK, P.O. Box 21,
41470 Gebze-Kocaeli, Turkey

G. ANGELOUSIS (175) Department of Food Technology, School of Food Technology and
Nutrition, T.E.I. of Athens, St. Spyridon Street, Egaleo, GR-122 10 Athens, Greece

D. APOSTOLOPOULOS (257) Kraft General Foods, General Foods U.S.A., Packaging
Evaluation Center, South Broadway, Tarrytown, NY 10591, U.S.A.

N. ARBELOT (75) Laboratoire AM3, URA 1411, Faculté des Sciences de Saint Jérôme,
Avenue Escadrille Normandie-Niemen, Case 561, F-13397 Marseille Cedex 13, France

P. AZARIO (75) Laboratoire AM3, URA 1411, Faculté des Sciences de Saint Jérôme,
Avenue Escadrille Normandie-Niemen, Case 561, F-13397 Marseille Cedex 13, France

A.S. BA-JABER (761) Department of Food Science, King Saud University, Riyadh,
Saudi Arabia

M.E. BAILEY (783) Department of Food Science and Nutrition, University of Missouri-
Columbia, Agriculture 21, Columbia, MO 65211, U.S.A.

R. BARONE (75) Laboratoire AM3, URA 1411, Faculté des Sciences de Saint Jérôme,
Avenue Escadrille Normandie-Niemen, Case 561, F-13397 Marseille Cedex 13, France

H. BEL-HAJ (526) Department of Food Science and Human Nutrition, Corlorado
State University, Fort Collins, CO 80523, U.S.A.

A. BELANGER (141) Agriculture Canada, Station de Recherches, St-Jean-sur-Richelieu, Québec, Canada J2S 8E3

J.M.R. BELANGER (141) Agriculture Canada, Food Research Centre, St. Hyacinthe, Québec, Canada J2S 8E3

B. BLACH (543) Colorado Cereals, Yuma, CO 80759, U.S.A.

M. BOURZEIX (437) Station Expérimentale de Pech Rouge-Narbonne, INRA, Bd. General de Gaulle, F-11100 Narbonne, France

R.J. BRADDOCK (571) IFAS, Citrus Research and Education Center, University of Florida, Lake Alfred, FL 33850, U.S.A.

P. BRUNERIE (163, 351) Centre de Recherche Pernod-Ricard, 120 Av. du Marechal Foch, F-94015 Créteil, France

M.D. CABEZUDO (451) Instituto de Fermentaciones Industriales (CSIC), Juan de la Cierva 3, E-28006 Madrid, Spain

K.R. CADWALLADER (571), Department of Food Science, Louisiana State University, Baton Rouge, LA 70803, U.S.A.

M.L. CAVALCANTE (643) Departamento de Nutriçao, Universidade Federal de Pernambuco, 50379 Recife, PE, Brazil

J.L. CAVALLO (651) General Foods U.S.A., 250 North Street, White Plains, NY 10625, U.S.A.

M. CHANON (75) Laboratoire AM3, URA 1411, Faculté des Sciences de Saint Jérôme, Avenue Escadrille Normandie-Niemen, Case 561, F-13397 Marseille Cedex 13, France

S. CHEVRIER (427) Cervac-Est, 1 Allée Chaptal, F-54630 Richardmenil, France

R.L. COLTON (341) BRAMCAFE International Ltd, 101 Tanglewood Drive, Lansdale, PA 19446, U.S.A.

K.L. CRIPPEN (183, 211) Southern Regional Research Center, U.S. Department of Agriculture, Agricultural Research Service, 1100 Robert E. Lee Blvd, New Orleans, LA 70124, U.S.A.

J. CROUZET (99) Génie Biologique et Sciences des Aliments, Institut des Sciences de l'Ingénieur de Montpellier, Université de Montpellier II - Sciences et Techniques du Languedoc, F-34095 Montpellier Cedex 05, France

H. DAUN (287, 303) Department of Food Science and the Center for Advanced Food Technology, Cook College, Rutgers University, P.O. Box 231, New Brunswick, NJ 08903, U.S.A.

P.G. DEMERTZIS (277, 287, 303, 313, 321) Laboratory of Food Chemistry, University of Ioannina, GR-451 10 Ioannina, Greece

L.F. DI CESARE (249) I.V.T.P.A., via Venezian 26, I-20133 Milano, Italy

S.J.B. DUFF (1) Energy, Mines and Resources Canada, Alternative Energy Division, Rm. 744, 580 Booth St., Ottawa, Ontario, Canada K1A 0E4

L. DWYER (723) Department of Food Science and Human Nutrition, Colorado State University, Fort Collins, CO 80523, U.S.A.

R.J. EVANS (27) KALSEC Inc., 3713 West Main St., Kalamazoo, MI 49007, U.S.A.

J.D. FLOROS (499) Department of Food Science, Purdue University, 1160 Smith Hall, West Lafayette, IN 47907, U.S.A.

H.-J. FU (347) Hangzhou Tea Processing Research Institute of the Ministry of Commerce, Hangzhou, Zhejiang, People's Republic of China

N. GIANNONITS-ARGYRIADIS (175) VIORYL, Kato Kifissia, GR-145 64 Athens, Greece

S.G. GILBERT (287, 303) Department of Food Science and the Center for Advanced Food Technology, Cook College, Rutgers University, P.O. Box 231, New Brunswick, NJ 08903, U.S.A.

A.E. GROSSER (123) Department of Chemistry, McGill University, 801 Sherbrooke St. West, Montreal, PQ, Canada H3A 2K6

A.A. GUILLOU (499) Department of Food Science, Purdue University, 1160 Smith Hall, West Lafayette, IN 47907, U.S.A.

W.F. GUO (347) Hangzhou Tea Processing Research Institute of the Ministry of Commerce, Hangzhou, Zhejiang, People's Republic of China

R.A. GUTHEIL (783) Department of Food Science and Nutrition, University of Missouri-Columbia, Columbia, MO 65211, U.S.A.

J.E. HARDWICK (595) Center for Crops Utilization Research, Iowa State University, Ames, IA 50011, U.S.A.

A. HOFFMANN (351) Gerstel GmbH, Aktienstrasse 232-234, D-4330 Mülheim a/d Ruhr, Germany

D.G. HOLM (537) San Luis Valley Research Center, Colorado State University, Center, CO 80759, U.S.A.

W.G. HUGHES (145) Department of Horticulture, Colorado State University, Fort Collins, CO 80523, U.S.A.

T. IIDA (153) Department of Industrial Chemistry, College of Engineering, Nihon University, Koriyama, Fukushima-ken 963, Japan

T. ISHIKAWA (153) Department of Industrial Chemistry, College of Engineering, Nihon University, Koriyama, Fukushima-ken 963, Japan

L. IZQUIERDO (451) Instituto de Agroquímica y Tecnología de Alimentos (CSIC), Jaime Roig 11, E-46019 Valencia, Spain

L.A. JOHNSON (595) Center for Crops Utilization Research, Iowa State University, Ames, IA 50011, U.S.A.

J.P. JOLY (427) Laboratoire de Chimie Organique 3, URA 486, B.P. 239, F-54506 Vandoeuvre Cedex, France

P.J. KALAOUZIS (321) Laboratory of Food Chemistry, Department of Chemistry, University of Ioannina, GR-451 10 Ioannina, Greece

M. KARAKUŞ (491) Department of Nutrition and Food Technology, TÜBITAK, P.O. Box 21, 41470 Gebze-Koacaeli, Turkey

V. KARATHANOS (329) Food Science Department and Center for Advanced Technology, Rutgers University, New Brunswick, NJ 08903, U.S.A.

S. KECK (351) Irish Distillers Group, Bow Street, Smithfield, Dublin 7, Republic of Ireland

S. KERMASHA (131) Food Science and Agricultural Chemistry Department, McGill University, P.O. Box 187, Macdonald Campus, Ste-Anne de Bellevue, Québec, Canada H9X 1CO

A.A. KHAN (679) Applied Research Inc., P.O. Box 1486, Hawthorne, CA 90250, U.S.A.

M. KIKUCHI (153, 469) Department of Industrial Chemistry, College of Engineering, Nihon University, Koriyama, Fukushima-ken 963, Japan

C.H. KIM (515, 519) Department of Food Science and Human Nutrition, Colorado State University, Fort Collins, CO 80523, U.S.A.

M.E. KOMAITIS (175) Department of Agricultural Industries, Agricultural University of Athens, Iera Odos 75, Votanikos, GR-118 55 Athens, Greece

M.G. KONTOMINAS (277) Laboratory of Food Chemistry, Department of Chemistry, University of Ioannina, GR-451 10 Ioannina, Greece

A.A. KOUTINAS (475) Department of Chemistry, University of Patras, GR-261 10 Patras, Greece

V. KOVAC (437) Faculty of Technology, University of Novi Sad, 21000 Novi Sad, Yugoslavia

M. LAGOUDAKI (313) Laboratory of Food Chemistry, Department of Chemistry, University of Ioannina, GR-451 10 Ioannina, Greece

M.L. LAW (565) Department of Bioscience and Biotechnology, University of Strathclyde, 131 Albion Street, Glasgow G1 1SD, Scotland, U.K.

C.L. LEDERER (371, 403) Sensory Science Laboratory, Department of Food Science and Technology, Wiegand Hall, Oregon State University, Corvallis, OR 97336, U.S.A.

L.M. LIBBEY (371, 403) Agricultural Chemistry Department, Oregon State University, Corvallis, OR 97331, U.S.A.

K. LORENZ (551) Department of Food Science and Human Nutrition, Colorado State University, Fort Collins, CO 80523, U.S.A.

N.V. LOVEGREN (183, 211) Southern Regional Research Center, U.S. Department of Agriculture, Agricultural Research Service, 1100 Robert E. Lee Blvd, New Orleans, LA 70124, U.S.A.

S.-J. LUO (347) Hangzhou Tea Processing Research Institute of the Ministry of Commerce, Hangzhou, Zhejiang, People's Republic of China

K. MacNAMARA (351) Irish Distillers Group, Bow Street, Smithfield, Dublin 7, Republic of Ireland

M.R. McDANIEL (371, 403) Sensory Science Laboratory, Department of Food Science and Technology, Oregon State University, Corvallis, OR 97336, U.S.A.

J.A. MAGA (145, 149, 515, 519, 526, 531, 537, 543, 551, 723, 761) Department of Food Science and Human Nutrition, Colorado State University, Fort Collins, CO 80523, U.S.A.

P. MAHESHWARI (595) Department of Food Science and Human Nutrition, Iowa State University, Ames, IA 50011, U.S.A.

E.L. MAIA (633) Departamento de Ciencia de Alimentos, Faculdade de Engenharia de Alimentos, Universidade Estadual de Campinas, C.P. 6121, 13081 Campinas, SP, Brazil

S.N. MAROUSIS (329) Central Engineering, Procter and Gamble Co., Cincinnati, OH 45232, U.S.A.

A.M. MARTIN (229, 239) Food Science Program, Department of Biochemisty, Memorial University of Newfoundland, St. John's, Newfoundland, Canada A1B 3X9

P.J. MARTIN-ALVAREZ (451) Instituto de Fermentaciones Industriales (CSIC), Juan de la Cierva 3, E-28006 Madrid, Spain

T. MATSUMOTO (153) Department of Industrial Chemistry, College of Engineering, Nihon University, Koriyama, Fukushima-ken 963, Japan

P. MAUGEAIS (163) Université du Havre, B.P. 540, Le Havre Cedex, France

P. METZGER (75) Laboratoire de Chimie Moléculaire, URA 1411, Faculté des Sciences de Saint Jérôme, Avenue Escadrille Normandie-Niemen, Case 561, F-13397 Marseille Cedex 13, France

D.B. MIN (617) Department of Food Science and Technology, The Ohio State University, 2121 Fyffe Road, Columbus, OH 43210, U.S.A.

B.S. MISTRY (617) Department of Food Science and Technology, The Ohio State University, 2121 Fyffe Road, Columbus, OH 43210, U.S.A.

Y.G. MOHARRAM (43) Food Science and Technology Department, Faculty of Agriculture, Alexandria University, Alexandria, Egypt

L. MOJOVIC (585) Biochemistry Engineering Department, Faculty of Technology and Metallurgy, P.O. Box 494, 11001 Belgrade, Yugoslavia

M. MOLL (427) Cervac-Est, 1 Allée Chaptal, F-54630 Richardmenil, France

N. MOLL (427) Laboratoire de Chimie Organique 3, URA 486, B.P. 239, F-54506 Vandoeuvre Cedex, France

P.A. MURPHY (595) Department of Food Science and Human Nutrition, Iowa State University, Ames, IA 50011, U.S.A.

W.D. MURRAY (1) Science and Technology Division, Library of Parliament, Ottawa, Ontario, Canada K1A 0A9

G.B. NICKERSON (371, 403) Agricultural Chemistry Department, Oregon State University, Corvallis, OR 97336, U.S.A.

Ž.L. NIKOLOV (595) Department of Food Science and Human Nutrition, Iowa State University, Ames, IA 50011, U.S.A.

Y. NODA (469) Department of Industrial Chemistry, College of Engineering, Nihon University, Koriyama, Fukushima-ken 963, Japan

J.R.J. PARÉ (141) Environment Canada, R.R.E.T.C., Ottawa, Ontario, Canada K1A 0H3

D.R. PATTON (731) Procter and Gamble Co., Miami Valley Laboratories, Cincinnati, OH 45239, U.S.A.

R. PEREZ (451) Instituto de Agroquímica y Tecnología de Alimentos (CSIC), Jaime Roig 11, E-46019 Valencia, Spain

J.R. PIGGOTT (565) Department of Bioscience and Biotechnology, University of Strathclyde, 131 Albion Street, Glasgow G1 1SD, Scotland, U.K.

N. RAMARATHNAM (141) Agriculture Canada, Food Research Centre, St. Hyacinthe, Quebec, Canada J2S 8E3

R.A. RENQUIST (531) Orchard Mesa Research Center, Colorado State University, Grand Junction, CO 81503, U.S.A.

E. REVILLA (437) Departamento de Química Agrícola, Geología y Geoquímica, Universidad Autónoma de Madrid, E-28049 Madrid, Spain

V. REYNE (99) Génie Biologique et Sciences des Aliments, Institut des Sciences de l'Ingenieur de Montpellier, Université de Montpellier II - Sciences et Techniques du Languedoc, F-34095 Montpellier Cedex 05, France

G.S. REYNHOUT (27) KALSEC Inc., 3713 West Main Street, Kalamazoo, MI 49007, U.S.A.

K.A. RIGANAKOS (277) Laboratory of Food Chemistry, Department of Chemistry, University of Ioannina, GR-451 10 Ioannina, Greece

M. RIVA (249) D.I.S.T.A.M., Sezione Tecnologie Alimentari, Università di Milano, via Celoria 2, I-20133 Milano, Italy

G.P. RIZZI (731) Procter and Gamble Co., Miami Valley Laboratories, Cincinnati, OH 45239, U.S.A.

D.B. RODRIGUEZ-AMAYA (633, 643) Departamento de Ciencia de Alimentos, Faculdade de Engenharia de Alimentos, Universidade Estadual de Campinas, C.P. 6121, 13081 Campinas, SP, Brazil

A.J. ST. ANGELO (711) Southern Regional Research Center, U.S. Department of Agriculture, New Orleans, LA 70124, U.S.A.

F.Z. SALEEB (651) General Foods U.S.A., 250 North Street, White Plains, NY 10625, U.S.A.

C. SALLES (99) Laboratoire de Recherches sur les Arômes, INRA, 17 rue Sully, F-21034 Dijon Cedex, France

M.D. SALVADOR (451) Facultad de Ciencias Químicas, Paseo de la Universidad 4, E-13071 Ciudad Real, Spain

N.B. SANCHEZ (371, 403) CIATI - Bartolomé Mitre y 20 de Junio, (8336) Villa Regina - Rio Negro, Argentina

T.H. SANDERS (183, 211) National Peanut Research Laboratory, U.S. Department of Agriculture, Agricultural Research Service, 1011 Forrester Drive S.E., Dawson, GA 31742, U.S.A.

G.D. SARAVACOS (329) Food Science Department and Center for Advanced Food Technology, Rutgers University, New Brunswick, NJ 08903, U.S.A.

A. SCHIRALDI (249) D.I.S.T.A.M., Sezione Tecnologie Alimentari, Università di Milano, via Celoria 2, I-20133 Milano, Italy

G.R. SCHMIDT (723, 761) Department of Animal Sciences, Colorado State University, Fort Collins, CO 80523, U.S.A.

S. SETO (153) Department of Industrial Chemistry, College of Engineering, Nihon University, Koriyama, Fukushima-ken 963, Japan

S. SHILER-MARINKOVITZ (585) Biochemistry Engineering Department, Faculty of Technology and Metallurgy, P.O. Box 494, 1101 Belgrade, Yugoslavia

J.N. SOFOS (743, 761) Departments of Animal Sciences and Food Science and Human Nutrition, Colorado State University, Fort Collins, CO 80523, U.S.A.

A.M. SPANIER (695) Food Flavor Quality - Meat Program, U.S. Department of Agriculture, Agricultural Research Service, Southern Regional Research Center, 1100 Robert E. Lee Blvd, New Orleans, LA 70124, U.S.A.

C.K. SQUIRE (145) Department of Food Science and Human Nutrition, Colorado Sate University, Fort Collins, CO 80523, U.S.A.

A.R. STEIMLE (731) Procter and Gamble Co., Miami Valley Laboratories, Cincinnati, OH 45239, U.S.A..

N.G. STOFOROS (665) National Food Processors Association, 6363 Clark Avenue, Dublin, CA 94568, U.S.A.

T. TAMURA (153) Department of Industrial Chemistry, College of Science and Technology, Nihon University, Kanda-ku, Tokyo 101, Japan

K. VAN EVEREN (551) Department of Food Science and Nutrition, Colorado State University, Fort Collins, CO 80523, U.S.A.

J.R. VERCELLOTTI (183, 211, 711) Southern Regional Research Center, U.S. Department of Agriculture, Agricultural Research Service, 1100 Robert E. Lee Blvd, New Orleans, LA 70124, U.S.A.

G. VERNIN (75) Laboratoire de Chimie Moléculaire, URA 1411, Faculté des Sciences de Saint Jérôme, Avenue Escadrille Normandie-Niemen, Case 561, F-13397 Marseille Cedex 13, France

S. VIDAL (651) General Foods U.S.A., 250 North Street, White Plains, NY 10625, U.S.A.

H. WETHERILT (15) Department of Nutrition and Food Technology, TÜBITAK, P.O. Box 21, 41470 Gebze-Kocaeli, Turkey

L.F.M. YONG (115) Aroma Biotech Pte Ltd, 6 Shenton Way, #29-01 DBS Building, Singapore 0106, Republic of Singapore

G. Charalambous (Ed.), Food Science and Human Nutrition
© 1992 Elsevier Science Publishers B.V. All rights reserved.

DEVELOPMENT OF A MICROBIALLY CATALYSED OXIDATION SYSTEM

S.J.B. Duff[1] and W.D. Murray[2]

[1]Energy, Mines and Resources Canada, Alternative Energy Division, Rm 774, 580 Booth Street, Ottawa, Ontario, CANADA K1A 0E4.

[2]Science and Technology Division, Library of Parliament, Ottawa, Ontario, CANADA, K1A 0A9.

SUMMARY

In the 1980's chemical food additives came under increasing public scruitiny. As a result, food and flavour companies became keenly interested in the development of naturally derived flavouring compounds. It was in this enviornment that an effort was undertaken to develop microbially-, or enzyme-catalysed reactions for the production of a range of important flavouring components of foods and beverages. This paper describes the inception, development and conclusion of a research program directed toward the development of a biotechnology-based flavour industry.

INTRODUCTION

In the early 1980's public concern over chemical food additives, led to more efforts on the part of the food industry to replace these artificial flavouring compounds with natural source compounds. As part of this trend, and with industrial cooperation, a small group at the National Research Council began to explore the practical potential for using microbes to produce a variety of flavouring compounds.

Initial efforts focused on the production of acetaldehyde, an ethereal and sharply pungent compound of which considerable quantities (147,678 kg) were used to impart a "freshness" to processed foods (1). A process for the was developed for the production of acetaldehyde and ethyl acetate using *Candida utilis*, a widely used food grade yeast (2). However, largely owing to the fact that these compounds were intermediates in the alcohol-dehydrogenase-catalysed pathway leading to ethanol, product yields were extremely low, and control requirements stringent (3). A search for more suitable organisms quickly led to a group of yeast which were able to grow using methanol as their sole carbon source. This unique ability was a result of alcohol oxidase, an inducible enzyme which catalyses the initial alcohol to aldehyde oxidation, the first step in a degrative pathway which eventually led to CO_2 and H_2O (Figure 1).

THE ALCOHOL OXIDASE ENZYME SYSTEM

Alcohol oxidase is an FAD-dependant enzyme consisting of a number of identical subunits (4). When some species of the

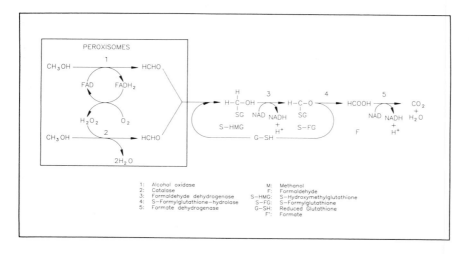

Fig. 1. The alcohol oxidase enzyme system of *Pichia pastoris*

genera *Pichia*, *Hansenula*, *Candida*, and *Torulopsis* are grown on limiting amounts of methanol, sub-cellular organelles known as peroxisomes, containing alcohol oxidase and catalase, are synthesized (5). These enzymes act in concert to oxidize methanol to formaldehyde. Peroxide produced in the regeneration of the cofactor is degraded by catalase. When whole cells are exposed to alcohols other than methanol, the alcohol oxidase-catalysed alcohol to aldehyde oxidation is carried out, however, further degradation of the aldehyde is prevented by the substrate specificity of the second enzyme in the pathway, formaldehyde dehydrogenase (6). As a result, the aldehyde product accumulates, and non-growing whole cells can be used as biocatalysts in a range of processes for the production of oxidized products (7-17).

INITIAL STUDIES

The broad alcohol substrate specificity of alcohol oxidase

indicated that methylotrophic yeast could be used in the development of a generic whole-cell process for the production of a wide range of flavour aldehydes. The use of non-growing whole cells as a biocatalyst had a number of advantages over the use of free alcohol oxidase. In whole cells the enzyme is co-immobilized with catalase and the necessary cofactor flavin adenine dinucleotide (FAD). A self-contained natural system ensured recycling the FAD and sustained activity. The intact cells maintained the proper environmental conditions of pH and ionic strength, protecting the enzymes from the potentially denaturing influences of an in vitro environment.

Initial studies centred on the development of a model system for the conversion of ethanol to acetaldehyde. Acetaldehyde is a highly volatile compound with a boiling point of 21·C. This characteristic necessitated the development of a closed-batch process so that product could be retained and quantified for determination of conversion efficiencies. The problem of end-product inhibition was mitigated by carrying out the whole-cell bioconversion in Tris buffer at pH 8.0. Alkaline Tris buffer has the ability to complex acetaldehyde in a 1:1 molar ratio. Following the bioconversion, dissociation of the acetaldehyde-Tris complex was accomplished by lowering the pH to 6.0.

Generally, tests for the conversion of ethanol to acetaldehyde were conducted in 160 ml serum vials containing 25 ml of cell suspension (5 g cells/litre 0.5 M Tris buffer, pH 8.0). The vials were flushed with oxygen, injected with the ethanol substrate (5% w/v), sealed, and pressurized with oxygen to 100 kPa. Vials were incubated at 30·C, with shaking, and were recharged with oxygen as required. Ethanol and acetaldehyde concentrations were quantified by gas chromatography, and specific activity calculations were expressed as the amount of acetaldehyde produced during the first hour of reaction per g cell dry weight.

Five methylotrophic yeasts, *Pichia pastoris*, *Pichia naganishii*, *Pichia angusta*, *Candida boidinii*, and *Hansenula polymorpha*, were compared for their ability to conduct the oxidation of ethanol to acetaldehyde (Fig. 2). Of these yeasts *P. pastoris* demonstrated the highest level of alcohol oxidase activity (1.22 g acetaldehyde produced per g cell dry weight per hour), and therefore was chosen for further study.

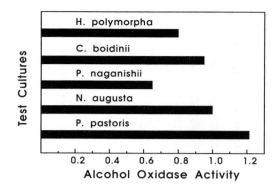

Fig. 2. Comparison of alcohol oxidase activity of five methylotrophic yeasts. Activity was measured at 30°C and is expressed as grams.

Medium composition and cell growth conditions for the induction of the alcohol oxidase enzyme system of P. pastoris have been described (9). The addition of 0.1% (w/v) yeast extract to the growth medium had the effect of increasing growth rate, and cell yield. Growth in the presence of yeast extract also had the beneficial effect of increasing both alcohol oxidase specific activity, and the total amount of acetaldehyde produced, by 20% (12). P. pastoris alcohol oxidase activity was highest during the logarithmic phase of growth (Fig. 3), and began to decline as soon as the culture entered the stationary phase of growth. Accordingly, cells were harvested during the late logarithmic phase to obtain the highest concentration of cells at maximum enzyme activity.

Figure 4 displays a typical ethanol to acetaldehyde conversion. Acetaldehyde was produced at a constant rate until approximately 22 g/litre or 0.5 M product had accumulated. At this point the binding capacity of the Tris buffer was exhausted, and free acetaldehyde restricted, and eventually stopped the oxidative activity. Since this bioconversion was mediated by nongrowing, metabolically active cells, substrate carbon was not lost to cell growth or maintenance. After 12 h of bioconversion, 30.2 g ethanol had been oxidized to 28 g acetaldehyde (97% carbon recovery). Even larger amounts of acetaldehyde could be accumulated if the bioconversion was conducted in the presence of higher molarity Tris buffer (Table 1).

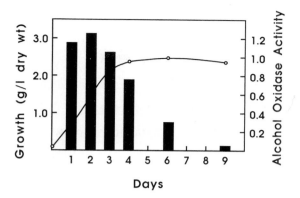

Fig. 3. Correlation of Pichia *pastoris* growth (o), and specific alcohol oxidase activity (bars) acetaldehyde per g cell dry weight per hour.

Even though Tris complexes acetaldehyde on an equimolar basis, it was observed that only 1.28 M acetaldehyde accumulated in the presence of 2.0 M Tris. This indicated that some mechanism other than end-product inhibition was limiting the full extent of the ethanol to acetaldehyde conversion. When cells from a 24-h bioconversion were harvested, washed, and used again, it was found that alcohol oxidase activity had been completely lost. Electron microscopy revealed that cells freshly grown in methanol contained peroxisomes but were devoid of these microbodies after the bioconversion.

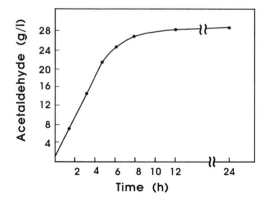

Fig. 4. Whole-cell bioconversion of ethanol to acetaldehyde by *Pichia pastoris*

TABLE 1.

Effect of Tris buffer molarity on total acetaldehyd production during a 24-h bioconversion.

Tris buffer (M)	Acetaldehyde (M)
0.5	0.64
1.0	1.08
2.0	1.28

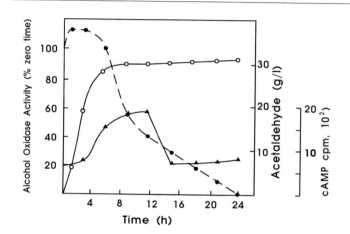

Fig. 5. Correlation of alcohol oxidase activity (o), intracellular cAMP level (▲), and acetaldehyde production (o) during the 24-h ethanol to acetaldehyde bioconversion.

INDUCTION AND REPRESSION: TOWARD SUSTAINED ACTIVITY

It has been demonstrated that when methylotrophic yeasts are transferred from a methanol medium to one containing a different carbon source, such as glucose or ethanol, a degradative inactivation of the alcohol oxidase system ensues (5). This type of degradative inactivation has been termed catabolite inactivation (18), and involves the proteolytic breakdown of the peroxisomes. Peroxisomes may comprise up to 30% of the total soluble protein (19), and contribute approximately 50% of the cytoplasmic volume (20). Accordingly, when the methylotrophic cells no longer require the enzyme system for methanol dissimilation the peroxisomes are degraded and the protein recycled to the amino acid pool. It therefore appeared that methanol-grown P. pastoris cells used for the oxidation of ethanol to acetaldehyde were subjected to the same factors that initiated catabolite inactivation in methylotrophic yeasts transferred from a methanol to an ethanol growth medium. Studies were initiated to determine the mechanism of catabolite inactivation in P. pastoris, with the goal of controlling this degradative event; thereby extending the useful life of the biocatalyst and increasing flavour aldehyde production.

By incubating P. pastoris in phosphate buffer in the presence of each of the substrates and product of the bioconversion, and in combinations of these, it was determined that acetaldehyde in the presence of oxygen was the effector of catabolite inactivation (21). This degradative event was initiated by the appearance of free acetaldehyde, and was characterized by an increase in the level of cyclic AMP (cAMP), which coincided with a rapid 55% drop in alcohol oxidase activity (Fig. 5). Subsequent enzyme inactivation proceeded at a constant but slower rate. This second phase was characterized by the disappearance of the peroxisomes, and was therefore due to proteolytic degradation.

The inactivation of alcohol oxidase in P. pastoris is very similar to the two-step sequence of catabolite inactivation that has been studied for fructose 1,6-bisphosphatase in a variety of yeast species (22-28). The close similarity between the data obtained in our studies and the sequence of events known to occur during the inactivation of fructose 1,6-bisphosphatase allowed the proposal of a possible mechanism of catabolite inactivation in P. pastoris. During the bioconversion, an increase in cAMP level occurs at the first appearance of free acetaldehyde in the presence of oxygen. It is proposed that cAMP activates a cAMP-dependent protein kinase that in turn phosphorylates protein residues on the peroxisomal enzymes. This phosphorylation correlates with the initial 55% drop in alcohol oxidase activity. Once phosphorylated, these proteins are marked for proteolytic degradation by proteases. During this second phase of catabolite inactivation, the loss of residual alcohol oxidase activity occurs at a slower constant rate.

Knowledge of the possible mechanism of catabolite inactivation allowed us to investigate means by which this phenomenon could be controlled. It had been noted that catabolite inactivation was temperature dependent, with little inactivation of cells held at 3·C in the presence of acetaldehyde and oxygen

(21). The effect of temperature on alcohol oxidase and protease activities were compared (Fig. 6). *P. pastoris* alcohol oxidase was found to be very psychrotolerant, with the specific activity at 3·C being 83% of that at 37·C. In contrast, protease activity was completely inhibited by temperatures below 15ºC.

The combination in *P. pastoris* of cold-sensitive proteases and a cold-tolerant alcohol oxidase system suggested that the ethanol-to-acetaldehyde bioconversion could be run at temperatures below 15·C without the occurrence of catabolite inactivation. By using increasing concentrations of Tris (up to 3.0 M) to prevent end product inhibition, a high concentration of 123 g of acetaldehyde per litre was achieved at 3·C, compared with only 58 g/litre at 30ºC (Fig. 7).

Acetaldehyde also was produced by a cyclic-batch procedure at 3ºC in 0.5 M Tris buffer. The bioconversion was stopped before the accumulation of free acetaldehyde, the acetaldehyde removed, and both the buffer and cells were recycled. Total acetaldehyde production of 140.6 g/litre was obtained by this cyclic-batch procedure. These results indicated that it should be possible to develop a low-temperature continuous bioconversion process for the production of flavour aldehydes.

PROCESS ENGINEERING

Elucidation of the mechanistic elements aspects involved in catabolite inactivation of the alcohol oxidase enzyme system enabled us to proceed with a rational process design for acetaldehyde production. Specifically, qualitative identification of oxygen levels, temperature and concentration of uncomplexed end product as the critical parameters led to an effort to quantify the influence of these factors. To this end, a modified Box-Behken [29] factorial design was used which examined each of the three parameters at three different levels. The parameters examined and the values chosen are shown in Table 2.

From this analysis, a design equation was derived which described the effect of each parameter examined, as well as the interactive terms between them. The fitted equation is given below for coded variables in terms of the initial (1 hour) rate of acetaldehyde production.

$$Y = 9.13 - X_1(1.29 - 0.87X_1) - X_2(2.18 - 0.55X_2) - X_3(2.32 - 1.52X_3) - 0.68X_1X_3 - 1.6X_1X_2 - 1.75 X_2X_3$$

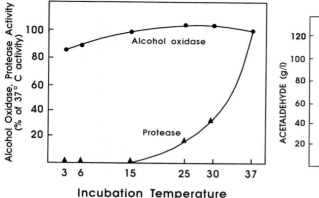
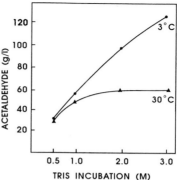

Fig. 6. Effect of temperature on *Pichia pastoris* alcohol oxidase and protease activities.

Fig. 7. Effect of Tris buffer concentration on the production of acetaldehyde by *Pichia pastoris* at 3 and 30°C.

The overall coefficient of determination $R^2 = 0.94$. An analysis of variance for the fitted data showed that the F test for the significance of the regression (ratio of mean square of factor effects to residuals) was 9.06, which is significant at the 99% confidence level.

This equation served to confirm and extend the earlier observations (12,21), namely that increasing oxygen concentration, temperature and acetaldehyde served to enhance catabolite inactivation and accelerate the rate of activity loss. As well, the synergistic interaction between oxygen and temperature, which resulted in enhanced catabolite inactivation under aerobic conditions at ambient temperatures, could be overcome through operation at lower (4°C) temperatures. The combined effect of all variables could be represented by a 3-dimensional diagram (Figure 8).

When the ethanol to acetaldehyde conversion is run at the optimum temperature for alcohol oxidase activity (ca. 30°C), acetaldehyde acts as a very strong effector of catabolite inactivation. As the concentration of acetaldehyde is increased from 0 to 4 g/l at 30°C, a decrease in reaction rate from approximately 16 g/l/h to 4 g/l/h is observed.

The role of oxygen can be illustrated by moving over the same acetaldehyde range at low (-1) oxygen concentration. Under these conditions, the rate of reaction decreased from 16 to ca. 9 g/l, a

TABLE 2.

Values of process parameters which correspond to the transformed variables.

VARIABLE	SYMBOL	CONCENTRATION LEVEL		
		-1	0	+1
Oxygen (psi)	x_1	0	15	30
Temperature (C)	x_2	5	17.5	30
Acet-aldehyde (g/l)	x_3	0	2	4

smaller decrease in rate than that observed at higher oxygen concentrations. To our knowledge this is the first quantified report of oxygen and acetaldehyde acting synergistically as co-effectors of catabolite inactivation in *Pichia pastoris*. It has been previously observed that the degradation of peroxisomes can be correlated with the metabolism of ethanol (5). Our work supports this contention, since it is under aerobic conditions in the presence of catabolite that the most pronounced effect on reaction rate is seen.

As suggested by preliminary results (12,21) the negative effects associated with catabolite inactivation can be reduced, even in the presence of high oxygen concentrations, by operating at lower temperatures. These observations are confirmed by the model equation. Over the same (0-4 g/l) range of acetaldehyde, the reaction rate is reduced by only 3 g/l when the reaction is run at 5°C. Finally, if the reaction is run under conditions of low temperature and low dissolved oxygen concentrations, over the range of acetaldehyde concentrations tested, there was no influence of acetaldehyde on reaction rate. This is better illustrated by examining the same figure from the back side (Figure 8b). The response volume essentially comes to a point at low oxygen concentrations and low temperature indicating that, under these conditions, the negative effects associated with acetaldehyde as an effector of catabolite inactivation of alcohol oxidase can be eliminated.

These studies are useful from the point of view of process design. By running fermenter-scale bioconversions at 5°C we have achieved acetaldehyde concentrations up to 130 g/l (3 M). Such high product concentrations are rarely achieved in biological processes, and serve to improve overall process economics. The influence of dissolved oxygen concentration can be easily seen by examining Figure 9. For low temperature reactions, there is generally an increase in reaction rate with increasing oxygen concentration, illustrating the physical constraint of limited oxygen solubility in 3 M aqueous Tris buffer. By using a closed aeration loop and maintaining constant oxygen overpressure, the dissolved oxygen concentration remained between 60 and 100% of saturation. Under these conditions, acetaldehyde rapidly accumulated, saturating the binding capacity of the Tris buffer within 4 hours. In reactors run at 30°C, there was a complete loss of activity after less than 2 hours as a result of catabolite inactivation. The concentration of acetaldehyde at this point was well below the binding capacity of the Tris buffer. This comparison provides a graphic illustration of the advantages associated with operation at lower temperatures.

CONCLUSIONS

This paper has described the development of the natural flavour program at the Division of Biological Sciences of the National Research Council of Canada, from its inception to its conclusion in early 1989. During this period of time, a rational screening program was undertaken, and yielded _Pichia pastoris_ as a practical candidate catalyst for a biological oxidation process. Shake flask experiments allowed the rapid evaluation of a range of reversible binding agents for the aldehyde product, and the selection of Tris buffer as a non-toxic reversible trapping agent for acetaldehyde. Factors influencing the sustained activity of the biocatalyst were elucidated, and the biochemical mechanism of

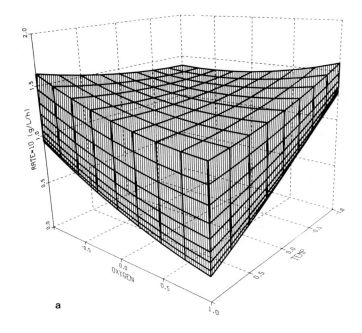

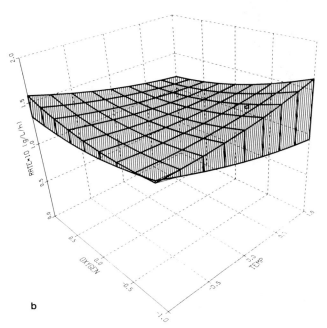

Fig. 8   Effect of oxygen, acetaldehyde and temperature on catabolite inactivation of _Pichia pastoris_.

catabolite inactivation was studied. The influence of the three major process variables (oxygen, temperature, and catabolite concentration) was modelled, and a low temperature bioprocess was designed to eliminate the influence of catabolite inactivation. A semi-continuous closed loop, pressurized bioreactor system was designed. The acetaldehyde production system was then successfully evaluated at the laboratory scale. Very high yields of acetaldehyde were obtained (up to 130 g/l in 4 hours) using the bioreactor system.

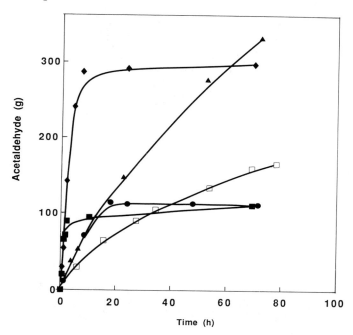

Fig.9. Reactor-scale batch conversion of ethanol to acetaldehyde as influenced by temperature and dissolved oxygen concentration. Reactor working volume was 2.5 litres. Symbols (temperature, °C/dissolved oxygen, % saturation): ● 5/0, + 5/10, ◊ 5/60, ✱ 30/0, □ 30/60.

REFERENCES

1. D.W. Armstrong, S.M. Martin and H. Yamazaki, Biotechnol. Letts. 6 (1984) 183-6.
2. J. Stofberg and F. Grundschober, Perfumer and Flavourist, 12 (1987) 27-56.
3. M.S.A. Wecker and R.R. Zall, Appl. Environ. Microbiol., 53 (1987) 2815-20.
4. R. Couderc and J. Baratti, Agric. Biol. Chem., 44 (1980) 2279-2289.
5. M. Veenhuis, J.P. van Dijken and W. Harder, Adv. Microb.

Physiol., 24 (1983) 1-82.
6   R.N. Patel, C.T. Hou, and P. Derelanko, Arch. Biochem. Biophys., 221 (1983) 135-142.
7   S.J.B. Duff and W.D. Murray, Biotechnol. Bioeng., 31 (1988a) 44-49.
8   S.J.B. Duff and W.D. Murray, Biotechnol. Bioeng., 31 (1988b) 790-795.
9   S.J.B. Duff and W.D. Murray, Biotechnol. Bioeng., 34 (1989) 153-159.
10 S.J.B. Duff, W.D. Murray and R.P. Overend, Enzyme Microb. Technol., 11 (1989) 770-775.
11 W.D. Murray, S.J.B. Duff, P.H. Lanthier, D.W. Armstrong, F.W. Welsh F.W. and R.E. Williams, Dev. Food Sci., 17 (1988) 1-18.
12 W.D. Murray, S.J.B. Duff and P.H. Lanthier, Appl. Microbiol. Biotechnol., 32 (1989) 95-100.
13 W.D. Murray, S.J.B. Duff and T.J. Beveridge, Appl. Environ. Microbiol., 56 (1990) 2378-2383.
14 Y. Sakai and Y. Tani, Agric. Biol. Chem., 50 (1986) 2615-2620.
15 Y. Sakai and Y. Tani, Appl. Environ. Microbiol., 54 (1988) 485-489.
16 Y. Sakai and Y. Tani, Agric. Biol. Chem., 51 (1987) 2617-2620.
17 Y. Tani, Y. Sakai and H. Yamada, Agric. Biol. Chem., 49 (1985) 2699-2706.
18 H. Holzer, Trends Biochem. Sci., 1 (1976) 176-181.
19 L. Dijkhuizen, T.O. Hansen and W. Harder, Trends Biotechnol., 3 (1985) 262-267.
20 M. Veenhuis, J.P. van Dijken, and W. Harder, Electron Microsc., 2 (1980) 84-85.
21 W.D. Murray, S.J.B. Duff and T.J. Beveridge, Appl. Environ. Microbiol., 56 (1990) 2378-2383.
22 T. Funaguma, Y. Toyoda and J. Sy, Biochem. Biophys. Res. Commun., 130 (1985) 467-471.
23 A.G. Lenz and H. Holzer, FEBS Lett., 109 (1980) 271-274.
24 P.M. Tortora, M. Birtel, A.G. Len, and H. Holzer, Biochem. Biophys. Res. Commun., 100 (1981) 688-695.
25 M.J. Mazon, J.M. Gancedo and C. Gancedo, J. Biol. Chem., 257 (1982) 1128-1130.
26 D. Muller and H. Holzer, Biochem. Biophys. Res. Commun., 103 (1981) 926-933.
27 E. Polnisch and K. Hofmann, Arch. Microbiol., 152 (1989) 269-272.
28 Y. Toyoda and J. Sy, Curr. Microbiol., 12 (1985) 241-244.
29 G.E.P. Box and N. Draper, Empirical model building and response surfaces, Chapter 7. John Wiley & Sons Ltd. N.Y., New York. (1987).

G. Charalambous (Ed.), Food Science and Human Nutrition
© 1992 Elsevier Science Publishers B.V. All rights reserved.

EVALUATION OF *URTICA* SPECIES AS POTENTIAL SOURCES OF IMPORTANT NUTRIENTS

H. WETHERILT

TÜBITAK, Dept. of Nutrition & Food Technology, Gebze-Kocaeli TURKEY

1. INTRODUCTION

The stinging nettle (common nettle) is consumed widely by people of the Northern and Eastern Anatolian Regions of Turkey. Its use as a vegetable is mentioned and praised in *Materia Medica* by Dioscorides and *Naturalis Historia* by Plinius, both works dating back to the 1st century A.D. In the middle ages, it was used as a component of soups and salads in Europe (1). Today, however, its popularity as a vegetable has declined and its common use confined virtually to Turkey, Scotland, and Finland (2) only.

The common nettle refers to several stinging varieties of *Urtica* species which belong to the family *Urticaceae*. This family comprises some 40 species and 500 varieties of monoic and dioic plants growing in tropical and subtropical regions. The main varieties identified under the *Urtica* species are *Urtica dioica* L., *Urtica urens* L., *Urtica cannabina* L., *Urtica pilulifera* L., *Urtica membranacea* Poir., and *Urtica kiovensis* Rogoff. Among these, *Urtica dioica* (dioic, perennial, 30-150 cm long), *Urtica urens* (monoic, annual, 15-45 cm long), and *Urtica pilulifera* (monoic, annual or rarely biannual, 30-90 cm long) are the varieties commonly used as spring vegetable in Turkey. The leaves of all three species have single-celled stinging hairs which come off at the slightest contact and secrete the sap contained in their vacuoles. This sap is a strong irritant due to its histamine and acetylcholine content and thus constitutes an effective defense system for the plant against animals.

Urtica dioica is used in Anatolian folk medicine as an expectorant, purgative, diuretic, tonic, galactagogue, hemostatic, vermifuge and panacea for the treatment of many ailments including eczema, rheumatism, sciatica, paralysis, oedema, hair loss, kidney infection, dismenorrhea, menorrhagia, nose bleeding, asthma, gastritis, hemorrhoids, hyperthyroidism, anemia, diabetes, gout, bronchitis, hepatitis, and cancer. Ingestion of a mixture of the crushed seeds of *Urtica pilulifera* and honey is also used widely to treat leukemia and various types of neoplastic disorders, in particular, hormone related cancers and tumours of the mouth, lung, and gastrointestinal system. Although some of these remedial applications can be traced to the ancient Greeks and Romans and therefore have a long history of practice, they are nevertheless based on folklore rather than scientific evidence and clinical observations.

Several studies have been reported on the pharmacological activity of *Urtica dioica* but not on *Urtica pilulifera*. Water extracts of dried leaves of *Urtica dioica* have shown inhibitory activity in *Paramecium* and *Lepidium* tests (3). The water soluble chlorophyllin from the leaves enter the preparation of a wound-healing antimicrobial ointment as the active principle (4). An alcoholic extract of the leaves is a component of a liquid preparation for treating psoriasis and seborrhoic eczemas (5). An aqueous alcohol extract of the roots is the active agent of some lotions and ointments for regenerating skin (6). The leaf extracts, owing to their antibleeding, antiplaque, anti-inflammatory, and antibacterial activities, enter toothpaste and mouthwash preparations (7).

In animal studies, extracts of the leaves have been shown to exhibit hypoglycemic and diuretic activity and also to improve the tonicity of the uterus and intestines. In tissue culture, the leaf extract has shown anticoagulant activity in a similar manner to that of heparin (8).

An aqueous alcohol extract of the *Urtica dioica* roots is sold as a diuretic in pharmacies in Germany. The aqueous alcohol extract has also been reported to inhibit nonmalignant hyperplasia of the prostate (9, 10). To treat this condition, the extracts are on sale in German pharmacies under the trade names of "Bazoton-Kapseln", "Prostagutt Tropfen", and "Prostatin Liquidum" (11).

From the water extract of the rhizomes, a very low molecular weight, monomeric, and heat resistant lectin (*Urtica dioica* agglutinin) has been isolated and shown to induce γ-interferon in human lymphocytes (12), stimulate proliferation of murine thymocytes and spleen-T-lymphocytes (13) and inhibit the growth of several phytopathogenic and saprophytic chitin containing fungi (14) in vitro. A polysaccharide isolated from the water extract of the roots reportedly exhibits immunological activity in the rat paw oedema, lymphocyte transformation, and complement tests (15).

Chemically, *Urtica dioica* foliage has been shown to contain chlorophyll a and b, coproporphyrin, protoporphyrin, β-carotene, violaxanthin, xantophyll, zeaxanthin, luteoxanthin, ascorbic acid, pantothenic acid, vitamin K_1, methylheptanone, acetophenone, acetylcholine, choline, histamine, serotonin, 5-hydroxytryptamine, nicotine, threono-1,4-lactone, and formic, acetic, butyric, citric, fumaric, glyceric, malic, oxalic, caffeic, p-coumaric, succinic, and threonic acids (16, 17). Tannin (18); a neutral and an acidic corbohydrate-protein polymer (19); a trigalactosyl diglyceride with antigenic activity (20); kaempferol, isorhamnetin, quercetin, and their glycosides (21); and lipase (22) have also been reported to be present in the leaves and infloresence.

The roots have been studied extensively and found to contain oleanol acid, 3β-sitosterin and its derivatives and glucosides, scopoletin, homovanillyl alcohol, secoisolariciresinol glucoside, neo-olivil and its derivatives and glucosides (16) as well as *Urtica dioica* agglutinin and the polysaccharide mentioned earlier. The analysis of the immunologically active polysaccharide fraction has yielded 35 % neutral sugars (glucose, galactose, rhamnose, mannose and xylose); 1 % protein; and 35 % uronic acid (15). The cytokinin type of compounds, namely zeatin, zeatin nucleotide, dihydrozeatin, isopentanyladenine, isopentenyladenosine, and isopentyladenine nucleotide have been detected in the xylem sap (23).

There have been very few reports on the chemical composition of the other varieties of *Urtica species*. However, the amine fraction (histamin, acetylcholin, cholin, and serotonin) is believed to be present in most of the varieties, if not in all (16). The hair and whole plant extracts of *Urtica urens* have been reported to contain high levels of leukotrienes LTB4 and LTC4, which suggests that the mechanism of urtication after contact with nettles is similar to that of insect venoms and cutaneous mast cells with regard to its spectrum of mediators (24). Stachydrine has been detected in *Urtica cannabina* (25) and the alkaloid bufotenin in *Urtica pilulifera* (26).

The leaves of *Urtica* species have been reported to be excellent sources of some important minerals and vitamins (27-29) and to have a higher level and better quality of protein when compared with many other green leafy vegetables (30). However, seasonal and regional variations in the nutrient contents of the plant can be large (1, 18). To our knowledge, there have been no reports on the nutritional value of the seeds of *Urtica pilulifera*.

The present work was thus undertaken to assess the nutritional properties of the fresh leaves and dried flowers of *Urtica dioica* L. and seeds of *Urtica pilulifera* L. grown in Turkey and to evaluate these commonly consumed varieties as potential sources of important nutrients.

2. MATERIALS AND METHODS

The fresh leaves of *Urtica dioica* were harvested during the months of April and May from plants growing wild in the Marmara Research Centre gardens in Gebze. The dried flowers of *Urtica dioica* and the seeds of *Urtica pilulifera* were purchased from four different herbalists in the Istanbul Spice Market and mixed before use.

Dry matter content was determined according to the AOAC method number 32.083 (31). Nitrogen was determined by the AOAC macro Kjeldahl method number 7.021-7.024. The results were multiplied by 5.30 to obtain % protein for foliage and by 6.0 to obtain % protein for seeds. Analyses for crude fiber and ash were carried out according to the AOAC Method number 7.070 and 22.027 respectively.

The petroleum ether soluble fraction was determined by the AOCS method A-a 4.38 (32) using light petroleum (b.p. 40-60°C). Gas chromatographic determination of fatty acids were conducted according to the AOCS Methods Ce 2.6 and 1.62 using a Pye Unicam PU 4500 Capillary Chromatograph instrument. Carbohydrate level was calculated by difference.

Amino acid profiles were determined with a Biotronik LC 5001 model analyser according to the AOAC method number 43.263-43.264. Sulphur amino acids (methionine and cysteine) were found to be the limiting amino acids; therefore, the ratio of their sum to the total of essential amino acids was used for the calculation of the chemical scores with egg protein as the standard of reference (33). Real protein values were found by multiplying protein level (as is) by chemical score value and percent digestibility (34).

Vitamin C level was measured by the Technicon Auto Analyser Method number 305-83 E; β-carotene by the AOAC method number 43.015-43.017 (31); α-tocopherol by the spectroscopic method of Lambertsen and Braekkan (35); thiamin by the Technicon Auto Analyser Method number 479-77A; riboflavin by the Technicon Auto Analyser Method number 140-71A; niacin by the Technicon Auto Analyser Method number 156-71A; and vitamin B_6 by microbiological assay based on the AOAC method number 43.229-43.234.

Iron, zinc, copper, calcium, magnesium, manganese, sodium, potassium, and selenium analyses were carried out according to standard atomic absorption methods using a HITACHI-50 model instrument. Phosphorous levels were determined by the AOAC method number 22.040-22.043 (31).

The analyses were conducted in duplicate and repeated when necessary.

3. RESULTS AND DISCUSSION

The chemical composition of the seeds, dried flowers, and fresh leaves are presented in Table 1. Literature values for the leaves of *Urtica dioica* are also given for comparison.

These findings showed that the seeds were, as expected, a good source of fat and protein. The dried flowers, when compared with the fresh leaves had a higher fat but lower protein and ash contents on a dry matter basis. The fat and protein contents of the leaves were in good agreement with literature values whereas the ash level was much higher than cited in earlier work. This difference can be attributed to the presence of higher levels of silicon in the Turkish plant. Although the content of this mineral was not determined in the present study, silicon dioxide levels in common nettle leaves were reported to vary between 1 and 12 % in Yugoslavia depending on the location of growth (18). As a green vegetable, the fresh leaves appeared to have exceptionally high levels of protein, ash, and fiber. When compared with levels in spinach and parsley, nettle leaves had three times as much ash and fiber and twice as much protein (39, 40).

TABLE 1
Macronutrient composition of seeds (*Urtica pilulifera*), dried flowers (*Urtica dioica*) and fresh leaves (*Urtica dioica*) (%).

Nutrients	Seeds a	Dried flower b	Fresh leaves b	Literature for leaves b	
Water	8.5	11.0	76.9	76.0	(36)
Fat	25.0	12.1	6.7	5.6	(1)
Protein	21.9	19.3	28.1	20.9-36.0	(1)
				19.7-37.3	(30)
				20.7-27.4	(37)
Nitrogen free extract	26.4	35.2	17.9	10.3	(38)
Fiber	11.4	16.6	23.2	39.6	(38)
Ash	6.8	16.8	24.1	14.8	(1)
				11.7-17.7	(18)

a   as is
b   dry matter basis except for water values

The amino acid composition of nettle leaf protein have been studied previously (1, 30). The results of the amino acid analyses for the seeds, dried flowers, and fresh leaves are presented in Table 2. The composition of the leaves are compared with those of *Urtica dioica* given in literature.
The protein quality of the *Urtica Pilulifera* seed, as displayed by its chemical score and real protein value is well above average when compared with other plants; however, due to its reputation as an antitumoural agent, it is sold at inflated prices and therefore cannot be considered as an economic source of protein.
Urtica dioica foliage has a strikingly high protein content (6.5%, as is) for a green vegetable and is naturally abundant. In comparison to literature values, the protein of the Turkish origin leaves was found to contain higher histidine but lower aspartic acid. With respect to their high lysine content and real protein value, the nettle leaves offer a better protein quality than all other greens used as vegetables. As lysine is the limiting amino acid in wheat, it is a specially important

essential amino acid for the balanced nutrition of the Turkish population whose staple diet is bread. Therefore, if the protein hydrolysates of the leaves could be produced at an industrial scale, this would afford an economic means of enriching bread and other cereal products.

TABLE 2
Amino acid composition of the protein hydrolysates (g/100 g protein), chemical score, and real protein value (%).

Aminoacids	Seeds	Dried flowers	Fresh leaves	Literature for leaves (30)	(1)
Phenylalanine	5.34	5.51	5.82	5.62	6.82
Lysine	5.82	4.67	5.53	6.97	13.88
Threonine	4.78	4.53	4.61	4.72	5.40
Valine	6.42	5.80	6.31	5.81	7.21
Methionine	1.62	1.39	1.76	1.89	0.87
Cysteine	2.21	0.35	0.85		
Isoleucine	4.56	4.10	4.78	4.25	4.91
Leucine	6.56	7.18	8.97	8.50	7.39
Tryptophan	0.97	1.91	1.28		
Histidine	4.30	4.52	4.10	1.90	2.92
Aspartic acid	9.20	13.15	9.07	12.78	10.78
Serine	6.75	6.87	6.19	6.05	4.61
Glutamic acid	14.73	12.32	13.30	12.73	13.09
Proline	4.78	4.21	4.87	4.91	4.83
Glycine	6.19	5.41	6.25	4.89	6.59
Alanine	3.15	6.27	6.54	6.07	6.67
Tyrosine	3.42	2.80	3.87	3.56	4.03
Arginine	9.20	6.13	5.90	6.48	
Total essential amino acids	38.28	35.44	39.21	37.76	
Chemical score	87	42	56		
Real protein value	15.5	6.3	3.1		

In Table 3, the fatty acid composition of the *U. Pilulifera* seeds are presented and compared with the reported values for the fatty acid composition in *Urtica Dioica* seeds. The percentage of oil in *Urtica pilulifera* seeds found in the present study (25.0%) was slightly higher than the reported level for *Urtica dioica* seed oil (23.5%) (41). The major component acid was found to be linoleic acid followed by oleic acid. However, when compared with the oil from *Urtica dioica* seeds, linoleic acid content was considerably lower whereas oleic and palmitic acid levels were higher. Oils from both varieties of seeds gave reasonable levels of the saturated long chain behenic acid which generally does not occur in quantity in common fats and oils.

TABLE 3
Fatty acid composition of the oil from *Urtica pilulifera* seed and comparison with reference values for *Urtica dioica* seed oil (%).

Fatty acids		U. pilulifera	U. dioica (41)
Propionic acid	C_{3-0}	2.39	–
Butyric acid	C_{4-0}	0.13	–
Caproic acid	C_{6-0}	0.21	–
Caprylic acid	C_{8-0}	0.10	–
Capric acid	C_{10-0}	0.09	–
Myristic acid	C_{14-0}	0.08	0.05
Pentadecanoic acid	C_{15-0}	Trace	0.01
Pentadecenoic acid	C_{15-1}	0.11	0.02
Palmitic acid	C_{16-0}	8.01	3.25
Palmitoleic acid	C_{16-1}	0.85	0.05
Heptadecanoic acid	C_{17-0}	0.1	0.02
Heptadecenoic acid	C_{17-1}	0.17	0.05
Stearic acid	C_{18-0}	3.11	0.68
Oleic acid	C_{18-1}	23.20	11.20
Linoleic acid	C_{18-2}	59.34	81.46
Linolenic acid	C_{18-3}	0.82	1.38
Arachidic acid	C_{20-0}	0.08	0.21
Eicosenoic acid	C_{20-1}	Trace	0.20
Eicosadienoic acid	C_{20-2}	–	0.03
Eicosatrienoic acid	C_{20-3}	–	0.14
Behenic acid	C_{22-0}	1.17	1.25

The results of the vitamin and mineral analyses for the seeds, dried flowers, and fresh leaves are shown in Table 4. Literature values reported for fresh leaves are also given for comparison when available.

Although the seeds did not exhibit any exceptional properties concerning micronutrients, their α-tocopherol and selenium levels were reasonably high. The dried flowers were found to be rich in α-tocopherol, riboflavin, iron, zinc, calcium, phosphorous and potassium. The results indicated that as a consequence of the drying process, total loss of vitamin C and a substantial decrease in provitamin A activity (β-carotene) were incurred. The high riboflavin level suggested that this vitamin was not affected substantially by drying.

TABLE 4
Vitamin and mineral contents of the seeds (*U. pilulifera*) dried flowers (*U. dioica*) and fresh leaves (*U. dioica*) (mg/100 g)

Nutrients	Seeds	Dried flowers	Fresh leaves	Literature for leaves	
Vitamin C	6a	0	238a	333a	(36)
				947b	(42)
β-Carotene	0.7a	1.9a	5.0a	20.2b	(38)
α-Tocopherol	20.2a	16.9a	14.4a	14.5a	(28)
Thiamin	0.13a	0.03a	0.02a	0.08a	(38)
Riboflavin	0.22a	0.76a	0.23a		
Niacin	1.79a	1.86a	0.62a		
Vitamin B6	0.15a	0.10a	0.07a	0.22a	(43)
Iron	33a	43a	13a	17-27b	(18)
			56b	15-25b	(29)
Zinc	4.3a	2.6a	1.0a	3.1-7.4b	(18)
			4.1b	4.3-5.5b	(29)
Copper	0.90a	1.2a	0.5a	1.0-2.6b	(18)
			2.3b	0.8-2.4b	(29)
Calcium	2170a	2980a	850a	2070-4430b	(18)
			3690b	2270-5090b	(29)
Phosphorous	642a	400a	75a	296-925b	(18)
			325b		
Magnesium	352a	325a	96a	458-1900b	(18)
			416b	2500b	(29)
Manganese	6a	19a	3a	3.1-7.2b	(18)
			13b	9.0-13.7b	(29)
Sodium	24a	24a	16a	140b	(38)
			69b		
Potassium	660a	1490a	530a	2091-3835b	(18)
			2300b	1080-1700b	(29)
Selenium	0.08a	0.002a	0.003a		
			0.012b		

a as is
b dry basis

In agreement with literature values, the fresh leaves proved to be one of the best natural sources of vitamin C, β-carotene and α-tocopherol. The Turkish origin leaves were found to be rich in riboflavin as well; however, their vitamin B_6 content was found to be less than a third of the level reported in literature.

As could be predicted from the ash content, the mineral concentrations of the leaves were remarkably high, especially with respect to the nutritionally important ones such as iron, calcium, and potassium. The potassium to sodium ratio, which is now considered as an index for the protective quality of the diet against cardiovascular (44) and neoplastic diseases (45), is noticeably high as well. These results clearly indicate the nutritional value of the fresh leaves with respect to both vitamins and minerals.

Particularly in Spring, when vitamin sources are scarce, consumption of fresh leaves can serve as a valuable food source for some very important vitamins. However, because the leaves are also known to contain oxalates which bind the minerals and therefore reduce their absorbance at the intestinal wall, it is not possible to make an estimate of the availability of these minerals to the organism. On the other hand, if the nutrients can be extracted free of oxalates from the nettles, their processing into supplementary drugs could yield nutritional and economic benefits. Indeed, a preparation from *Urtica dioica* foliage is already being processed into water soluble tablets (urtriphyllin) in Russia (46).

ACKNOWLEDGEMENT

The author is grateful to Prof. M. Pala for auspicious support, Prof. A. Baysal for helpful discussions and Dr. O. Devres for technical assistance.

REFERENCES

1   R.E. Hughes, P. Ellery, T. Harry, V. Jenkins, and E. Jones, J. Sci. Food Agric., 31 (1980) 1279-1285.
2   P. Peura and J. Koskenniemi, Acta Pharm. Fenn., 94 (1985) 67-70.
3   M. Oswiecimska, Z. Komala, and B. Liszka, Folia Biol. 28 (1980) 245-251.
4   M. Pop, L. Georgescu, D. Breazu, N. Maier, and E. Andronescu, Rom. RO 87,148 (Cl. A61K9/06), 29 Jun 1985.
5   I. Janosik, Czech. 185,262 (Cl. A61K35/78), 15 Sept. 1980.
6   G. Verzzar, S. Nyiredy, P. Babulka, K. Mikita, S. Meszaros, A. Gulyas, B. Galambosi, and J. Vincze, Ger. Offen DE 3,504, 355 (Cl. A61K7/48), 14 Aug 1985.
7   G. Voerman, Eur. Pat. Appl. EP 341,795 (Cl. A61K7/26) 15 Nov 1989.
8   E. Atasu and V. Cihangir, FABAD Far. Bil. Der. 2 (1984) 73-81.
9   H. Ziegler, Fortsch. Med., 101 (1983) 2112-2114.
10 U. Dunzerhofer, Z. Phytother, 5 (1984) 800-804.
11 N. Chaurasia and M. Wichtl, Dtsch. Apoth. Ztg., 126(1986) 81-83.

12 W.J. Peumans, M. De Ley, and W.F. Broekart, FEBS. Lett. 177 (1984) 99-103.
13 A.M. Le Moal and P. Truffa-Bachi, Cell. Immunol. 115 (1988) 24-35.
14 W.F. Broekart, J. van Parijs, F. Leyns, H. Joos, and W.J. Peumans, Science, 245 (1989) 1100-1102.
15 H. Wagner, F. Willer, and B. Kreher. Planta Med. 55 (1989) 452-454.
16 N. Chaurasia. Inaugural-Dissertation zur Erlangung der Doctorwürde. Pachbereichs Pharmazie und Lebensmittelchemie der Philipps-Universitat, Marburg/Lahn, 1957.
17 S.E. Kudritskaya, G.M. Fishman, L.M. Zagorodskaya and D.M. Chikovani. Khim. Prir. Soedin. 5 (1986) 640-641.
18 N. Krstic-Pavlovic and R. Dzamic, Agrohemija 3 (1985) 191-198.
19 S. Anderson and J.K. Wold, Phytochemistry 17 (1978) 1885-1887.
20 A. Radunz, Z. Naturforsch., C: Biosci. 31C (1976) 589-593.
21 M. Ellnain-Wojtaszek, W. Bylka, and Z. Kowalewski, Herba Pol., 32 (1986) 131-137.
22 L.N. Korchagina, V.F. Rudyuk, and V.T. Chernobai, Rast. Resur. 9 (1973) 577-581.
23 A. Fusseder, B. Wagner, and E. Beck, Bot. Acta 101. (1988) 214-219.
24 B.M. Czarnetzki, T. Thiele, and T. Rosenbach, Int. Arch. Allergy Appl. Immunol. 91 (1990) 43-46.
25 O.V. Vishnevskii and D.V. Proshunina, Farm. Zh. 2 (1989) 50-53.
26 I. Regula, Acta Bot. Croat. 31 (1972) 109-112.
27 E.P. Trofimova, Izv. Akad. Nauk Tadzh. SSR, Otd. Biol. Nauk. 1 (1977) 43-48.
28 V.H. Booth and M.P. Bradford, Brit. J. Nutr., 17 (1963) 575-581.
29 R. Adamski and J. Bieganska, Herba Pol. 26 (1980) 177-180.
30 I. Ullrich and W. Jahn-Deesbach, Angrew. Botanik 58 (1984) 255-266.
31 AOAC, Official methods of Analysis of the Association of Official Analytical Chemists. Thirteenth edition, S. Williams (ed.), Washington D.C., 1984.
32 AOCS, Official and Tentative Methods of the American Oil Chemists Society. Vol. 1 and II., Third edition, W.E. Link (ed.) Illinois, 1973.
33 H. Scherz and G. Kloos, Food Composition and Nutrition Tables 1981/1982. Wissenschaftliche Verlagsgesellschaft, Stuttgart, 1981.
34 Amino-acid Content of Foods and Biological Data on Proteins, Food and Agriculture Organization of the United Nations, Rome, 1970, p 5.
35 G. Lambertsen and O.R. Breakkan, Analyst, 84 (1959) 706-711.
36 W. Franke and A. Kensbock, Ernaehr. Umsch., 28 (1981) 187-191.
37 R. Adamski and J. Bieganska. Herba Pol. 30 (1984) 17-26.
38 J.A. Duke, Handbook of Medicinal Herbs, CRC, 1987, pp. 501-502.
39 Food Composition Tables, Turkish Dietetics Association, Ankara, 1985.
40 Food Composition Tables for the Near East, Food and Agriculture Organization of the United Nations, Rome, 1982.
41 G. Lotti, C. Paradossi, and F. Marchini, Riv. Soc. Ital. Sci. Aliment. 14 (1985) 263-270.
42 V.I. Senchilo, Mater. S'ezda Farm. B. SSR, 3 (1977) 156-157.

43 G. Slapkauskaite and R. Varnaite, Liet. TSR Mokslu Akad. Darb. Ser. C 4 (1988) 25-28.
44 F.C. Luft and M.H. Weinberger, Am. J. Clin. Nutr. 45 (1987) 1289-1294.
45 G.A. Kune, S. Kune and L.F. Watson, Nutr. Cancer 12 (1989) 351-359.
46 I.A. Muravev, L.P. Lezhneva, and A.V. Kuznetsov, Farm. Zh. (Kiev) 1 (1990) 47-49.

ALTERNATES TO SYNTHETIC ANTIOXIDANTS

R.J. EVANS and G.S. REYNHOUT

KALSEC, Inc., Kalamazoo MI 49005

The use of BHA, BHT, TBHQ or propyl gallate has limits. Use of these synthetic antioxidants to protect quality in processed foods is more severely restricted in the EC and the Far East than it is in the U.S.A. In all these markets, there is an increasing preference for, and competition in, further processed foods. The result is a need for improved, acceptable methods of protecting these foods during process stress and extended shelf life.

Recent developments have increased the number of useful, naturally occurring compounds that inhibit oxidative attack in foods. Selecting the optimum performer from these new inhibitors for a specific food system is not always easy. In dealing solely with an oil of known fatty acid composition, the choice of inhibitor is relatively simple. To optimize the shelf life of a formulated food product, evaluation of combinations of two or more inhibitors may be required.

These mixtures can be screened by a number of accelerated tests. Shelf life estimates based on these studies need to be confirmed by evaluation under the actual conditions in the marketplace.

The needs of the food processor for stability may soon become secondary to consumer demand for "antioxidants" in their diet. A series of papers presented at a recent American Chemical Society symposium (1) reported significant physiological benefits from natural foodstuffs containing free radical inhibitors.

Other new technology is impacting antioxidant needs. Consumer concerns relating to trans acid formation in partially hydrogenated fats are already being heard. Unless new, directing catalysts are found to eliminate the formation of trans acids, partially hydrogenated fat declarations on product labels may have a negative effect.

Proper packaging of further processed food is essential. Additives will not help for long if the food package is a poor barrier to oxygen or light or if its volatile components introduce off flavors. Conversely, a good barrier package with an inert atmosphere can augment the benefits of the appropriate inhibitors. The need for good barrier characteristics is not always compatible with the broad demand for recyclable materials.

In the past, cost differentials and limited needs have not supported aggressive development work with natural materials. Now, the trends to further processing, consumer "chemophobia", and publicized challenges to the safety of synthetics have been responsible for an abrupt change in the level of interest in the natural systems. This is true in the U.S. and the EC. Japan has always had a strong preference for the natural inhibitors.

Market needs have focused development efforts on natural systems that provide a level of protection to lipids, pigments and flavors similar to, and even superior to, that of synthetic antioxidants. These changes have shifted the economics. Many companies are currently engaged in intensive searches for new functional natural compounds and new combinations of established naturally derived inhibitors.

The search is identifying effective natural systems that inhibit oxidation and maintain the desirable flavor, color and aroma of these sophisticated foods. The recent literature and symposia include more frequently such things as tea, carob pods, vanillin, oats and other potential candidates. In this decade, we will see one or more of these become commercially significant.

However, the technologist already has a substantial shopping list of technically recognized "natural", functional candidates available. While not all are truly natural products, in the Far East certain reacted materials are considered "natural" or in the EC are considered as "soft" additives. Multinational marketers need to recognize that attitudes differ greatly. As of today, new label laws are being formulated in the U.S. and the resolution of what will be acceptable additives in the various countries in the EC is somewhat unclear. Table I lists those candidates that are likely to survive.

ascorbic acid	phytic acid
ascorbyl palmitate	sage extracts
carob	spices (whole or ground)
carotene	rosemary extracts
citric acid	tea extracts
enzymes	tocopherols
lecithin	vanillin
malic acid	wood smoke
phosphates	

Table 1

This list can be shortened by restricting it to those materials that have proven relatively cost effective, are generally available, reasonably stable, enjoy broad use and are approved for food use in one or more major markets. Some of the survivors may be unsuited for use in certain systems. There may be color reactions, flavor development, a pro-oxidant situation, or solubility limitation. Some are too volatile or thermally degrade. Comments on these limitations will be provided below.

There is another important aspect in evaluating the list of candidates. Some of the terms in this list are generic. There are dramatic difference in behavior among the "tocopherols" and also in the various spice preparations. These differences will be discussed.

LaBuza (2) has established a classification system which will help to group the survivors by mechanism. Class I, primary inhibitors, covers the phenolics, which intercept and neutralize the propagating free radicals. Included are tocopherols, extracts of sage, tea, and rosemary, and wood smoke. Class II, secondary inhibitors, includes the acid chelating agents which inactivate the metal inciters. Class III encompasses environmental factors like heat and light which incite or accelerate oxidation and must be managed.

Phenolics (Class I)
Any of the natural Class I products is a mixture of molecules

having variations of the basic phenolic structure shown in Figure 1.

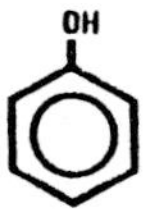

Phenol

Figure 1

The hydrogen of the OH is readily donated to neutralize the highly reactive free radicals developed in the early stage of oxidation. This is the mechanism that stifles the chain reaction of oxidation. The free radicals generated in foods by the oxidation mechanism are widely suspected of being involved in tumor development (3). The intense interest of the press in reports (1) that green tea extracts, beta carotene, spice extracts etc. can inactivate these free radicals is understandable.

Inactivation of the free radical (R$^\bullet$) by a phenolic (PH) is simply expressed as R$^\bullet$ + PH -> RH + P$^\bullet$. The phenolic radical created does not normally propagate further oxidation.

The first of the phenolics to be reviewed are the four tocopherol homologs shown in Figure 2.

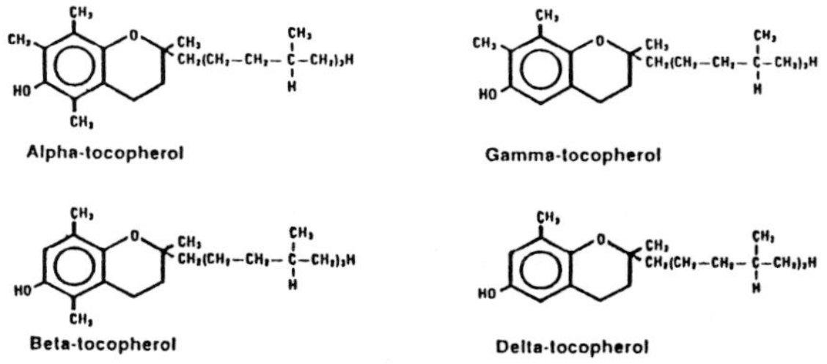

Alpha-tocopherol   Gamma-tocopherol

Beta-tocopherol   Delta-tocopherol

Figure 2

The tocopherols differ among themselves mainly in the number and placement of methyl groups. The natural concentrates are effective antioxidants. The typical phenolic structure, again, is common to the Class I food grade antioxidants. Performance differs greatly and here, especially, the generic term should be avoided.

The homolog of tocopherol most widely mentioned in the literature of the fifties and sixties is "alpha tocopherol". Not all papers specified whether the synthetic "dl" or natural "d" alpha tocopherol was used.

The alpha forms are rarely used for food stabilization. Producers caution that when added to certain substrates, the synthetic dl alpha can become pro-oxidant at levels as low as 200 ppm. Similar pro-oxidant behavior with the d alpha has been reported when measured under accelerated test conditions. This poor performance has been attributed to the influence of the free radical addition product formed by the alpha derived phenoxy radical and an alkoxy radical. In contrast, "spent" gamma and delta radicals form dimers that function as inhibitors (4).

In the more complex physiological systems, d alpha tocopherol (vitamin E) is the most potent antioxidant of the various tocopherols.

The most commonly used tocopherol systems are the "mixed tocopherols", offered in 50 or 70% concentrates. Of the tocopherols present, gamma and delta predominate. Modest amounts of beta, which has little activity, are present. As of today, no synthetic version of these is being marketed. Higher purity natural concentrates of gamma and of delta are under commercial development.

Animal fats are generally devoid of tocopherols and therefore benefit from tocopherol stabilization. The oxidized tocopherol radical, in the presence of iron can become pro-oxidant by the Haber-Weiss reaction. Therefore, the use of a chelating acid with tocopherol is suggested to complex the metals in these fats.

Most crude vegetable oils contain tocopherol mixtures. In crude soy they are present at up to 1500 ppm. In refining, these levels are deliberately reduced. Frankel (5) has suggested that the optimum is between 400 and 600 ppm. If higher levels are left in the refined oils, they demonstrate a pro-oxidant effect (2,5).

If oils are to be stabilized with mixed tocopherol concentrates, it's important to monitor the total level of naturally occurring tocopherol in the refined oil so as to not exceed any pro-oxidant threshold.

The oil solubility of tocopherol and its low flavor level accommodate broad usage. In most systems, its low color level is also advantageous. (A possible exception is in high stress systems like spray drying where oxidation of tocopherol can yield quinones with a characteristic pink color.)

Mixed tocopherol concentrates have broad food approvals and have been used effectively for decades.

Another group of Class I compounds is spices and spice extracts. Whether the ancients first added sage to oils to preserve them or to impart flavor is academic. Through the centuries, certain spice flavors have become characteristic of sausage and preserved meats and these flavorful phenolic systems have continued to serve both purposes.

Of the spices with practical levels of phenolic inhibitors, Table 2 shows those those are most commonly cited.

Rosemary	Peppermint
Sage	Oregano
Thyme	Mace
Turmeric	Nutmeg

Table 2

Spices have the typical cellular structure of the vegetable kingdom. This cellular structure impairs rapid release of flavor, aroma and phenolics. Grinding of spices enhance release of these components and, when freshly ground, their effectiveness. More recently, commercial extraction with food grade solvents has concentrated these fractions into volatile oils and oleoresins. The phenolic are released from the cell and become very efficient. Cort (6) has shown the enhanced efficiency of several extracts as opposed to use of the whole spice in an emulsion system. Data from her study, which was catalyzed by hemoglobin, are shown in Figure 3.

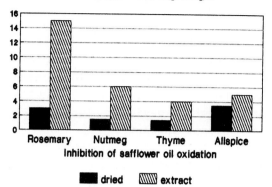

Figure 3

The superior performance of the extracted phenolics may well allow for lower total usage of spices and herbs to achieve any desired physiological effects.

Economo (7) has shown the relationship between addition levels of various oleoresins and onset of rancidity in lard in Figure 4.

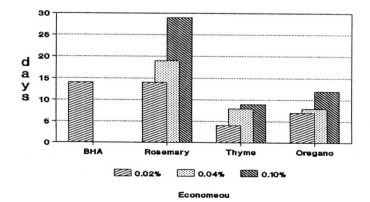

Figure 4

Oleoresins of rosemary have become popular in protecting foods against lipid oxidation, pigment breakdown, color fade and flavor washout. They also affect flavor in several ways. At very low subliminal levels, the harsh acidic high notes of low pH products are smoothed out. With the "burn" minimized, natural flavors of the protected food are emphasized. At slightly higher levels, rosemary can, in many systems, be likened to the rounding benefits of vanilla added to chocolate. The rosemary flavor is not easily perceived but neither is it truly subliminal. Where a pronounced rosemary flavor is desired, higher levels can be used without fear of pro-oxidant problems.

Accelerated screening of natural phenolics is practical. There are various methods for measuring the resistance to oxidation inhibitors impart. Good correlation is often seen between the improvement in shelf life of lipid containing foods and measurements obtained in accelerated studies using the Rancimat (8). This instrument stresses lipids with heat and bubbled air. The volatile by-products of oxidation are collected in water and the increase in conductivity in the water is measured. The rate of increase accelerates suddenly and the time to reach this "induction time" is reported. This method correlates well with the Active Oxygen Method (Swift's Stability Method) which requires frequent peroxide analysis. The Rancimat inflection points are measured in minutes where the slower AOM takes hours. A newer system is being introduced called the Oxidograph (9). This measures oxygen absorption by the sample with computerized manometric chip technology.

There are many phenolics in rosemary. Some that have been identified by Brieskorn, (10) Inatani (11), and Houlihan (12) are shown in Figure 5.

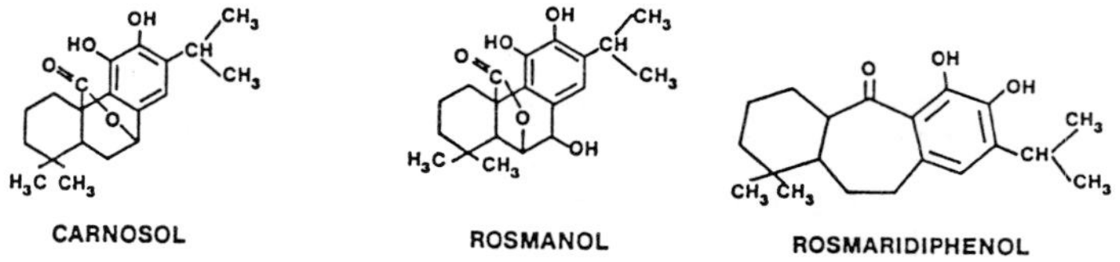

CARNOSOL   ROSMANOL   ROSMARIDIPHENOL

Figure 5

In evaluating rosemary, again, use of generic terms in defining compounds can result in unproductive studies. There are at least four types of "oleoresin rosemary". The first is a simple extractive, produced by procedures that leave much of the phenolics behind. These are primarily flavor concentrates and fall into the commodity class.

The second is one that concentrates the resinous fraction into powders with a significant, but erratic, phenolic content. These powders are poorly soluble in fats and oils unless heated to high temperature.

The third type is produced by supercritical extraction. The extraction procedure has been found to be quite expensive in terms of activity when compared with alternates.

The forth type of oleoresin rosemary encompasses those made by the Chang (13) and Todd (14) patents. Their rapid commercial adoption is the result of several unique factors. These extracts are available as liquids that are soluble in oils at room temperature. Water dispersible and water miscible forms are also available. This greatly simplifies their incorporation when compared with other phenolics. Also, the water miscible version is better able to penetrate the cell wall barrier in seeking out lipids in processing of breakfast cereal, dehydrated potatoes etc.

Required levels of oleoresin rosemary produced under the procedures of Chang and Todd are potent enough to be effective at what ordinarily would be called subliminal flavor levels. At higher levels, its pleasant flavor becomes more perceptible. These extracts, in addition to unique solubility, are effective at levels that pose no problems of color or aroma. In figure 6,

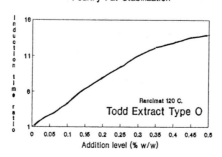

Figure 6

improvement in stability of refined poultry fat is plotted versus addition levels of the extract produced under Chang and Todd. Panelists generally do not detect the rosemary flavor below 1,000 ppm in poultry. Good stabilization is achieved at 500 ppm or lower. Again, note there is no pro-oxidant effect, even at 1,000 ppm level suggested for spray drying, or even at 5,000 ppm. Depending on desire, the flavor can be held at subliminal or significant levels.

Figure 7 shows another unusual property of the Todd rosemary extracts (Type O). Their thermal stability. When held at 200 degrees C., slightly above deep fat frying temperatures, in open vessels, loss through volatilization is modest.

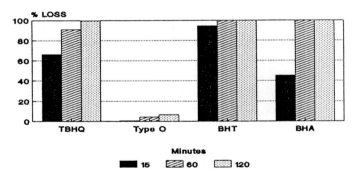

Figure 7

Most important, the inhibiting activity of each of these extracts produced under the Chang and Todd methods is standardized, eliminating the performance variations ordinarily associated with other extracts and, indeed, with many natural products.

Typical benefits in lard stabilization and in inhibiting oxidation in soybean oil that are provided by these extracts are shown in figures 8 and 9.

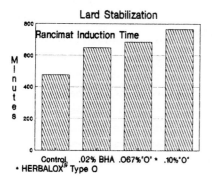
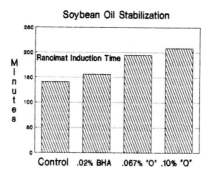

Figure 8   Figure 9

Rosemary, sage and tea extracts may be labeled as such, or as is more common, "natural flavoring added" in most areas. Where a statement of function is required, "to inhibit rancidity" should be acceptable.

The last in the group of approved phenolics is wood smoke. This ancient technology remains an effective technique for inhibiting oxidation. Its use is restricted to those where its characteristic flavor is desirable. No pro-oxidant problems have been reported. Approval for use in the EC is pending and a plant is being constructed within Europe in anticipation.

Chelators (Class II)
This category of aids to retarding rancidity includes the acids. Many function by complexing with trace metals to form chelates. Ohlson (15) has shown inactivation or removal of reactive metals like copper and iron is essential since, in their active state, they accelerate the oxidation reaction. A high free fatty acid content tends to enhance solubility of metals in fats. As discussed above, iron can react with a phenolic by the Haber-Weiss-Fenton mechanism and convert certain phenolics themselves to troublesome free radicals.

Judicious use of organic acids to inactivate metals is often desirable. Choices include malic, citric, phosphoric, and ascorbic acid. Phytic acid is approved for use in Japan. With its 6 chelating sites, it is very reactive. Although it occurs in many crops, regulators are moving cautiously until its effect on mineral metabolism is clarified.

Borenstein reports ascorbic acid reduces iron, enhancing iron assimilation (16). Fe^{++} also can initiate the Fenton reaction.

Lecithin, due to its phosphoric acid content can also chelate metals. Phosphatidyl ethanolamine in lecithin can act as a pro-oxidant in the presence of iron at significant levels according to Brandt (17). While lecithin has excellent fat solubility, when heated it tends to darken. It may also develop a detectable flavor.

Phosphates are often used in foods for various reasons and can function as chelators.

Oxygen Absorbers
Ascorbic acid also has the ability to absorb oxygen. In packages with limited headspace, this can be an effective way to inhibit oxidation. It has good solubility in aqueous systems but is insoluble in lipids. An ester, ascorbyl palmitate has limited solubility in lipids and is also an oxygen absorber.

Oxygen absorption ability has also been attributed to the tocopherols and to beta carotene. These molecules react with singlet oxygen and absorb its tremendous (and highly troublesome) energy.

The packets of oxygen absorbing material sometimes included in food containers are helpful. They, of course, provide no protection of foods during processing. The results of oxidation are not reversible. The use of aluminum in the construction of some of these packets raises a question.

In using absorbers, the importance of proper packaging and package integrity is obvious.

Warmed Over Flavor
No discussion of the flavor impact of oxidation is complete without considering a major problem in meat and poultry. A specific flavor problem in muscle foods results in formation of

noxious compounds that leave no doubt in the consumer's mind about total loss in quality. It is described in the literature by a misleading term, "warmed over flavor".

If muscle tissue is sliced, ground or otherwise comminuted, the ruptured muscle cells release iron and enzymes to react with the unsaturated phospholipids present in the muscle. Peculiar breakdown products result. They generate strong odors when the food is heated in cooking. This type of oxidation continues even at freezer temperatures unless stored at minus 40 degrees C. or lower.

Perhaps it should be called "muscle lipid oxidation" since it does not require either precooking or reheating to develop. The off-flavor and the offensive odors are emphasized by heating. A recent survey by a consumer publication tested a number of frozen entrees. Panelists reported the presence of "warmed over flavor" in both high and low cost product lines, especially beef.

TBA values reported by Gray (18) corresponded well with sensory findings in an evaluation of warmed over flavor using phosphates which chelate and the Todd rosemary extract as the phenolic inhibitor. His findings are shown in Figure 10.

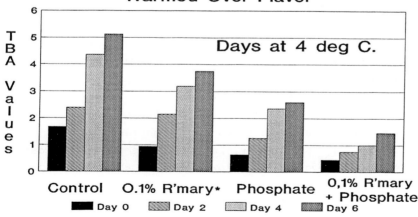

*HERBALOX® Type O Rosemary, Kalsec Inc.

Figure 10

When TBA values are above 2, "warmed over flavor" is generally detectable.

More recently, StAngelo (19) reported on studies of warmed over flavor in cooked beef patties. He reports sensory scores using "cooked beef brothy" as desirable and "painty" and "cardboardy" as detrimental. Results from sequential studies are shown in Figure 11.

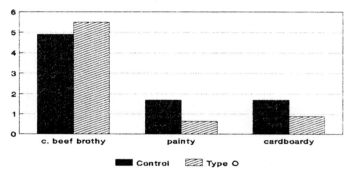

Figure 11

Environmental (Class III)
A PET plastic film metalized on one side can transmit enough light energy to generate singlet oxygen (20). Light transmission is a problem with many types of packaging.

Heat accelerates the oxidative reaction.

Reduction of water content can concentrate reactants and accelerate oxidation. Conversely, LaBuza (21) showed water can inactivate metals by hydration at low levels of water activity.

New Technology
The effectiveness of ascorbic acid in aqueous systems has long been recognized. The introduction of ascorbyl palmitate was an effort to enhance the solubility of ascorbic in lipid systems. This esterification resulted in substantial increases in cost and

provided limited solubility. Extensive research by various organizations has sought ways to enhance the performance of unesterified ascorbic acid in fats. Performance data on a system developed by Todd (22) for use in anhydrous products are shown in Figure 12.

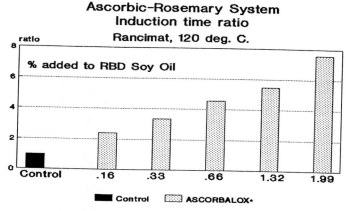

Figure 12

Cautions

In evaluating natural inhibitors or synthetic antioxidant systems, a number of causes for error have been seen often.
1. Frozen material cannot be thawed for use as day 1 or "fresh samples". Oxidation continues in the freezer above minus 40 C.
2. Incorporation of the additive as early as possible in the process is essential. Oxidative damage can't be reversed.
3. Confirmation of accelerated testing data with room temperature data and sensory evaluation is essential.

Conclusion

Obviously, there is far more to managing oxidation than use of an additive. It starts with checking process water for trace metals like copper and iron and ends with an expiration date on the package. The many other factors needing to be managed are reviewed in excellent texts edited by Allen and Hamilton (23) or Min and Smouse (24).

There are indeed many naturally derived inhibitors of oxidation that can be employed in protecting the flavor of processed foods.

Performance data confirms they can match or exceed the synthetics. Of the natural inhibitors discussed here, three have already achieved vitamin status, C, E, and beta carotene as pro-vitamin A. The marketplace had shown that natural materials are desirable and existing regulations insure broad acceptance.

References
1. Symposium, Phenolic Compounds in Food and Health, 8/91, in press, Am. Chem Soc.
2. LaBuzza, T.P. et al, J. Am. Oil Chem. Soc. 46(1969) 409.
3. Symposium, Antioxidants in Foods, IFSc, 10/91, in press, Elsevier Applied Science Pub.,NY,NY
4. Kiyomi, K., Food Antioxidants, Hudson, B.J.H. ed., Elsevier Science Publishers Ltd., Essex, England(1990) 73
5. Frankel, E.N., et al, Fette-Seifen-Anstrichmettel 61(1959) 1036.
6. Cort, W. M., Fd. Technol., Champaign, 28(1974) 60
7. Mikrolab, Aarhus Denmark
8. Metrohm AG, Herisau, Switzerland
9. Economou, K.D. et al, J. Am. Oil Chem. Soc. 68(1991) 109.
10. Brieskorn, C. H.,et al, J. Org. Chem. Soc. 29(1964) 2293.
11. Inatani, R.,et al, Agric. Biol. Chem. 46(1982) 1661
12. Houlihan, C.M.,et al, J. AM. Oil Chem. Soc. 62 (1985) 96.
13. U.S. Patent 3,950,266 (Chang, S. et al).
14. U.S. Patent 4,283,429, 4,877,635, (Todd, P.) and others.
15. Ohlson, R. "Symposium on Metal Catalyzed Oxidation", Paris, Sept. 1973.
16. Borenstein, B., Food Technology 41:6 (1987) 98.
17. Brandt,P., Lebensmittel Ind, 20 (1983) 21.
18. Gray, J.I., Third Int'l. Conf. on Food Additives, Food Ingredients Europe, London 1988.
19. StAngelo, A.J.et al, J. Food Sci. 55(1990) 1501.
20. D.B. Min, Flavor Chemistry of Foods, Min, D.B. and Smouse, T.H., (eds) The Am. Oil Chem. Soc.,Champaign IL (1989)92.
21. LaBuza, T.P, Crit. Rev. Food Technol. 2:355 (1971)
22 U.S.Patent pending, (Todd, P., Kalsec, Inc.)
23. Allen,J.C. and Hamilton, R.J.(eds) Rancidity in Foods, 2nd edition (1989) Elsevier Applied Sci.Pub. NY,NY.
24. Flavor Chemistry of Foods, Min, D. B. and Smouse, T.H., (eds) The American Oil Chemists Society, Champaign IL,

UTILIZATION OF COTTONSEED PROTEIN IN PREPARING NEW EDIBLE FOOD PRODUCTS

Y.G. MOHARRAM[1] and N.S. ABU-FOUL[2]

1. Food Science And Technology Department, Faculty of Agriculture, Alexandria University, Alexandria, Egypt.

2. Gaza Palestine, Omar El-Mokhtar Street, El-Remal, 54-163.

1. INTRODUCTION.

An adequate supply of low cost, high quality protein food is needed to break the vicious cycle of poverty, malnutrition and disease. The objected world protein deficit by 2000 is expected to be 4.314.000 metric tons (Ridlehuber and Gardner, 1974). Oilseeds such as cottonseed in the form of refined edible flour can offer a partial solution to this problem. The annual production of cottonseed is around 34 million tons (FAO, 1989). It contains ca 20% protein. So, it can participate by ca. 6% of world's total supply of edible protein. On other side, there are a number of factors, both economic and technical, have combined to prevent the use of any significant quantity of cottonseed flour for human food. Therefore most of this flour is used currently as cattle feed where is a conversion ratio from plant to animal protein of 6 or 7 to 1 (Ridlehuber and Gardner, 1974).

The main problem of the utilization of cottonseed in food purpose is a gossypol, a toxic pigment unique to plants of the cotton tribe (Smith and Clawson, 1970). But gossypol can be inactivated by cooking or by chemical treatments, extracting with selective solvents, separating the pigment glands by liquid or air classification or bred out of the plant by genetic or radiative means. Each of these procedures has advantages and disadvantages. But generally the technology of their applications is still not widely known. The biological value and digestibility of cottonseed are somewhat lower than soybean, resulting lower net protein utilization (NPU). On the other hand, the protein efficiency ratio (PER) and the chemical score of cottonseed and soybean are comparable (Anon, 1970). The consumption of glandless cottonseed flour in human nutrition is still limited comparing with soybean, peanut and sesame oil seeds. It is only being employed as an additive in bakery products (Khan et al. 1976 and El-Sayed et al. 1978 a,b), as a filler in meat products (Lawhon et al. 1974; Ziprin et al. 1981 and Abdel-Aal 1988). and supplement to cereal based diet as an Incaparina vegetable protein mixtures (Bressani, 1965).

2. COTTONSEED CHARACTERISTICS:

2.1 Physical properties.

Cottonseed is processed into four major products, approximately 16 % crude oil, 45% meal, 9% linters and 26% hull (cater et al. 1979). According to Bhatt et al. (1961) no significance differences were noticed in the kernel percent (50.1-53.2%) between the cottonseed varieties. The hull percent was significantly higher in *Gossypium arbareum* and *G. herbaceum* than in *G. hirsutum*. The hull, kernel and the seed index (the weight of 1000 g seed) of the Egyptian cottonseed varieties were 32.4-44.1%, 58.3-67.6% , and 9.07-10.39 g (Abdel Rahman 1961, Osman et al. 1981 and Helmy, 1985). Lusas and Jividen (1987) reported that the percent and weight of 100 kernel of glanded and glandless cottonseed were 61.4 and 59.6, 6.5 and 7.0 g, respectively. Wan et al. (1979) suggested the removing of both hull and pigment glands to improve the colour of the glandless and liquid cyclone process (LCP) cottonseed flour. The Hunter "L" lightness value of the colour of the dry hexane-extracted glanded and glandless cottonseed flour was 84.3 and 89.8 , respectively (Lusas and Jividen, 1987). The light tan colour of LCP cottonseed flour had L. (lightness) 87.3, and b (yellowish) 14 (Blouin and Cherry, 1980). Lovibond colour of glanded and glandless cottonseed were 29.5 and 29.6 yellow, 5.9 and 5.9 red, 6.8 and 6.9 blue, respectively. After defatting with hexane the blue colour was disappeared and the red colour was reduced to 0.2-0.9. The colour of the flour was described as white in case of glandless varieties and yellow in glanded types. The bulk density of the whole, flour, defatted , and degossypolized cottonseed was 0.62, 0.63, 0.52, and 0.72 g/cm^3 (Abu-Foul , 1990). Rahma and Narasinga Rao (1983 b) found that the bulk density of cottonseed flour increased after chemical and enzymatic modification.

The hull, the protective tissue of cottonseed, forms from two integuments of several layers of cottonseed empty and lignified palisade cells containing pigments. The cotyledon consists of cellular cytoplasmic including, nuclei, spherosomes, aleurone layer, and other particular important components to the physiological of the seeds in addition to gossypol glands in glanded cottonseed varieties. The oil is usually stored in an intracellular organs cells called spherosomes with a 2 μ diameter. Part of protein is located in aleurone grains with a diameter ranges from 9-20 μ as storage protein. The other is distributed among the cells of cotyledon and known as non storage protein. Within the protein bodies, there is a globoids, the storage site of the phytin and phytates. Gossypol glands consist of a rigid cell wall with 5-8 closely fitting thick curved plates. It has a large size, 100-400 μm, and net work like internal structure (Yatsu, 1965; Englemen, 1966; Dieckert and Dieckert, 1976 and Osman et al. 1987). According to Abu-Foul (1990) no variations were observed in the ultrastructure of the cotyledons of the kernels of glanded , Giza 76, and glandless, Alex. IV, cottonseed varieties except the gossypol glands (Fig. 1 A). The latter are located only in the cotyledons of the glanded cottonseed type (Fig. 1 B). Each gossypol gland is enclosed by a double rings of an elongated thin wall, It is strongly coloured visually and appeared perfectly clear under light

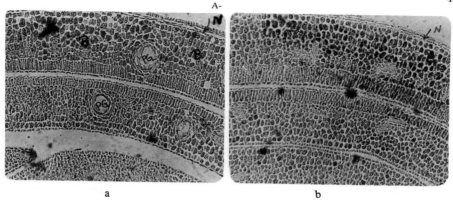

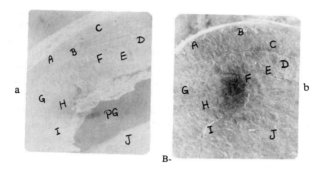

Fig. 1 A. Light micrograph of cottonseed (2.5 x 0.08 x) stained with Sudan black B.
(a), Glanded, Giza 76, variety (b) Glandless, Alex IV, variety.
B. Scanning electron micrograph of cottonseed (45x, 10 Um).
A. Hull or cell wall, B. Mitochondria,
C. Endoplasmic retinculum, D. Aleurone layer,
E. Globoid, F. Nucleus, G. Spherosome,
H. proptasid, I. Plasmodesmate, J. Dicytosome,
PG. Pigment gland

microscopy. This is an indication that their contents are homogeneous and are in state of single phase solution or solid. Also, the outer structure of these glands appeared as a rigid and not membraneous wall (Fig. 2A, B) consisting of distinct spherical particles embedding in a net work like structure (Yatsu et al. 1974 and Abu-Foul, 1990).

Dehulling of the cottonseed did not affect the ultrastructure of cottonseed. Defatting with hexane led to disorganize the cytoplasmic membranes of the cytoplasm. The oil bodies became empty and also intact after this process (Hensarling et al. 1970). The protein bodies and gossypol glands did not influence with this process (Abu-Foul, 1990). Only solvents containing water caused disruption for the gossypol pigment gland intracellular structure (Jacks et al. 1974). Degossypolization of cottonseed with organic solvents (Fig. 3A,B) led to remove the gossypol, disappear the internal structure of the pigment glands, disrupt the intercellular structure and rupture the cell wall of the gossypol gland (Abu-Foul, 1990).

2.2. Chemical properties. The major components of cottonseed is the carbohydrate followed by protein and oil. Dietary fibers represents the main part of the cottonseed carbohydrates. It consists of 25.9% lignine, 11.42% hemicellulose, 2.5% cellulose (Abu-Foul, 1990) According to Abdel-Aal (1988) the Canadian dehulled glandless cottonseed contained 14.5% dietary fiber. Lawhon et al. (1977) showed that no variation in sugar content was observed between 16 varieties of cottonseed. The total sugars form from 11.95% rafinose, 2.62 % sucrose, 0.68% stachyose and traces of glucose (Cegla and Bell, 1977). The level of oil, crude protein, crude fiber and free gossypol are varied from 17.1-23.2, 36-46, 1.2-1.7 and 0.004-0.27 %, respectively between glandless cottonseed varieties (Pandey and Thejappa, 1976 and Green et al. 1977). The range of moisture, crude protein, crude oil, ash, crude fiber, carbohydrate and free gossypol are 7-10, 17.4-24.3, 18.4-23.8, 2.2-2.6, 18.7-19.3, 28.5-39.5 and 1.03-1.31%, respectively in glanded varieties (Lopes, 1970; Osman et al. 1981, Helmy, 1985, and Ikurior and Fetuga, 1988). According to Gad et al. (1961) and Osman et al. (1981) significant differences are only observed in gossypol and flavonoids contents between glanded and glandless cottonseed varieties. The minerals of cottonseed can be arranged according to their concentrations in the following decreasing order, P, K, Ca, Na, Fe, Cu, Mn, Ni, Co, Pb and Cd, respectively (Abu-Foul, 1990).

Dehulling reduces 35% of the nitrogen free extract, 89% of the crude fiber, 80% of neutral detergent fiber(NDF) , 88% of acid detergent fiber (ADF) , 60% of the hemicellulose, 62% of the cellulose, 91.5% of lignine and 29.5% of Na and increases the other components (Damaty and Hudson, 1975; Osman et al. 1981; Helmy, 1985; Sun Shankang et al. 1987; Ikurior and Fetuga, 1988 and Abu-Foul, 1990). Defatting with hexane reduces the oil to 0.8-1.15 % and increases the protein, gossypol , total flavonoids and minerals (Canella and Sodini, 1977; Rahma and Narasinga Rao 1984; El-Fishawy, 1986; Lusas and Jividen, 1987 and Abu-Foul, 1990). Table (1) shows the effect of oil extraction methods on gossypol content. Generally, the level of moisture, crude protein, oil, ash , crude fiber, carbohydrate and free gossypol are ranged from 3.1-4.8 , 48.01-65.4, 0.32-1.9, 7.1-9.3, 3-4.4,

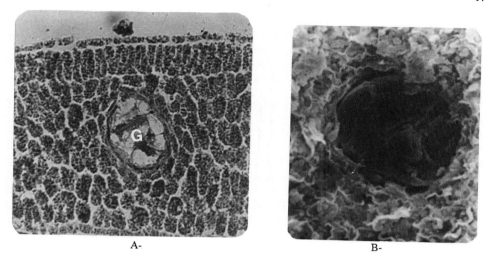

Fig. 2. Light (A) (6.3 x 016x) and scanning electron micrograph
(B) (x 200) of gossypol pigment glands of glanded, Giza 76, variety.

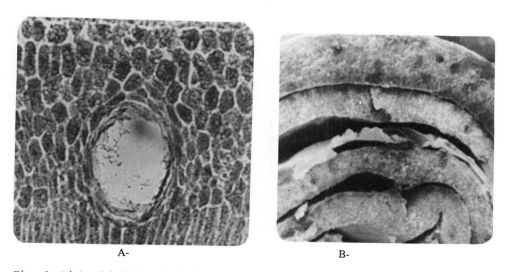

Fig. 3. Light (A) (6.3 x 0.16x) and scanning electron micrograph
(B) (10Um) of glanded cottonseed cotyledon after degossypolization
with 70% acetone 99.5% acetone.

Table 1
Effect of oil extraction methods on free, bound and total gossypol

Oil extraction method	% Gossypol			Reference
	Free	Bound	Total	
1- Direct solvent extraction.	0.05-1.45	0.08-0.88	0.29-1.93	Relich et al. 1968; Shaheen et al. 1973; Mayorga et al. 1975; Canella and Sodini, 1977; Cherry and Gray,1981;Osama et al. 1981;Anon. 1982; Rahma and Narasinga Rao, 1983 a and 1984 and Abu-Foul, 1990
2- Screw press solvent extraction.	0.007-0.045	0.905-1.08	0.95-1.12	Milner, 1960; Mayorga et al. 1975 and Anon. 1982
3- Pre-press solvent extraction.	0.05-0.2	0.88-1.08	0.95-1.13	Milner, 1960; Mayorga et al. 1975 and Anon. 1982
4- Cooking solvent extraction.	0.12-0.31	1.097-1.41	1.217-1.72	El-Sayed et al 1978a;Rahma and Narasinga Rao,1983 a, b and El-Fishawy, 1986.
5- Azeotropic solvent extraction using Hexane, acetone, water.	0.1-0.164	0.232-0.268	0.332-0.432	El-Sayed et al 1978a and El-Fishawy, 1986
6- Successive solvent extraction :				
a- Hexane, 85% isopropanol alcohol.	0.069	0.58	0.649	Rahma and Narasinga Rao, 1984
b- Acetone-85% isopropanol alcohol.	0.15	0.27	0.42	Rahma and Narasinga Rao, 1984
c- Hexane-70% acetone, 99.5% acetone.	0.011—0.021	0.186	0.197	Cherry and Gray, 1981 and Abu-Foul, 1990
d- Hexane-75% acetone, methylene chloride	0.014—0.039	0.158	0.172	Cherry and Gray, 1981 and Abu-Foul, 1990
e- Hexane-30% H2o, methylene chloride.	0.075—0.14	0.13	0.144	Cherry and Gray, 1981 and Abu-Foul, 1990
I- Liquid cyclone process(LCP) :				
Over flow flour	0.031-0.07	0.014-0.3	0.045-0.95	Smith, 1971; Wan et al 1979; Blouin et al 1981 and Cherry and Gray, 1981.
Under flow flour	2.6	0.82	3.42	
7- Hexane followed by flotation technique (Hexane-perchloroethylene).	0.144	0.244	0.388	El-Fishawy, 1986.
8- Glandless cottonseed meal	0.002-0.064	0.01-0.11	0.015-0.174	Bui-xuan Nhuan,1970; Lawhon et al 1972 ; Wan et al 1979; Blouin et al 1981 and Blankenship; Alford, 1983 and Abu-Foul, 1990

11.4-16.9 and 1.38-1.72%, respectively in cottonseed meal (Bressani et al. 1964; Braham et al. 1965; Bui-xuan Nhuan, 1970; Canella and Sodini, 1977; Osman et al. 1981; Rahma and Narasinga Rao, 1984, Lusas and Jividen, 1987 and Abu-Foul, 1990).

2.3. Functional properties. Lawhon and Cater (1971) showed that the foam capacity and foam stability after 0.0, 10 min. and 4 hrs. at pH 4 of the glandless cottonseed protein were 64-82, 11.3-32.5 and 4-29.3 ml, respectively. According to Lawhon et al. (1972) the glandless cottonseed flour produced foams of higher viscosity and greater volume when whipped in various liquid media than had been obtained from whipped protein isolate. The results of Crenwelge et al. (1974) showed that the oil addition in the range of 0.4-2 ml /sec. did not appreciably affect the rate of emulsification capacity. The optimum pH for obtaining a good emulsification capacity from cottonseed flour were 8.9 and 0.884. g/100 ml. Lawhon et al. (1974) stated that the foams of egg albumin were less stable than foams from cottonseed protein. The data of Childs and Park (1976) indicated that the water and oil holding capacities, emulsification and foaming capacities of glandless cottonseed flour were 3.5, 2.6, 456.6 and 126.67 ml/g. The acetylation of glandless cottonseed flour caused an increase in the specific viscosity of the flour and its functionality and a decrease in heat coagulability of the protein isolate. They noted that emulsification capacity of a protein depends upon the level of solubilized protein (Kinsella 1976 and Rahma and Narasinga Rao, 1984). On the other side, the partial succinylation of cottonseed flour increased the yield of protein isolate at pH 4.5 and gave protein isolate with higher water soluble, lighter in colour, higher in oil absorption, emulsion capacity, gel strength, water hydration, water retention, viscosity and lower in bulk density as compared with non succinylated protein isolate. The same observations were reported by Choi et al. (1982) for protein isolates from succinylated, maleylated and dimethylglutarylated flours. The effect of enzymatic modification of cottonseed flour with a protease enzymes on the functional properties was studied by Rahma and Narasinga Rao (1983a). The results showed a decrease in holding capacity (30%), increase in emulsification capacity (90%), foam capacity (40%) and bulk density. However, foam stability and oil absorption capacity did not improve. They also reported that the degossypolization of cottonseed flour with a mixture of 1:1 of 85% isopropanol and hexane reduced the fat absorption capacity. El-Refai et al. (1987) found that nitrogen solubility index and emulsion stability were higher for Egyptian glandless cottonseed flour than glanded one, while the water capacity was nearly similar in both flours. Osman et al. (1987) found that the foaming capacity and viscosity of storage protein (SP) were superior than of NSP. On the other hand, the foam stability for the SP was inferior to non storage protein (NSP). According to Zarins and Marshall (1988) the water capacity of glandless cottonseed flour was 204. The study of Abu-Foul (1990) showed that slight variations were observed in the functional properties, water absorption, fat absorption, emulsification capacity, foaming capacity, foaming stability and nitrogen solubility index between cottonseed flour of glanded and glandless varieties. Removing of the cottonseed hull improved from these properties. Water and fat absorption were increased after degossypolization of glanded cottonseed with organic solvents, while other properties were decreased. On the other side, marked increase in the viscosity was noticed only with the increase of the protein content from 0.5-2% of the free fat of glanded, glanded degossypolized and glandless cottonseed flour suspensions. A sharp increase in turbidity in free fat flour suspension of cottonseed varieties was observed up to 70°C and especially at 90°C. The changes in turbidity, heat denaturation of the protein at the last temperature were more noticed in glandless than glanded varieties, especially after dehulling and degossypolization processes (Abu-Foul, 1990).

2.4 <u>Nutritional value</u>. Several investigators determined the amino acids of cottonseed meal and protein (Tables 2 and 3). The biological value (BV), net protein utilization (NPU) and digestibility of cottonseed meal are somewhat less than those of soybean, while the protein efficiency ratio (PER) and chemical score are comparable (Anon, 1970). El-Sayed et al. (1978a) reported that the protein digestibility of Egyptian glandless cottonseed flour was 90.7% compared to 100.6 % for casein and 73.6% for wheat flour. Martinez and Hopkins (1975) found that PER's and lysine values were ranged from 1.26-1.82 and 3.6-4% in commercially processed glanded cottonseed meals. PER and epsilon amino free lysine (EAF available lysine) decreased from 2.34 to 2.3 and 3.82 to 3.76% after cooking the glandless cottonseed meal at 108.9°C. Abu-Foul (1990) showed that the degossypolization of glanded cottonseed with organic solvent, acetone and methylene chloride, with percolation technique increased the content and the availability of lysine, improved the PER, digestibility and the chemical score to the level similar to that found in glandless cottonseed protein.

The non storage protein isolate (NSP) of cottonseed contains higher level of lysine, methionine, leucine, isoleucine and arginine than storage protein isolate (SP) (Osman et al. 1981 and Abu-Foul, 1990). The PER of the total, storage and non storage protein isolates of defatted glandless cottonseed are 2.22, 1.4 and 2.4, respectively (Martinez and Hopkins, 1975).

3. REMOVAL THE COTTONSEED GOSSYPOL

Several procedures were suggested to solve the cottonseed gossypol problem. It includes:-

3.1 <u>Inactivation by cooking</u>. According to Bailey (1948) cooking of cottonseed meals prior to hydraulic or screw pressing serves to inactivate gossypol. It converts the gossypol from the free to the bound form (Bressani et al. 1964) Cater and Lyman (1969) stated that during cooking the free gossypol reacts with the free amino group of cottonseed protein. The free gossypol content of cooked meal is about 0.04-0.1% after hydraulic pressing and 0.02-0.06% after screw pressing (Berardi and Goldblatt, 1980). At these levels, the meal is suitable as feed not only for cattle, sheep and goat but also for non ruminant such as swine, horse, mule and poultry when it applied to 9% of total ration (Bailey, 1948). Extrusion cooking of full fat kernels of cottonseed in a Brady low cost extruder gave product with a low nutritional value (PER. 1.43, NPU. 30.9) and high free gossypol content

Table 2.
Amino acids content of cottonseed meal prepared by different methods.

Amino acids (g./ 100 g. protein)

Cottonseed genotype:	Cystine	Glycine	Lysine	Available lysine	Tryptofan	Threonine	Valine	Methionine	Leucine	Isoleucine	Phenylalanine	Histidine	Arginine	Aspartic acid	Serine	Glutamic acid	Proline	Alanine	Tyrosine	References
Glanded	1.62-4.8	3.94-4.68	2.3-5.6	3.23	1.22-1.69	2.25-4.4	3.45-5.51	0.7-2.71	3.65-8.8	2.45-5.0	3.19-6.8	2.7-5.29	9.28-15.9	6.36-10.42	2.31-5.33	16.76-20.78	1.42-4.4	3.01-6.24	1.59-4.05	Martinez and Frampton, 1962; Krishnamoorthi, 1965 ; Rooney et al. 1972; Harden and Yang, 1975; Kadan et al. and Abu-Foul, 1990
Glandless	2.22-2.8	4.36-4.7	4.4-6.6	3.8-4.5	1.22-2.05	3.1-4.47	4.5-5.1	0.6-7.2	6.7-6	3.1-3.6	3.1-6.6	2.6-4.13	10.01-11.93	9.11	3.9-4.88	18.02-20.7	1.19-4.6	3.13-6.8	2.09-3.9	1980; Osman et al. 1981; Zarins and Cherry, 1981; Blankenship and Alford, 1983; El-Bary et al. 1985 Zhuge et al. 1988 and Abu-Foul, 1990
Oil extraction methods:																				
1- Successive solvent extraction:																				
A-Liquid cyclone process (LCP)	2.2	4	4.2	3.6	1.4	3.1	4.1	1.5	5.7	3.3	5.7	2.7	12	9	4.2	21.1	3.7	3.7	3.1	Castro et al. 1976 and Lusas and Jividen, 1987
B- 70% acetone, 99.5% acetone. a:		4.65	4.16-4.44		1.67	3.13-3.86	4.41	1.12-2.67	5.67	3.16	5.86	3.42	9.45	9.29	4.33	19.80		4.5	2.89	Cherry and Gray, 1981 and Abu-Foul, 1990
b:		4.64	4.26		1.65	1.88	4.48	1.16	6.51	3.46	5.86	3.41	9.88	9.35	4.39	19.26		4.17	2.91	Abu-Foul, 1990
C- 75% acetone, methylene chloride. a:		4.61	4.15-4.62		1.69	1.44-1.92	4.49-5.27	1.16-3.1	6.16	3.2	5.85	3.42	9.27	9.7	4.40	20.07		4.16	2.91	Cherry and Gray, 1981 and Abu-Foul, 1990
b:		4.66	4.22		1.68	1.92	4.47	1.17	6.62	3.9	6.88	3.41	9.51	9.06	4.30	19.92		4.18	2.90	Abu-Foul, 1990
D- 30% H2O, Methylene chloride a:		4.60	4.11-4.35		1.68	4.26-4.90	4.46-4.7	1.6-3	6.05	3.19	5.87	3.46	9.81	9.34	4.18	20.12		4.16	2.91	Cherry and Gray, 1981 and Abu-Foul, 1990
b:		4.61	4.21		1.80	3.94	4.18	1.15	6.58	3.10	5.86	3.41	9.95	9.22	4.4	20.08		4.18	2.96	Abu-Foul, 1990
E- Hexane - acetone - water			4.2		1.67	3.78	5.67	1.41	9.37		5.02	2.83	11.82							El-Fishawy, 1986
2- Cooking solvent extraction	3.5	3.2-3.52			0.67	2.7-3.2	3.72-4.2	1.01-1.41	7.36-8.90	2.16-3.39	4.16-4.27	2.22-2.67	9.03-9.61	8.03	3.44	16.07	3.14	3.30	2.22	El-Bary et al. 1985 and El-Fishawy, 1986
3- Gland flotation			4.51		1.45	3.9	5.41	1.35	9.07		4.96	2.7	11.74							El-Fishawy, 1986
4- Expelled air classification	1.61	4.6	4.18			3.46	3.53	1.84	5.81	2.36	5.94	4.95	10.78	10.50	5.27	20.56	4.05	4.58	3.84	Zhuge et al. 1988

Dessolventization methods:-

a - Blending

b - Percolation

Table 3.

Amino acids content of cottonseed protein isolates prepared by different methods.

	Amino acids (g./ 100 g. protein)																	
	Cystine	Glycine	Lysine	Available Lysine	Tryptohan	Threonine	Valine	Methionine	Leucine	Isoleucine	Phenylalanine	Histidine	Arginine	Aspartic acid	Serine	Glutamic acid	Proline	Alanine	Tyrosine	References
Glanded cottonseed flour:																			
Acid precipitation total protein isolate			4.26		1.15	3.94	5.47	1.32	9.12	9.12	5.11	2.73	10.04							El-Fishawy , 1986
Azeotropic protein isolate.			4.15		1.16	3.82	5.64	1.44	9.38	9.38	5.04	2.77	9.28							El-Fishawy , 1986
Protein isolate heated precipitate.			3.15		0.64	3.30	4.25	0.98	8.86		4.92	2.72	9.01							El-Fishawy , 1986
Glandless cottonseed flour:																			
Acid precipitate:																			
Storage protein isolate (SP)	1.3	1.53	4.19	2.93 1.13	2.8	1.16	2.63 02	4.64 69	1.11 45	5.66 34	3.3 67	6.38 35	3.10	12.67	9.46	5.0	21.29	1.08	3.73	3.88	Zarins and Cherry, 1981; Lusas and Jividen (1987) and Abu-Foul, 1990
Nonstorage protein isolate (NSP)	3.1	3.25	4.52	6.28 09	5.8	1.6	3.44 65	2.99 46	1.59 19	4.33 64	3.44 47	4.14 69	2.48	8.53	10.5	4.14	19.35	4.78	6.03	3.15	Zarins and Cherry, 1981; Lusas and Jividen (1987) and Abu-Foul, 1990
Ultrafiltration :																			
Storage protein isolate (SP)	1.0		3.3	2.9	1.6	3	4.7	1.6	5.9	3.1	5.9									Lusas and Jividen (1987)
Nonstorage protein isolate (NSP)	3.9		6.7	3.1	1.7	3	4.1	1.7	5.6	3	3.9									Lusas and Jividen (1987)
IIS protein isolate.	0.18	5.15	2.67		1.78	2.84	5.27	0.58	6.57	4.64	6.32	2.73	14.20	10.10	4.0	22.46	3.3	4.45	1.53	Reddy and Narasinga Rao (1988b)

(0.11%) (Jansen et al. 1978). In contrast, extrusion of solvent extracted cottonseed flour through a Wanger extrusion cooker at temperature 115 to 175°C reduced the free gossypol content three to five fold. The extruded meal had a good functional and nutritional properties with biological value 55-57 (Vs 56 for texturized soybean protein) and 3.6% available lysine (Cabrera et al. 1979). Osman et al. (1981) found that traditional cooking process at 220-230°F for 20 min. for cottonseed flakes containing 10% moisture reduced 47 % of the free gossypol. The increasing of the moisture content of the flakes to 18% before cooking and using 180°F and 40 min. for cooking lowered 18% of free gossypol. According to Shah et al. (1986) the free gossypol content of cottonseed meal was reduced to 0.045% by soaking in boiling water for 15 min. Zhuge et al. (1988) developed a process based on extrusion, drying, fine grinding and air classification to reduce the gossypol. The free, bound and total gossypol were changed from 0.28, 0.067 and 0.95 % in whole meal to 0.03 , 0.49 and 0.52 % in coarse fraction and 0.04, 0.92 and 0.96 % in fine fraction , respectively.

3.2 <u>Chemical treatment</u>: According to Rice (1952) the treatment of hexane defatted cottonseed flakes with aniline and water for 20 min. at 100°F (38°C) in a Jacketed mixing unit then drying at 230°F (110°C) for 20 min. gave a bright golden yellow meal containing 0.04% or less free gossypol. The dianilino-gossypol product formed through this process is non toxic and could be left in the meal. Bressani et al. (1964) reported that the addition of iron in the presence of calcium salts reduced the concentration of free gossypol in food mixtures containing cottonseed flour. According to Calrk et al. (1965) the treatment of cottonseed meal with a primary aliphatic amine caused a reduction of total and free gossypol of cottonseed. The soluble gossypol-amine derivative was removed upon extraction with hexane leaving meal with a total gossypol content of 0.3% (Calrk, 1966). They also reported that iron salts, such as ferrous sulfate, are effective in an activating gossypol when added to swine and poultry rations, probably by forming a complex that is not readily absorbed from the digestive tract. This treatment turns the meal colour to the brownich-black (Clawson and Smith 1966). Aslam et al. (1970) found that a combination of 1.5% calcium hydroxide + 0.2 % ferrus sulfate reduced gossypol to 0.04 % but gave a meal with a dark colour. Bressani et al. (1980) showed that cooking of cottonseed meal with calcium hydroxide and ferrous sulfate reduced the free gossypol to 0.04%. The irradiation of solvent extracted cottonseed meal with gamma radiation reduced 80% of total gossypol content (Jaddou et al. 1983). Rahma and Narasinga Rao (1983a and b) indicated that both chemical and enzymatic modification of cottonseed meal reduced free gossypol by 33-50% and by 40%, respectively. Bound gossypol was reduced only by 10-15 % after chemical modification.

3.3 <u>Extraction methods</u>: According to Bailey (1948) the preliminary rupture of the walls of the glands by moistening or grinding permits rapid extraction of gossypol by any organic solvents such as chloroform or diethylether. Vaccarino (1961) reported that a 50 ton/day commercial plant for the production of gossypol free cottonseed meal by acetone extraction has been operated by G. and S Vaccarino company in Sicily since

1957. The process is similar to the pre press hexane extraction process but requires a rectifying tower to remove the water extracted with the oil and gossypol. The obtained meal is used in feed for chickens, laying hens and pigs. Vix *et al.* (1969) used mixture of acetone, hexane and water in direct extraction of cottonseed flakes. The nutritional value of the obtained meal was high but their colour and flavour were objectionable. The lingering, bitter after taste characteristic of these feeds, was ascribed to interaction of sulfhydryl compound, such as cysteine, with mesitly oxide present in the acetone or formed during processing. According to Krishnamoorthi (1965) the use of a mixture of hexane acetone and water removed part of the free gossypol from cottonseed meal to the extracted oil. Cater and Lyman (1969) prepared low gossypol-cottonseed meal by using successive extraction with hexane-2-butanone and ether, respectively at room temperature. Cottonseed flour with 0.01-0.03% free and 0.2-0.36% total gossypol was prepared by Damaty and Hudson (1975) using sequential extraction, first with aqueous, and then with anhydrous acetone. The flavour of this product was not acceptable and described as catty odour due to the reaction between the hydrogen sulfide resulted from the decomposition of the sulfur-containing amino acids and the mesitly oxide in acetone. The results of Cherry and Gray (1981) showed that using 70% acetone followed by 99.5% acetone; 75% acetone followed by methylene chloride; 30 % moisture followed by methylene chloride lowered the free gossypol of cottonseed meal from 1.083 to 0.011; 0.014 and 0.014 %, respectively. Rahma and Narasinga Rao (1984) extracted cottonseed flakes with one of the following solvents: (A) hexane; (B) 1:1 mixture of 85% isoporopanol and hexane ; and (c) acetone followed by 1:1 mixture of isopropanol and hexane. They found that meal (B) had the lowest free gossypol content (0.069%). Abu-Foul (1990) degossypolized defatted hexane cottonseed meal with three selective solvent systems, 70% acetone followed by anhydrous acetone, 75% acetone followed by methylene chloride and increasing the moisture of the meal to 30% followed by methylene chloride. These solvents reduced both gossypol from 0.781 to 0.017-0.073% and flavonoids from 0.925 to 0.05-0.17 %, nitrogen free extract from 33.61 to 25.5-28.6% and increased from protein, crude fiber and ash. No much differences were osberved as a result of applying these solvents either by percolating and/or blending methods.

3.4 <u>Gland removal methods</u>. The resistance of the pigment glands to rupture led to the development of several methods for removing of gossypol glands by mechanical methods (Bailey 1948). The gland flotation process including the suspension of the fine ground meal in a flotation liquid of a 1.378 g/ml density such as hexane/perchloroethylene, agitating violently to detach the glands from adhering tissues, centrifugation and removing the pigment glands from the meal (Boatner and Hall, 1946; Vix *et al.* 1947 and 1949; El-Fishawy, 1986 and Osman *et al.* 1987). The disadvantages of the gland flotation process led to the development of the Liquid Cyclone Process (LCP) (Vix et al. 1971 and Horn *et al.* 1982). In this process differential settling of meal components in a single liquid, hexane, with the centrifugal force, a liquid cyclone, was used to accentuate the separation. The products are a gland free overflow slurry containing 13-15% high protein solid and a gland rich coarse meal under flow slurry containing 43-45% solids (Gardner *et al.* 1976). Hensarling and Jacks (1982) suggested the following points to improve the results of this process , (1) addition of acetic acid to hexane to aid oil separation, (2) extraction with mixed solvents to improve the colour, (3) extraction of the under flow with propylene glycol/methylene chloride to remove the gossypol and (4) sonication to increase the recovery of LCP protein from 25.9% to over 60%. Generally, the LCP flour had much nitrogen solubility, high available lysine, good colour, 2.34 to 2.67 PER value and a good functional properties. (Hensarling and Jacks, 1982). According to Martinez *et al.* (1970) USDA's Southern Regional Research Center developed a process based on employing a spiral classifier to separate coarse particles from fine. The yield of the edible flour produced by this process was 44% and was similar to the LCP product in its contents of free and total gossypol, nitrogen solubility, available lysine, colour and flavour (Freeman *et al.* 1979). Shemer (1980) separated the defatted glanded cottonseed flour into particles of an average diameter greater or smaller than 0.8 mm. The fine particles fraction had 0.0% free and 0.9-1.3% total gossypol, 58-62% protein with 1.6 PER value. This process was called the Physical Fractionation Process (PFP), and the obtained flour was named Milou-Pro. The flour was added to certain type of soups, souces, minced beef, turkey meat and backed products in Israel and in tortillas in Mexico. The products were acceptable and palatable but had a brown colour (Trostler *et al.* 1983).

3.5 <u>Glandless cottonseed</u>. The development of edible cottonseed occurred in 1959 when McMichael succeeded in breading glandless cottonseed by crossing cultivated Acala cotton strains with the a primitive Hopi strain from Arizona. A different approach was used in Egypt to produce *G. barbadense* cotton with glandless seeds called Bahtim 110. This strain was derived from a glanded Giza 45 variety which subjected to irradiation with radioactive phosphorus (Afifi *et al.* 1966). The glandless cottonseed flour had a lighter colour and bland flavour than glanded one (Wan *et al.* 1979). Until now the production of these varieties is scanty and is not economically competitive with glanded cottonseed types.

4. COTTONSEED EDIBLE PRODUCTS.

Until now the cottonseed meal is used mainly as a feed for ruminants, where there is a conversion ratio from plant to animal protein of 6 or 7 to 1., and as a fertilizer. According to Gillham (1969) one-quarter of the flour potentially available from world production of cottonseed could alleviate the protein shortages of under developed nations. A primary technical objective in the processing of edible cottonseed flour is the reduction of the toxic impact of gossypol. The previous part showed that this problem could be solved by selecting the proper degossypolizing process and its efficient application. Abu-Foul (1990) stated that the degossypolization of cottonseed meal with 70% acetone followed by anhydrous acetone led to:-

1. Removal the free gossypol to level less than the 0.045%, the permissible limit by FAO(1973).

2. Producing a new product in addition to the known four of cottonseed, gossypol. This product can be used in the production of antiseptic, pharmaceuticales, plastic and explosive industries.

3. Improving the colour of cottonseed flour by reducing its content of flavonoids.

4. Yielding flour containing 54.72-62.01 % protein, with solubility greater than 50% in Nacl solution, 1.1% lipid, 2.6-3% crude fiber, 7.98-9.3% ash, 3.9% available lysine, bland flavour, light yellow colour, high water and fat absorption , good emulsification capacity and viscosities, excellent foam properties with high stability, a considerable gelation characteristics and good heating denaturation characteristics.

Generally, these properties meet FDA approved in USA, the guidelines established by the Protein Advisory Group (PAG) (1971) and nearly similar with those of glandless one. These advantages help to wide the utilization of the flour of glanded cottonseed varieties in food applications. Generally there were a limited uses for this flour comparing with glandless one which is not produced economically at the present time. Also the levels of uses of the later flour, glandless cottonseed, in food preparation did not more than 25% except in case of Tamunut. Generally, the following points were suggested by Abu-Foul (1990) to prepare vegetable protein mixture edible products based on cottonseed flour.

1. Containing approximately 30% protein with more essential amino acids than those reported in FAO (1973).

2. Having 25-100% level of cottonseed flour.

3. Free from foreign matter, microorganisms and toxic substances.

4. With a bland flavour, light colour, and functionally desirable.

5. Stable under processing, marketing and stroage conditions.

6. Useful as additives in traditional as well as new food formulations.

7. Processing at competitive costs.

4.1. <u>Glanded cottonseed flour</u>: According to Altschull *et al.* (1950) a food grade cottonseed flour has been produced commercially in United State, under the name Proflo. The manufacture of this product differs from that of meal in several respects, the seed is selected more carefully, the hulls are essentially all removed , more oil is left the press cake, and the press cake is pulverized and classified until 97% of it passes through a 200 mesh screen. Anon (1963) reported that Proflo contains 58.4% protein with 62.5% solubility in 0.02 N NaoH, 5.1% lipids, 2.4% fiber, 0.03% free gossypol, 0.92% total gossypol, 2.9% phytic acid, 3.5% available lysine, dark yellow colour and slight flavour. The substituion of up to 10% of wheat flour by Proflo in bread, biscuits, carakers, doughnuts and prepared food mixes increased the protein content and quality with no secrifice in appearance, flavour, texture, or eating quality. Several blends were prepared by Bresseani (1965) containing from 9 to 38% cottonseed flour. Protein content, protein digestibility and PER of these blends were 27% , 70% and 2.3, respectively. Bressani et al. (1969) stated that a vegetable protein mixture was developed in the 1950 by Institute of Nutrition of Central America and Panama (INCAP), Guatemale, called Incaparina, to use as dietary supplement for protein defecicent low income population. The original product contained 29.4% corn flour, 29% sorghum, 38% cottonseed flour, 3% torula yeast, 1 % $CaCO_3$ and vitamin A (45000 I.U./100 g.). The specification for the use cottonseed flour were, the free gossypol content being no more than 0.06 % and 1.2% total gossypol. In India, weaning foods called Ball-Ahar and Ball-Amur used the Incaparina prenciples (Scrimshaw, 1980). Cooking foods containing Incaparina reduced the free gossypol level by 53% owing to the interaction of gossypol with $CaCO_3$ present in formula (Bressani et al., 1980). The results of the nutritional studies carried out on weanling rats and dogs showed that both Proflo and Incaparina are not only high in nutritional value but also their levels of free and bound gossypol were not high enough to interfere with reproduction (Bressani et al. 1980). Matthews et al. (1970), Green et al. (1976) and Blouin et al. (1981) evaluated the LCP cottonseed flour as a substitute for wheat flour in bread, biscuit, cake, doughnuts, sugar cookies, macaroni, wafers, chapatis, peanut butter cookies and salting cracker's for corn flour in muffins and tortillas (Mc Pherson and Ou, 1976) for rice in breakfast cereals (Spadaro and Gardner, 1979) for milk in cream cake filling, for non fat dry milk in soft serve frozen deserts (Martinez et al. 1970) for beef in ground patties and frankfurters (Terrell et al. 1979). According to Cater et al. (1977) LCP cottonseed flour can be texturized by thermoplastic extrusion and the product is comparable with textured soy flour. The results of Harden and Yang (1975) indicated that up to 25% of wheat flour could be repalced by LCP cottonseed flour in bread making by straight-dough method but the product had a rough texture and dark colour. In Egypt, Abu-Foul (1990) prepared:-

1. Six extruded products from degossypolized glanded cottonseed flour (Fig. 4). He found that the products made from 1:1 cottonseed to rice or corn had nearly the same physical properties of that prepared from 100% corn or rice. The extrusion process lowered 70% of the gossypol, did not affect the proximate composition and slightly improved the nutritional properties of the extruded products. Generally, the utilization of cottonseed increase the protein content and improved the nutritional value of such products.

2. Six suggested food gruel blends from degossypolized glanded cottonseed flour. The gruels were high in protein, excellent in nutritional value and with a good organoleptic characteristics. The consistency of these food gruels was based on the type and source of starch, protein content, temperature and the ratio of the dry blend to water. Only the colour of these gruels was less acceptable than that containing glandless cottonseed flour (Fig. 5).

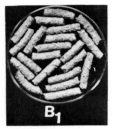

40% GCS
40% RF
17% Balady chick pea
3% casein (free fat)

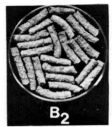

40% GCS
40% CF
17% Balady chick pea
3% casein

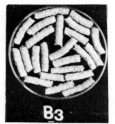

40% GCS
20% RF
20% CF
17% Balady chick-pea
3% casein

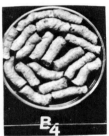

40% DGCS
40% RF
17% Balady chick pea
3% casein

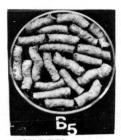

40% DGCS
40% CF
17% Balady chick pea
3% casein

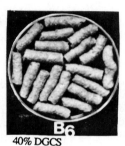

40% DGCS
20% RF
20% CF
17% Balady chick pea
3% casein

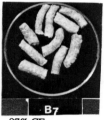

97% CF
3% casein

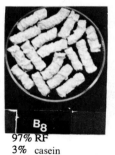

97% RF
3% casein

Fig.(4): Ingredients and appearance of the cottonseed extruded products.
GCS = Defatted glandless cottonseed flour; DGCS = Defatted glanded degossypolized cottonseed flour;
RF = Rice flour; CF = Corn flour.

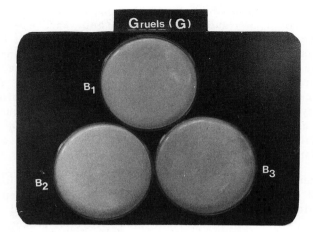

Degossypolized cottonseed, Giza 76 variety

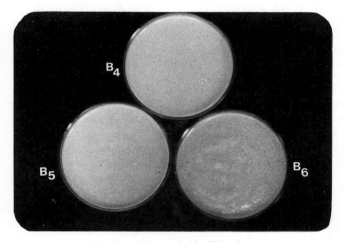

Glandless Cottonseed, Alex.IV variety

Fig. (5)
Appearance of the food gruels based on cottonseed protein.

3. Nine types of high protein biscuits. He found that these products were high in protein, excellent in nutritional value, and had a good acceptability compared with that made from 100% wheat flour. The physical properties, thickness, weight index and dimensions, of these types of biscuits were affected according to the presence or absence of gluten, type and source of starch, and protein content. Generally, the panelists preferred the products containing glandless cottonseed flour than glanded degossypolized one. Also, biscuits could be prepared without wheat flour and also from 100% cottonseed flour. Coating of biscuits with chocolate led to avoid the discolouration problem and improved from the platability of this product (Fig. 6).

4. Ten types of doughnuts from degossypolized glanded cottonseed flour. The results showed that the products had a good organoleptic properties. The coating of this products with chocolate instead of immersion in sugar solution improved from their sensoric properties. Generally the panelists preferred the products containing glandless than glanded degossypolized flour (Fig. 7).

5. Ten vegetable blends to use as a fried products (Fig. 8). The obtained data indicated that these products had a technological properties, weight loss, shrinkage, oil absorption, and frying time, comparable with the control, 100% decorticated faba bean. The panelists accepted all products either containing glandless or degossypolized glanded cottonseed flour.

6. Vegetable cottonseed dairy products (Figs. 9, 10 and 11). He found that the blending of reconstituted Nido milk with degossypolized glanded and or glandless cottonseed milks at a ratio of 3:1 and 1:1 after addition the butter flavour gave excellent dairy products. These products were equal in its physiochemical properties and sensoric properties with reconstituted Nido milk. The milk made from 3:1 Nido reconstituted to glandless cottonseed milk gave acceptable curd and yoghurt products.

7. Acceptable cottonseed butter and chocolate (Figs. 12 and 13). The butter was prepared from either whole or defatted glandless cottonseed flour after roasting at 160°C for 20 and 7 min., respectively. The chocolates prepared from the butter of both type of cottonseed were acceptable especially that made from mixing one part of cottonseed butter to three part of cocao chocolate.

4.2. Glandless cottonseed:

4.2.1. Kernel uses: The discovery of glandless cottonseed led to the development of Tamunuts (TAMUS = acronym of Texas A and M University) in 1968, whole undefatted kernels for use in snack food and other's applications (Anon, 1978). Toasted cottonseed kernels had a bland nutty flavour that is highly pleasing in snacks especially in candies, baked goods, cracked wheat-type breads (containing 60% protein), pecan-type pies, dessert toppings and ice cream in USA (Rosenblum, 1980). A mixture of 1:1 white rice and Tamunuts gave a tasty product with triple the protein content of rice. Grinding the toasted Tamunut in equipment used for peanut

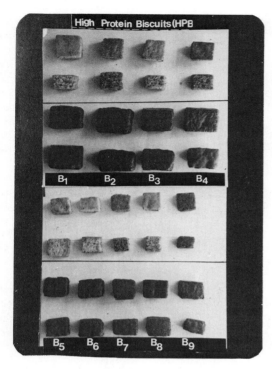

Fig. (6) Appearance of high protein biscuit based on cottonseed protein.

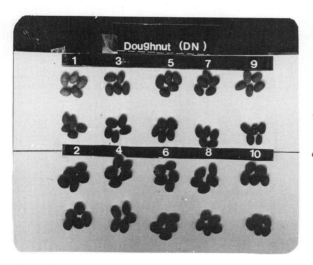

Fig. (7) Appearance of doughnut based on cottonseed protein.

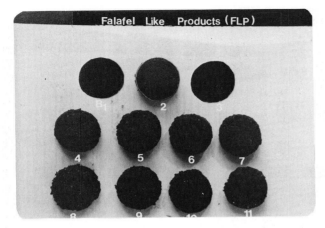

Fig. (8) Appearance of falafel like products based on cottonseed protein.

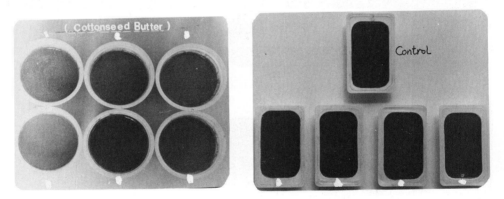

Fig. (12) Appearance of cottonseed butter.

Fig. (13) Appearance of cottonseed chocolate.

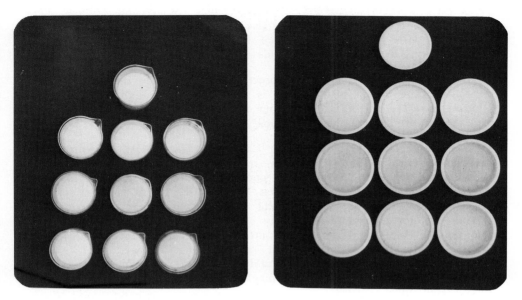

Fig. (9) Appearance of milk made from cottonseed milk, soybean milk and Nido Nestle milk blends.
Fig. (10) Appearance of Yoghurt made from cottonseed milk, soybean milk and Nido Nestle milk blends.

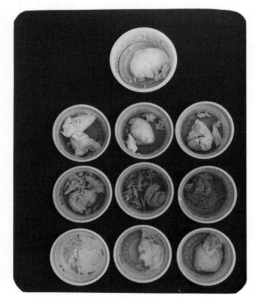

Fig. (11) Appearance of curd made from cottonseed milk, soybean milk and Nido Nestle milk blends.

butter gave a highly acceptable Tamunut butter (Staats and Tolman, 1974). Combinations of cooked long grain rice, wild rice, bulgur, wheat and white corn grits with glandless cottonseed kernel prepared as side dishes gave attractive products rich in amino acids (Anon, 1978 and Reber et al. 1983).

4.2.2. Flour uses: It can be processed in the same manner as glanded cottonseed. The colour of the flour is white and much lighter than those of glanded one. The flavour of this flour is bland and equivalent in bladness to milk based protein supplement (Anon, 1978).

4.2.2.1. Meat products: Lawhon et al. (1974) found that meat leaves containing 25% partially rehydrated wet-processed cottonseed concentrate had 55% less loss of cook-out juices than control loaves. El Sayed et al. (1978 a,b) showed that however the meat sausage containing 20% glandless cottonseed flour had better texture than the control. Its flavour did not acceptable. Generally cottonseed flour can substitute 10% of the sausage meat without greatly affecting the acceptance taste and the nutritive value of sausage. Ziprin et al. (1981) showed that glandless cottonseed concentrate was considerably more effective than soy or peanut products for retarding the development of oxidative ranciditiy in cooked refrigerated meat patties.

4.2.2.2. Cereal and baked products. Martinez et al. (1970) produced high protein wheat breads with an excellent characteristic by replacing 15% of wheat flour by cottonseed flour. Generally, the maximum successful wheat flour replacement level was approximately 10%. Castro et al. (1976) recommended the use of full fat glandless cottonseed flour for replacement of wheat flour by 10% in white bread and 100% in browness and some cookies and confectioneries. Khan et al. (1976) reported that glandless cottonseed concentrate was similarly to glandless cottonseed flour when used to fortify bread by 30% protein. In Egypt, the study of El-Sayed et al (1978 a,b) indicated that protein content of the bread can improved by adding 7.5-10% glandless cottonseed flour. This addition did not affect the bread acceptability and increased its protein content to 30-42 %. Also they found that the replacing of 5% of the semolina with glandless cottonseed flour gave macaroni product similar in its technological and sensoric propeties to the control.

The sugar cookies prepared with 6% 100 mesh glandless cottonseed flour by Lawhon et al. (1972) were highly acceptable, and preferred over 100% wheat flour controls. The sensory acceptable replacement for glandless cottonseed flour in quick breads, biscuits, muffins, coffee cakes, and nut breads was found to be approximately 25 % of the wheat flour (Milner, 1969; Harden and Yang, 1975; Blouin et al, 1981). According to the results of El-Sayed et al. (1978a,b) biscuits containing 5% glandless cottonseed flour had better organoleptic quality than control. Results of Lawhon et al. (1975) showed that doughnuts fortified with glandless cottonseed flour were judged statistically equivalent to doughnuts fortified with high solubility soy flour. Green et al. (1976) fortified corn tortillas with glandless cottonseed flour, and high solubility soy flour to achieve 11, 13 and 15% protein in the blends. They found that tortillas fortified with glandless cottonseed flour were slightly preferred over the soy flour fortified product. In 1977, Green *et al.* reported that incorporation of up to 18% glandless cottonseed kernels in corn tortillas gave acceptable organoleptically product similar to control and preferred over soy-fortified one. Also it increased the protein content by 62% (from 11.1 to 18 %) and appreciably improved the protein efficiency ratio (PER) of the protein. Abu-Foul (1990) prepared acceptable high protein biscuits and doughnut products from blends containing 25-100% glandless cottonseed flour.

4.2.2.3. <u>Dairy products and beverages</u>: El-Soda *et al.* (1979) studied the effect of adding cottonseed flour to cow's milk in zabadi making. They found that the chemical and sensory properties of product containing 5, 10 and 15 g. cottonseed flour per 100 g. milk were similar to those of the control. Increasing the cottonseed level to 25 g gave product with a salting flavour, weak consistency, yellow colour and weak acidity. Tamucurd, a tofu-like product, from glandless cottonseed kernels was prepared by Kajs *et al.* (1979). The obtained curd had a bland flavour and used as a cream cheese substitute in cooking and in preparing of a link-sausage type meat substitute product. Abou-Donia *et al.* (1983) prepared acceptable processed cheese containing 5.4% of glandless cottonseed flour. Glandless cottonseed flour has been evaluated as a substitute for 5, 10 and 15% of non fat dry milk in ice cream by El-Deeb and Salam (1984). Results indicated that the possibility of replacing milk non-fat solids with up to 10% defatted cotton flour in vanillin mixes and up to 15% in chocolate mixes. Abu-Foul (1990) prepared a good acceptable milk, curd and zabadi by mixing 1:3 of glandless cottonseed milk and Nido reconstituted milks (Fig. 14).

4.2.2.5. <u>Frozen desserts</u>. Simmons *et al.* (1980) reproted that no statistical differences in overall acceptability of soft-serve frozen desserts at up to 20% replacement of their solids by glandless cottonseed flour, and 60% replacement by SP isolate.

4.2.2.5. <u>Vegetable protein mixtures</u>. In Egypt, El-Sayed *et al.* (1978a) formulated three baby food using glandless cottonseed flour at 25% level with wheat and rice flours. The protein content was generally high (22.4-25.8%) and contained balanced amino acids. Also, they prepared soup containing 80% glandless cottonseed flour and 5% skim milk powder, 1% fresh carrots, 3% fresh potato, 1% tomato juice, 1% dried onion, 1 % dried garlic, 1% cumin and 1% salt. In Haiti, a corn -based blend of glandless cottonseed flour and cottonseed oil for pre school age children was found to be comparable in nutritional quality, acceptability and gastroin testinal tolerance to the US food for Peace blend, corn-soy-milk (CSM) (Hayes *et al.* 1983). A study of various corn-based formulation showed that glandless cottonseed flour gave a better quality protein than soybean or peanut flour. The blends without dairy products had the best colour and flavour stability (Hayes *et al.* 1984). Abu-Foul (1990) found that the blend containing 40% glandless cottonseed flour, 40% rice or corn, 17% chick pea and 3% casien was rich in nutritional value and suitable to prepare acceptable food gruels, high protein biscuits , doughnut and fried bean paste like products.

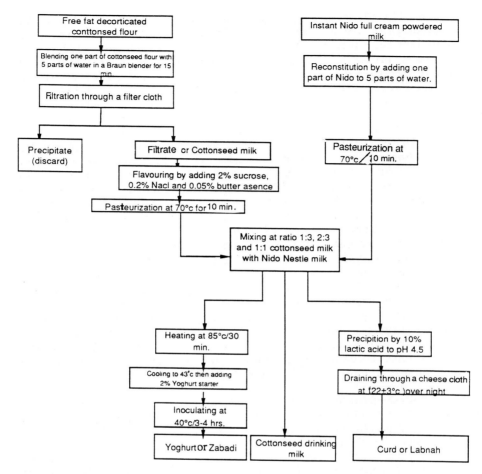

Fig (14)   Schematic diagram for producing cottonseed dairy products

4.2.2.6. Extrudate products. The extrusion of defatted native glandless and glanded cottonseed flours (CS and LCP) produced extrudates with highly puffed, expanded structures and low bulk densities (Taranto et al. 1975 and Gegla et al. 1977a, b). The addition of cereals to cottonseed flours before extrusion improved the physical and sensory properties of the extrudates and reduced the production costs (Cegala et al. 1977c, and Abu Foul, 1990).

The results of Jansen et al. (1978) showed that the extrusion inactivated 52% of antitrypsin activity, improved the PER, lowered the free and total gossypol in extruded blends of whole corn and glanded cottonseed (70/30) and of sorghum / glandless cottonseed mixtures. The extruding for the glanded cottonseed alone reduced the level of free gossypol from 0.65% to 0.21 % and increased the protein quality to that of casein (Taranto et al. 1978). Taranto and Rhee (1979) reported that the microscopic examination of glandless cottonseed extrudate products showed that they are not fibrous but sheated polymer matrices interspersed with insoluble carbohydrate in a brick and mortar structure. Del Valle et al. (1986) prepared extrudate products from a blend of cottonseed / soybean (50/50) using a Brady low cost extruder. They found that the obtained product was comparable in quality to soy products and had a good nutritional value. Abdel-Aal (1988) prepared acceptable extrudate products by blending glandless cottonseed with rice and faba bean flours at a ratio of (1:8:1 w/w). The extrusion conditions of these products were 15-20 % feed moisture, 180-200°C barrel temperature and 180 rpm screw speed. The extrusion process improved the protein digestibility of the product. Abu-Foul (1990) prepared acceptable extrudate products by blending 40% glandless cottonseed with 20-40% rice or corn flour, 17% chickpea , 3% casien, 1.5 salt, 1% ammonium bicarbonate, 1% calcium carbonate , 2% dry yeast, 0.5 % dry cheese and traces of anato dye (Fig. 4).

4.2.3. Protein isolate uses. Lawhon et al. (1974) showed that the orange-flavoured "ade" beverages and the orange-flavoured fruit drinks containing up to 3% glandless cottonseed protein isolate were organoleptically acceptable. Berardi and Cherry (1980) reported that suspended total glandless protein isolate in 0.3% NaCl at pH 4-9 can be texturized by heating to 90°C with continuous agitating. The meat loaves containing up to 10% of the textured protein isolate had acceptable texture, colour and flavour. Increasing the level of texturized protein to 30% resulted non acceptable product even with added oil and flavour. Choi and Rhee (1984) found that glandless cottonseed protein isolate was preferred as soybean isolate at levels up to 40% repalcement for sodium caseinate in imitation. Mozzarella cheese analogs According to El-Fishawy (1986) the nutritional value of the biscuits containing 20% cottonseed protein isolate was superior than control.

5. REFERENCES

1. E.M. Abdel-Aal, Formulation and evaluation of novel, nutritious and economical products from cereal, legume and oilseed blends, ph. D.

Thesis, 1988, Food Science and Technology Department, Faculty of Agriculture. Alexandria University, Alexandria, Egypt.

2. A.Y. Abdel-Rahman, Technological and chemical studies on cottonseed and cottonseed oil, M.Sc. Thesis, 1961, Food Technology Department, Faculty of Agriculture. Alexandria University, Egypt.

3. S.A. Abou-Donia, A.E. Salem and K.A. El-Sayed, Indian Dairy Sci. 36, 1983, 119.

4. N.S. Abu-Foul, Physico-chemical, nutritional and technological studies on food uses of glanded and glandless cottonseed protein, ph. D. Thesis, 1990. Food Science and Technology Department. Faculty of Agriculture. Alexandria University, Alexandria, Egypt.

5. A. Afifi, A.A. Abdel-Bary, S.A. Kamel and I. Heikal, The Emire cotton Growing Rev. 34, 1960, 112.

6. A.M. Altschull, G.M. Lyman and F.H. Thurber, in : A. M. Altschull (Ed), Processed Plant Protein Stuffs: Cottonseed Protein, Academic Press, New Yourk, 1950, pp. 469-534.

7. Anon, Proflo. Data Sheet No. 102, 1963, Traders Oil Mill Co., fort. Worth, Texas, U.S.A.

8. Anon,FAO Nutritional studies , No. 24, 1970, FAO, Roma, x+ 285 pp.

9. Anon, Nutritional cottonseed products. Assoc. Memphis, Tenn, 8th (ed.), 1978, 22pp.

10. Anon, J.A.O.C.S. 59, 1982, 752-766 A.

11. M. Aslam, M. Arshad and A.S. Magsood, Pakistan Journal of Scientific and Industrial Research. 13, 1970, 271.

12. A.E. Bailey (Ed), Cottonseed and cottonseed products, "Their chemistryu and chemical technology" Intersience publishers, INC, New York, 1948.

13. L.C. Berardi, and J.P. Cherry, J.Fd. Sci. 45, 1980, 377.

14. L.C. Berardi, and L.A. Goldblatt, in: L.A. Liener (Ed), Toxic constituents of plnt food stuffs: Gossypol, 2nd. Edn., Academic Press, New York, 1980, pp. 183-237.

15. J.Y. Bhatt, K.S. Bhujag and R.L. Lyengar, Indian cotton. Growing. Rev. 15, 1961, 374.

16. D.C. Blankenship and B.B. Alford, "Cottonseed; The new staff of life, 1983, TWU Press, Denton; TX.

17. F.A. Blouin, and J.P. Cherry, J.Fd. Sci. 45, 1980 953.

18. F.A. Blouin, Z.M. Zarins and J.P. Cherry, J.Fd. Sci. 46, 1981, 266.

19. C.H. Boatnar and C.M. Hall, Oil and Soap, 23, 1946, 123.

20. J.E. Braham, L.G. Elias and R.L. Bressani, J.Fd. Sci. 30, 1965, 531.

21. R.L. Bressani, Fd. Technol. 14, 1965, 1655.

22. R.L. Bressani, J. E. Braham and L.G. Elias, Fd. Nutr. Bull. 2, 1980, 24.

23. R.L. Bressani, L.G. Elias, J.E. Braham and M. Erales, J. Agric. Fd. Chem. 17, 1969, 1135.

24. R.L. Bressani, L.G. Elias, R. Jarquin and J.E. Braham, Fd. Technol. 18. 1964, 95.

25. Bui-Xuan-Nhuan, Oleagineux. 26, 1970, 713.

26. J. Cabrera, L.E. Zapata, T.S. DeBuckle, I. Ben-Gera and A.M. De Sandoval, J. Fd. Sci. 44, 1979, 826.

27. M. Canella and G. Sodini, J.Fd. Sci. 42, 1977, 1219.

28. C.E. Castro, S.P. Yang and M.L. Harden, Cereal Chem. 53, 1976, 291.

29. M.L. Cater, J.P. Cherry and P.A. Moller, Oil Mill Gaz. 83, 1979, 22.

30. C.M. Cater, and C.M. Lyman, J.A.O. C.S. 46, 1969, 649.

31. C.M. Cater, K.F. Mattil, W.W. Meinke, M.V. Taranto and J.T. Lawhon, J.A.O.C.S. 54, 1977, 90A.

32. G.F. Cegla, and K. R. Bell, J.A.O.C.S. 54, 1977, 150.

33. G.F. Cegla, W.W. Meinke and K.F. Mattil (Ed), Comparison of properties of texturized extrusions of native and denature cottonseed flours. Proceeding of 37th. Annual Meeting of the Institute of Food Technologists, Philadelphia, PA, June 5-8, 1977a, U.S.A. paper # 407.

34. G.F. Cegla, W.W. meinke, D..A. Suter and K.F. mattil, (Ed), Some critical parameters for the extrusion texturization of cottonseed flours. Proceeding of 37th Annual meeting of the Institute of Food Technologists, Philadelphia , PA, June 5-8, 1977 b, U.S.A. Paper # 428.

35. G.F. Cegla, D.A. Suter , W.W. Meinke and K.F. mattil (Ed), Texturization and evaluation of fortified glandless and glanded cottonseed flours. Proceeding of 37th Annual Meeting of the Institute of Food Technologists, Philadelphia , PA, June 5-8, 1977 c, U.S.A. Paper # 408.

36. J.P. Cherry and M.S. Gray, J.Fd. Sci. 46, 1981, 1726.

37. E.A. Childs and K.K. Park, J. Fd. Sci. 41, 1976, 713.

38. Y.R. Choi, E.W. Lusas and K.C. Rhee, J.Fd. Sci. 47, 1982, 1713.

39. Y.R. Choi and K.C. Rhee, Annual report to the natural fibers and food protein commission, 1983-1984. Food protein research and developing center, Texas A and M University, College Station, Tx, 1984, pp. 263-274.

40. S.P. Clark (Ed), Inactivation of gossypol with mineral salts: National Cottonseed Products, Association, Memphiss, Tenn., U.S.A., 1966, pp. 178-182.

41. S.P. Clark, B.D. Deacon and J.T. Lawhon, Oil Mill Gas. 69, 1965, 16.

42. A.J. Clawson and F.H. Smith, J. Nutr. 89, 1966, 307.

43. D.D. Crenwelge, C.W. Dill, P.T. Typor and W.A. Landman, J. Fd. Sci. 39, 1974, 175.

44. M.S. Damaty and B.J. Hduson, J.Sci. Fd. Agric. 26, 1975, 109.

45. F.R. Del Valle, M. Escobedo, P. Ramos, S.De Santiago, R. Becker, H. Bourges, K.C. Rhee, Y.R. Choi, M. Vega and J. Ponce, J.Fd. Sci. 51, 1986, 1242.

46. J.W. Dieckert and M.C. Dieckert, J. Fd. Sci. 41, 1976, 475.

47. A.A. El-Bary, M.A. Bisher and K.A. El-Sayed, Alex. Sci. Exch. 6, 1985, 123.

48. S.A. El-Deeb and A.E. Salam, Alex. Sci. Exch. 5, 1984, 87.

49. F.A. El-Fishawy, Chemical and technological studies on cottonseed proteins, M.Sc. Thesis, 1986, Food Science and Technology Department, Faculty of Agriculture. Assuit University, Egypt.

50. A.A. El-Refai, Studies on proteins and enzymes in fruits and cottonseed. Ph. D. Thesis, 1978. Institute of Food Technology and Dairy Science, Technical Univ., Munich, Federal Republic of Germany.

51. A.A. El-Refai, M.A. Owon, K.A. Ammar and A.M. Harras, Chemie Mikrobiologie Technologie der Lebensmittel. 11, 1987, 13.

52. K.A. El-Sayed, E.A. Salem and A.A. Abdel-Bary, Alex. J. Agric. Res. 26, 1978a, 327.

53. K.A. El-Sayed, E.A. Salem and A.A. Abdel-Bary, Alex. J. Agric. Res. 26, 1978b, 609.

54. M. El-Soda, K.A.. El-Sayed, A.A. El-Bary, A. Abou-Donia and R.I. Mashaly, J. Dairy Sci. 62, 1979, 61.

55. E.M. Englemen, Am. J. Bot. 53, 1966, 231.

56. Food and Agriculture Organization , FAO Nutrition Meetings Report Series. 52, 1973.

57. Food and Agriculture Organization, Production Yearbook, 42, 1989, Fd. and Agric. Org., United Nations, Rome.

58. D.W. Freeman, R.S. Kadan, G.M. Ziegler and J.J. Spadaro, Cereal Chem. 56, 1979, 452.

59. A.M. Gad, M.N. Hafez and A.Khier Eldin, J. Chem. (U.A.S.) 4, 1961, 273.

60. H.K. Gardner, R.J. Horn and L.E. Vix, Cereal Chem. 53, 1976, 549.

61. F.E. Gillham, S.Afr. J. Sci. 65, 1969, 173.

62. J.R. Green, J.T. Lawhon, C.M. Cater and K.F. Mattil, J.Fd. Sci. 41, 1976, 656.

63. J.R. Green, J.T. Lawhon, C.M. Cater and K.F. Mattil, J.Fd. Sci. 42, 1977, 790.

64. M.L. Harden, and S.P. Yang, J. Fd. Sci. 40, 1975, 75.

65. R.E. Hayes, P.H. Carolyn, J.I. Wadsworth and J.J. Spadaro, Fd. Nutr. Bull. 5, 1983, 23.

66. R.E. Hayes, J.J. Spadaro, J.I. Wadsworth and D.W. Freeman, AR S-S. 18, 1984, US Dep. of Agric. , Washington D. C., IV+24 pp.

67. H.E. Helmy, Factors affecting colour fixation of cottonseed oil, ph. D. Thesis 1985. Food Technology Department, Faculty of Agriculture. Ain Shams University, Egypt.

68. T.P. Hensarling and T.J. Jacks, J.A.O.C.S. 59, 1982, 516.

69. T.P. Hensarling, L.Y. Yatsu and T.J. Jacks, J.A.O.C.S. 47, 1970, 224.

70. R.J. Horn, S.P. Koltun and A.V. Graci, J.A.O.C.S. 59, 1982, 233.

71. S.A. Ikurior and B.L. Fetuga, Fd. Chem. 26, 1988, 307.

72. T.J. Jacks, L.Y. Yatsu and T.P. Hensarling,. J.A.O.C.S. 51, 1974, 169.

73. H. Jaddou, M.M. Al-Hakim, L.Z. Al-Adamy and Mhasisen, J. Fd. Sci. 48, 1983, 988.

74. R.S. Kadan, D.W. Freeman, G.M. Ziegler and J.J. Spadaro, J.Fd. Sci. 45, 1980, 1566.

75. T.M. Kajs, J.T. Lawhon and K.S. Rhee, Fd. Technol. 33, 1979, 82.

76. M.N. Khan , J.T. Lawhon, L.W. Rooney and C.M. Cater, Cereal Chem. 53, 1976, 388.

77. J.E. Kinsella, Fd. Sci. and Nutr. 7, 1976, 219.

78. V. Krishnamoorthi, Fd. Technol. 19, 1965, 1085.

79. J.T. Lawhon and C.M. Cater, J. Fd. Sci. 36, 1971, 372.

80. J.T. Lawhon, C.M. Cater and K.F. Mattil, J.Fd. Sci. 37, 1972, 317.

81. J.T. Lawhon, C.M. Cater and K.F. Mattil, Fd. Prod. Dev. 9, 1975, 110.

82. J.T. Lawhon, S.U. Lin, L.W. Rooney, C.M. Cater and K.F. Mattil, J. Fd. Sci. 39, 1974, 183.

83. J.T. Lawhon , D. Mulsow, C.M. Cater and K.F. Mattil, J. Fd. Sci. 42, 1977, 389.

84. M.H. Lopes, Agron. Mocambican. 4, 1970, 199.

85. E.W. Lusas and G.M. Jividen. J.A.O.C.S. 64, 1987, 839.

86. W.H. Martinez, L.C. Berardi and L.A. ; Goldblatt. J. Agric. Fd. Chem. 18, 1970, 961.

87. W.H. Martinez, and V.L. Frampton, J. Agric. Chem. 10, 1962, 410.

88. W.H. Martinez and D.T. Hopkins, in : M. Friedman (Ed), Cottonseed protein products. Variation in protein quality with product and process: Part II. Quality factors plant breeding, composition, processing and anti nutrients, Marced Dekker, New York, 1975, pp. 355-374.

89. R.H. Matthews, E.J. Sharpe and W.M. Clark, Cereal Chem. 47, 1970, 81.

90. E. Mayorga, J. Gonzaler, J. Menchu and C. Rolz, J. Fd. Sci. 40, 1975, 1270.

91. C.M. Mc Pherson and S.L. Ou, J. Fd. Sci. 41, 1976, 301.

92. M. Milner, USDA Southern Regional Research Laboratory, New Orleans, 1960, 66.

93. M. Milner (Ed), Protein -enriched cereal foods for world needs: Status of development and use of some unconventional proteins, Assoc. Cereal Chem., St. Paul, Minn, 1969, pp. 97-104.

94. H.O. Osman, E.K. Moustafa, A.R. El-Mahdy and Y.G. Moharram, Alex. J. Agric. Res. 29, 1981, 620.

95. S.N. Pandey and N. Thejappa, Indian Journal of Agricultural Sciences, 46, 1976, 15.

96. Protein Advisory Group of the United Nation, PAG. "Protein rich mixtures for uses as weaning foods" FAO/WHO/Unicef, New York. Guidline No. 8, 1971.

97. E.H. Rahma and M.S. Narasinga Rao, J. Agric. Fd. Chem. 31, 1983a, 356.

98. E.H. Rahma and M.S. Narasinga Rao, J. Agric. Fd. Chem. 31, 1983b, 352.

99. E.H. Rahma and M.S. Narasinga Rao, J. Fd. Sci. 49, 1984, 1057.

100. E.F. Reber, L.Ebon, A. Aladeselu, W.A. Brown and D.D. Marshall, J. Fd. Sci. 48, 1983, 217.

101. M.I. Reddy, and M.S. Narasinga Rao, J. Agric. Fd. Chem. 36, 1988, 241.

102. H.G. Reilich, J. O'Neill, R.S. Levi and J. Yamauchi, J.A.O.C.S. 5, 1968, 185.

103. J.V. Rice, Chemical Abst. 46, 1952, 11503.

104. J.H. Ridlehuber, and H.K. Gardner, J.A.O.C.S. 51, 1974, 153.

105. L.W. Rooney, C.B. Gustafson, S.P. Clark and C.M. Cater, J. Fd. Sci. 37, 1972, 14.

106. D. Rosenblum, Fd. Prod. Develop. 14, 1980, 34.

107. N.S. Scrimshaw, Fd. Nut. Bull. 2, 1980, 1.

108. F.H. Shah, W.H. Shah, M. Yasin and N. Abdullah, Pakistan Journal of Scientific and Industrial Research 29, 1986, 380.

109 A.B. Shaheen, M.El-Gindy, M.S. Raouf and A.M. Galal, Agric. Res. Rev. 51, 1973, 187.

110. M. Shemer, Israeli. Patent 50612, 1980, to Milouot Haifa Bay Sehlements Development Co. Ltd.

111. R.G. Simmons, J.R. Green, C.A. Payne, P.J. Wan and E.W. Lusas, J. Fd. Sci. 45, 1980, 1505.

112. A.K. Smith, J.A.O.C.S. 48, 1971, 38.

113. F.H. Smith, and A.J. Clawson, J.A.O.C.S. 47, 1970, 443.

114. J.J. Spadaro and H.K. Gardner, J.A.O.C.S. 56, 1979, 422.

115. L.G. Staats, and M.M. Tolman, J. Fd. Sci. 39, 1974, 758.

116. Sun Shankang, Chen Jianhua, Xiang Shikang and Wei Shoujun, Scientia Agricultura Sinica 20, 5, 1987, 12-16.

117. M.V. Taranto, G.F. Cegla and K.C. Rhee, J. Fd. Sci. 43, 1978, 973.

118. M.V. Taranto, W.W. Meinke, C.M. Cater and K.F. Mattil, J.Fd. Sci. 40, 1975, 1264.

119. M.V. Taranto, and K.C. Rhee, J. Fd. Sci. 44, 1979, 628.

120. R.N. Terrell, J.A. Brown, Z.L. Carpenter, K.F. Mattil and C.W. Monagle, J. Fd. Sci. 44, 1979, 865.

121. N. Trostler, T. Cohen and V. Brener, Proceeding of the Congr. Food Sci. Technol. 3, 1983, 89.

122. C. Vaccarino, J. A.O.C.S. 38, 1961, 143.

123. H.L. Vix, H.P. Dupuy and M.G. Lambou, Protein -rich food products from oilseeds. ARS, US Department of Agric. Washington, DC., 1969, pp. 62-76.

124. H.L. Vix, P.H. Eaves, H.K. Gardner and M.G. Lambou, J.A.O.C.S. 48, 1971, 611.

125. H.L. Vix, J.J. Spadaro, C.H. Murphy, R.M. Presell, E.F. Pollard and E.A. Gastrock, J.A.O.C.S. 26, 1949, 526.

126. H.L. Vix, J.J. Spadaro, R.D. Westbrook, A.J. Crovetto, E.F. Pollard and E.A. Gastrock, J.A.O.C.S. 42, 1947, 228.

127. P.J. Wan, J. Green , C.M. Cater and K.F. Mattil, J. Fd. Sci. 44, 1979, 475.

128. L.Y. Yatsu, J. Cell. Biol. 25, 1965, 193.

129. Z.M. Zarins and J. P. Cherry, J. Fd. Sci. 46, 1981, 1855.

130. Z.M. Zarins and W.E. Marshall, Cereal Chem. 65, 1988, 359.

131. Q. Zhuge, E.S. Posner and C.W. Deyoe, J. Agric. Fd. Chem. 36, 1988, 153.

132. Y.A. Ziprin, K. S. Rhee, Z.L. Carpenter, R.L. Hostetler, R.N. Terrell and K.C. Rhgee, J. Fd. Sci. 46, 1981, 58.

G. Charalambous (Ed.), Food Science and Human Nutrition
© 1992 Elsevier Science Publishers B.V. All rights reserved.

COMPUTER-AIDED ORGANIC SYNTHESIS APPLIED TO THE STUDY OF FORMATION OF AROMA COMPOUNDS. THERMAL DEGRADATION OF DIALLYL DISULFIDE.

G. VERNIN[1] and J. METZGER[1], P. AZARIO[2], R. BARONE[2], M. ARBELOT[2] and M. CHANON[2]

[1]Laboratoire de Chimie Moléculaire, URA 1411, Chimie des Arômes-Oenologie, Faculté des Sciences et Techniques de Saint-Jérôme, Avenue Escadrille Normandie-Niémen, Case 561, France 13397 Marseille Cédex 13.

[2]Laboratoire AM3, URA 1411, Faculté des Sciences de Saint-Jérôme, Avenue Escadrille Normandie-Niémen, Case 561, France 13397 Marseille Cédex 13.

SUMMARY

Barone et al.(J. Org. Chem., 1988, 53, 720) developed the program SOS (Simulated Organic Synthesis) for the retrosynthesis of organic compounds and recently adapted SOS to Macintosh, and it works also in the forward direction (Vernin et al., J. Agric. Food Chem., 1987, 35, 761). In this approach the program predicts the compounds which could be formed from starting material. Thus one may predict by products of a reaction or propose mechanisms for a reaction. We present in this paper a new version of SOS specifically developed for the prediction of aroma compounds in model reactions. The program may help the analysis of complex mixtures by indicating the potential products expected from a given reaction. The program was applied to predict the products formed during the pyrolysis of diallyl disulfide. This reaction was experimentally studied by Block et al. (J. Amer. Chem. Soc., 1988, 110, 7813). Starting from the set of reactions proposed by Block the program not only found the products identified by this author but proposed several new products not yet identified. Some of these supplementary products could originate from the unability of SOS to attach rate constants to every considered step, but some could simply have been missed in the analytical study of these complex mixtures.

1. INTRODUCTION

We developed the program SOS (Simulated Organic Synthesis) for the retrosynthesis of organic compounds (1) and we recently adapted SOS for the Macintosh (2). SOS may also be used in the forward direction. It has been applied to the synthesis of volatile heterocyclic compounds in food flavors (3). In this approach the program predicts the compounds which could be formed from starting products. This approach makes it possible to predict the by-products of a reaction, to study the mechanism of a reaction or to predict all the products which could be formed during a complex reaction. In the present case it means of sulfide compounds arising from the thermal degradation of diallyl disulfide. The program may help the analytical chemist by suggesting all the products expected to be formed during this reaction.

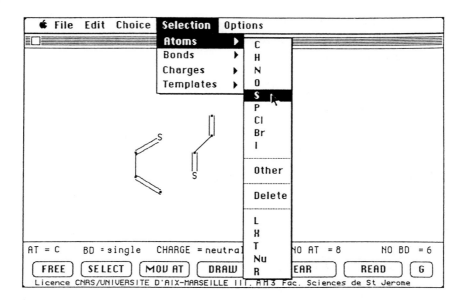

Fig. 1. View of the screen (input of structures)

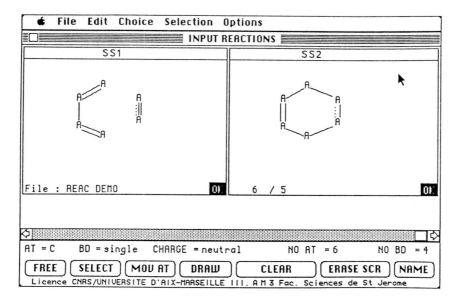

Fig. 2. View of the screen (input of a reaction)

2.   DESCRIPTION OF SOS

SOS is running on a Macintosh; its use is very friendly : the input of structures and reactions is done graphically by means of mouse and scrolling menus.

Figure 1 shows a view of the screen during the input of starting materials. When the user draws the structure, the computer stores all the informations about this structure : namely nature and number of atoms and bonds.

The input of a reaction is done by drawing it on the screen. The chemist uses the same subroutine as the one used in the input of the starting structure. Figure 2 shows a view of the screen during this part of the program.

In the left part of the screen, the chemist draws the substructure characteristic of the reaction. This substructure is to be searched in the starting materials and if it is found the program replaces it by the substructure which is in the right window. In this scheme the letter A stands for any atom. This feature provides a generalized representation of the reaction.

For example, if the starting materials are : $CH_2=CH-CH=S + CH_2=CH-CH=S$ the program perceives the possibility of the Diels-Alder reaction and proposes the solutions of Figure 3.

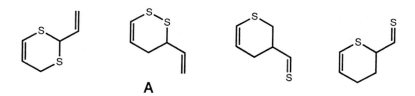

A

Fig. 3. The four solutions given by SOS for the Diels-Alder reaction of thio-acrolein.

Figure 4 shows the screen when the program displays one solution. In this case the structure is correctly drawn. When the program displays the solutions it keeps the coordinates of the atoms as they are in the starting materials, so, solution N°A is somewhat distorted (Figure 5).

An option allows to redraw the structure. This option uses the method developed by Carhart (4) to recalculate the coordinates of the structures. Figure 6 shows the new drawing obtained for structure of Figure 5 by this option.

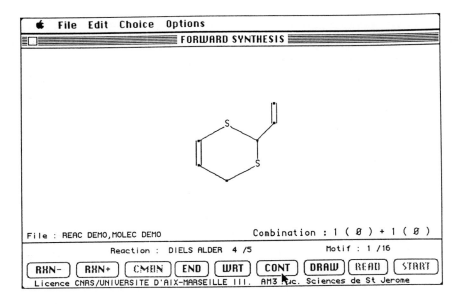

Fig. 4. Output of a solution.

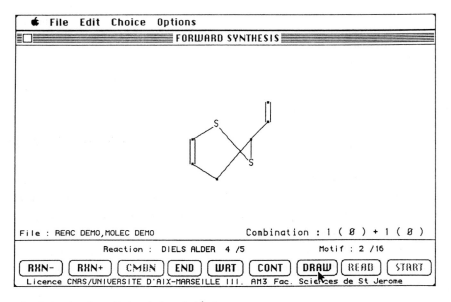

Fig. 5. Output of a distorded solution.

In the previous version of the program (3) the combinations were made by the chemist : for example, there were two starting materials 1 and 2. From them the program proposed the formation of 3,4,5 and 6. The chemist was the one deciding that 1 had to react with 3 to 6, then 2 had to react with 3 to 6 and so on.

This manual version is still present in the new version. We added an option which allows the computer to make all the combinations two by two for a number of levels fixed by the user.

Figure 7 shows the window which allows the user to select the number of levels to perform the study.

3.   EXAMPLE

In the course of several investigations on garlic essential oils (5,6,7) numerous unidentified compounds were found. Block *et al.* (8) have rencently shown that most of these compounds arise mainly from the thermal degradation of diallyl disulfide (that we write Al_2S_2 = $CH_2=CH-CH_2-S-S-CH_2-CH=CH_2$) the main component of garlic essential oils. Identified compounds are reported in Figure 8. The authors proposed that only two kinds of reactivity : Diels-Alder and radicalar reactions were sufficient to rationalize the experimentally identified products.

3.1   Products from Diels-Alder Reaction

Figure 9 displays new products predicted by the Diels-Alder reaction. Most of these products involve a reaction with the cyclic double bond of compound such as 13. Block *et al.*(8) did not describe such products : the exo double bond must be the most reactive.

The problem which arises is to decide up to which level we have to analyze the combinations : the starting compound defines the level 0. Upon thermolysis two products are formed (level 1). Then in the medium there are compounds which may react : those of level 0 and those of level 1, they give products of level 2; those of level 1 + level 1 ⟶ level 3 and again we may imagine new combinations : level 0 + level 2, level 0 + level 3, level 1 + level 2, level 1 + level 3, level 2 + level 2, level 2 + level 3, level 3 + level 3, and so on. In the program there is an option which allows the user to define the number of levels to explore automatically (Figure 7).

Since we based our study from Block's work we may use the yields given (8) : compound 5 is formed in a sufficient amount to allow further reactions. By Diels-Alder reaction it could react with CH_2=CH-CH=S (thioacrolein) to form structures of Figure 10, which in turn could react by Diels-Alder, but we do not display these new products because the yield should be very low.

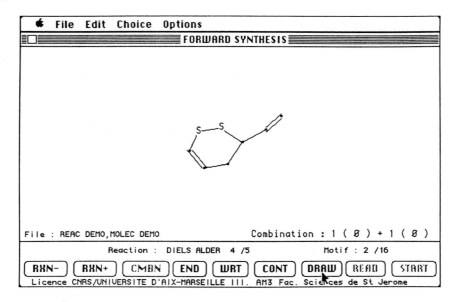

Fig. 6. Solution of Figure 5 redrawn by the program.

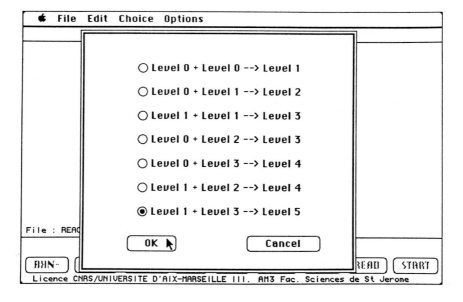

Fig. 7. Selection of the levels to be analyzed.

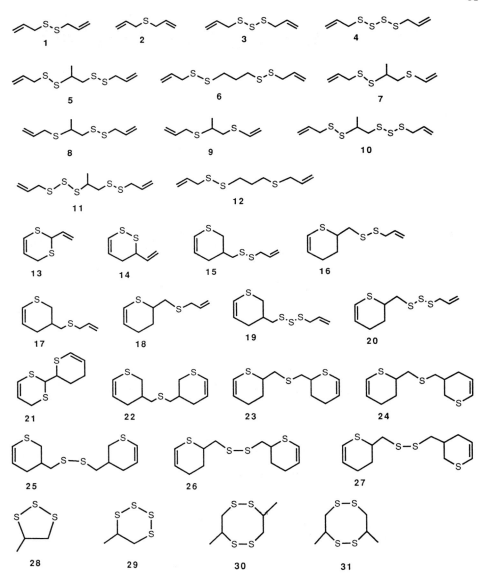

Fig. 8. Structures identified by Block et al. (8) by thermal degradation of diallyl disulfide.

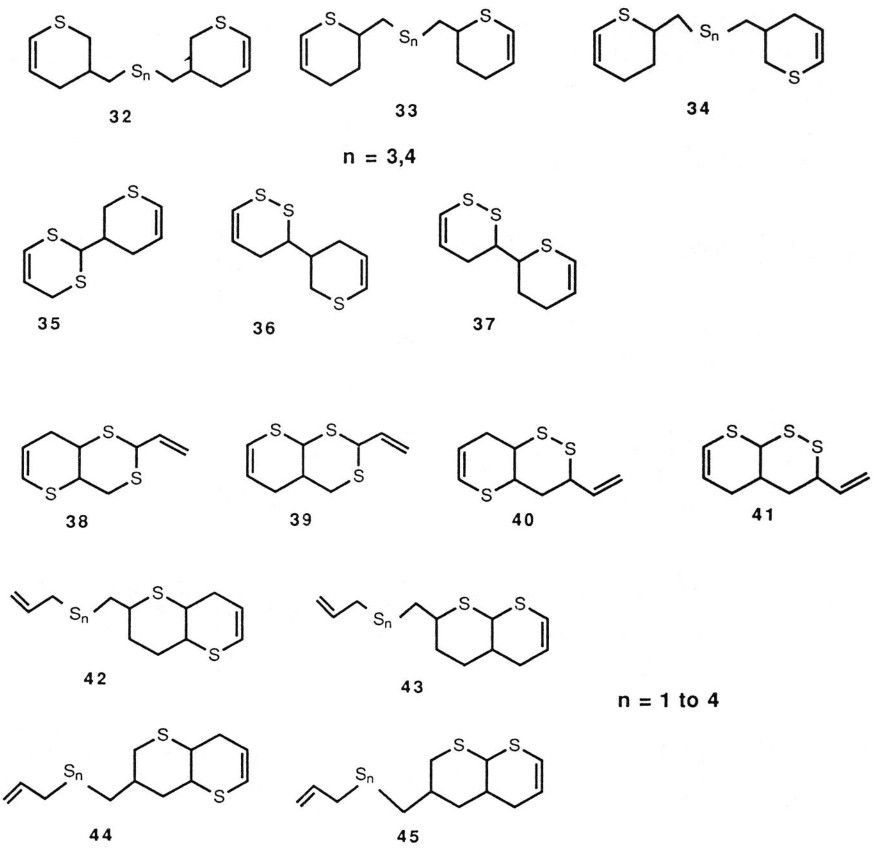

Fig. 9. New structures proposed by the Diels-Alder reaction.

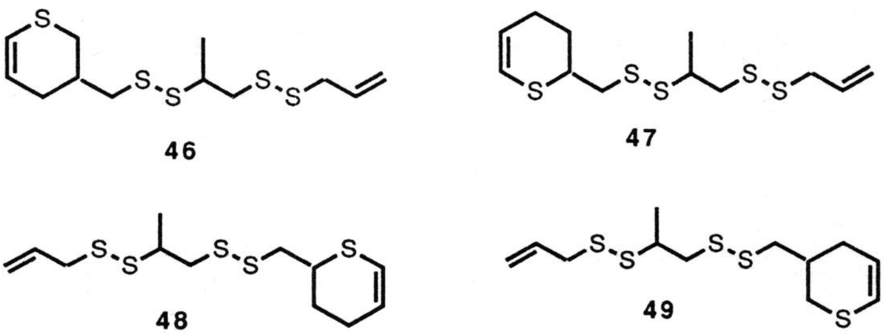

Fig. 10. Compounds from structure 5 arising by the Diels-Alder reaction.

3.2 Products from radicalar reactions

From Block's study the reactions of Scheme 1 explain the formation of the linear compounds of Figure 8.

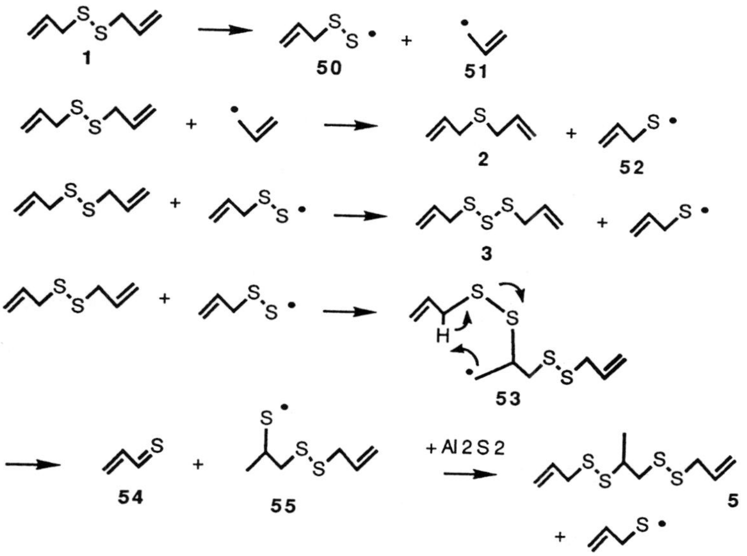

Scheme 1. Basic reactions explaining the formation of structures of Figure 8.

These reactions are coded in SOS by the general Scheme 2.

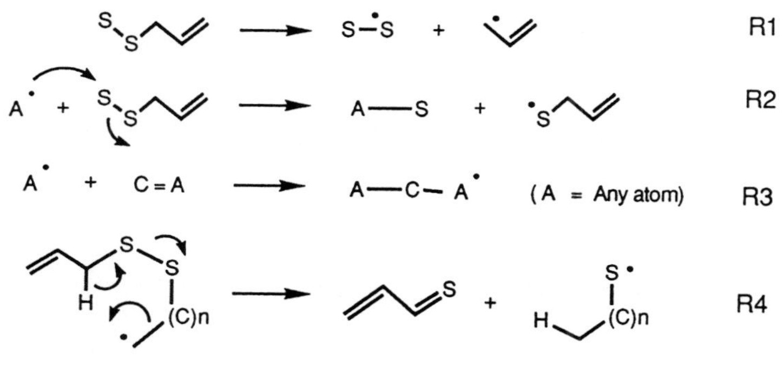

Scheme 2. Basic reactions coded in the program

From these reactions and the starting materials presented in Figure 11 SOS finds the products identified by Block and proposes new structures.

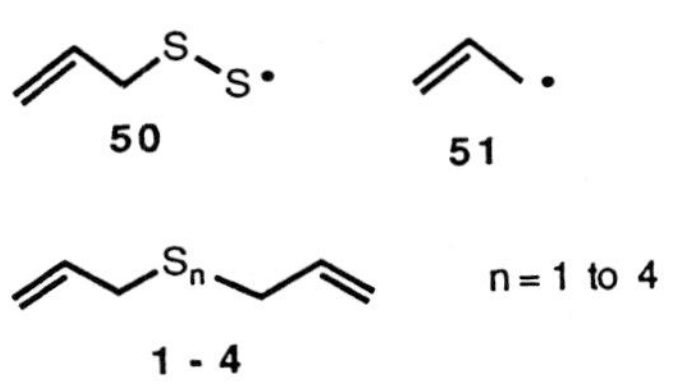

Fig. 11. Starting materials for SOS.

We present in Schemes 3 to 6 these new structures and the mechanism proposed.

For radicals 51 and 52 we select only the solutions involving a Markovnikov attack of the double bond, since the anti-Markovnikov is not favoured (8). (Schemes 5, 6).

In the reactions proposed by Block there is only one termination reaction, reaction of type R2 (Fig. 12).

Classical reaction in the field of radicalar chemistry is not envisaged, such as R· + R'H → RH + R'·.

If we introduce this reaction we obtain new structures which are displayed in Figure 12. The number of each structure indicates its origin. Another possibility is given in Scheme 7.

These structures could further react by Diels-Alder reaction and new structures could be proposed.

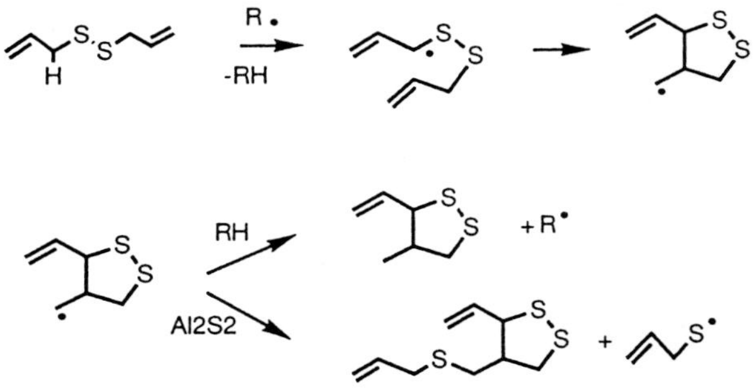

Scheme 7. New structures proposed for intramolecular cyclization of diallyl disulfide.

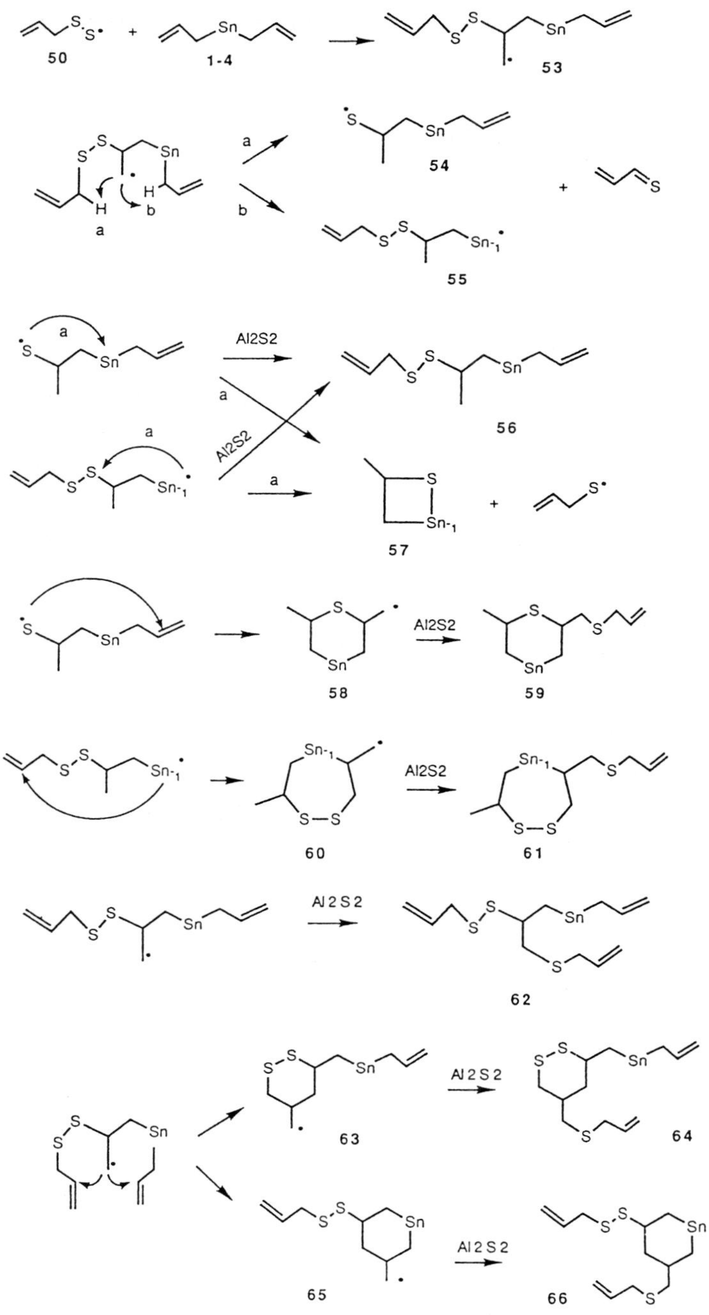

Scheme 3. New structures proposed by SOS.

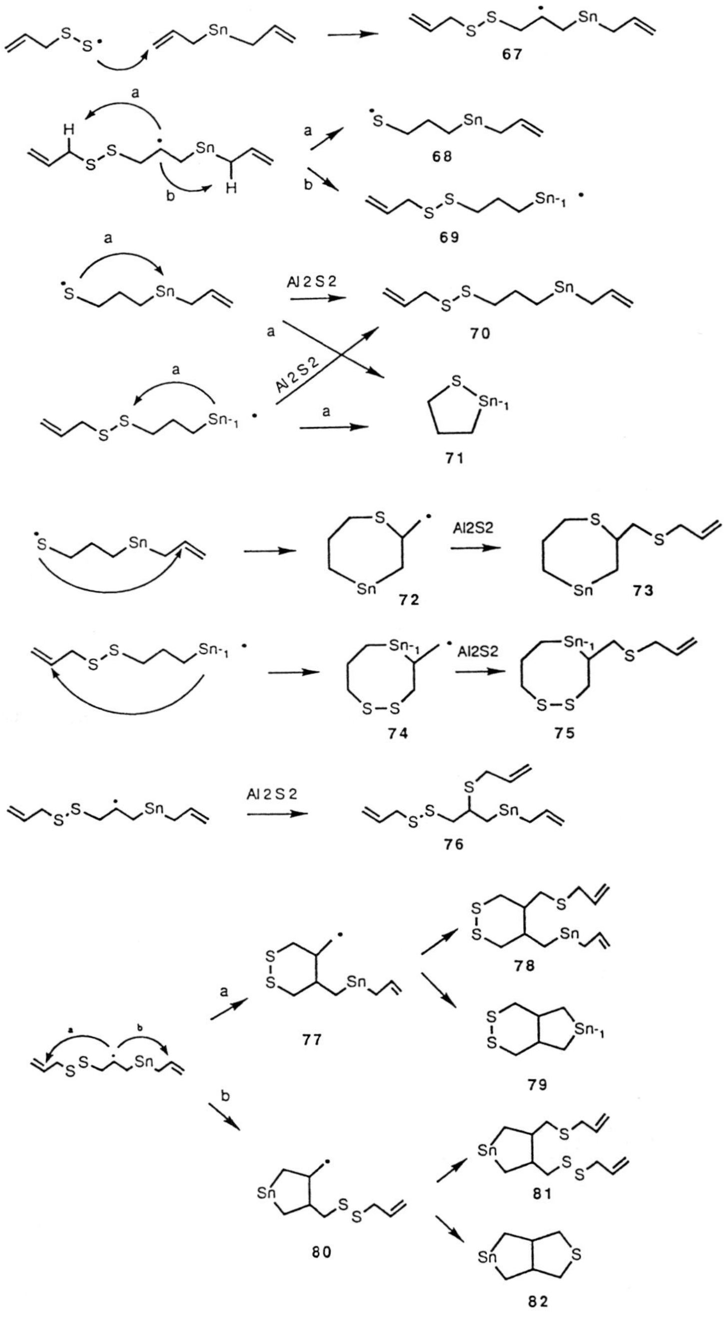

Scheme 4. New structures deriving from the initial anti-Markovnikov addition.

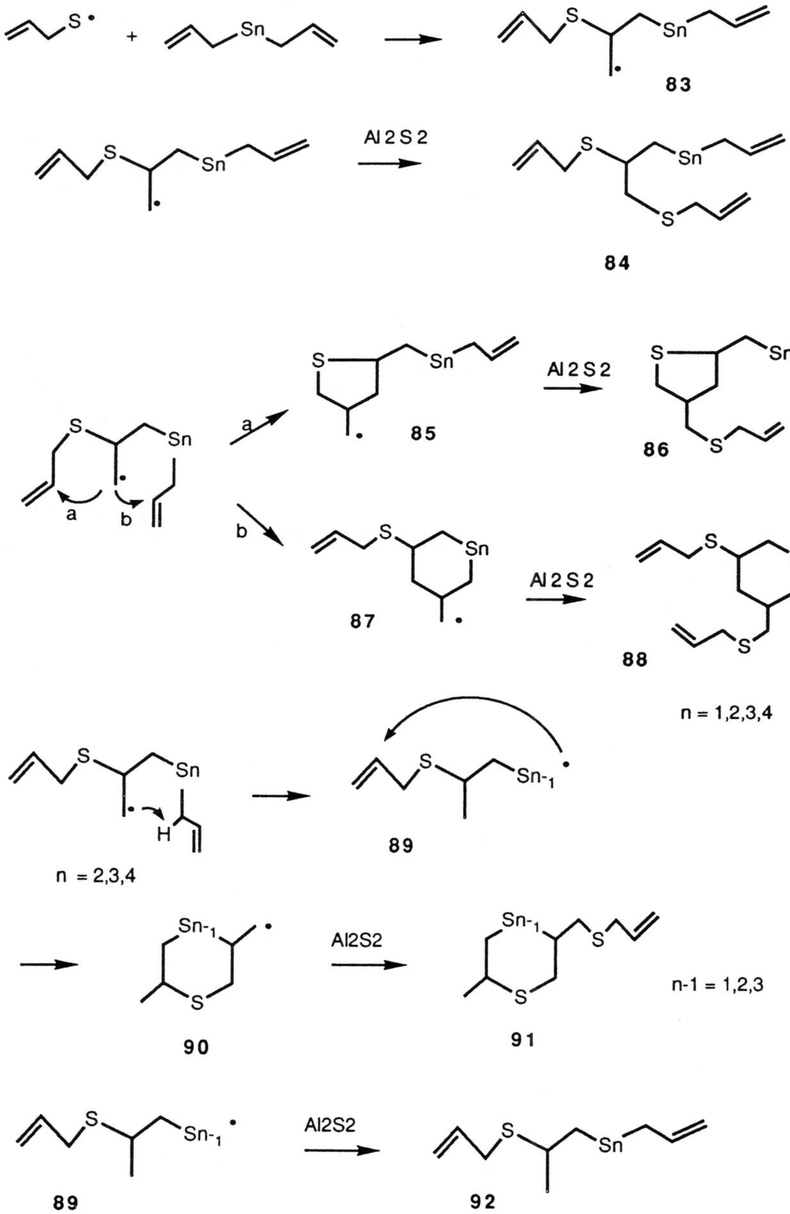

Scheme 5. New structures proposed by SOS from the AlS° radical.

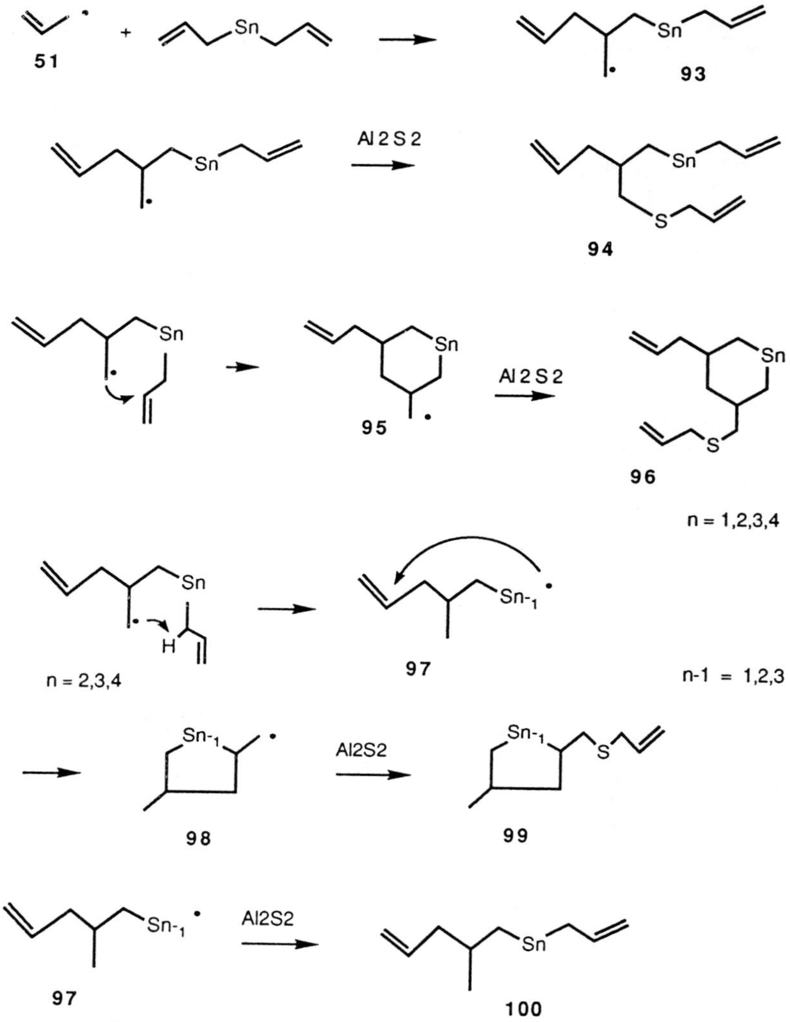

Scheme 6. New structures deriving from the allyl radical.

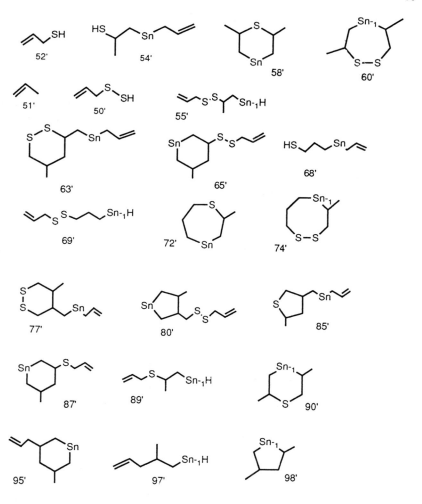

Fig. 12. Structures obtained by hydrogenation of the corresponding radical (i.e. radical 52 → 52').

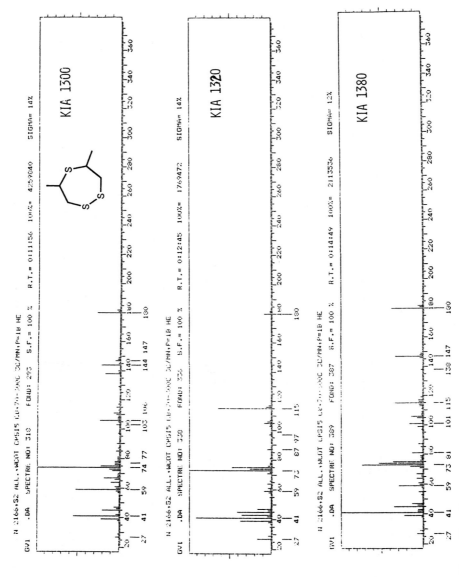

Fig. 13a. Mass spectra of sulfur-containing compounds (MW : 180).

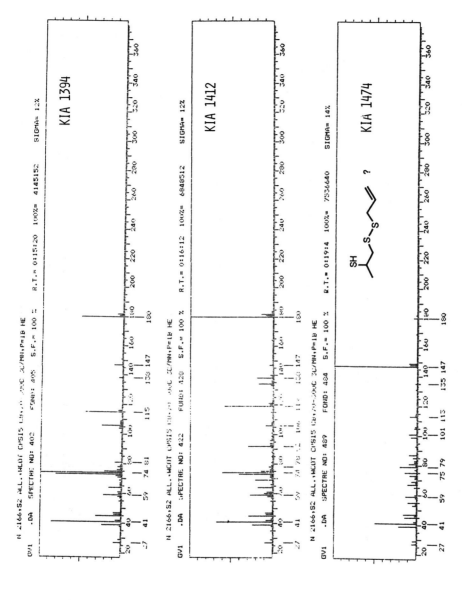

Fig. 13b. Mass spectra of sulfur-containing compounds (MW : 180).

4. EXPERIMENTAL STUDY

Diallyl disulfide was thermally decomposed 24 h at 110°C and the reaction mixture was analyzed by GC/MS on a WCOT CPSIL 5 CB apolar column at programmed temperature from 70°C to 300°C with $\Delta T = 3°C/min$. *A Ribermag R-10-10 apparatus was used and 100 mass spectra were recorded showing the complexity of the reaction.*

Among all mass spectra recorded we found not only those reported by Block et al. (8) but also a great number of others not previously described. Among them we identified two series of compounds of molecular weight 180 and 202 respectively.

4.1 Compounds of molecular weight 180

Six compounds of molecular weight 180 may agree with the empirical formula $C_6H_{12}S_3$ from which the isotopic abundances are $M + 1 = 9.3\%$ and $M + 2 = 13.7\%$, respectively. The mass spectra of such compounds are reported in Figures 13a and 13b. Their analytical data are shown below :

Compounds	T_R (min)	KIA	M + 1	M + 2	m/z
1	11.56	1300	8	13.4	74,41,59,106,144
2	12.45	1320	11,25	12.5	73,41,115,75
3	14.49	1380	8.8	14.4	41,73,74,75,115,147
4	15.20	1394	7.65	12.7	74,73,41,115,180
5	16.12	1412	8.5	13.3	180,41,119,74,73,119,92,106
6	19.4	1474	6.7	15.5	147,41,79,59

The presence of three sulfur atoms in a ring is highly probable according the M + 2 values.

A radicalar attack of an allyldithio radical upon diallyl disulfide may be considered. The following scheme is suggested (Scheme 8).

The two isomers 58' and 72' can also be formed according to Scheme 8bis.

Another ring at 9 links D can also be considered from the radical.

It is difficult in the absence of other analytical data (^{1}H-NMR) to definitely attribute the good structures to mass spectra.

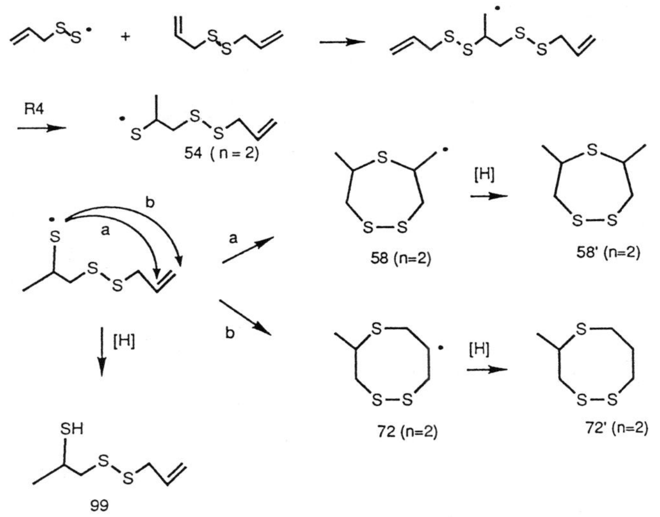

Scheme 8. Suggested formation for compounds 58' and 72' of molecular weight 180.

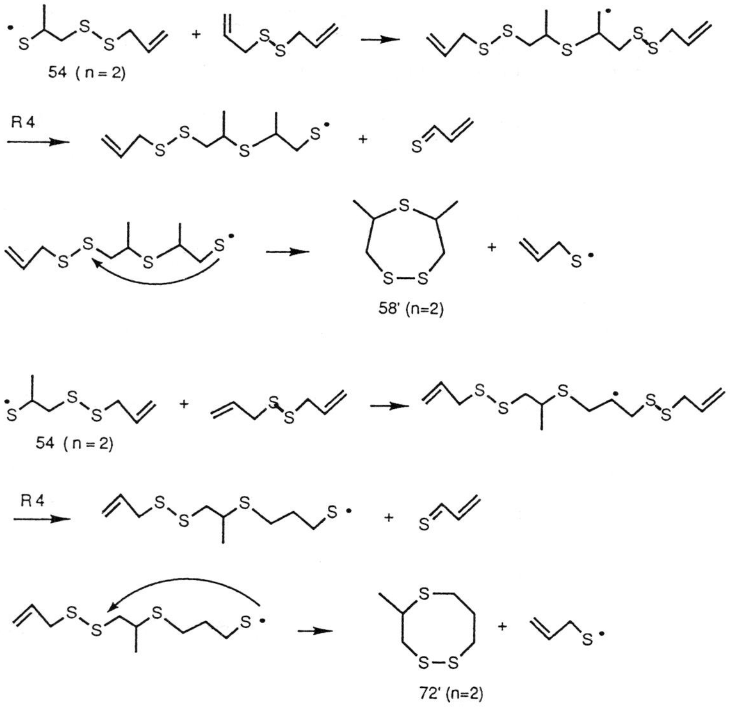

Scheme 8bis. Other mechanism proposed for compounds 58' and 72'.

4.2 Compounds of molecular weight 202

Four compounds of molecular weight 202 were also found. Their mass spectra are reported in Figure 14. The most probable empirical formula is $C_3H_6S_5$ (M + 1 = 7.46% and M + 2 = 22.45%). Their analytical data are reported below :

Compounds	T_R (min)	KIA	M + 1	M + 2	m/z
1	23.48	1610	7	21.9	138,73,74,41,
2	23.59	1615	8.3	20.2	138,115,73,41
3	24.07	1618	-	-	178,115,75,73,45,41
4	24.26	1625	-	-	178,138,75,73,41

These compounds may be formed by attack of the allyldithio radical upon allyl tetrasulfide according to the following schemes 9 and 9bis.

The base peak at m/z 138 in the compound (KIA 1610) corresponds to the loss of two sulfur atoms from the molecular ion. This later is also the base peak of the methyl-1,2,3-trithiopentane (KIA 1177).

The Kovats index difference KID = 1610 - 1177 = 433 is in good agreement with the presence of two additional sulfur atoms in the ring.
The minor fragments at m/z 64, 96, 128 and 160 agree with $S_2^{+\bullet}$, $S_3^{+\bullet}$, $S_4^{+\bullet}$ and $S^{+\bullet}$ radical cations. The fragments at m/z 73 and 74 correspond to :

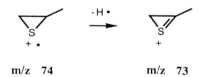

The three other compounds are characterized by fragments at m/z 115, 99, 59 and 41.

CH_3CS^+ $C_3H_5^+$

m/z 115   m/z 99   m/z 59   m/z 41

Finally, a compound MW 106 predicted by the computer as the 1,2-dithiocyclopentane 71 (n = 2) (See Scheme 4) was recently reported by chinese authors (7) and also found by us.

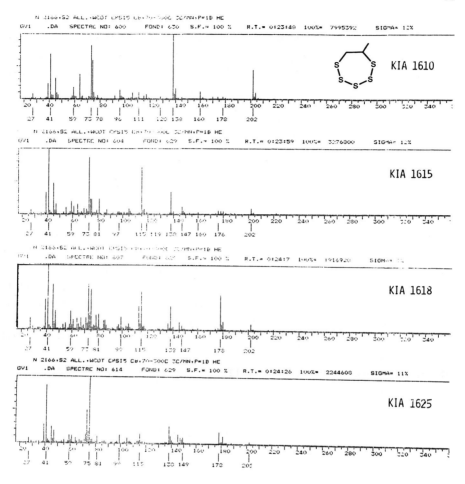

Fig. 14. Mass spectra of sulfur-containing compounds (MW : 202).

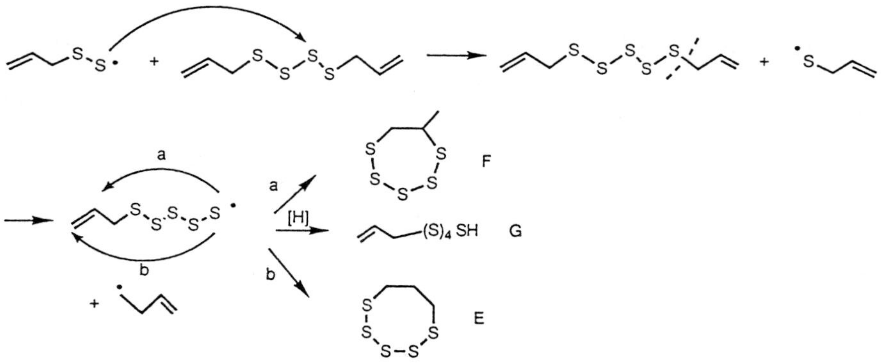

Scheme 9. Suggested formation of compounds (MW : 202). First hypothesis.

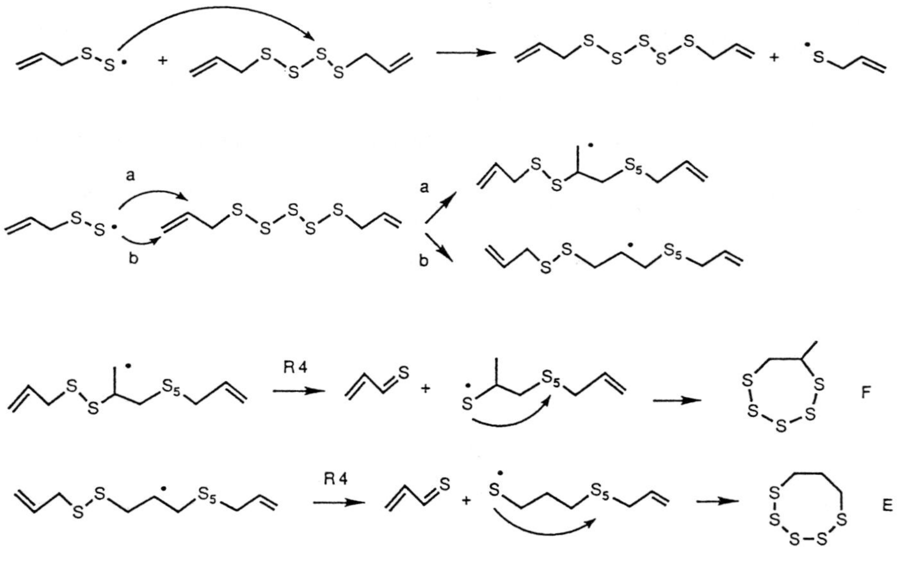

Scheme 9bis. Other suggested mechanism for the formation of compounds (MW 202) Second hypothesis.

CONCLUSION

Not only all the compounds identified in the study of Block et al.(8) were correctly found by the SOS program, but in addition, many new sulfur-containing compounds were also predicted by thermal degradation of diallyl disulfide. This paper also shows what help experimental chemists can expect from this approach. But, numerous unidentified compounds require further attention and analytical data (G.C. coupled with FTIR).

REFERENCES

1a R. Barone, M. Chanon and J. Metzger, Revue IFP, 1973, 771;
1b R. Barone and M. Chanon, Nouveau J. Chimie, 2(6) (1978) 659;
1c R. Barone, M. Chanon, P. Cadiot and M. Cense, Bull. Soc. Chim. Belges, 91 (1982) 333.
1d R. Barone and M. Chanon, in : Computer Aids to Chemistry (G. Vernin and M. Chanon Eds) Ch. I, Ellis Horwood Publisher, Chichester, England, 1986, pp. 19-102.
2a P. Azario, R. Barone and M. Chanon, J. Org. Chem., 53 (1988) 720;
2b P. Azario, M. Arbelot, A. Baldy, R. Meyer, R. Barone and M. Chanon, New. J. Chem., 14 (1990) 951.
3   G. Vernin, C. Párkányi, R. Barone, M. Chanon and J. Metzger, J. Agric. Food Chem., 35 (1987) 761.
4   R.E. Carhart, J. Chem. Inf. Comput. Sci., 16 (1976) 82.
5   G. Vernin, J. Metzger, D. Fraisse and C. Scharff, Planta Medica, 1986, 96-101
6   G. Vernin and J. Metzger, in : Modern Methods of Plant Analysis (H.F. Linskens and J.F. Jackson Eds.), Ch. X, Springer Verlag, Heidelberg (1991), in press.
7   Tung Hsi Yu and Cung-Mau Wu, Shih P'in k'o Hsueh (Taipei), 15(4) (1988) 385-393.
8   E. Block, R. Iyer, S. Grisoni, C. Saha, S. Belman and F.P. Lossing, J. Amer. Chem. Soc., 110 (1988) 7813-7827, and references herein.

FORMATION OF AROMA BY HYDROLYSIS OF GLYCOSIDICALLY BOUND COMPONENTS

V. Reyné, C. Salles[x] and J. Crouzet
Génie Biologique et Sciences des Aliments
Institut des Sciences de l'Ingénieur de Montpellier
Université de Montpellier II-Sciences et Techniques du Languedoc
34095 Montpellier Cédex 05
France

SUMMARY

Acid hydrolysis has been used in order to establish the presence of glycosidically bound components in fruits. During this treatment, rearrangement reactions of free monoterpene alcohols generally occur. This inconvenient may be avoided using enzymatic hydrolysis, however the specificity of enzymes requires the previous knowledge of the structures of compounds used as substrates in order to control the reaction. Several glycosidically bound components, glucosides, rutinosides and arabinoglucosides present in grapes and apricot were isolated, separated and identified using non destructive methods, MS-MS low energy CAD spectra and HPLC. ß-D-glucosidase, α-L-rhamnosidase, α-L-arabinase activities were purified from several enzyme preparations. The kinetic studies of α-L-rhamnosidase were performed using different substrates and more particularly glycosidically bound terpenic alcohols. Catalytic efficiency may be a criteria for the choice of preparations able to hydrolyse glycosidically bound components. For example the catalytic efficiency of the rhamnosidase activity present in hesperidinase is more important towards linalyl ß-D-rutinoside than towards geranyl ß-D-rutinoside, this substrate is efficiently hydrolyzed by naringinase.

INTRODUCTION

The presence of glycosidically bound terpene compounds in plants is known since the begining of the century , Bourquelot and Bridel have suggested in 1913 the occurrence of geranyl ß-D-glucoside in *Pelargonium*.

Concerning the fruits, Cordonnier (2) found in grape Muscat of Alexandria a fraction able to release terpenic alcohols through hydrolysis. Glycosidically bound aromatic, and terpenic alcohols as well as polyols were isolated and identified by Williams et al and Gunata et al (3,4).These non volatile compounds were subsequently identified in several fruits: passion fruit, papaya, tomato, pineapple, mango....(5-9)

Acid hydrolysis has been used in order to establish the presence of glycosidically bound components in fruits (9,10). However during this treatment, rearrangement

---

x Present adress: Laboratoire de Recherches sur les Arômes, INRA, 17 Rue Sully 21034 Dijon Cedex,France

reactions of free monoterpene alcohols may occur (11,12).This inconvenient may be avoided by the use of enzymatic hydrolysis (13,14). Gunata et al (14) have shown that the hydrolysis of monoterpenyl glycosides was a sequential phenomenom. In the first step the (1→ 6) linkage between terminal sugar : arabinose or rhamnose and ß-D-glucose unit was cleaved with the release of ß-D-glucoside which was substrate of a ß-D-glucosidase.

According to the specificity of enzymes required for sequential hydrolysis the knowledge of the structure of compounds used as substrates is necessary in order to control the reaction. More recently Shoseyev et al (15) reported the production of an endo-ß-glucosidase when a strain of *Aspergillus* was grown on a medium containing grape monoterpene glycosides as the sole carbon source.

The aim of the present paper is the determination of several glycosidically bound components present in grape and apricot using non destructive methods as well as the isolation and the characterization of some enzymatic activities able to hydrolyse these compounds.

Table 1
Volatile components in free and bound forms present in different cultivars of apricot and muscat grapes expressed in mg of linalool per kg of pulp

Cultivar	Free components	Bound components	Total	Ratio bound/free
Apricot				
Bergeron	1.9	3.2	5.1	1.6
Canino	2.8	3.6	6.4	1.3
Rouge du Roussillon	1.5	7.6	9.1	5.2
Précoce de Tyrinthe	0.6	3.1	3.7	5.4
Grapes				
Muscat of Alexandria (a)	1.1	5.6	6.7	5.1
Muscat de Hambourg (b)	1.4	6.3	7.7	5.2
Canada muscat (a)	0.96	4.1	5.06	4.3

(a) Dimitriadis and Williams (10)
(b) Essaied (19).

EVIDENCE FOR GLYCOSIDICALLY BOUND VOLATILES IN APRICOT

If the presence of glycosidically bound volatile components in grapes is well established, the data concerning apricot are scarce (16-18). The use of the rapid analytical technique of estimation of free and potentially volatil components (10) has shown that bound volatile components were present in the different apricot cultivars studied (Table 1). However the quantities of the two forms and their ratio vary from one cultivar to the other. In the case of Rouge du Roussillon which is a very aromatic cultivars, and of Precoce de Tyrinthe the ratio between bound and free forms is the same as the ratio given by Dimitriadis and Williams and Essaied (10,19) for different Muscat grape cultivar. However the quantities of free and bound components are about three times higher in Rouge du Roussillon than in Precoce de Tyrinthe. In these conditions the former cultivar was used for this work.

The volatile compounds isolated after acid hydrolysis of the heterosidic pool obtained from apricot by adsorption on hydrophobic adsorbant (3) are reported table 2.

Table 2

Volatile components identified after acid and enzymatic hydrolysis of heterosidic fraction isolated from apricot c.v. Rouge du Roussillon

Volatile components	Acid hydrolysis	Enzymatic hydrolysis Pectinol VR 40°C 12 h
trans-linalool oxide, furanoid	++	+
cis-linalool oxide, furanoid	++	+
linalool	++++	++
α-terpineol	++++	+++
nerol	++	
geraniol	+	++++
benzyl alcohol	+++	+++
2-phenylethanol	+	+

These results show clearly that the nature and the quantity of volatile compounds identified are dependent of the hydrolytic procedure used. As previously reported rearrangement reactions of free monoterpene alcohols occur when acid hydrolysis is used as indicated by the high level of α-terpineol and the presence of linalool oxides. On the other hand it is evident that the results obtained by enzymatic hydrolysis are dependent of the specificity of the enzyme towards the different glycosides present in the extract and of the hydrolysis rates of these compounds (16, 20). In these conditions the controlled regeneration of aroma from bound volatile compounds present in fruits requires the previous knowledge of :

- the structure of glycosidically bound components,
- the kinetic characteristics of enzyme using these compounds as substrates.

As far as possible, non destructive methods were used for the structural study of grape and apricot glycosidically bound compounds. However some partial or total enzymatic hydrolysis were used, more particularly for purified fractions, in order to confirm the identifications or the tentative identifications obtained.

ISOLATION OF GLYCOSIDICALLY BOUND COMPONENTS

The grape and apricot glycosidically bound volatile components were isolated as indicated by Salles et al (21). The diagram of the process used is given figure 1.

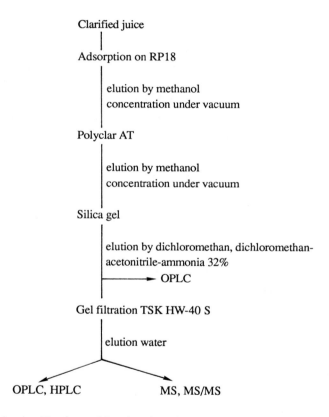

Fig.1 Isolation, purification and fractionation of grape and apricot glycosidically bound components.

MASS SPECTROMETRY STUDIES

The use of conventional mass spectrometry for the structural study of non volatile glycoconjugated compounds may allow the determination of the molecular weights, of the number and the mass of the different sugars and aglycons and their sequences.

According to Domon and Hostettmann (22), the use of field desorption (FD) for the structural study of polyphenolic glycosides gives only informations concerning the molecular weight of the compounds. The fragments obtained after cleavage of the sugar units are present in low intensity and don't give any information on the structure of the molecule.

In good agreement with this report only the $M^{+\circ}$ ion is present in the FD mass spectra of neryl, and geranyl ß-D-glucosides and geranyl ß-D-rutinoside as well as of different fractions isolated from apricot or grapes.

When Fast Atom Bombardment (FAB) in positive ion mode was used the determination of the molecular weight was impossible, none protonated or cationized molecule being detected, as indicated for neryl ß-D-glucoside (Figure 2). An ion m/z 163 $(MH-154)^+$ in the case of neryl and geranyl glucoside may be attributed to an enoxonium ion produced by cleavage of the osidic linkage with loss of the aglycon moiety.

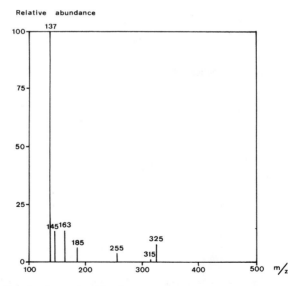

Fig. 2 Fast Atom Bombardment (positive ion mode) spectrum of neryl ß-D-glucoside.

Fragment ions m/z 145, m/z 127 and m/z 109 result from the deshydratation of the enoxonium ion whereas fragment ions m/z 153 and m/z 137 are characteristic of the aglycon moiety.

The results obtained using FAB in positive ion mode are in desagreement with those obtained with polyphenolic glycosides or with cardioglycosides (22,23) where molecular species are always present.

In the contrary the molecular ion m/z 461 (M-H)⁻ is present when FAB in negative ion mode was used (Figure 3), moreover informations concerning the saccharidic sequence may be obtained, m/z 325 (Rut~O)⁻, 163 (Rha~O)⁻.

Negative ion chemical ionization (NICI) for monoglucosides and desorption chemical ionization in negative ion mode (NI-DCI) for glycosides allow the determination of the molecular weight of the molecule (M-H)⁻, the nature of the sugars constitutive of the saccharidic moiety and their sequence : m/z 163 (Rha ~ O)⁻, m/z 325 (Rut ~ O)⁻ and m/z 315 (O ~Glu ~ O-Agl)⁻ in the case of geranyl ß-D- rutinoside (Figure 4) (24).

However in some cases the fragment ions are weakly abundant or absent, m/z 149 (Arab ~O)⁻ and m/z 311 (Ar-Gluc ~O⁻) as shown on the linalyl arabinoglucoside spectrum (Figure 5)

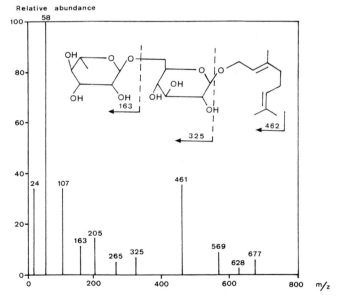

Fig.3 Fast Atom Bombardment (negative ion mode) spectrum of neryl ß-D-rutinoside.

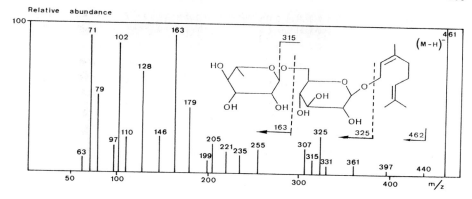

Fig. 4 Negative Ion Desorption Chemical Ionization (NI-DCI) spectrum (NH_3/NH_2^-) of geranyl ß-D-rutinoside

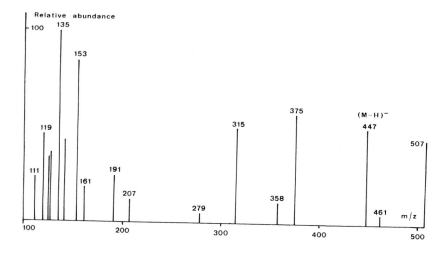

Fig.5 Negative Ion Desorption Chemical Ionization (NI-DCI) spectrum (NH_3/NH_2^-) of linalyl arabinoglucoside

As previously reported (16,21) more important informations are given by DCI spectra in positive mode. According to (22,25,26), informations about molecular weight: m/z 334 (M+NH$_4$)$^+$ and structure of the molecule, m/z 180 (Glu~O~NH$_3$)$^+$, 198 (Glu ~OH+NH$_4$)$^+$, 137 (Agl)$^+$, 154 (Agl~NH$_3$)$^+$ are obtained (Figure 6).

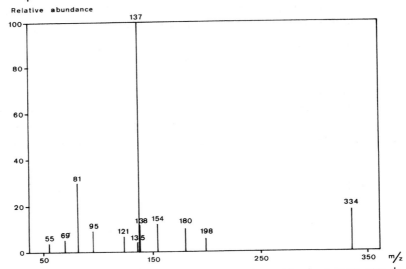

Fig.6 Desorption Chemical Ionization (DCI) spectrum, in positive mode (NH$_3$/NH$_4^+$) of geranyl ß-D- glucoside.

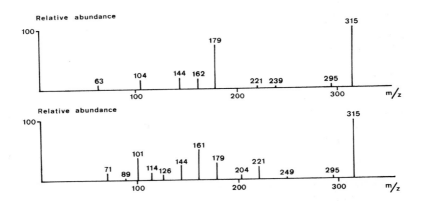

Fig.7 Negative Ion Chemical Ionization (NI-DCI) spectra of neryl and geranyl glucosides.

However, whatever the ionisation mode used, it is not possible to distinguish between isomers constitutive of the aglycon moiety of the molecule (Figure 7).

Finally glycosidically bound volatile compounds may be characterized using NICI or NI-DCI MS/MS (24, 27-29). The relative abundance of the ionic species detected in the low energy CAD spectra varies according to the nature of the aglycone moiety. From these findings, experimental rules, usable for the tentative identification were established.

The use of these rules, the use of shift technic with ($^2H_3$) ammonia reagent gas in NI-DCI mass spectrometry as well as the determination of retention time in OPLC and HPLC have allowed the identification or the tentative identification of several glycosidically bound volatile components in apricot and grapes (table 3) (16, 18, 30). Glucoside derivatives are the most important components isolated at this time from apricot, only linalyl arabinoglucoside was identified among saccharidic derivatives. In grapes rutinoside and arabinoglucoside derivatives are more abundant than glucosides.

Table 3

Glycosidically bound volatile components identified or tentatively identified in apricot and grapes

Identification	Apricot	Grapes	
Linalyl glucoside	+		I
α-terpinyl glucoside	+		I
neryl glucoside	+		I
geranyl glucoside	+		I
benzyl glucoside	+ (four isomers)	+ (two isomers)	T
enediol glucoside		+ (five isomers)	T
dienediol glucoside	+ (four isomers)	+ (six isomers)	T
linalyl rutinoside		+	I
geranyl rutinoside		+	I
α-terpinyl rutinoside		+	I
enediol rutinoside		+	T
linalyl arabinoglucoside	+	+	I
α-terpinyl arabinoglucoside		+	I
geranyl arabinoglucoside		+	I
2-phenylethyl arabinoglucoside		+	I
neryl arabinoglucoside		+	I
enediol arabinoglucoside		+	T

I identified by MS, MS/MS and HPLC
T tentatively identified by MS and MS/MS

In these conditions according to the sequential enzymic hydrolytic mechanism described by Gunata et al (4) the use of ß-D-glucosidase, α-L-arabinofurosidase, α-L-rhamnopyranosidase is necessary in order to obtain the hydrolysis of the bound component identified in apricot and grapes.

EVIDENCE FOR α-L-RHAMNOSIDASE ACTIVITY.

The presence of ß-D-glucosidase and α-L-rhamnosidase activities in enzyme preparations obtained from *A. nigerr* such as naringinase, hesperidinase or pectolytic enzyme is well established (31-36). On the other hand an α-L-arabinofuranosidase was detected in several commercial crude enzymatic preparations (36) and more particularly in Hemicellulase REG 2 from *Aspergillus niger* (37). ß-glucosidase activity is also present in sweet almond emulsin (38, 39).

α-L-rhamnosidase activity was detected in several commercial preparations by estimation of the quantity of rhamnose released by action of these enzymes on rutin (1,7 mM) during 6 h at different temperatures and pH (table 4)

Table 4
Characterization of α-L-rhamnosidase activity in different commercial preparations

Preparation	Optimum temperature	Optimum pH
Pectinol C	20	2.2
Pectinol VR	37	5.0
Rohament P	45	4.0
Pectinase *A. niger*	25	4.0
Cellulase	60	5.8
Pectinase fungal	50	4.5
Naringinase	45	6.8

The best results were obtained using optimal conditions for hydrolysis for Pectinol C., *A. niger* pectinase and naringinase. Hesperidinase preparation was also used.

SEPARATION OF GLYCOSIDASE ACTIVITIES

A. niger pectinase and hesperidinase were partially purified according to the following process (Fig 8).

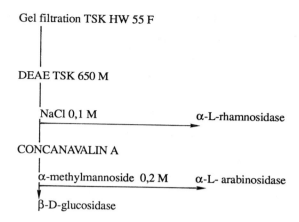

Fig. 8 Process used for α-L rhamnosidase, α-L-arabinase and ß-D glucosidase activities from *A.niger* pectinase and hesperidinase preparations.

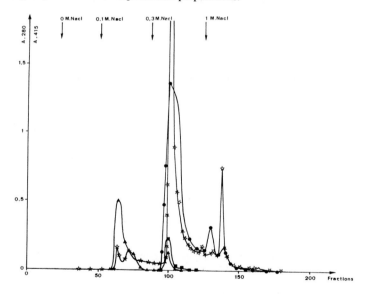

Fig.9 Ion exchange chromatography of active fractions isolated by gel chromatography on DEAE TSK 650M. Fractions of 5 ml were assayed for proteins (☆) at 280nm and for α-L-rhamnosidase (▲), α-L-arabinase (■) and ß-D-glucosidase (●) activities at 415 nm.

In a first step of the work the α-L-rhamnosidase was more particularly studied, this enzyme was obtained without any ß-D-glucosidase or a-L-arabinosidase activities after gel filtration on TSK HW 55 F and ion exchange chromatography on DEAE TSK 650 M (fig 9).

Two preparations of α-L-rhamnosidase were respectively obtained from *Aspergillus niger* pectinase and hesperidinase after gel filtration and ion exchange chromatography with 50 % yield, the overall purification factor were respectively 7.2 and 2.2.

In the case of *Aspergillus niger* pectinase preparation the purification factor was multiplied by 2.9 after affinity chromatography on Concanavalin A (table 5).

Table 5

Purification of α-L-rhamnosidase from *Aspergillus niger* pectinase.

	Total activity ($\mu M\ min^{-1}$)	Proteins (mg)	Specific activity ($\mu M\ min^{-1} mg^{-1}$)	Yield %	Purification factor
Crude enzyme	4200	53.25	78.87	100	1
gel filtration TSK HW 55 F	3600	46	78.26	86	0.99
DEAE TSK 650 M	2000	3.55	563.4	47.6	7.2
Concanavalin A	1125	0.69	1630	26.7	20.6

KINETIC STUDIES

Kinetic studies of α-L-rhamnosidase obtained after the ion exchange chromatography step from *Aspergillus niger* pectinase and hesperidinase commercial preparations were realized using Lineweaver and Burk method with different substrates : p-nitrophenylrutinoside (PNPR), naringin, hesperidin, linalyl and geranyl rutinoside.

When PNPR was the substrate the kinetic was followed by the increase of absorbance at 415 nm resulting of the formation of phenate ion in basic medium, for the other substrates the quantities of glucosides liberated after partial hydrolysis were determined by HPLC using a C_{18} reversed phase. The values obtained for V_{max}, K_M and catalytic efficiency : V_{max}/K_M for the different substrates and for the two enzymes are given in tables 6 and 7

Table 6

Kinetic characteristics of a-L-rhamnosidase isolated from *Aspergillus niger* pectinase for different substrates.

Substrate	V_{max} ($\mu M\ min^{-1}$)	K_M (mM)	Catalytic efficiency(min-1)	Catalytic efficiency(%)[a]
PNPR	137	0.215	0.64	43.8
naringin	66	0.045	1.46	100
hesperidin	624	0.96	0.65	44.5
linalyl ß-D-rutinoside	316	1.25	0.25	17.1
neryl ß-D-rutinoside	1083	7.90	0.14	8.4
geranyl ß-D-rutinoside	1379	9.96	0.14	8.4
α-terpinyl ß-D-rutinoside	333	5.0	0.06	4.5
methyl α-L-rhamnoside		not substrate		

a- relative to naringin.

Table 7

Kinetic characteristic of a-L-rhamnosidase isolated from hesperidinase for different substrates.

Substrate	V_{max} ($\mu M\ min^{-1}$)	K_M (mM)	Catalytic effeciency (min^{-1})	Catalytic efficiency (%)[a]
PNPR	659	20	0,03	1.2
naringin	67.6	0.30	0.23	9.2
hesperidin	847.5	0.34	2.49	100
linalyl ß-D-rutinoside	113	0.1	1.13	45.3
geranyl ß-D-rutinoside	333	4.8	0.07	2.8

a. relative to hesperidin

More high is the value of the ratio V_{max}/K_M more efficient is the enzyme towards the substrate.

In the case of α-L-rhamnosidase isolated from *Aspergillus niger* pectinase it is clear that naringin is the better substrate. Good efficiency was obtained for its isomers hesperidin and the non natural substrate PNPR. The catalytic efficiencies found for glycosidically bound terpenic compounds was only 50 to 20 % of that obtained for naringin. As previously reported by Kurosawa et al (33) methyl α -L-rhamnoside was not substrate of the α-L-rhamnosidase isolated from *Aspergillus niger* pectinase.

In the case of α-L-rhamnosidase isolated from hesperidinase, a preparation obtained from *Aspergillus niger* by induction with hesperidin, having α (1→6) linkage between rhamnose and glucose units, only compounds possessing this linkage such as hesperidin and linalyl ß-D-rutinoside are good substrates, the better being hesperidin. Low catalytic efficiencies were found for compounds possessing α (1 → 2) linkage between rhamnose and glucose units as well as for geranyl ß-D-rutinoside.

For the two enzymatic preparations, the value of catalytic efficiency for geranyl (or neryl) ß-D-rutinoside is lower than that determined for linalyl ß-D-rutinoside whereas the values found for V_{max} are higher for geranyl than for neryl derivative. The value of the catalytic efficiency of α -terpenyl rutinoside is only the half of that obtained for geranyl ß-D-rutinoside when α-L-rhamnosidase from pectinase is used.

The results related to the hydrolysis of terpenyl glucosides concerning the kinetic show that velocity determination are inadequate for the choice of a preparation able to hydrolysate glycosidically bound compounds. The velocity curves obtained for terpenyl glucoside production by action of maringinase on geranyl and linalyl rutinosides are very similar (fig 10) whereas the catalytic efficiencies for these two are always different.

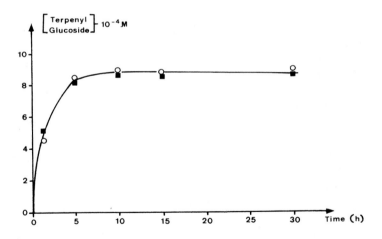

Fig.10 Hydrolysis of linalyl (○) and neryl (■) rutinosides by *A. niger* naringinase preparation.

In the present case the α-L-rhamnosidase from hesperidinase is perfectly suitable for the sequential hydrolysis of linalyl ß-D-rutinoside whereas it is not efficient for breaking the glycosidic linkage present in neryl and geranyl rutinosides.

In these conditions catalytic efficiency of enzymatic preparations for the different components present in the heterosidic pool of fruits must be tested and different enzyme coktails used according to the nature of glycosidically bound components identified in order to obtain generation of aroma.

REFERENCES
1 E. Bourquelot and M. Bridel, Comptes Rendus Acad. Sci. , 157 (1913) 72-74.
2 R. Cordonnier, Ann. Tech. Agric., 1 (1956)75-110.
3 J.P. Williams, C.R. Strauss, B. Wilson and R.A. Massy-Westropp, Phytochemistry, 21 (1982) 2013-2020.
4 Z. Gunata, C. Bayonove, R. Baumes and R. Cordonnier, J. Chromatogr., 331 (1985) 83-90.
5 K.H. Engel and R. Tressl, J. Agric. Food Chem., 31 (1983) 998-1002.
6 J. Heidlas, M. Lehr, H. Idstein and P. Schreier, J. Agric. Food Chem., 32 (1984) 1020-1021.
7 R.G. Buttery, G. Takeoka, R. Teranishi and L.C. Ling, J. Agric. Food Chem., 38 (1990) 2050-2053.
8 P. Wu, M.C. Kuo, T.G. Hartman, R.T. Rosen and C.T. Ho, J. Agric. Food Chem., 39 (1991) 170-172.
9 A. Koulibaly, M. Sakho and J. Crouzet, Lebensm. Wissen. Technol. submitted.
10 E. Dimitriadis and P.J. Williams, Am. J. Enol. Vitic., 35 (1984) 66-71.
11 P.J. Williams, C.R. Strauss, B.S. Wilson and R.A. Massy-Westropp, J. Agric. Chem., 28 (1982) 1219-1223.
12 W.F. Erman, Chemistry of the monoterpenes: an encyclopedic handbook, part A , M. Dekker, New York, 1985, pp. 329-479.
13 Z. Gunata, S; Bitteur, J.M. Brillouet, C. Bayonove and R. Cordonnier, Carbohydr . Res., 184 (1988) 139-149. 14
14 W. Schwab and P. Schreier, J. Agric. Food Chem., 36 (1988) 1238-1242.
15 O. Shoseyov, B.A. Bravdo, R. Ikan and I. Chet, Phytochemistry, 27 (1988) 1973-1976.
16 C. Salles, H. Essaied, P. Chalier, J.C. Jallageas and J. Crouzet, in P. Schreier (Ed.), Bioflavour'87, Walter de Gruyter, Berlin, 1988, pp 145-160.
17 G. Krammer, P. Winterhalter, M.Schwab and P. Schreier, J. Agric. Food Chem. ,39 (1991) 778-781.
18 C. Salles, J.C. Jallageas, F. Fournier, J.C. Tabet and J. Crouzet, J. Agric. Food Chem.,39 (1991) in press.

19 H. Essaied, DEA Sciences des Aliments. Université de Montpellier II, 1985.

20 Z. Gunata, C.Bayonove, C. Tapiero and R. Cordonnier, J. Agric. Food Chem., 38 (1990) 1232-1236.

21 C. Salles, J.C. Jallageas and J. Crouzet, J. Chromatogr., 522 (1990) 255-265.

22 B. Domon and K. Hostettman , Phytochemistry, 24 (1984) 575-580.

23 R. Isobe, T. Komori, F. Abe and T. Yamauchi, Biomed. Environ. Mass Spectrom., 13 (1986) 585-594.

24 C. Salles, J.C. Jallageas, F.Fournier, J.C. Tabet and J. Crouzet in Y. Bessière and A.F. Thomas (Eds.) Flavour Science and Technology, J. Wiley &Sons, Chichester, 1990, pp. 233-236.

25 K. Hostettman, J. Doumas and M. Hardy, Helv. Chim. Acta, 64 (1981) 297-303.

26 N. Takeda, K. Harada, M. Suzuki and A. Tatematsu, Biomed. Mass Spectrom., 10 (1983) 608-613.

27 R.B. Cole, J.C. Tabet, C. Salles, J.C . Jallageas and J. Crouzet, Rapid Commun. Mass Spectrom.,3 (1989) 157-160.

28 R.B. Cole, J.C. Tabet, C. Salles, J.C. Jallageas and J. Crouzet in P. Longevialle (Ed.), Adv. Mass Spectrom., 11B (1989), 1020.

29 F. Fournier, L. Ma , J.C. Tabet, C. Salles, J.C. Jallageas and J. Crouzet presented at the 2nd International Symposium on Applied Mass Spectroscopy in Health Sciences. Barcelona, 1990.

30 C.Salles Ph. D. Thesis, Université de Montpellier II. 1989.

31 W.J. Dunlap, R.E. Hagen and S.H. Wender, J. Food Sci., 27 (1962) 597-601.

32 S. Kamiya, S. Essaki and M. Hama, Agr. Biol. Chem., 31 (1967) 133-136.

33 Y. Kurosawa, K. Ikeda and F. Egami, J. Biochem., 73 (1973) 31-37.

34 M. Roitner, T.Schalkhammer and F. Pittner, Monat. für Chemie, 115 (1984) 1255-1267.

35 M.A Sanchez, C. Romero, A. Manjon and J.L. Iborra, Biotech. Lett., 9 (1987) 871-874.

36 R. Cordonnier, Z. Gunata, R. Baumes and C. Bayonove, Conn. Vigne Vin, 23 (1989) 7-23.

37 Z. Gunata, J.M. Brillouet, S. Voirin, R. Baumes and R. Cordonnier, J. Agric. Food Chem., 38 (1990) 772-776.

38 P. Lalegerie, Biochimie, 56 (1974) 1297-1303.

39 A.K. Grover and R.J. Cushley, Biochem. Biophys. Acta, 482 (1977) 109-124.

G. Charalambous (Ed.), Food Science and Human Nutrition
© 1992 Elsevier Science Publishers B.V. All rights reserved.

THE EFFECT OF CARBON AND NITROGEN SOURCES ON THE GROWTH AND AROMA PRODUCTION OF PENICILLIN ITALICUM

Leslie F. M. Yong

Aroma Biotech Pte Ltd, 6 Shenton Way, #29-01 DBS Building, Singapore 0106, Republic of Singapore.

SUMMARY

An isolate of Penicillium italicum obtained from the soft-rot of an orange was found to produce an orange-like aroma when grown on potato dextrose agar. Linalool was detected as the main volatile component in the pentane extract of the culture broth of the fungus. It was observed that the accumulation of linalool by P. italicum was significantly affected by the carbon source present in the growth medium; the sensory quality of the aroma was relatively unaffected. However, both the sensory profile of the aroma produced and the amount of linalool accumulated in the culture broth were affected by the nitrogen sources examined. This investigation was carried out under liquid surface cultivation of the fungus.

1. INTRODUCTION

A strain of Penicillium italicum which was isolated from the soft-rot of an orange was found to produce an orange-like aroma when cultured on potato dextrose agar. P. italicum had been reported by Raper and Thom (1949) to produce a fragrant odour; whereas Smith (1969) described its odour as nauseating. A literature search showed that practically no work has been conducted on the biochemical aspects of its aroma production. In this paper we report on the detection of linalool as the major component of the volatiles produced by the P. italicum isolate and how its production is affected by the carbon and nitrogen sources in the liquid media during surface cultivation.

2. MATERIALS AND METHODS

Either Analar grade or the purest bacteriological or chemical grade materials were used.

The strain of P. italicum Wehmer was isolated from the soft-rot of an orange by Dr Leslie F M Yong and was identified by Dr G Lim of the National University of Singapore. It was maintained on potato dextrose agar (PDA) slants under a layer of paraffin oil and stored at 4°C. One-week old PDA slope cultures incubated at 24 ± 2°C were used to prepare inocula containing 10^5 ± 10^6 spores/mL of suspension. The inocula (1 mL aliquots) were added into 50 mL aliquots liquid media contained in 250 mL Erlenmeyer flasks. The flasks were incubated at ambient temperature, i.e. 24 ± 2°C without agitation. The mineral salts composition of the medium is as reported in Yong et al. (1985). The carbon and nitrogen sources were varied according to the experimental design, and they were autoclaved separately at 121°C for 15 minutes and added to the sterilized mineral salts media before inoculation.

The culture broth after removal of mycelial growth by filtration was extracted with n-pentane in a J & W Liquid-liquid extractor as reported in Kok et al. (1987). The gas liquid chromatographic (GLC) conditions used for qualitative and quantitative analyses of the n-pentane extracts of P. italicum cultures were as described in Kok et al. (1987); 1-heptanol was used as the internal standard.

A Hewlett-Packard (Model HP 5988A) combined gas chromatograph-mass spectrometer (GC-MS) was used for linalool identification by mass spectroscopy. The GC-MS was equipped with a HP 59970C work station installed with a combined Wiley/NBS mass spectral library. The mass spectral data were obtained with a cross-linked methyl silicone fused silica column as well as Carbowax 20M column (20m x 0.2 mm i.d.) using a temperature programme same as that for GLC analysis of the pentane extract; He carrier gas flow was 1.0 mL/min; temperature of ion source and all connection parts 200°C, and electron energy was set at 70 eV.

Mycelial dry weight was determined gravimetrically as described in Yong and Lim (1986) and pH values were determined using a Corning Model 7 pH meter.

Sensory evaluation of the orange aroma in the culture broth or GLC effluent was conducted by sniffing (Yong et al. 1985).

3. EXPERIMENTAL: RESULTS AND DISCUSSION

3.1 Identification of Linalool

The sensory characteristics of a concentrated pentane extract of P. italicum culture broth were found to be similar to that of the broth before extraction. Capillary GLC examination of the extract with a 20m x 0.2mm i.d. Carbowax 20M column and also a 20m x 0.2mm i.d. cross-linked methyl silicone column showed the presence of one predominant peak. This peak was found to be linalool by examination of its mass spectrum and Kovat's indices on both Carbowax 20M and methyl silicone columns. Its identity was further confirmed by co-chromatography with an authentic sample of linalool on both the polar and non-polar columns, and by comparing the sensory characteristics of this peak with that of authentic linalool peak as it eluted from the GLC column. Linalool has a pleasant, sweet, slight-rose-like odour.

3.2 Effect of carbon & nitrogen sources on growth & linalool production

A single point assay method was used to study the effect of various carbon and nitrogen sources on the growth and linalool production of P. italicum. The effect was observed on the 8th day of incubation since preliminary experiments showed that (1) the orange aroma of the cultures was most intense based on sensory-evaluation and (2) GLC analysis showed linalool accumulation peaked at this time.

3.3 Effect of carbon sources

The type of carbon source (with glutamic acid as the sole nitrogen source) did not have any significant effect on the odour quality of P. italicum cultures. Except for 1,5-gluconolactone, all other carbon sources which supported growth enabled the production of an orange-like aroma (see Table 1 which shows the effect of carbon sources on the odour profile of P. italicum cultures). Table 2 shows the quantity of linalool accumulation in media containing different carbon sources. There was a direct relationship observed between the intensity of the orange aroma as determined by sniffing and the amount of linalool assayed by GLC. It was observed that glucose and sucrose in combination with glutamic acid as the nitrogen source gave better accumulation of linalool when compared to other carbon sources. When "vitamin-free" casamino acids was used as the nitrogen source, glucose gave the highest level of linalool accumulation (see Table 3). With casamino acid present as the sole nitrogen source in the media, the pH value was higher than those with glutamic acid; the initial pH was 5.2 for casamino acids media and 3.2 for glutamic acid media (see Table 4).

TABLE 1

Effect of carbon sources on odour profile of P. italicum cultures
(Nitrogen source: glutamic acid)

Carbon source	Aroma profile
MONOSACCHARIDES	
Hexoses	
Fructose	Sweet, orange
Galactose	Sweet, orange
1,5-gluconolactone	N.D.
Glucose	Sharp, orange peel-like
Pentoses	
Arabinose	Sweet, orange
Xylose	Mouldy, orange
DISACCHARIDES	
Maltose	Mouldy, orange
Lactose	Sour, orange
Sucrose	Sour, orange
POLYHYDROXYL ALCOHOLS	
Glycerol	Cooling, sour, orange
Mannitol	Sour, mouldy, orange
Sorbitol	N.D.
ACIDS	
Pyruvic acid	Cooling, sour, orange

TABLE 1 (continued)

Carbon source	Aroma profile
Acetic acid	N.D.
CONTROL	N.D.

Note: N.D.: Odour not detected by sniffing.

TABLE 2

Effect of carbon sources on linalool accumulation, pH, and growth of P. italicum (Nitrogen source: glutamic acid)

Carbon source	Linalool ±s.d.* (μg/L)	pH** Initial	pH** Final	Dry wt. ±s.d.* (g/L)
MONOSACCHARIDES				
Hexoses				
Fructose	30 ± 5	3.2	3.3	2.20 ± 0.44
Galactose	35 ± 10	3.2	3.2	1.60 ± 0.02
1,5-Gluconolactone	N.D.	3.0	2.8	1.20 ± 0.10
Glucose	57 ± 5	3.2	3.6	3.10 ± 0.40
Pentoses				
Arabinose	25 ± 1	3.1	3.2	0.60 ± 0.04
Xylose	40 ± 5	3.1	3.4	0.90 ± 0.09
DISACCHARIDES				
Maltose	Trace	3.2	3.5	0.40 ± 0.04
Lactose	Trace	3.2	3.4	0.60 ± 0.12
Sucrose	50 ± 1	3.2	3.6	3.30 ± 0.86
POLYHYDROXYL ALCOHOLS				
Glycerol	Trace	3.2	3.5	0.40 ± 0.12
Mannitol	Trace	3.2	3.3	0.50 ± 0.01
Sorbitol	N.D.	3.2	3.3	N.G.
ACIDS				
Pyruvic acid	20 ± 1	4.0	4.4	0.60 ± 0.02
Acetic acid	N.D.	3.1	3.1	N.G.
CONTROL	N.D.	3.2	3.2	N.G.

* Standard derivation derived from 6 replicates.
** pH: Initial: After autoclaving and before inoculation.
        Final: At end of incubation period.
Trace: Less than 10 μg/L culture broth.
N.D.: Not detected.
N.G.: No growth.

TABLE 3

Effect of glucose and sucrose on linalool accumulation by P. italicum in media with different nitrogen sources

Nitrogen source	Amt. of Linalool ± s.d.* (µg/L)	
	Glucose	Sucrose
Aspartic acid	41 ± 5	60 ± 10
Glutamic acid	98 ± 10	50 ± 5
Vitamin-free casamino acids	122 ± 20	47 ± 5

* Standard deviation derived from 6 replicates.

TABLE 4

Effect of nitrogen sources on linalool accumulation, pH, and growth of P. italicum (Carbon source: glucose)

Nitrogen source	Linalool ±s.d.* (µg/L)	pH** Initial	Final	Dry wt. ±s.d.* (g/L)
AMINO ACIDS				
Alanine	28 ± 5	5.1	5.2	44 ± 5
Arginine	20 ± 5	7.2	4.6	47 ± 6
Asparagine	Trace	4.6	6.3	35 ± 2
Aspartic acid	40 ± 10	3.1	3.3	77 ± 10
Citrulline	15 ± 2	5.5	4.1	29 ± 2
Creatine	N.D.	5.6	5.6	N.G.
Cysteic acid	N.D.	2.3	2.3	N.G.
Cysteine	N.D.	4.7	2.9	21 ± 1
Cystine	N.D.	5.0	3.0	N.G.
Glutamic acid	57 ± 5	3.2	3.8	112 ± 20
Glutamine	10 ± 2	5.0	4.1	98 ± 20
Glycine	25 ± 5	5.0	4.7	43 ± 6
Histidine	Trace	6.5	6.2	15 ± 3
4-Hydroxyproline	N.D.	4.9	4.8	N.G.
Iso-leucine	Trace	5.0	3.9	20 ± 5
Leucine	N.D.	5.1	3.7	34 ± 3
Lysine	N.D.	9.0	8.3	Trace
Methionine	N.D.	4.8	3.4	Trace
S-Methyl-L-cysteine	N.D.	5.2	3.8	Trace
Ornithine monochloride	Trace	5.1	3.3	28 ± 4
Phenylalanine	N.D.	5.0	4.1	30 ± 3
Phenylglycine	N.D.	4.8	3.4	N.G.
Proline	Trace	5.0	4.2	52 ± 3
Serine	18 ± 5	5.2	5.1	63 ± 3
Threonine	10 ± 4	5.2	4.2	37 ± 9
Tryptophan	N.D.	4.9	3.9	Trace
Tyrosine	N.D.	5.2	3.8	16 ± 1
Valine	N.D.	5.3	3.7	19 ± 1
AMIDE				
Urea	20 ± 10	5.8	6.0	30 ± 5
PEPTIDE				
Glycylglycine	10 ± 1	5.2	5.1	10 ± 3

TABLE 4 (continued)

Nitrogen source	Linalool ±s.d.* (μg/L)	pH** Initial	Final	Dry wt. ±s.d.* (g/L)
PROTEIN				
Vitamin-free Casamino acids (Difco)	127 ± 4.5	5.2	4.2	192 ± 30
Technical grade Casamino acids (Difco)	130 ± 50	5.2	4.1	188 ± 30
Casein	35 ± 5	5.0	3.6	60 ± 20
INORGANIC NITROGEN				
Ammonium sulphate	N.D.	4.6	3.0	36 ± 5
Sodium nitrate	10 ± 2	4.6	5.0	14 ± 2
CONTROL	N.D.	4.6	4.6	N.G.

* Standard deviation derived from 6 replicates.
** pH: Initial: After autoclaving and before inoculation.
    Final: At end of incubation period.
Trace: Less than 10 μg Linalool/L or less than 1 g mycelial dry wt./L.
N.D.: Not detected.
N.G. No growth.

3.4 Effect of nitrogen sources

The effect of nitrogen sources was investigated by varying the nitrogen source in culture media containing glucose. Nitrogen sources exerted a greater influence on the aroma profile of P. italicum than carbon sources (see Table 5). P. italicum grown in either alanine, aspartic acid, glutamic acid, or glycine (with glucose as the carbon source) exhibited a very strong orange aroma. The "arginine", "citrulline", "glutamine", "serine", "threonine" and "tyrosine" cultures produced an orange aroma of moderate intensity. "Leucine" culture gave a strong over-ripe banana-like odour with a trace of orange aroma. With "iso-leucine", "histidine", "proline", and "tyrosine" cultures, a weak orange aroma was observed. "Valine" culture produced a faint orange aroma with a detectable banana note. When grown in phenylalaine, a honey-like aroma was distinctly evident, and in lysine, P. italicum produced a non-descript sweet fragrant odour. With the flasks containing sulphur amino acids (i.e. cysteine, cystine, methionine, and S-methyl-L-cysteine) a rotten egg or cooked cabbage odour which differed from that of the uninoculated controls was detected. In the di-peptide glycylglycine P. italicum produced a moderately strong orange aroma, whereas in urea (which is an amide) a sweet, alcoholic, orange aroma was observed. When complex nitrogen sources such as casamino acids and casein were used, an orange peel-like odour was definitely evident; the intensity of the odour in P. italicum cultures was stronger with "vitamin-free" and "technical grade" casamino acids as nitrogen sources than with casein (see Table 4). Inorganic nitrogen sources also affected aroma profile production; "ammonium sulpahte" culture produced a moderately strong milk-like odour and "sodium nitrate" culture gave a sour orange aroma of moderate strength.

TABLE 5

Effect of nitrogen sources on odour profile of P. italicum cultures (Carbon source: glucose)

Nitrogen source	Aroma profile
AMINO ACIDS	
Alanine	Sour, orange
Arginine	Sweet, orange
Asparagine	Mouldy, orange
Aspartic acid	Sour, citrus, orange
Citrulline	Citrus, sour, orange
Creatine	N.D.
Cysteic acid	N.D.
Cysteine	Rotten egg
Cystine	Cabbage
Glutamic acid	Sharp, orange peel
Glutamine	Sweet, orange
Glycine	Sour, citrus, orange
Histidine	Mouldy, orange
4-Hydroproline	N.D.
Iso-Leucine	Sour, orange
Leucine	Over-ripe banana, slight orange
Lysine	Sweet, fragrant
Methionine	Cabbage
S-Methyl-L-cysteine	Rotten egg
Ornithine monochloride	Sweet, orange
Phenylalanine	Honey
Phenylglycine	N.D.
Proline	Fresh, orange
Serine	Sweet, orange
Threonine	Sweet, orange
Tryptophan	Skatol-like
Tyrosine	Orange
Valine	Orange
AMIDE	
Urea	Alcoholic, sweet, orange
PEPTIDE	
Glycylglycine	Orange
PROTEIN	
Vitamin-free Casamino acids	Sharp, orange peel
Technical-grade Casamino acids	Sharp, orange peel
Casein	Sharp, orange peel
INORGANIC NITROGEN	
Ammonium sulphate	Milky
Sodium nitrate	Sour, orange
CONTROL	N.D.

N.D.: Not detected.

On GLC examination, it was found that the linalool peak was absent in all cultures which did not possess an orange aroma. Table 4 shows the amount of linalool accumulated by P. italicum in various nitrogen sources. Nitrogen sources not only affected the qualitative aroma profile produced by P. italicum but also the quantitative amount of linalool accumulation. "Vitamin-free" and "technical-grade" casamino acids gave about the same value for linalool accumulation, which was far better than those of the other nitrogen sources examined. This superior effect on linalool production may possibly be explained by better growth in casamino acids combined with a more favourable pH environment (see Table 4).

4. CONCLUSION

Based on the above-reported findings, the type of nitrogen and carbon sources used in fermentation media would have an important bearing on the development of a process for the biotechnological production of natural aroma extracts by P. italicum. Whereas carbon sources mainly affected the quantitative aspect of the aroma production, nitrogen sources affected the aroma production not only quantitatively but also qualitatively. Similar effects by carbon and nitrogen sources on the aroma production by Trichoderman viride had also been reported by Yong et al. (1985) and Yong and Lim (1986).

The qualitative effect of nitrogen sources which are amino acids could be explained by the fact that upon metabolism of amino acids by P. italicum, a variety of carbon skeletons are produced. These carbon skeletons could then be the origin of different small volatile organic molecules possessing different aroma characteristics. For example, Yu et al. (1968) reported that 3-methylbutanol and 3-methylbutanal which are the major components of banana aroma, were formed by incubating tomato extract in the presence of leucine.

In quantitative terms, "technical-grade" or "vitamin-free" casamino acids gave the best accumulation of linalool by P. italicum in media containing glucose as the carbon source. This also indicates that the presence of any vitamins in casamino acids would not have a significant effect on aroma production of P. italicum.

5. REFERENCES

1. M.F. Kok, F.M. Yong and G. Lim, J. Agric. Food Chem., 35 (1987) 779-781.
2. K.B. Raper and C. Thom, in: K.B. Raper and C. Thom (Eds), Manual of Penicillin, William and Wilkin Co., USA, 1949, pp. 526.
3. G. Smith, in: J.E. Smith (Ed.), An Introduction to Industrial Mycology, Edward Arnold, London, 1969, p. 207.
4. F.M. Yong and G. Lim, MIRCEN J.,2(1986) 483-488.
5. F.M. Yong, H.A. Wong and G. Lim, Appl. Microbial Biotechnol., 22(1985) 146-7.
6. M.H. Yu, D.K. Salunkhe and L.E. Olson, Plant Cell Physiol., 9(1968), 633-8.

The Computer Simulation of the Chemical Kinetics of Flavor Compounds in Heated Foods

ARTHUR E. GROSSER

Department of Chemistry, McGill University, 801 Sherbrooke St. W., Montreal, PQ H3A 2K6 CANADA

SUMMARY

The computer simulation of the kinetic behavior of the production and destruction of flavor compounds is presented. In particular, a model is considered for foods which are heated in a constant-temperature bath. The variation of the concentrations of these compounds as a function of time is explored. The experimental quantities which are needed for a successful simulation are evaluated for systems which may polymerize.

INTRODUCTION

As the materials and processes available to the food technologist multiply, the scientific problems quickly become too complex to be solved by obvious or even direct experiments. The multiplicity of choices becomes so vast that proposing a new process or formulation either will involve too many possible experiments or the unsatisfactory but frequently employed invocation of "scientific intuition".

It is therefore useful to have a theoretical framework which allows the computation of sufficient food parameters to at least direct the researcher toward the most fruitful avenues of endeavour. This paper will propose a simple model for such a computation.

I   ISOTHERMAL REACTIVE CASE (MODEL I):

It is assumed that the chemical changes which are of interest have been studied to an extent such that the rate laws governing these changes are known. For a process in which reactants, R and S, are transformed into products, P and Q, in the presence of catalytic material, C,

$$R + S \xrightarrow{C} P + Q \qquad [1]$$

the rate law can be a function of any of these species to any power. We will assume that the rate laws are simple functions of only the reactant concentrations,

$$-d[R]/dt = k\,[R]^\alpha\,[S]^\beta \qquad [2]$$

where k is the rate constant and α and β are the orders with respect to the reactants, R and S.

Kinetic experiments are most often performed in an isothermal system so that the rate constant does not change with time. The simulation of such an experiment to determine the composition, or extent of reaction as a function of time is straightforward, dependent only on a knowledge of k, α, β, and the initial concentrations of the reactants and products.

For example, for reactions where one reactant forms one product in the absence of a catalyst:

R ⟶ P [3]

and where the overall orders, n, are 1, 2 and 3, the behaviour of the concentrations of reactants and products is shown in Figure 1, assuming the initial reactant concentration, $[C]_0$, is 1.0 and the initial product concentration, $[P]_0$, is zero.

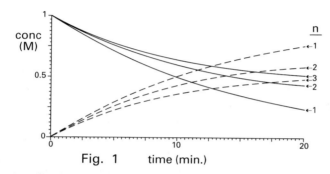

Fig. 1. Concentration versus time for Model 1. Solid lines are for reactants; dashed, for products. (This convention is observed in all subsequent Figures.) The order, n, is given on the right hand side.

The rate constant for the first-order reaction has been chosen to be 6.93×10^{-2} min^{-1} which corresponds to a half-time, $t_{1/2}$, of 10 minutes. For orders n = 2 and 3, k = 6.93×10^{-2} M^{1-n} min^{-1}. Note that in the system under consideration, where the concentration is set at unity, the <u>initial</u> rates are identical.

II. TEMPERATURE GRADIENT NON-REACTIVE CASE (MODEL II)

In the heat treatment of food, however, an object at an ambient temperature, T_a, is subjected to heating, perhaps by immersion in a "bath" at a higher temperature, T_b. A temperature gradient is soon set up throughout the volume of the food, the periphery of the object warming quickly while the center preserves its ambient temperature for some time. Thus, for reactions with a finite energy of activation, at short times the rate constant for the reaction under consideration has a large value at the periphery and a much smaller one at the center. The extent of the chemical transformations at the periphery are therefore greater than at the center at every stage of the heating. At long times, of course, the temperature of the food becomes ultimately uniform and equal to that of the bath. The decomposition of reactant flavour compounds or the production of them is therefore a function of time *and* position in the food.

In setting up a hypothetical model to calculate these chemical transformations, the principle that we will follow is to make the first model as simple as possible. This is necessary to keep control over the simulation by preserving an intuitive picture of the direction of the expected results. Once one is assured that the simple simulation is calculating correctly, it is easy to add complexities one-by-one and verify that the changed output varies in the appropriate manner.

This model of a food will assume spherical symmetry and uniform composition. The radial distance from the center is r and the outer radius is a. The bath is assumed to be at constant temperature, T_b, and the temperature of the food object is initially and uniformly at the ambient temperature, T_a.

The equation for heat flow in a sphere (1,2) leads to the equation

$$T(r,t) - T_a = (T_b - T_a) \{1 + (2a/\pi r) \sum_{n=1}^{\infty} [(-1)^n/n][\sin(n\pi r/a) \exp(-\kappa n^2 \pi^2 t/a^2)]\} \quad [4]$$

where $T(r,t)$ is the temperature of the food at radial distance, r, and time, t, and κ is the thermal diffusivity which is given by $\kappa = K/C_p$, where C_p is the volumetric heat capacity and K is the thermal conductivity.

Let the input parameters for this model be arbitrarily set as follows: $a = 1$ cm, $T_a = 20.0°C$, $T_b = 100.0°C$, $\kappa = 1 \times 10^{-2}$ cm^2 min^{-1}, $[R]_o = 1$ M, $[P]_o = 0$ M. (Table 1, at the end of this paper, summarizes the input parameters for all the Models.)

The solutions to these and subsequent numerical integrations were performed by a fourth-order Runge-Kutta technique. Equation [2] does not converge quickly at small times, especially for r close to a. In such cases, $T(r,t)$ is set equal to T_a for $0 \le t \le 0.1$ or 0.5. The summation is carried out to twelve terms. The dependence of $T(r,t)$ is shown in Figure 2 as a function of t for a family of curves in r. It should be noted that these and subsequent Figures may be equivalently interpreted in a more general sense by identifying r with the reduced radius, r/a. The qualitatively expected behavior is observed: the periphery of the food gets hotter first and stays hot longest, and the center has the shortest exposure to high temperatures.

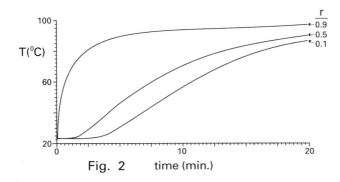

Fig. 2. Temperature (°C) versus time for Model II. The radial distance, r, is indicated.

III. TEMPERATURE GRADIENT, REACTIVE CASE, FIRST ORDER (MODEL III)

We may now proceed to combine Models I and II to obtain a reactive system which has temperature gradients. Let us assume reaction [3] obeys the Arrhenius equation,

$$k(T) = A \exp(-E_a/RT) \qquad [5]$$

where A is the pre-exponential factor; E_a, the energy of activation; R, the universal gas constant; and T, the absolute temperature.

Let the parameters be those of the temperature gradient non-reactive case (Model II) where n = 1 and let the Arrhenius parameters be such that k_{333}, the rate constant at T = 333 K, is 0.0693 min^{-1}, namely: E_a = 20.00 kcal mole^{-1} and A = 9.262 x 10^{11} min^{-1}.

Before a simulation is run using these simple equations, the qualitative result is clearly foreseen. The periphery of the food is subject to large rate constants (and large rates of reaction) quickly and for the longest time. Any chemical transformations will occur mostly at the periphery and unless the starting reagent is exhausted at some region, the percent conversions of reactant to products will always be greatest at the periphery and will decrease in a regular way as the radius decreases. The simulations bear out these ideas as is seen in Figure 3.

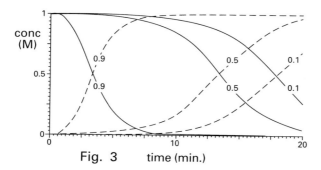

Fig. 3. Temperature (K) versus time for Model III. r is indicated on the appropriate curve.

IV. TEMPERATURE GRADIENT, SECOND-ORDER REACTION (MODEL IV):

At this stage, it may be instructive to consider what effects would be expected from a different rate law. What if, for example, the reaction was second order in R rather than first order? Intuitively, we would expect the rate to diminish more quickly as the reactant concentration is reduced.

This model will be the same as Model III except that the rate law will be second order, and k_{333}, the rate constant at T = 333 K, is set equal to 6.93 x 10^{-2} M^{-1} min^{-1}, which sets equal the initial rates of Models III and IV. The results of the simulation are shown in Figure 4. The general dependence of the concentration on t is qualitatively unchanged as seen in Fig. 4a. The quantitative differences are negligible until times close to the half-time of the reaction, as can be seen in Figure 4b which compares the concentration versus time behaviours for Models III and IV at r = a/2.

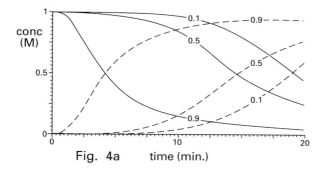

Fig. 4a   time (min.)

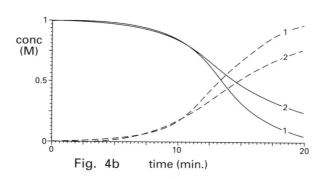

Fig. 4b   time (min.)

Fig. 4. (a) Concentration versus time for Model IV. r is indicated on the right-hand side. (b) Models III and IV are compared for r = 0.5 a, to show sensitivity to the order, n, which is indicated.

V. TEMPERATURE GRADIENT, FIRST- ORDER REACTION, VARIABLE E_a (Model V)

A more striking result will surely be apparent with reactions with different energies of activation, E_a. Let us compare Model III with a system of the same parameters, save only that E_a will be either 50% greater or 50% less than the reference value of 20 kcal mole^{-1}, that is E_a will be 10 or 30 kcal mole^{-1} with A chosen so that the rate constants are the same at 333 K as the reference case.

Prediction of the qualitative behaviour of these systems is clear. For a low value of E_a, the rate constants are not strongly temperature-dependent and k does not increase greatly from its value at 293 K. The extent of reaction is small even at the periphery. For a high value of E_a, the rate constants are strongly temperature-dependent and the extent of reaction is a dramatic function of r and t.

Figure 5 shows the quantitative results which bear out these presuppositions. Fig. 5a shows the substantially different behaviour for the Model with E_a equal to 10 and 30 kcal mole^{-1}. Figure 5b compares the concentration versus time behavior at r = a/2 for various E_a's.

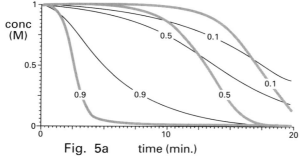
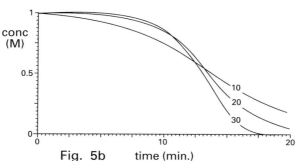

Fig. 5. (a). Concentration versus time for Model V. r is indicated. narrow line: $E_a = 10$ kcal mole^{-1}; wide line: $E_a = 30$ kcal mole^{-1}. (b). To show the sensitivity to E_a, Models III and V are compared for r = 0.5 a. E_a in kcal mole^{-1} is indicated on the curves.

The concentration is clearly highly sensitive to this parameter and this can lead to very different spatial distributions of the concentrations of the flavor compounds within the food at any given heating time which is not too long. This effect may be particularly important when two or more flavor compounds, present in the same food sample have transformations governed by different E_a's.

VI. TEMPERATURE GRADIENT, FIRST ORDER REACTION, E_a = 20 kcal mole^{-1}, VARIABLE THERMAL DIFFUSIVITY

The last problem we will consider is the variation in thermal diffusivity, κ. To estimate this effect, we will return to Model IV, but specify that κ be either 50% greater or 50% less than its reference value in that Model, namely 1×10^{-2}. The result is shown in Figure 6.

Not unexpectedly, the effect of the thermal diffusivity is marked. The highest rate of reaction corresponds to the largest value of κ, corresponding to the most rapid transfer of heat.

An added complication is that κ may change as heating progresses. This can be due to the temperature dependence of the material (including phase changes) or changes in its chemical composition, or both. This necessary input is complicated by the fact that the composition and the temperature are changing simultaneously.

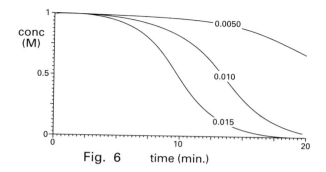

Fig. 6. To show the sensitivity of κ, concentration versus time is plotted for Models III and VI. the values of k, in cm² min⁻¹, are indicated on the curve.

One expects the thermal conductivity to be less sensitive to these changes than the heat capacity. If the foodstuffs under consideration have a high water content and can be compared to dilute aqueous solutions, chemical changes should not affect K. Even phase changes should not change K greatly, since it depends on average molecular vibrational frequencies.

On the other hand, there is the expectation that aqueous solutions of organic molecules are subject to large variations in the heat capacity. Hydrophobic moieties on monomeric peptides that would otherwise not be in contact with a solvent can be exposed upon heating and/or via chemical reaction (especialy cross-linking to form an extended structure), promoting the structured arrangement of solvent molecules around the hydrophobic groups (3). This "iceberg state" formation leads to a higher heat capacity and a lower value of κ.

TABLE 1

Input Parameters of the Models

Model	Figure	n	T	reaction	k_{333}[a]	E_a kcal/mole	$\kappa \times 10^{-2}$ cm²/min
I	1	1,2,3	isothermal	yes	6.93×10^{-2}	0.0100	---
II	2	-	gradient	no	0	-	1
III	3	1	gradient	yes	6.93×10^{-2}	20	1
IV	3	2	gradient	yes	6.93×10^{-2}	20	1
V	5	1	gradient	yes	6.93×10^{-2}	10,20,30	1
VI	6	1	gradient	yes	6.93×10^{-2}	20	0.5,1,2

For all Models: $a = 1.00$ cm, $T_a = 293K$, $T_b = 373K$, $[R]_0 = 1.00$ M, $[P]_0 = 0$.

[a] Units of k are min⁻¹ for first-order reactions and $M^{(1-n)}$ min⁻¹ for nth order reactions ($n \neq 1$).

CONCLUSION

Simulations of the kinetic behavior of the chemical transformations in a heated food can be fully carried out if

1. The geometry of the food can be approximated by a simple geometric shape.
2. The rate law does not change (alternate pathways of decomposition do not become important) during the heating.
3. The Arrhenius equation is obeyed (with no temperature dependence of the pre-exponential factor, A, and a constant value of E_a.)
4. The thermal diffusivity remains constant or is known as a function of temperature and composition.

Of these constraints, the first and the last seem to offer the most uncertainty, but one expects the results to be more sensitive to item 4. On the other hand, any number of reagents, their initial concentrations, their rate laws and energies of activation under any combination of ambient and bath temperatures may easily be simulated to yield quantitative predictions of the concentration gradients of flavor compounds.

One may alternatively regard these parameters, not as quantities whose values must be rigorously determined, but rather as opportunities to create and modify food fabrications. For example, one could compensate a non-uniform spatial distribution of a flavor compound by changing the spatial distribution of the initial concentration of the precursor, by modifying the spatial density to influence κ, or even by changing the shape of the food. A suitable simulation can then lead to a quantitative specification of the necessary properties.

ACKNOWLEDGEMENTS

The author wishes to thank the V.K. Krieble Foundation and the Department of Chemistry for their continued support, and Joanne Marentette for helpful advice.

REFERENCES

1. H.S. Carslaw and J.C. Jaeger, Conduction of Heat in Solids, 2nd ed., Oxford, London, 1959, p. 233.
2. S.W. Benson, The Foundations of Chemical Kinetics, McGraw-Hill, New York, 1969, p. 427 ff.
3. C. Tanford, The Hydrophobic Effect: Formation of Micelles and Biological Membranes, 2nd ed., Wiley, New York, p. 22 ff.

FLAVOR COMPOUNDS IN MAPLE SYRUP

by

Inteaz Alli, Emmanuel Akochi-K. and Selim Kermasha

Food Science and Agricultural Chemistry Department
McGill University
P.O. Box 187 Macdonald Campus
St-Anne de Bellevue, Québec
Canada H9X 1C0

Abstract

Maple syrup is characterized by an unique "maple" flavor. There is presently no definite compound or compounds which have been identified as the "maple" flavor. However, numerous flavor compounds have been identified in maple syrup. These include primarily phenolic compounds, pyrazines and carbonyl compounds. The existence of these flavor compounds is related to both the presence of certain compounds (sucrose, reducing sugars, nitrogen containing compounds, soluble lignins) in the maple sap as well as the heating of the sap at elevated temperatures for its conversion to syrup.

Introduction

Maple syrup is the characteristic product resulting from thermal processing of maple sap, the exudate tapped from the trunk of mature sugar maple trees (*Acer Saccharum* MARSH). The initial maple sap which represents a solution in which sucrose is the major component (minor quantities of reducing sugars, and traces of nitrogenous compounds and minerals and soluble lignins also present) is converted to syrup by extended heating at elevated temperatures. It is likely that, during this heating process, numerous chemical reactions involving not only sucrose but also the minor components of the sap take place. Undoubtedly, these chemical reactions contribute immensely to the development of the characteristic flavor of the syrup which is formed. However, they have not been studied in the maple system. Although the flavor of maple syrup is very characteristic of the product, the exact chemical compound or compounds which are responsible for this characteristic flavor is yet to be established, in spite of the fact that there are commercially available "maple" flavors.

This paper will address the identification of flavor compounds in maple syrup and the factors which could influence the presence, the formation, and the development of these compounds when maple is converted to syrup.

Identified volatile compounds in maple syrup

Table 1 shows a list of volatile compounds which to date have been reported to have a role in maple flavor. On the basis of their structures, most of these compounds can be gouped as phenolics, pyrazines and carbonyl compounds.

Phenolic compounds:

Filipic *et al.* (1965) reported the presence of the volatile phenolic compounds vanillin, syringaldehyde, dehydroconiferyl alcohol, 2,6-dimethoxyphenol and syringoyl methyl ketone among the volatiles of maple syrup. These compounds are considered as degradation products of lignin; however it has not been established which lignin compounds are present in the initial maple sap.

Pyrazine compounds:

There have been sporadic reports either dealing with the presence of pyrazines in maple syrup or associating pyrazines with the flavor of maple syrup. Winter et al (1972) suggested that 2,5-dimethyl-3,6-diisobutylpyrazine demonstrated maplelike flavor characteristics. More recently, Masuda and Mihara (1986) reported that 5-isopropyl-2,3-dimethylpyrazine gave a "sweet, maplelike, brown odor." In these reports however, the pyrazine compounds where not actually identified in the maple syrup. In a systematic study of pyrazines in maple syrup, Alli et al (1990) reported the presence of at least seven pyrazine compounds; these included methyl pyrazine, 2,3-dimethylpyrazine, 2,5-dimethylpyrazine, 2,6-dimethylpyrazine, ethylpyrazine, trimethylpyrazine, and 2-ethyl-6-methylpyrazine. These pyrazine compounds, in addition to a large number of other pyrazines contribute flavor and are present in various thermally processed foods (Maga, 1982), and are therefore not unique to maple syrup. Kallio (1988) reported the presence of the 2,6-dimethylpyrazine, along with several other volatile compounds in the pentane-diethyl ether extract of birch syrup, a product similar to maple syrup but obtained from the sap of birch trees (*Betula pubesceus* Enrh).

Carbonyl compounds:

Filipic et al (1965) reported the presence of 2-hydroxymethylcyclopent-2-en-1-one as a minor component of maple syrup and suggested that this carbonyl compound contributed to the characteristic maple flavor. Several other carbonyl compounds (3-hydroxybutanone, 3-hydroxy-2-pyranone, 3-methy-2,5-furandione) were identified in the dichloromethane extracts of maple syrup (Alli et al 1990). Bean and Setser (1992) listed 3-hydroxy-4-methyl-5-ethyl-2(5*H*)-furanone and propionaldehyde as flavor compounds of maple syrup identified with the maple like syrup flavor; however, these compounds were not actually identified in maple syrup. Kallio (1988) reported the presence of various carbonyl compounds in the volatiles of maple syrup; these include 2-hydroxy-3-methyl-2-cyclopenten-1-one, 3-hydroxybutanone, 2,5-dimethyl-4-hydroxy-3(2H)-furanone, 2,3-dihydro-3,5-dihydroxy-6-methyl(4H)-pyran-4-one, 2-methyl-2-cyclopenten-1-one, 2-methyl-2,5-cyclohexadien-1,4-dione and 3-methyl-3-buten-2-one.

Other compounds:

In addition to the groups of compounds described above, several other volatile compounds have been reported (Kallio, 1988) in maple syrup; these include: alcohols (2-ethyl-1-hexanol, 2-furanmethanol, 2-hydroxymethylcyclopenten-2-en-ol); organic acids (2-ethyl-1-hexanoic acid, n-hexanoic acid, n-nonanoic acid); this author suggested that aliphatic alcohols and carboxylic acids might be due to antifoaming agents used during the processing of maple sap to syrup.

Maple sap components that contribute to syrup flavor

In order to explain the origin of some of the flavor compounds which have been reported in maple syrup, it is perhaps convenient to start with an investigation of the sap components which could potentially contribute to flavor. Although the sap is considered "flavorless", the presence of certain compounds (organic acids, minerals) can contribute some flavor; however, it is unlikely that chemical induced flavor compounds which are found in the syrup would be found in the sap before processing to syrup. In fact, we have found (unpublished results) the absence of pyrazines in maple sap but their presence in the syrup resulting from the same sap. Table 2 lists chemical components which have been reported to be present in maple sap. Sucrose represents the dominant component and its concentration by thermal processing is responsible for many of the properties of maple syrup. However, several of the minor components (nitrogenous compounds and soluble lignins) contribute directly both flavor and color attributes, because of their involvement in thermally induced reactions.

Effects of processing conditions on maple syrup flavor compounds

Undoubtedly, the thermal processing of maple sap contribute immensely to the development of flavor compounds in the syrup. The principal reactions which occur are caramelization reactions (Kallio, 1988), reactions between reducing sugars and amino acids or Maillard reaction (Kallio, 1988) and alkaline degradation of lignin derived compounds (Filipic *et al.*, 1965).

Caramelization reactions:

These represent mainly dehydration and/or fragmentation reactions of sugars, and include furans, pyrones, cyclopentens, carbonyl compounds and acids (Bean and Setser, 1992). Caramelization reactions can be expected during the heating of maple sap which contains sucrose and small amounts of reducing sugars (Jones and Alli, 1987). These reactions occur under both acidic and basic conditions, with acidic conditions promoting dehydration reactions which result in production of furfurals, and alkaline conditions favoring isomerization and fragmentation of sucrose (Feather, 1982; Monte and Maga, 1981). It is likely that most of the cyclopentene compounds, furan and pyran derivatives, and carbonyl compounds listed in Table 1 result mainly from caramelization reactions. Among these, is the 2-hydroxymethylcyclopent-2-en-1-one which is reported to contribute to the characteristic maple flavor (Filipic et al., 1965). However, it may prove difficult to describe the characteristic maple flavor resulting from caramelization reactions, since Herz and Shallenberger (1959) describe a "caramel" aroma when glucose only was heated to 180°C. In addition, commercial "caramel" color contain a large number of pyrazine compounds which are products from reactions between sugars and nitrogen containing compounds (Tsuchida *et al.*, 1986), suggesting that there is much more to the "caramel" reaction attribute than reaction involving sugars only.

Reducing sugar-amino acid reactions

There is extensive information on the role of reactions involving reducing sugars and amino acids (as well as other nitrogen containing compounds) in the development of characteristic flavor compounds. The presence of both reducing sugars and amino acids in maple sap (Kallio, 1988; Jones and Alli, 1987; Morselli and Whelan, 1986) implicates reactions involving these compounds during thermal processing of sap to syrup. In addition, the identification of various pyrazine compounds in maple syrup(Alli et al, 1990; Kallio, 1988) confirms that these reactions take place during heating of the sap. Thus, the pyrazine compounds listed in Table 1 would all be expected to result from thermally induced amino acid-reducing sugar reactions. There are numerous reports on the mechanisms which are involved in the formation of pyrazine compounds. Wang and Odell (1973) reported that several pyrazine compounds were formed from the thermal treatment of amino-hydroxy compounds; however, pyrazines were not formed when the amino acids (aspartic acid, glutamine, aspargine) which were identified in maple sap (Morselli and Whalen, 1986; Kallio, 1988) were heated.

Alkali degradation of lignin derived compounds

Filipic *et al* (1965) demonstrated the presence of several flavor contributing phenolic substances in maple syrup. It is postulated (Filipic *et al*, 1965) that as maple sap is converted to syrup by boiling, the solution passes through an alkaline pH and reaches a maximum pH of about 9. Under these conditions, small quantities of soluble lignins which may be present in the sap could result in the formation of phenolic substances such as vanillin, syringaldehyde, syringoyl methyl ketone, 2,6-dimethoxyphenol (Table 1).

Conclusion

Numerous volatile flavor compounds have been identified in maple syrup, these include pyrazines, phenolic compounds and carbonyl compounds. None of these compounds have been reported to be present in maple sap from which the syrup is prepared. However, many of the compounds present in the sap could be regarded as precursors or reactants that are involved in the formation of the various flavor compounds. Sucrose and reducing sugars are involved in caramelization reactions resulting primarily in carbonyl compounds, reducing sugars and nitrogenous compounds are involved in reactions which result in pyrazine compounds, and alkali degradation of soluble lignins resulting in formation of phenolic compounds. The exact contribution of these flavor compounds to the characteristic flavor of maple syrup is still uncertain.

Table 1 : Identified flavor compounds of maple syrup

Phenolic compounds

vanillin[1]
syringaldehyde[1]
dehydroconiferyl alcohol[1]
syringoyl methyl ketone[1]
2,6-dimethoxyphenol[1]

Pyrazine compounds

methylpyrazine[2]
2,3-dimethylpyrazine[2]
2,5-dimethylpyrazine[2]
2,6-dimethylpyrazine[2]
ethylpyrazine[2]
trimethylpyrazine[2]
2-ethyl-6-methylpyrazine[2]
2,5-dimethyl-3,6-diiso butylpyrazine[3]
5-isopropyl-2,3-dimethylpyrazine[4*]

Carbonyl compounds

2-hydroxymethylcyclopent-2-en-1-one[1]
2-hydroxy-3-methyl-2-cyclopenten-1-one[6]
2-methyl-2-cyclopenten-1-one[6]
2-methyl-2,5-cyclohexadien-1,4-dione[6]
2,3-dihydro-3,5-dihydroxy-6-methyl(4H)-pyran-4-one[6]
2,5-dimethyl-4-hydroxy-3(2H)-furanone[6]
3-methyl-3-buten-2-one[6]
3-methyl-2,5-furandione[2]
3-methyl-2-cyclopenten-2-ol-1-one[1]
3-hydroxybutanone[2,6]
3-hydroxy-2-pyranone[2]
3-hydroxy-4-methyl-5-ethyl-2(5H)-furanone[5]
propionaldehyde[5]

Other compounds

2-ethyl-1-hexanol[6]
2-hydroxymethylcyclopenten-2-en-ol[6]
2-furanmethanol[6]
2-ethyl-1-hexanoic acid[6]
n-hexanoic acid[6]
n-nonanoic acid[6]

---

*not actually identified in maple syrup
[1]Filipic et al., 1965; [2]Alli et al., 1990; [3]Winter et al., 1972
[4]Masuda and Mihara, 1986; [5]Bean and Setser, 1992; [6]Kallio, 1988

Table 2 : Identified chemical components of maple sap

Sugars

sucrose[1]
glucose[1]
fructose[1]
galactose[1]
raffinose[2]

Organic acids

oxalic acid[3]
glyconic acid[2]
fumaric acid[3]
tartaric acid[3]
malic acid[3]
cis-aconitic acid[3]
citric acid[3]
shikimic acid[3]
succinic acid[3]

Nitrogenous compounds

aspartic acid[4]
aspargine[4]
glutamine[4]
ammonia[4]
proline[4]
urea[4]

Minerals

calcium[2]
potassium[2]
sodium[2]
magnesium[2]
manganese[2]

Other compounds

soluble lignin[5]

---

[1]Jones and Alli, 1987; [2]Kallio, 1988; [3]Molica and Morselli, 1984; [4]Whalen and Morselli, 1980; [5]Filipic et al., 1965

References

Alli, I., Bourque, J., Metusin, R., Liang, R. and Yaylayan V., 1990. Identification of pyrazines in maple syrup, J. Agric. Food Chem., 38: 1242.

Bean, M. M. and Setser, C. S., 1992. Polysaccharides, Sugars and Sweeteners. In: Food Theory And Applications. 2nd Ed. J. Browers (Ed), pp. 69-198, Macmillan pub. Co., N.Y.

Feather, M. S. 1982. Sugar Dehydration Reactions. In: Food Carbohydrate. Lineback D. and Inglett G. E. (Eds) pp. 113-133, AVI, Westport, CT.

Filipic, V. J., Underwood, J. C. and Willits, C. O., 1965 The indentification of methylcyclopentenolone and other compounds in maple syrup flavor extract, J. Food Sci., 30: 1008.

Herz, W. J., and Shallenberger, R. S., 1959. Some aromas produced by simple amino acid,sugar reaction. Journal paper No. 1177, N.Y. State Agricultural Experiment Station, Cornell Uni. Geniva, New York.

Jones, A. R. C., and Alli, I., 1987. Sap yields, sugar content, and soluble carbohydrates of saps and syrup of some Canadian birch and maple species. Can. J. For. Res., 17, 263.

Kallio, H., 1988. Comparison and characteristics of aroma compounds from maple and birch syrup. Proceedings, 5th In ternational flavor conference; Charalambos, G., Ed., pp. 241-248, Elsevier, Amsterdam.

Maga, J. A., 1982. Pyrazines in food: An update. CRC Crit. Rev. Food Sci. Nutr. 16, 1.

Masuda, H. and Mihara, S. 1986. Synthesis of alkoxy (alkylthio)-, phenoxy-, and (phenylthio) pyrazines and their olfactive properties. J. Agric. Food Chem. 34: 377.

Mollica, J. N. and Morselli, M. F., 1984. Sugars and sugar products: Gaz Chromatographic determination of nonvolatile organic acids in sap of sugar maple (*Acer saccharum* Marsh). J. Assoc. Off. Anal. Chem., 67: 1125.

Monte, W. C. and Maga, J. A., 1981. Flavor chemistry of sucrose. Sugar Thecnol. Rev. 8: 181.

Morselli, M. F. and Whalen, M. L., 1986. Amino acid increase in xylem sap of Acer saccharim prior to bud break. Am. J. Bot. 73, 722, Abstr. 329.

Tsuchida, H., Morinaka, K., Fujii, S., Komoto, M. and Mizuno, S. 1986. Identification of novel non-volatile pyrazines in commercial caramel colors. In: Amino-Carbonyl Reactions In Food And Biological Systems. Fujimaka, M. and Namiki, M. (Eds) pp. 85-94, Elsevier, Amsterdam, Oxford, New York, Tokyo.

Wang, P. and Odell, V. G., 1973. Formation of pyrazines from thermal treatment of some amino-hydroxy compounds, J. Agric. Food Chem. 21: 868.

Winter, M., Gautschi, F., Flament, I., Stoel, M. and Goldman, I. M., 1972. Flavor modified soluble coffee. U.S. Patent 3 702 253.

G. Charalambous (Ed.), Food Science and Human Nutrition
© 1992 Elsevier Science Publishers B.V. All rights reserved.

A RAPID METHOD FOR MONITORING FOOD VOLATILES

J. R. Jocelyn Paré[*1], Jacqueline M. R. Bélanger[2], André Bélanger[3], and N. Ramarathnam[2]

[1]Environment Canada, R. R. E. T. C., Ottawa, ON, Canada   K1A 0H3
[2]Agriculture Canada, Food Research Centre, St. Hyacinthe, QC, Canada   J2S 8E3
[3]Agriculture Canada, Station de Recherches, St-Jean-sur-Richelieu, QC, Canada   J3B 3E6

SUMMARY

The qualitative compositions of aroma concentrates of lemon obtained by conventional steam distillation and by a novel microwave irradiation technique are similar as evidenced by gas chromatography data. This comparative study also shows that such aroma concentrates can be prepared much more rapidly and efficiently using the microwave-assisted process (MAP). This method can be used as a rapid screening technique for determining the pre-processing qualitative aromatic value of native foodstuff such as fresh plant material.

1.   INTRODUCTION

The odor and the overall flavor character of a fresh or processed food has been not only a fascinating topic of research to flavor chemists but also an equally frustrating one. This is due mainly to the complications involved in the isolation and the characterization of volatile components that are present in trace amounts. This frustration has been partly resorbed in the last two decades as a result of the remarkable development of analytical techniques that are far more sensitive, accurate and well suited for the analysis of trace volatile components. Despite these advances in analysis, the methods for their extraction and their isolation have remained traditional. The physical principles behind the extraction processes used to date were always the same until the recent developement of a novel microwave-assisted process (MAP) used to extract a variety of natural products from various materials (1).

Distillation, liquid-liquid extraction, adsorption (as in headspace) and other procedures are commonly used for the isolation of aromatic constituents from specific food materials. The method used to isolate these components can have profound effects on the resulting aromagram. Thus, there is a need to improve the existing methods and/or to develop innovative isolation techniques to make use fully of the rapid progress and the improvement in both, the efficiency and the accuracy, of analytical tools.

The classical procedures for the isolation and the concentration of volatiles have been reviewed by several workers (2-6). Those reports state that steam distillation, at atmospheric pressure, is still the most commonly used method for isolating volatiles.

Although the latter has advantages, especially when volatiles from large volumes of samples are to be extracted, it also has intrinsic disadvantages for qualitative analysis. The first one is the long period of time required to perform a single distillation. Secondly, the subsequent steps, such as the extraction with relatively large volumes of organic solvents and the concentration procedures can lead to the introduction and/or the production of considerable artefacts, *e.g.* severe thermal degradation processes producing artefacts in the case of garlic (7).

For food processing purposes, where qualitative aromatic properties of starting materials, intermediate products and the finished foodstuffs are to be evaluated on the basis of their relative flavour compositions, steam distillation is indeed costly and time consuming. To overcome this problem we expanded on our recently patented microwave-assisted extraction process (1, 8) and we now report on a novel method whereby food aromas can be generated, collected and concentrated from a food system within 10 minutes. This technique involves the use of microwave technology. The latter is becoming widely popular both in household and in various commercial food processing applications (9, 10). The case of lemon is presented as an example although the method is applicable to a wide variety of food systems.

2. EXPERIMENTAL

2.1 Lemon

Fresh lemons (Sunkist, CA) were purchased commercially from a local food store and used as obtained without any treatment.

2.2 Microwave-assisted aromas collection

One whole lemon was sliced into small cubes and placed in a 500 mL air-tight nalgene container (Nalge, U.S.A.) equipped with a two-outlet lid which was bearing two small Eppendorf pipette tips. The first one of them was packed with glass wool to act as a safety vent whereas the second one acted as a receiver for a Florisil Sep-Pak (Waters, MA). This assembly was placed in a domestic microwave oven (Kenmore, model 300 Auto recipe) of 42,5 dm^3 and operating at 2450 MHz and 625 watts. The irradiation sequence was as follows: 60s irradiation - 60s pause - 30s irradiation. Volatiles were generated inside the chamber, along with water vapors, and were trapped onto the Florisil cartridge. The latter was allowed to cool down for one minute and was subsequently eluted with two portions of distilled diethyl ether (1,5 and 2,0 mL). The eluate was carefully concentrated to 1.0mL under a mild stream of nitrogen (UHP) prior to the gas chromatographic analysis.

2.3 Steam distillation

For comparison purposes a steam distillation experiment was carried out on one sliced lemon in a 1-L two-necked flask for one hour at which time *ca.* 250 mL of the aqueous distillate was collected. The distillate was extracted with distilled diethyl ether (2 X 25 mL) and the combined ethereal fraction was dried over anhydrous Na$_2$SO$_4$ and concentrated to a final volume of one mL prior to gas chromatographic analysis.

2.4 Gas chromatography

The concentrated eluate from above was analyzed by gas chromatography (Hewlett-Packard, OH, model 5890) using a DB-5 capillary column (0,32 mm o.d., 30 m, J&W Scientific, CA). The temperature program ranged from 60 to 100°C at 3°C.min^{-1}, then from 100 to 240°C at 6°C.min^{-1}. Helium was used as carrier gas at a flow rate of 1,5 mL.min^{-1}. The injector and detector temperatures were set at 225 and 250°C respectively.

2.5 Gas chromatography/mass spectrometry

Mass spectral analyses were performed on a medium resolution double focusing normal geometry mass spectrometer (VG 7070-EHF) coupled to a gas chromatograph identical to that above. The mass spectrometer was operated under electron impact conditions with an ionization energy of 70eV and an accelerating potential of 6000 V.

3. RESULTS AND DISCUSSION

A comparison of typical gas chromatograms of aromatic concentrates isolated by the two methods under investigation shows that the composition of the two concentrates is similar for the first 25 minutes. This region includes all low boiling alcohols, esters, carbonyl compounds, terpene hydrocarbons and a few short-chain acids. The fraction beyond 25 minutes, for the present analytical conditions, contains mainly higher hydrocarbons and long-chain fatty acids that are released from the lemon peel. A preliminary mass spectrometric analysis (data not shown) indicated that the main aromatic component, namely $\underline{d}$-limonene, was present at a retention time of ca. 14,5 minutes.

The qualitative extraction of the aromatic components by the microwave-assisted technique took less than 10 minutes and consumed small volumes of organic solvents (3,5 mL). On the other hand, the overall steam distillation process required well over two hours and used a much larger quantity of the extracting solvent. These results suggest that extraction of aromatic concentrates from food materials can be obtained faster by the microwave-assisted technique. This should result in a reduction in the formation of artefacts usually found in extracts prepared by conventional processes making use of long exposure to heat, such as in steam distillation (7). Furthermore, this microwave-assisted technique requires very little power. This factor, along with the reduced solvent consumption, could lead to operational costs that are more in line with respect to other current methodologies.

The reduced processing time and artefact formation result from the two different modes of action taking place for the two extraction methods. The microwave technique involves a quasi-instantaneous disruption of the internal structure of the plant material whereas steam distillation involves a slow, heat-induced, diffusion of the contents of the plant material through the various walls and membranes that constitute its internal structure. We have reported elsewhere on electron microscopy (1, 8) and on chemical (11) studies that established these modes of action.

Further work is in progress in our laboratories to evaluate the range of applications of this novel process and to assess its potential for quantitative analysis. As it stands, however, this method can be used directly in the research laboratory without any special requirement not readily available. Furthermore, upon some development, it could prove useful in receiving areas or in distribution centers or wherever there is a need for a rapid screening and monitoring of the aromatic profile of a given material. This is mainly due to the relative ease with which it can be performed, to the low processing costs associated with it and to its extremely rapid response time.

4. ACKNOWLEDGEMENTS

We acknowledge the technical assistance of J. Lapointe, M. Sigouin and R. Laing during the course of these investigations. One of us (NR) acknowledges the award of a Visting Fellowship from the Natural Sciences and Engineering Research Council of Canada.

5. REFERENCES

1. J. R. J. Paré, M. Sigouin, and J. Lapointe, U. S. Patent number 5 002 784, Mrch 26, 1991, and related pending applications.
2. C. Weurman, *J. Agric. Food Chem.* **17** (1969), 370.
3. R. Teranishi, P. Issenberg, I. Hornstein, and E. Wick, (Eds.), *Flavor Research: Principles and Techniques*, Marcel Dekker, New York, 1971, p. 37.
4. R. A. Flath, *J. Agric. Food Chem.* **25** (1977), 439.
5. W. G. Jennings, (Ed.). *Gas Chromatography with Glass Capillary Columns*, Academic Press, New York, 1978, p. 105.
6. H. Sugisawa, in: R. Teranishi, R. A. Flath and H. Sugisawa (Eds.) *"Flavor Research: Recent Advances"*, Marcel Dekker, New York, (1981), p. 11.
7. E. Block, R. Iyer, S. Grisoni, C. Saha, S. Belman, and F. P. Lossing, *J. Am. Chem. Soc.* **110** (1988), 7813.
8. J. R. J. Paré, Continuation-in-Part Patent Applications (3) pending in the USA and related pending applications.
9. F. J. Smith, *Res. Dev.* (1988) (1) 54.
10. R. F. Heinze, *Cereal Foods World* **34** (1989), 334.
11. A. Bélanger, B. Landry, L. Dextraze, J. M. R. Bélanger, and J. R. J. Paré, *Riv. Ital. EPPOS* **2** (1991), 455.

G. Charalambous (Ed.), Food Science and Human Nutrition
© 1992 Elsevier Science Publishers B.V. All rights reserved.

BRAMBLE DRIED LEAF VOLATILES

J.A. MAGA[1], C.K. SQUIRE[1] and H.G. HUGHES[2]

[1]Department of Food Science and Human Nutrition, Colorado State University, Fort Collins, Colorado 80523 (United States)

[2]Department of Horticulture, Colorado State University, Fort Collins, Colorado 80523 (United States)

SUMMARY

Leaves from named cultivars of red raspberry (Rubus idaeus), black raspberry (R. occidentalis) and blackberry (R. laciniatus) from plants grown in a greenhouse environment were harvested, air dried and extracted in a Likens-Nickerson apparatus. The resulting volatiles were analyzed by GC/MS. A total of 20 peaks was observed with blackberry, whereas red and black raspberry had 10 and 12 peaks, respectively. The major volatiles in all three cultivars were 1-octene-3-ol, linalool and (Z)-3-hexen-1-ol. Other compounds identified included hexanal, n-butanol, myrcene, α-terpinene, (E)-2-hexenal, (E)-8-ocimene, octanal, terpinolene, decanal, benzaldehyde, dihydrolinalool, 6-methylheptanol, octanol and (E)-2-nonenal.

INTRODUCTION

Herbal teas have been brewed for thousands of years, primarily for medicinal purposes rather than for refreshment. Most have characteristic and unique aromas whose quality is dependent upon plant variety and climatological conditions during plant growth.

Various portions (leaves, roots, fruits) of bramble plants have a long history of use as herbal tea components in North America, and during the last decade, their popularity has increased. However, few studies appear in the literature describing the volatile composition of such products. One such study (2) reported that dried raspberry leaves contained trans-2-hexenal, cis-3-hexenol, citral, hexanal, octanal, phenylacetaldehyde, linalool, methyl salicylate, α-terpineol, pulegone, nerol, geraniol, dodecanal, β-ionone and tetradecanal. Most of these compounds have also been reported to be present in the leaf portions of many other plants including pears, tomatoes, walnuts, figs, alfalfa and red clover (3-7).

In contrast to leaf analyses, many researchers have reported upon the volatile composition of bramble fruits (8-15), with well over 100 compounds being identified. In the case of raspberry fruit, the compounds α- and β-ionone and 4-(p-hydroxyphenyl-2-butanone ("raspberry ketone") are thought to be mainly responsible for its aroma, while 3,4-dimethoxyalybenzene is most characteristic of blackberry fruit aroma.

Therefore, the objective of this study was to identify and compare the volatile leaf composition of various types of bramble plants that were grown under the same conditions in hopes of providing a better understanding as to the actual compounds that are present along with their relative amounts.

MATERIALS AND METHODS
Leaf Material Source

Leaves were manually picked from the canes of red raspberry (Rubus idaeus variety Titan), black raspberry (R. occidentalis variety Black Hawk) and blackberry (R. laciniatus variety Black Satin) from one-year-old plants that were grown in individual pots in a greenhouse environment during July, 1990, in Fort Collins, Colorado.

Leaf Drying and Storage

Harvested leaves from each variety were permitted to air dry at 30°C in the absence of sunlight for approximately 24 hours. At this point, their moisture had been reduced to approximately 7-9%. The dried leaves were placed in moisture proof plastic bags and stored at 20°C in the dark until evaluated approximately two weeks later.

Volatile Extraction and Concentration

Five grams of dried leaf were added to 250 ml of distilled water in a 500 ml round bottom distillation flask and attached to a Likens-Nickerson continuous distillation apparatus that was operated at atmospheric pressure. A total of 200 ml of freshly distilled diethyl ether was added to the 250 ml solvent recovery flask. Extraction on each sample was performed for 1.5 hours. Another series of samples was extracted in the same manner as described above and the solvents from the two extractions combined. To minimize oxidative/thermal changes within the extracted samples, the solvent extracts were then concentrated under nitrogen flow to 25 ml, and then dried on Type 4A molecular sieve (Union Carbide, New York, NY). Finally, the samples were concentrated to 0.4 ml under nitrogen flow.

GC/MS Analyses

A Hewlett-Packard model 5890A gas chromatograph equipped with a flame ionization detector and connected to a Hewlett-Packard Model 5995 mass spectrometer were utilized for volatile analysis/identification. The GC was equipped with a 30 meter by 0.32 mm i.d. Supelcowax 10 capillary column (Supelco, Inc., Bellefonte, PA). A 0.3 μl sample of concentrate was injected onto the column which was at 40°C. This temperature was held for 2 min. and then increased 2°C/min. to a final temperature of 220°C, which was held for 10 min. The injection port temperature was 140°C and the flame ionization detector was operated at 280°C. The carrier gas was helium at a flow rate of 40 ml/min. The mass spectrometer was operated at 70 eV ionizing voltage. Spectra generated for each peak were automatically compared with stored data bank spectra, and once peaks were tentatively identified, authentic compounds were injected for reverification of identification. GC peak data were converted to relative percent distribution.

RESULTS AND DISCUSSION

Compounds identified in the dried leaves, and their relative amounts, among the three bramble varieties evaluated are summarized in Table 1.

TABLE 1

Compounds Identified, and Their Percent Relative Amounts, in Dried Bramble Leaves			
Compound	Red Raspberry	Black Raspberry	Blackberry
Hexanol	---	---	0.10
n-Butanol	1.26	1.13	3.94
Myrcene	1.65	1.51	2.22
α-Terpinene	---	---	0.43
(E)-2-hexenal	2.71	2.37	4.28
(E)-β-Ocimene	5.72	4.65	2.58
Octanal	3.72	2.21	1.24
Terpinolene	---	0.51	1.21
(Z)-3-Hexen-1-ol	6.94	11.61	19.33
1-Octene-3-ol	28.54	23.30	18.95
Unknown	1.55	2.00	2.81
Decanal	---	3.54	9.92
Benzaldehyde	---	---	0.71
Dihydrolinalool	---	---	1.06
6-Methylheptanol	---	---	0.31
Octanol	---	---	0.76
(E)-2-Nonenal	---	---	1.02
Unknown	---	---	2.86
Linalool	21.79	18.34	9.36
Geraniol	26.12	28.83	16.91

In comparing the two raspberry varieties in Table 1, it can be seen that they have very similar volatile profiles. The major components in both red raspberry and black raspberry were 1-octen-3-ol, linalool and geraniol, which account for approximately 75% of total volatiles. The only apparent difference between the two varieties of raspberries is that two additional compounds, terpinolene and decanal were detected in the black raspberry varietal.

When the blackberry sample was compared to the raspberry samples, the first significant observation was the greater number of volatiles present in blackberry leaves. Also, in blackberry leaves, the predominant compound was found to be (Z)-3-hexen-1-ol (19.33%), which was approximately two to three times the amount associated with the raspberry varietals.

Relative to the literature, five of the compounds identified in raspberry leaves identified in this study (hexanal, (E)-2-hexenal, octenal, (Z)-3-hexen-1-ol, geraniol) were previously identified in dried raspberry leaves (2). The remainder are apparently newly identified. Also, apparently, this is the first report on the volatiles associated with blackberry leaves.

In conclusion, a series of common volatiles were found in the three varieties of dried bramble leaves evaluated in this study, but their relative proportions were found to be different. Among the two raspberry and one blackberry varietals evaluated, blackberry had the most complex volatile profile.

REFERENCES

1. M. Marlin, The Complete Book of Herbal Teas, Congdon and Weed (Eds.), St. Martin's Press, New York, 1983.
2. M. Kirsi, R. Julkunen-Tiitto and T. Rimpilainen, in: G. Charalambous (Ed.)., Flavors and Off-Flavors '89, Dev. Food Sci. 24, Elsevier, Amsterdam, 1990, pp 205-211.
3. R.G. Buttery, J.A. Kamm and L.D. Ling, J. Agric. Food Chem., 30 (1982) 739-742.
4. R.G. Buttery, J.A. Kamm and L.C. Ling, J. Agric. Food Chem., 32 (1984) 254-256.
5. R.G. Buttery, R.A. Flath, T.R. Mon and L.C. Ling, J. Agric. Food Chem., 34 (1986) 820-822.
6. R.G. Buttery, L.C. Ling and D.M. Light, J. Agric. Food Chem., 35 (1987) 1039-1042.
7. R.L. Miller, D.D. Bills and R.G. Buttery, J. Agric. Food Chem., 37 (1989) 1476-1479.
8. D.N. Georgilopoulos and A.N. Gallois, Z. Lebensm. Unters. Forsch., 184 (1987) 374-380.
9. D.N. Georgilopoulos and A.N. Gallois, Z. Lebensm. Unters. Forsch., 185 (1987) 299-306.
10. D.N. Georgilopoulos and A.N. Gallois, Food Chem., 28 (1988) 141-148.
11. E. Guichard and S. Issanchou, Sci. Aliments, 3 (1983) 427-438.
12. E. Guichard, Sci. Aliments, 4 (1984) 459-472.
13. M. Houchen, R.A. Scanlan, L.M. Libbey and D.D. Bills, J. Agric. Food Chem., 20 (1972) 170.
14. E. Honkanen, T. Pyysalo and T. Hirvi, Z. Lebensm. Unters. Forsch., 171 (1980) 180-182.
15. H. Kallio, J. Food Sci., 41 (1976) 555-562.

INFLUENCE OF VARIETY AND LOCATION OF GROWTH ON RESULTING BRAMBLE DRIED LEAF VOLATILES

J.A. MAGA[1], C.K. SQUIRE[1] and H.G. HUGHES[2]

[1]Department of Food Science and Human Nutrition, Colorado State University, Fort Collins, Colorado 80523 (United States)

[2]Department of Horticulture, Colorado State University, Fort Collins, Colorado 80523 (United States)

SUMMARY

Leaves from named cultivars of red raspberry (Rubus idaeus) and black raspberry (R. occidentalis) from plants grown both in the field and in a greenhouse environment were harvested, air dried and extracted in a Likens-Nickerson apparatus. The resulting volatiles were analyzed by GC/MS. With red raspberry, 20 peaks were noted for the field grown sample while only 10 peaks were observed with the greenhouse sample. In both red raspberry samples, the major volatile components were 1-octene-3-ol, geraniol and linalool. With field grown red raspberry, decanal was also a major component while no decanal was detected in the greenhouse grown sample. With the black raspberry samples, 20 compounds were observed in each with the major volatiles being (Z)-3-hexen-1-ol, 1-octene-3-ol and geraniol.

INTRODUCTION

The use of raspberry leaves in medicinal drinks in North America has a long history (1). With the increased popularity of herbal teas, more products are appearing that include various bramble leaves as part of their formulation. In spite of this, few studies have appeared on the volatile composition of bramble leaves (2).

As demand for these products continues to grow, a year round supply of freshly dried leaves becomes of economic concern and thus in northern climates, greenhouse production is a possible alternative.

Therefore, the objective of this study was to evaluate the dried leaf volatile composition of both red and black raspberries as influenced by internal (greenhouse) and external (field) conditions of growth. Data of these type would be useful in determining if one variety could be substituted for another, and if growing plants in a greenhouse setting would result in a similar leaf volatile composition as field grown plants.

MATERIALS AND METHODS
Leaf Material Source

Leaves were manually picked from the canes of red raspberry (Rubus idaeus variety Titan) and black raspberry (R. occidentalis variety Black Hawk) from one-year-old plants that were grown in individual pots in a greenhouse environment during July 1990 in Fort Collins, Colorado. The same named varieties of the same age were also grown outdoors within 100 meters of the greenhouse and served as the source of field grown leaves.

Leaf Drying and Storage

Harvested leaves from each variety and location were permitted to air dry at 30°C in the absence of sunlight for approximately 24 hours. At this point, their moisture content had been reduced to approximately 7-9%. The dried leaves were placed in moisture proof plastic bags and stored at 20°C in the dark until evaluated approximately two weeks later.

Volatile Extraction and Concentration

Five grams of dried leaf were added to 250 ml of distilled water in a 500 ml round bottom distillation flask and attached to a Likens-Nickerson continuous distillation unit that was operated at atmospheric pressure. A total of 200 ml of freshly distilled diethyl ether was added to the 250 ml solvent recovery flask. Extraction on each sample was performed for 1.5 hours. Another series of samples was extracted in the same manner as described above and the solvents from the two extractions combined. To minimize oxidative/thermal changes within the extracted samples, the solvent extracts were then concentrated under nitrogen flow to 25 ml, and then dried on Type 4A molecular sieve (Union Carbide, New York, NY). Finally, the samples were concentrated to 0.4 ml under nitrogen flow.

GC/MS Analysis

A Hewlett-Packard Model 5890A gas chromatograph equipped with a flame ionization detector and connected to a Hewlett-Packard Model 5995 mass spectrometer were utilized for volatile analysis/identification. The GC was equipped with a 30 meter by 0.32 mm i.d. Supelcowax 20 capillary column (Sulpelco, Inc., Bellefonte, PA). A 0.3 µl sample of concentrate was injected onto the column which was at 40°C. This temperature was held for 2 min. and then increased 2°C/min. to a final temperature of 220°C, which was held for 10 min. The injection port temperature was 140°C and the flame ionization detector was operated at 280°C. The carrier gas was helium at a flow rate of 40 ml/min. The mass spectrometer was operated at 70 eV ionizing voltage. Spectra generated for each peak were automatically compared with stored data bank spectra and once peaks were tentatively identified, authentic compounds were injected for reverification of identification. GC peak data were converted to relative percent distribution.

RESULTS AND DISCUSSION

Several facts are obvious from viewing the data shown in Table 1.

TABLE 1

Influence of Bramble Variety and Location of Growth on the Relative Percent Dried Leaf Volatiles				
Compound	Red Raspberry (Titan)		Black Raspberry (Black Hawk)	
	Field Grown	Greenhouse Grown	Field Grown	Greenhouse Grown
Hexanal	0.13	---	1.10	0.10
n-Butanol	0.48	1.26	10.45	3.94
Myrcene	1.94	1.65	1.79	2.22
α-Terpinene	0.24	---	0.40	0.43
(E)-2-Hexenal	3.94	2.71	3.33	4.28
(E)-3-Ocimene	2.15	5.72	4.80	2.58
Octanal	1.63	3.72	1.74	1.24
Terpinolene	1.36	---	0.73	1.21
(Z)-3-Hexen-1-ol	10.90	6.94	17.97	19.33
1-Octene-3-ol	19.80	28.54	16.62	18.95
Unknown	---	1.55	2.30	2.81
Decanal	16.38	---	7.40	9.92
Benzaldehyde	0.75	---	0.32	0.71
Dihydrolinalool	1.56	---	0.64	1.06
6-Methylheptanol	0.37	---	0.30	0.31
Octanol	1.51	---	0.24	0.76
(E)-2-Nonenal	1.54	---	0.42	1.02
Unknown	---	---	---	2.86
Linalool	16.27	21.79	11.82	9.36
Unknown	0.15	---	0.41	---
Geraniol	19.65	26.12	17.22	16.92
Unknown	0.25	---	---	---

In the case of the red raspberry varietal, the field grown sample had significantly more detectable volatiles, 20 versus 10 for the greenhouse grown equivalent. Also, the field grown sample had four major peaks accounting for approximately 72% of the total volatiles (1-octene-3-ol, geraniol, linalool and decanal), whereas the greenhouse grown sample only had three major volatiles that accounted for 76% of its total volatiles. The compound decanal, at 16.38%, was only found in the field grown sample of red raspberry. This would suggest that its formation/presence was perhaps photochemically influenced since the field grown plants were exposed to greater light intensity than the greenhouse grown plants.

In viewing the more extensive assortment of volatiles associated with field grown red raspberry, it would appear that, in contrast, the greenhouse grown red raspberry did not have as complex a volatile profile; which would probably influence its overall aroma profile in an herbal tea, even though it would still possess the overall characteristic aroma of raspberry leaves. Therefore, some subtle aroma differences would be detectable to the trained individual when comparing field grown versus greenhouse grown red raspberry dried leaves.

However, dramatically different results were observed in the case of black raspberry. As seen in Table 1, the volatile compositions of both the field grown and greenhouse grown samples were nearly identical, with 20 compounds being detected in both. The major volatile compounds present in dried black raspberry leaves were the same as those identified in red raspberry, and included decanal. Also, the n-butanol levels in black raspberry were significantly higher than those found in red raspberry.

From the black raspberry data obtained in this study, it would appear that, purely from a volatile composition standpoint, it is more tolerant to a greenhouse setting and thus could be effectively grown in this type of environment.

REFERENCES

1 M. Marlin, The Complete Book of Herbal Teas, London and Weed (Eds.), St. Martin's Press, New York, 1983.
2 M. Kirsi, R. Julkunen-Tiitto and T. Rimpilainen, in: G. Charalambous (Ed.), Flavors and Off-Flavors '89, Dev. Food Sci. 24, Elsevier, Amsterdam, 1990, pp 205-211.

G. Charalambous (Ed.), Food Science and Human Nutrition
© 1992 Elsevier Science Publishers B.V. All rights reserved.

STEAM VOLATILE CONSTITUENTS FROM SEEDS OF *MOMORDICA CHARANTIA* L.

M. KIKUCHI[1], T. ISHIKAWA[1], T. IIDA[1], S. SETO[1], T. TAMURA[2] and T. T. MATSUMOTO[2]

[1] Department of Industrial Chemistry, College of Engineering, Nihon University, Koriyama, Fukushima-ken, 963 (Japan)

[2] Department of Industrial Chemistry, College of Science and Technology, Nihon University, Kanda-ku, Tokyo 101 (Japan)

ABSTRACT

Steam distillates from seed oils and seeds, except for the crusts(embryos), of *Momordica charantia* L. (Japanese name: Nagareishi and Futoreishi) under reduced pressure (250-310 mmHg) by using a cold trap connected to a receiver and by the SDE method, were extracted with a mixed solvent (C_5H_{12}-Et_2O, 2:1). In the case of steam distillates from seed oils, seven acidic compounds, nineteen n-paraffins (C_{12}-C_{20}), a compound $C_{10}H_{16}O$ (M^+ 152) with a unique fragrance, p-cymene, l-menthol, nerolidol, pentadecanol, hexadecanol and squalene were identified. In the case of seeds, except for the crusts (embryos), nine aldehydes (mainly pentanal, *trans*-2-hexenal, t-2-heptenal and $2(E),4(E)$-nonadienal), six alcohols, four acids (mainly valeric acid), four esters (mainly amyl formate and amylvalerate), four acetals, 2-butylfuran and 2-hexanone were identified.

INTRODUCTION

Studies on steroids and triterpenoids in seed oils of *Cucurbita-ceae* plants have been carried out for analysis of a characteristic unsaponifiable constituents in the oils as well as from the point of view of their biogenesis.[1~8] However, no study on volatile constituents of the seed oils and seeds except for the crusts (embryos) has been made. Small amount of volatile oils with unique fragrances from steam distillates of the seed oils and the seeds except for the crusts (embryos) were obtained.

The present work was undertaken in order to identify the characteristic constituents contributing to the unique smell of the volatile oils of *Momordica charantia* L. (Nagareishi and Futoreishi in Japanese name).

METHODS

Materials(Seeds)

Nagareishi(1) and (4), and Futoreishi(2),(3) and (5) stored for a half year after they were harvested in Aichi-prefecture, were used.

Extraction of the seed oils

Extraction of seed oils was carried out by the following two methods. 1. The seeds crushed by a meat chopper were extracted with methylene chloride by a soxlet extractor for 10 h. 2. The crushed seeds were further finely powdered by a homogeneizer, and was extracted with hexane first and then methylene chloride with stirring for 10 min three times, respectively.

Collection of the volatile oil

1. The seed oil was added to water(500 ml per 100 g of the seed oil), and was then steam distilled under reduced pressure (250-310 mmHg), by using a cold trap connected to a receiver. The resulting distillate with a unique smell was saturated with sodium chloride and extracted with pentane. After drying of the extract over anhydrous sodium sulfate, the extract was concentrated to leave the volatile oil. 2. Likens-Nickerson Steam Distillation Liquid-Liquid Extraction (SDE system) was applied to the seeds except for the crusts (embryos) using C_5H_{12}-Et_2O (2:1) as the solvent. Embryos (200-300 g) was put into a 2 litre round flask of the SDE apparatus with 2 litre of water. After a one hour distillation, the extract was dried over anhydrous sodium sulfate and was concentrated to leave the volatile oil.

Fractionation of the volatile oil

The volatile oil of the seed oil was separated by 10 % Na_2CO_3 into its acidic and neutral fractions. The neutral fraction was further fractionated into six fractions by column chromatography, using a 12 mm x 280 mm column packed with silica gel. This column was eluted successively with the following solvent systems (v/v): pentane, pentane-ethyl ether (10:1, 5:1, 3:1, 1:1),ethyl ether; hexane, hexane-ethyl ether (10:1,5:1,3:1, 1:1), ethyl ether. The acidic fraction was esterified with diazomethane. This mixture of methyl esters and concentrated effluents of neutralfraction were analyzed by gas chromatography (GC) and gas chromatography-mass spectrometry (GC-MS), respectively.

GC condition

A Shimazu Model GC-5A gas chromatograph with a flame ionization detector (FID) and 3 mm i.d. x 3 m glass columns packed with 5 % PEG 20M/Uniport HP (60-80 mesh) and with Unisol 3000/Uniport C (80-100 mesh) were used for the analyses of steam volatile oils and the neutral fractions, and the methyl esters and effluent by column chromatography, respectively. Also, a Hewlett Packard Model 5970 gas chromatograph equipped with 0.2 mm i.d. x 25 m SCOT glass capillary column coated with VFA was used for the analyses of fractions by column chromatography of neutral fractions. The column temperature was programmed from 80 to 200 °C at a rate of 3°C/min, and flow rate of the nitrogen carrier gas was 50 ml/min. The volatile oils from the embryos of the seeds were directly analyzed by GC, Model 5970 gas chromatograph equipped with 0.2 mm i.d. x 25 m SCOT glass capillary column coated with Carbowax 20M. The column temperature was programmed from 55 to 210 °C at a rate of 4°C/min, and flow rate of the nitrogen carrier gas was 50 ml/min.

GC-MS condition

A Hitachi M-80 mass spectrometer connected a Hewlett Packard Model 5970 gas chromatograph equipped with a SCOT glass capillary column (0.25 mm i.d. x 20 m) coated with VFA was used. Ionizing voltage was 70 eV.

Authentic compounds

n-Paraffins ($C_{12}-C_{30}$) and a mixed of liquid paraffins purchased from Gasukuro Kogyo Co., Ltd. were used. Methyl esters of fatty acids $C_{12}-C_{18}$ and $C_{18:1}-C_{18:3}$ were prepared from the corresponding acids with diazomethane in ether at room temperature. The other authentic samples were kindly provided by Professor Hiroshi Kameoka of Kinki University.

RESULTS AND DISCUSSION

Steam volatiles under reduced pressure

The yields of volatile oils are shown in Table 1. The volatile oils have strong a characteristic unique smell. Also, gas chromatograms of these volatile oils and their neutral fractions are shown in Fig. 1. From Fig. 1, main peaks in the volatile oil (a) of Nagareishi (1) were not observed in its neutral fraction (b). So, it seems that the main constituents of the volatile oil of Nagareishi (1) are acids. Futoreishi (2) and (3)'s peak 5 in the volatile oils was also an acid because peak 5 disappeared in (2) and (3) in neutral fractions. Furthermore, peak 10 in the neutral fraction of Nagareishi (1), peak 4 and 8 in the neutral fractions

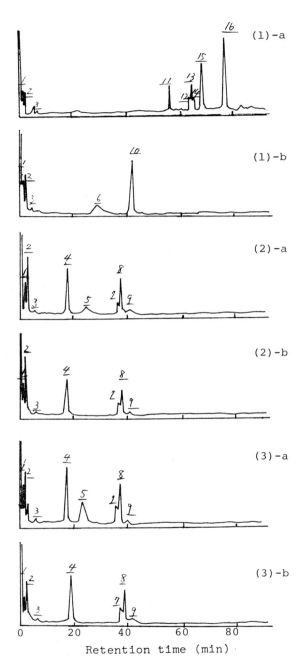

Fig. 1 Gas Chromatograms of Steam Volatile Oils(a) and Neutral Fractions(b)
   column : 5% PEG 20M, 3m
   temperature : 80～200 °C at a rate of 3 °C/min

Table I
Steam volatile oils from the seed oils of *Momordica charantia* L.

Seed Oil	Weight of Seed Oil (g)	Steam Volatile Oil (g)	(%)
(1)	668	0.358	0.05
(2)	572	0.123	0.02
(3)	280	0.561	0.20

of Futoreishi (2) and (3) are characteristic constituents of these volatile oils.

Acidic constituents were identified as their methyl esters by comparing their GC-RRT [relative retention time: relative retention time for methyl lauriate (retention time, 43 min) was taken as 1.00] and mass spectra (GC-MS) with those of authentic compounds.[9,12] Gas chromatograms of methyl esters of Nagareishi and Futoreishi are shown in Fig. 2. From GC-RRT of these methyl esters, C_{12} (lauric acid), C_{14} (myristic acid), C_{16} (palmitic acid), C_{18} (stearic acid), and unsaturated C_{18} fatty acids (oleic acid, linolic acid and linolenic acid) were identified. In addition, branched fatty acids containing over 18 carbons were also detected. The composition percentage of these acids estimated by GC peak areas are shown in Table II.

Table II
Composition percentage of acids

Seed Oil	Carbon Number of Acids						
	C_{12}	C_{14}	C_{16}	C_{18}	$C_{18:1}$	$C_{18:2}$	$C_{18:3}$
Nagareishi (1)	4.7	1.3	4.8	4.4	7.0	28.3	4.7
Futoreishi (2)	0.6	2.6	11.9	7.8	11.5	6.8	8.2
" (3)	—	0.2	0.9	3.8	7.1	5.7	9.7

The fractions obtained on silica gel column chromatography are shown in Table III. From these Fr-1, n- paraffins of C_{12}-C_{30} were identified. Gas chromatograms of Fr-1 of (1)-(3) and authentic liquid paraffins (A) are shown in Fig. 3. Thus, although the paraffins identified are shown in Table III, it was difficut to estimate these relative quantities.

Steam volatiles by the SDE method

The yields of volatile oils are shown in Table IV. Gas chromato-

Table III
Column chromatography of neutral fractions

Seed Oil	Fr-1		Fr-2		Fr-3		Fr-4		Fr-5		Fr-6	
	(mg)	(%)	(mg)	(%)	(mg)	(%)	(mg)	(%)	(mg)	(%)	(mg)	(%)
(1)[*1]	8.3	(11)	—	—	15.2	(20)	—	—	13.0	(17)	13.5	(18)
(2)[*2]	64.5	(62)	19.1	(18)	7.9	(8)	2.4	(2)	—	—	10.9	(10)
(3)[*2]	32.9	(20)	15.1	(9)	6.4	(4)	11.8	(7)	31.7	(13)	46.6	(29)

[*1] Fr-1(pentane), Fr-2-Fr-5(pentane-ethyl ether, 10:1, 5:1, 3:1, 1:1), Fr-6(ethyl ether)

[*2] Fr-1(hexane), Fr-2-Fr-5(hexane-ethyl ether, 10:1, 5:1, 3:1, 1:1), Fr-6(ethyl ether)

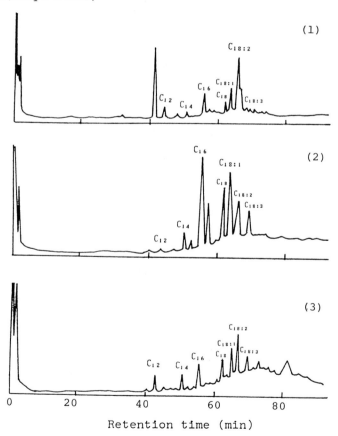

Fig. 2 Gas Chromatograms of Methyl Esters of Acidic Fraction of Volatile Oils
  column : Unisole 3000, 3m
  temperature : 80〜200 °C at a rate of 3 °C/min

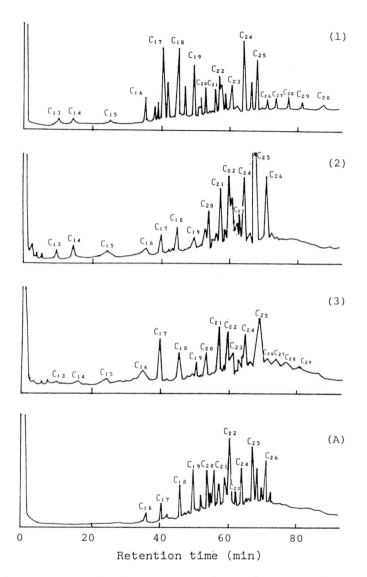

Fig. 3 Gas Chromatograms of Fr-1 (1～3) and a Mixture of
        Authentic Liquid Paraffins (A)
   column : Unisole 3000, 3m
   temperature : 80～200°C at a rate of 3 °C/min

grams of these volatile oils without separation into acidic and
neutral fractions, were run directly. The constituents identified
from these GC were shown in Table V.

Table IV

Steam volatile oils from the embryos of *Momordica charantia* L.

Seed Embryo	Weight of Embryo (g)	Steam Volatile Oil (g)	(%)
Nagareishi (4)	4281	7.08*	—
Futoreishi (5)	4334	8.64*	—

* There is contained the extracted solvent in quantity.

Conclusion

It can be summarized that fragrant terpene compounds were of low content in both steam volatiles of seed oils under reduced pressure and by the SDE method of seeds except for the crusts (embryos) of *Momordica charantia* L. contrary to our expectation. Since fragrant compound $C_{10}H_{16}O$ is especially intersting for smell, urgent elucidation of its structure is desirable.

ACKNOWLEDGMENT

The authors wish to thank Mr. Takaaki Toyoda of Takasago Perfumery Industrial Co., Ltd. for measurements of the GC-MS spectra and analysis by library search system. Thanks are also, due to Professor Hiroshi Kameoka of Kinki University for his kind gift of authentic paraffins.

REFERANCES

1 T.M.Jeong, T.Itoh, T.Tamura, T.Matsumoto, Lipids, 9 (1974) 921
2 T.Iida, J.M.Jeong, T.Tamura and T.Matsumoto, Lipids 15, (1980) 66-68
3 T.Itoh, T.Tamura, T.M.Jeong, T.Tamura and T.Matsumoto, Lipids 15, (1980) 122-123
4 T.Itoh, Y.Kikuchi, T.Tamura and T.Matsumoto, Phytochemistry 20 (1981) 761-764
5 T.Itoh, Y.Kikuchi, N.Shimizu, T.Tamura and T.Matsumoto, Phytochemistry 20 (1981) 1929-1933
6 T.Iida, T.Tamura and T.Matsumoto, Phytochemistry 20 (1981) 857
7 T.Itoh, K.Yoshida, T.Tamura and T.Matsumoto, Phytochemistry 21 (1982) 727-730
8 T.Itoh, T.Shigemoto, N.Shimizu, T.Tamura and T.Matsumoto, Phytochemistry 21 (1982) 2414-2415
9 A.G.Sharkey, J.L.Shultz and R.A.Friedel, Anal. Chem. 31 (1959) 87-94
10 J.H.Beynon, R.A.Saunders and A.E.Williams, Anal. Chem. 33 (1961) 221-225
11 D.H.Williams, H.Budzikiewicz and C.Djerassi, J. Am. Chem. Soc 86 (1964) 284-287
12 R.E.Kourey, B.L.Tuffey and V.A.Yarborough, Anal. Chem. 31 (1959) 284-287

Table V
Identified compounds from volatile oils from embryos

	Rt	Compound	Composition percentage (%)
Nagareishi (4)	2.246	Pentane	2.39
	2.292	Ether	2.46
	2.716	Butanal	0.61
	2.895		0.34
	3.246	Pentanal	49.42
	4.170	Hexanal	1.73
	4.683	Amyl formate	0.25
	4.725		0.40
	4.851	Butanol	4.36
	6.231		1.12
	6.419	trans-2-Hexenal	0.45
	6.849	Amyl alcohol	13.90
	8.141		0.38
	8.604	trans-2-Heptenal	3.89
	9.327	Hexanal	0.32
	11.379	Amyl valerate	0.90
	12.914		0.70
	13.093	Pentanal dibutyl acetal	0.36
		Pentanal amyl propyl acetal	
	15.842	Pentanal amyl butyl acetal	2.21
	17.990	2(E),4(Z)-Nonadienal	1.01
	18.549	Pentanal diamyl acetal	3.72
	19.079	2(E),4(E)-Nonadienal	6.79
	20.032	Valeric acid	1.45
	23.418		0.84
Futoreishi (5)	2.234		1.20
	2.290		0.39
	2.373	Heptane	1.20
	2.546	Octane	1.38
	2.721	Butanal	0.85
	2.896	EtOH	0.68
	3.237	Pentanal	13.67
	3.532	Butyl formate	1.01
	4.136	2-Hexanone	0.50
	4.684	Amyl formate	4.00
	4.847	Butanol	3.00
	5.530		0.38
	6.229		0.64
	6.416	trans-2-Hexenal	2.06
	6.831	Amyl alcohol	9.51
	7.668		0.99
	8.595	trans-2-Heptenal	2.72
	8.699	Butyl valerate	1.35
	11.391	Amyl valerate	4.29
	12.913	Pentanal dibutyl acetal	0.58
		Pentanal amyl propyl acetal	
	15.829	Pentanal amyl butyl acetal	1.32
	16.960		0.85
	18.523	Pentanal diamyl acetal	0.98
	19.639		1.27
	19.979	Valeric acid	26.15
	22.212		14.48
	22.876	Caproic acid	0.67
	24.638		0.80
	25.880		0.63
	26.176	trans-2-Hexenoic acid	0.66
	28.971	trans-2-Heptenoic acid	

COMPARISON OF VOLATILE COMPONENTS IN TWO NARANJILLA FRUIT (SOLANUM QUITOENSE LAM.) PULP FROM DIFFERENT ORIGIN

P. BRUNERIE[1] and P. MAUGEAIS[2]

[1]CENTRE DE RECHERCHE PERNOD RICARD, 120 Avenue du Maréchal Foch 94015 CRETEIL (FRANCE)

[2]UNIVERSITE DU HAVRE, B.P. 540 LE HAVRE CEDEX (FRANCE)

SUMMARY :

Aroma volatiles from the frozen pulps of naranjilla fruit (Lulo) from two origins (Colombia and Costa Rica) were studied by GC/MS and GC/sniffing analysis after solvent extraction and concentration. The comparison of the volatiles of the two pulps showed important qualitative and quantitative differences. In this study 150 components were identified, among them about 50 were newly found in this fruit. Futhermore methyl 3-acetoxy butyrate found in the Lulo pulp had not been reported to the best of our knowledge to occur in nature.

INTRODUCTION :

Naranjilla or Lulo is a tropical fruit which grows on the Amazonian part of the Andes. It looks like a small orange growing on 1 to 2,5 meters high trees, between 1300 and 2300 meters elevation.

At maturity the fruit is yellow and its pulp is nearly green and very juicy. The green juice extracted from the pulp is used to make refreshing beverages which are very popular in the Andes (1-4). The fruit, easy to handle, contains high quantities of pulp, grows very quickly and is available on an industrial scale, but unfortunately the pulp is very sensitive to oxydation.

This fruit nearly unknown in Europe possesses a complex flavor which seems to be a mixture of banana, pineapple and strawberry. Its use in food might be developped with success in Europe as these aromatic notes are well accepted by the consumers.

Few analysis have been published on the composition of the aroma of the fruit (5,6) but some differences in the volatiles composition of fruits from different origins were detected.

We report in this paper our work on the volatile components analysis of two frozen pulps of Naranjilla fruit, one from Colombia and the other one from Costa Rica, not only by GC/MS analysis but also by GC/sniffing technique in order to evaluate the contribution of each identified compound to the total fruit's flavor and to detect traces of typical components of Naranjilla.

MATERIAL AND METHODS :
The frozen fruit pulp was obtained by air freight from Colombia and Costa Rica and stored a - 20°C. All solvents used were freshly distilled.

- SAMPLE PREPARATION

Solvent extraction. 200 g of friezed pulp were weighed and diluted with 200 ml of distilled water. 100 µl of an ethanolic solution of Ethyl nonanoate (1 µg/ml) were added as internal standart for quantification.

The mixture obtained is submitted to solvent extraction with 3 times 400 ml of a mixture of pentane and ether (2:1). The extract was then dried on Na_2SO_4 and concentrated to 1 ml in a Kuderna Danish evaporator. The crude and concentrated extract was analysed by Capillary GC for quantification.

- PREFRACTIONATION

The crude extract was subjected to chromatography on activated silica gel in a 10 x 2 cm column. The extract was fractionated by a stepwise gradient of ether in pentane (100 ml of 0, 10 and 100 % ether). The collected fractions were dried on Na_2SO_4 and concentrated to 1 ml in the Kuderna Danish evaporator before GC, GC/MS and GC sniffing analysis.

- HRGC ANALYSIS

A 50 m long FFAP Column (Hewlett Packard) with a 0,32 mm i.d. and a 0,53 film thickness was used in a Hewlett Packard 5890 equiped with a split/splitless injector and a FID detector, the both at a temperature of 250°C. The carrier gas was helium at 2 ml/min and the temperature programm was isothermal at 50°C during 3 min, then heated at 3°C per min to 120°C and then at 2°C per min to 220°C and finally isothermal a 220°C during 60 min.

The signal obtained from the FID was integrated by a 3393 A **Hewlett Packard integrator.**

- HRGC/MS ANALYSIS

A Carlo Erba Fractovap 4160 coupled by an interface at 250°C with a Kratos MS25 magnetic sector mass spectrometer was used. The temperature of the ion source was 150°C, the electron energy 70 ev, the injected volumes were 1 µl in the splitless mode.

The chromatographic conditions were the same as for GC analysis.

- HRGC SNIFFING ANALYSIS

The same column was fitted in a Girdel serie 30 gas chromatograph equipped with a split/splitless injector and a 3393 A integrator. The effluent was splitted at the end of the column approximately 90 % to a sniffing mask (SGE) and 10 % to a FID. Each fraction of the extracts were sniffed twice by trained panelist during a period not exceding 20 to 25 min. The odor impressions were recorded and correlated with the GC/MS analysis.

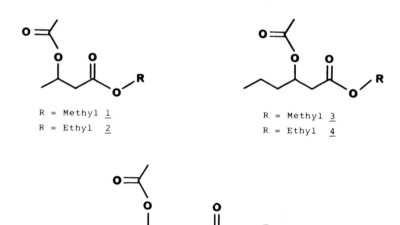

FIGURE 1

<u>1</u> Methyl 3-acetoxy butyrate, <u>2</u> Ethyl 3-acetoxy butyrate
<u>3</u> Methyl 3-acetoxy caproate, <u>4</u> Ethyl 3-acetoxy caproate
<u>6</u> Methyl 5-acetoxy caproate, <u>7</u> Ethyl 5-acetoxy caproate

- SYNTHESIS OF THE ACETOXY ESTERS (1-4, Fig 1)

The hydroxy esters purchased from Aldrich were mixed with an equimolar quantitie of acetyl chloride in redistilled ether as solvent. The medium was then stirred half an hour under agitation. The organic phases were then washed with a 5 % bicarbonate solution, seperated by decantation, dried on Na_2SO_4, concentrated and analysed by GC/MS. The spectras and retention indices of the acetoxy esters thus obtained were compared with those recorded during GC/MS analysis of the Lulo pulp extract.

RESULTS AND DISCUSSION

The GC profiles of the crude extracts (fig 3 and 4) show a great number products and illustrate the complexity of this fruit's flavor. We have identified about 150 different components (Table 1) some of them having a very important aromatic contribution as revealed by GC sniffing analysis such as furaneol, linalol, acids, lactones, sulfur compounds and esters.

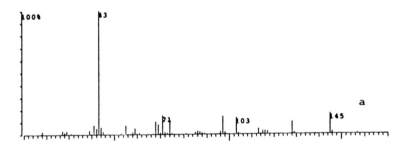

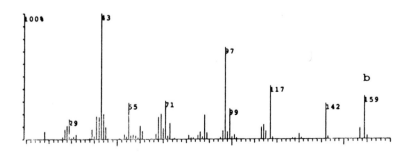

FIGURE 2A
a) Methyl 3-acetoxy caproate
b) Ethyl 3-acetoxy caproate

Among these components ethyl and methyl 3-acetoxy caproate 3 and 4 (fig 2A) methyl and ethyl 5-acetoxy caproate 6 and 7 (fig 2C) were found before only in pineapple (7, 11), grape and red wine (8-10) respectively but not in Lulo and methyl 3-acetoxy butyrate 3 (fig 2B) never been found as yet in nature.

The 3 hydroxy acids and derivatives being major constituents in various tropical fruits (11) and their formation from fatty acids metabolism having been well studied (12,13) it was not surprising to find these kind of products in the Lulo pulp. The extracts containing high quantities of acetic acid and 3-hydroxy esters, esterification reactions can have occured either in the fruit or during the extraction concentration procedure giving rise to the formation of the corresponding acetoxy esters. The mass spectras of these components showed a major m/z = 43 ion corresponding to (CH3-CO+) ion and m/z = M-43 ion from which the molecular weight of the corresponding acetoxy ester was obtained. The identification has been then confirmed by chemical synthesis.

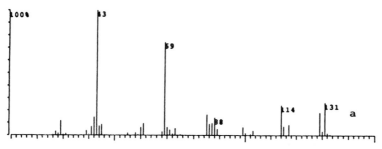

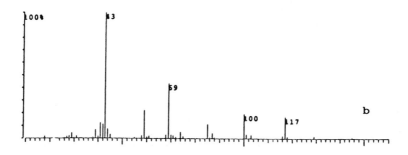

FIGURE 2B
a) Ethyl 3-acetoxy butyrate
b) Methyl 3-acetoxy butyrate

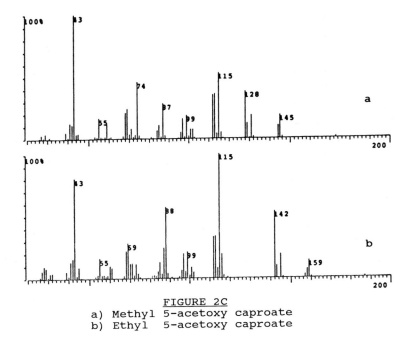

FIGURE 2C
a) Methyl 5-acetoxy caproate
b) Ethyl 5-acetoxy caproate

The fruit from Columbia (fig 3) is particularly rich in esters wich give fruity and often strong notes and in acetic acid responsible for the acidity of the pulp. The sulfur compounds occur mainly in this fruit. methyl (methyl thio) propionate, with a strong potatoes like odor, was already reported to be present in the Lulo (5) and methyl (methyl thio) acetate found for the first time in this fruit was not found in the fruit from Costa Rica.

Phenyl acetaldehyde, with a strong floral odor, hyacinth like, geraniol wich gives rose and citronella notes, ß ionone, geranyl acetone with floral odors were only found in the fruit from Costa Rica. Linalol which gives at the extract a floral and sweet note and 3-hydroxy 2,5-dimethyl 4 (5H) furanone with a "caramel like" odor were found in the fruit from Costa Rica (fig 4).

The both extracts contain high quantities of free acids such as butyric acid with a strong cheese like perception in sniffing.

In conclusion, the extracts of the fruit pulp contain many volatile components with strong and important aromatic properties explaining the complex flavor perception of the pulp. Furthermore high variations in the aroma composition and in the taste of the pulp exist, probably due to either climatic differences, between the geographical countries of origin or different varieties of the tree. Despite these aromatic difference, this fruit is very interesting and might be introduce with success in European Countries.

ACKNOWLEDGMENT

We thank particularly :
P. DESMAREST and A. FIOC who give us the frozen pulp,
A. ROZENBLUM, B. DECARPENTRIE and Y. KOZIET for their technical assistance.

TABLE 1

COMPONENTS IDENTIFIED IN LULO PULP
A : FROM COLUMBIA AND B : FROM COSTA RICA
AMOUNTS IN PPM RELATIVE TO THE INTERNAL STANDARD

	A	B	ODOR		A	B	ODOR
ALCOOLS				**ACIDES**			
2-PROPANOL	0,013	0,024		ACIDE ACETIQUE	11,4	0,5	vinegar; +++
ETHANOL	0,107	0,078		ACIDE FORMIQUE	8,4x10-3	0,293	
1-PROPANOL	-	0,01		ACIDE ISOBUTYRIQUE	0,058	0,058	
2-METHYL 3 BUTEN-2-OL	-	0,111		ACIDE BUTYRIQUE	2,376	10,7	cheesy; +++++
ISOBUTANOL	0,13	0,093		ACIDE ISOVALERIQUE	0,061	0,071	cheesy, roasted; +++
3-PENTANOL	0,091	0,154		ACIDE 2-METHYL BUTYRIQUE	-	+	
2-PENTANOL	0,61	0,350		ACIDE VALERIQUE	-	0,04	animal; ++
1-BUTANOL	0,0515	0,045		ACIDE 2-BUTENOIQUE	0,022	0,225	
1-PENTEN-3-OL	-	<0,01		ACIDE CAPROIQUE	0,877	0,671	animal; +++
2-METHOXY ETHANOL	0,012	0,058		ACIDE HEPTANOIQUE	8x10-3	0,015	
2-ETHOXY ETHANOL	-	0,01		ACIDE 3-HEXENOIQUE	0,034	0,113	
CIS2-PENTEN-1-OL	-	0,968		ACIDE 2-HEXENOIQUE	0,033	0,01	
ALCOOL ISOAMYLIQUE	0,673	-	chemical, solvent; ++	ACIDE CAPRYLIQUE	0,072	0,037	
1-PENTANOL	0,016	-		ACIDE 2,4-HEXADIENOIQUE	-	0,054	
2-HEPTANOL	6,7x10-3	-		ACIDE PELARGONIQUE	-	0,02	
2-PENTENOL	6,7x10-3	-		ACIDE DECANOIQUE	0,01	0,01	
2-METHYL 2-BUTEN-1-OL	-	+		ACIDE BENZOIQUE	0,515	0,387	
1-HEXANOL	0,67	0,046		ACIDE PHENYL ACETIQUE	-	-	
CIS3-HEXENOL	1,02	0,429	green (grassy); +++				
2-HEXENOL	+	+		**ESTERS**			
2-ETHYL 1-HEXANOL	-	0,034	banana skin; +	ETHYL FORMATE	-	+	
2-ETHYL HEXANOL	0,037	-		ETHYL ACETATE	1,284	+	
ALCOOL BENZYLIQUE	0,088	0,04		METHYL BUTYRATE	+	0,647	cheesy
2-PHENYL ETHANOL	0,299	0,02	rose; ++	ETHYL BUTYRATE	3,785	0,15	fruity, cheesy; ++
2,6-DIMETHYL 3,7-				ISOBUTYL ACETATE	0,023		
OCTADIENE 2,6-DIOL	0,062	0,081		METHYL ISOVALERATE	0,024	-	
1-DODECANOL	-	9.10-3		BUTYL ACETATE	0,052	0,064	
3,7-DIMETHYL 1,7-				METHYL VALERATE	0,08		
OCTADIENE 3,6-DIOL	0,018	0,04		METHYL 2-BUTENOATE	0,609	0,350	fruity, green
				ISOAMYL ACETATE	0,111	-	
CETONES				ETHYL 2-BUTENOATE	0,058	-	
ACETONE	0,103	-		METHYL CAPROATE	1,84	0,164	fruity, pineapple ++
PROPANONE	+	-		METHYL 2-METHYLENE			
2-BUTANONE	0,013	0,021		BUTYRATE	0,238	-	
2-PENTANONE	0,503	0,931		ETHYL CAPROATE	0,928	0,04	fruity, sweet pineapple; ++
3-PENTEN-2-ONE	-	0,02		ETHYL 2-METHYL			
3-HYDROXY 2-BUTANONE	1,832	0,038		2-BUTENOATE	0,019	-	
6-METHYL 5-HEPTEN 2-ONE	0,023	0,026	fruity, green slightly metallic	METHYL 3-HEXENOATE	0,085	-	
4-HYDROXY 4-METHYL				HEXYL ACETATE	0,053	0,05	fruity
2-PENTANONE	8,4x10-3	9x10-3		METHYL (2-HYDROXY			
4-HYDROXY 4-METHYL				2-METHYL) BUTYRATE	0,017	-	
PENTANONE	9x10-3	-		METHYL 2-HEXENOATE	0,62		
ACETOPHENONE	0,061	0,071		ETHYL 2-ETHOXY ACETATE	0,014	0,130	
METHYL ACETOPHENONE	-	0,05		3-HEXENYL ACETATE	0,131	0,968	green, fruity weak
				METHYL LACTATE	0,023	-	
ALDEHYDES				2-HEXENYL ACETATE	0,022	-	fruity, pear
HEXANAL	0,130	+		ETHYL LACTATE	0,117	-	
BENZALDEHYDE	0,811	0,168		METHYL (3-HYDROXY			
PHENYL ACETALDEHYDE	-	0,136	floral hyacinth; ++ (+)	3-METHYL) BUTYRATE	7x10-3	-	

	A	B	ODOR		A	B	ODOR
ETHYL OENANTHATE	-	0,020		**LACTONES**			
METHYL CAPRYLATE	0,034	0,025	fruity, soap	ɣ-HEXALACTONE	1,085	3,301	fruity, slightly coconut; ++
HEXYL BUTYRATE	0,164	-		δ-HEXALACTONE	0,017	+	
ETHYL CAPRYLATE	0,097	0,140	fruity; ++	ɣ-HEPTALACTONE	0,017	-	
ETHYL ACETYL ACETATE	0,027	-		ɣ-OCTALACTONE	0,01	0,04	alliaceous coconut; ++
METHYL 3-HYDROXY.BUTYRATE	0,128	0,069	mouldy	δ-OCTALACTONE	+	<0,01	
DIMETHYL MALONATE	8x10-3	-		ɣ-DECALACTONE	-	0,054	
ETHYL 3-HYDROXY BUTYRATE	0,557	0,095		δ-DECALACTONE	-	0,01	
BUTANEDIOL DIACETATE	0,012	-		ɣ-UNDECALACTONE	0,015	0,081	fruity, peach; ++
METHYL 3-ACETOXY BUTYRATE	0,461	-					
OCTYL ACETATE	0,024	-		**COMPOSES SOUFRES**			
ETHYL 3-ACETOXY BUTYRATE	0,263	0,072		METHYL (METHYLTHIO) ACETATE	0,023	-	
ETHYL (2-HYDROXY 4-METHYL) VALERATE	0,027	-		METHYL (METHYLTHIO) PROPIONATE	0,05	-	potatoes, alliaceous; ++
DIMETHYL SUCCINATE	0,015	-		BENZOTHIAZOLE	0,033	0,035	
METHYL BENZOATE	2,725	0,265	fruity; ++				
METHYL 3-HYDROXY CAPROATE	1,101	0,191		**PHENOLS**			
ETHYL BENZOATE	0,355	-	fruity, heavy; ++	PHENOL	0,014	0,041	
ETHYL 3-HYDROXY CAPROATE	1,09	0,114		CRESOL	-	+	
METHYL 3-ACETOXY CAPROATE	0,115	0,164					
ETHYL 3-ACETOXY CAPROATE	1,085	0,301		**COMPOSES FURANIQUES**			
BENZYL ACETATE	0,046	0,056	floral, fruity	METHYL FUROATE	0,015	-	
ISOPROPYL BENZOATE	0,015	-		FURFURAL	-	0,01	
METHYL 5-ACETOXY CAPROATE	0,102	-		3-METHYL 2,5-FURANEDIONE	-	+	
ETHYL 5-ACETOXY CAPROATE	0,01	-		3-HYDROXY 2,5-DIMETHYL 4 (5H) FURANONE	0,185	0,240	caramel; +
ETHYL PHENYL ACETATE	0,063	-	honeyed slightly rose; +				
METHYL 5-HYDROXY CAPROATE	0,014	0,015					
METHYL CINNAMATE	0,071	0,058	strawberry; +				
ETHYL CINNAMATE	+	-					
THYMYL ACETATE	-	0,038					
METHYL 3-HYDROXY CAPRYLATE	-	0,01					
COMPOSES TERPENIQUES							
TERPINENE	-	0,014					
FENCHONE	0,024	-					
LIMONENE	-	0,341	slightly lemon				
TERPENE	-	0,045	zest, orange				
LINALOL	0,461	2,046	floral sweet; +++				
BORNYL ACETATE	-	0,049					
TERPENE DIOL (U. Struct)	+	-					
4-TERPINEOL	-	0,058	earthy				
α-TERPINEOL	0,118	0,476					
NEROL	0,012	0,130					
P-CYMEN-8-OL	0,014	-					
TERPENE DIOL (U. Struct)	0,049	-					
7-HYDROXY LINALOL	0,033	0,035					
EUGENOL	0,08	0,019					
ISOEUGENOL	0,026	0,04					
METHOXY EUGENOL	0,089	-					
VANILLINE	0,08	0,213					
VERATRALDEHYDE	0,08	-					
GERANIOL	-	0,671	rose, citronella; ++				
GERANYL ACETONE	-	0,028	floral, slightly rose				
β-IONONE	-	0,019					
β-IONONE 5,6-EPOXY	-	0,02					
CARVACROL	-	0,025					

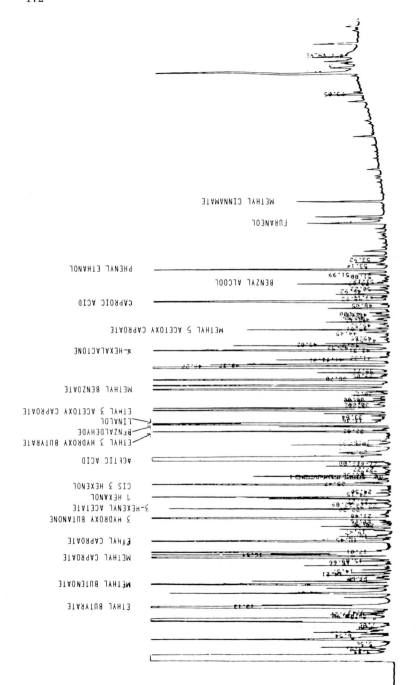

FIGURE 3
GC profile of the pulp extract of Lulo from Colombia

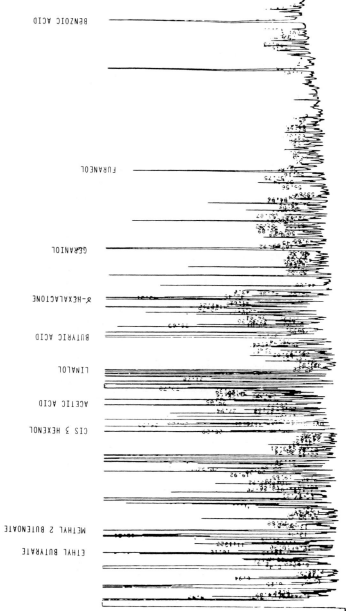

FIGURE 4
GC profile of the pulp extract of Lulo from Costa Rica

REFERENCES

1   DUKE J.A.
    Econ. Bot. (1970), $\underline{4}$, 344-366
2   LEHMAN G., PAREDES A., CHIRIBOGA MA
    Fruchtsaft ind. (1964), $\underline{9}$, 307
3   HERMANN, K
    Lebensm. Unters. und Forsch (1981), $\underline{173}$, 47-60
4   BENK, E.
    Verbraucherdienst (1973), $\underline{18}$, (10) 229
5   BRUNKE E.J., MAIR P. HAMMERSCHMIDT
    J. Agric. Food. Chem. (1989), $\underline{37}$, 746-748
6   SUAREZ M., DUGUEC C., WINTOCH, H. SCHREIER P.
    in press
7   NAF MULLER
    Helv. Chim. Acta (1971), $\underline{54}$, 1880
8   SCHREIER P.
    Can. Inst. food, Sci. Technol. J. (1981), $\underline{14}$, 112
9   SCHREIER P.
    Lebensm. Wiss. Technol (1980), $\underline{13}$, 312
10 SCHREIER P.
    J. Agric Food Chem. (1980), $\underline{28}$, 926
11 MAARSE, H., CA VIISHER (1989)
    Volatives in Food - qualitative data CIVO-TNO Zeist
12 PEREIRA, W., V.A. BACON, H. PATTON, B. HOLPERN
    Anal. Lett. (1970), $\underline{3}$, 23
13 R. TRESSL, J. HEIDLAS, W. ALBRECHT, K.H. ENGEL
    in Bioflavor 87 WALTER DE GRUYTER (1988),
    Editor P. SCHREIER

ANALYSIS OF THE VOLATILE CONSTITUENTS OF A SPECIAL TYPE OF WHITE BREAD

MICHAEL. E. KOMAITIS , GEORGE AGGELOUSIS and NIKI GIANNONITS-ARGYRIADIS.

1. Department of Agricultural Industries, Agricultural University of Athens, Iera Odos 75, Votanikos, Athens 118 55, Greece.

2. Department of Food Technology, School of Food Technology and Nutrition, T.E.I. of Athens, Saint Spyridon Str., Egaleo, 122 10 Athens, Greece.

3. VIORYL, -Kato Kifisia- 145 64- Athens- Greece.

SUMMARY

The volatile constituents of a special type of white bread containing anise were investigated. The flavour components were collected in a dichloromethane-diethylether 2:1 v/v solution and identified by combined gas chromatograrhy-mass spectroscopy.
38 compounds were identified. Some of them had not been reported previously. Several of the components that contribute to the characteristic aroma of this type of bread are attributed to anise.

These components are: Anethole, carvacrol, p-methoxy-propyl-benzene, fatty acid esters, acetophenone, o-and p-methoxy-cinnamaldehyde and p-methoxy-benzaldehyde.

1. INTRODUCTION

A great volume of literature has been published in recent years concerning the composition of volatile components of bread (Collyer, de Figueiredo, Mulders et al, Nago, Voudouris al al, Schierlebe and Grosch, Folkes and and Gramshaw),(1-11).
Most of the investigations concerned the qualitative composition and as a consequence the number of the volatile compounds now exceeds 250.
Folks and Gramshaw (11) identified a total 190 volatile compounds in a aroma concentrate prepared from white bread crust. Mulders and his co-workers (3-6) determined the composition of white bread aroma. The first three papers (3,4,5) covered the qualitative composition and the fourth the quantitative gas chromatographic analysis of the main componets of the vapour above the bread. Schierlebe and Grosch (9,10) studied the flavour compounds of different bread types.
The aim of this study was to identify the volatile components responsible for the aroma of a different type of bread prepared in Greece with addition of anise. The latter is added to improve the bread flavour and make it more attractive to the consumer.

2. MATERIALS AND METHODS

2.1. Breadmaking process

The breadmaking process had as follows: 300g of flour, 4,5g of sodium chloride, 6g of yeast and 1.2g of anise were blended in a farinograph (Brabender) for 1 minute.
Enough water was added to give a dough consistency of 500 B.U. The produced mass was left to ferment, at $30\,°C$ and relative moisture 80%, for 75 minute. The loaves were baked

for 45 minutes at an oven temperature of 220°C.

2.2. Isolation of volatile components.

The vapour developing during the baking of 6 kg of bread was collected with the help of a specially built apparatus. High purity nitrogen passed though the oven (10 ml per min, for 45 min.) and carried the vapour into a series of four cooled conical flasks containing dichloromethane-diethyl ether 2:1 v/v. The mixture was dried over anhydrous sulphate at 4°C and was stored at -18°C until used.

2.3. Vapour analysis.

The solvents were concentrated under reduced pressure using a thin film evaporator. The light yellow oil obtained was used for further analysis.

2.4. Gas Chromatography Mass Spectroscopy.

The collected vapour was analysed by gas chromatography-mass spectroscopy using a NERMAG R1010-C apparatus. The operation parameters were as follows:
Carrier gas helium, column SE-30, column length 25m, quadropole elecrton impact 70 eV, ion source temperature 150°C. The column temperature was held at 50°C for 4 minutes after the injection of the sample, then increased to 250°C and held at this temperature for 10 minutes. The rate of temperature increase was 2°C/min.

3. RESULTS AND DISCUSSION.

The qualitative characteristics of the flour used are shown in Table 1.
The identified compounds are listed in Table 2. The gas chromatogram revealed 59 components. 31 components were positively identified by comparing their retention times and mass spectra with those of known compounds. Some formulae

were deduced from mass spectra only. The tentatively identified compounds were 7. Two other peaks were artifacts.

It is interesting to note the presence of hydrocarbons p-cymene (a well characterised oxidation product of γ-terpinene) squalene, octadecane, tricosane, pentacosane, and nonacosane. p-Cymene and squalene are normally found in bread and anise.

The presence of high molecular weight hydrocarbons may be attributed to yeast constituents. In yeast triglycerides and phospholipids, fatty acids range from C8 (or lower) to C24 and since lipases and phospholipases are present in yeast this could explain the presence of high molecular weight hydrocarbons (Ames and MacLeod 1985; Hunter and Rose 1972), (12,13).

Components that contribute to the aroma of this type of bread and come from the added anise are:
a. Carbonylic compounds: acetophenone, p-methoxy-benzaldehyde o-methoxy-cinnamaldehyde, p-methoxy-cinnamaldehyde.
b. Esters-Ethers: fatty acid methylesters, p-methoxy-propylbenzene and anethole.
c. Phenols: carvacrol.

Some interesting compounds not reported previously in bread aroma studies are: 2-ethyl-4-methyl-1- pentanol, 3-methyl-2-methoxy-pyrazine and 2-(4-isoproryl-phenyl) propenal.

Preliminary experiments to determine the percentage of the various constituents in the bread vapour revealed that the major component was anethole (almost 30%).

Anethole is largely responsible for the characteristic flavour of this particular type of bread that makes it very attractive to many consumers.

TABLE 1.

Qualitative characteristics of flour.

Variety	Type of flour	Wet gluten % w/w	Moisture % w/w	Ash % w/w	Protein % Nx5.7
Yecora	70%	30	12.1	0.5	12.4

TABLE 2.
Components identified in the vapour of white bread with anise.

Components	RT min	m/e
Phenol ***	2:27:8	94,40,65,66,50,55,74
Benzyl alcohol ***		108,77,79,107,91
p-Cymene ***		119,77,134,89,104
Butyl-pentanoate ***	3:01:2	85,73,91,56,57
Phenyl acetaldehyde ***		121,91,77
2-Ethyl-4-methyl-1-pentanol ***		57,43,41,55,83,73,70,112
Ethanoic acid ***	3:16:4	43,45,60,42
Phenyl-methyl ketone ***		105,77,120,43,28,15

Compound	Time	Ions
3-Methyl-2-methoxy-pyrazine ***	3:23:3	124,123,95,93,98,106
2-Phenyl-ethyl alcohol ***	5:14:9	91,92,122,65,51,77,31,104
Naphthalene ***		128,51,64,102,63,127,129
Ethyl benzoate ***	7:33:6	51,77,105,150,45
p-Methoxy-propyl benzene ***	8:54:0	148,147,77,121,117,91,107,133
p-Methoxy-benzaldehyde ***	10:36:6	135,136,77,92,107,63,65,39
cis-anethole ***		148,147,117,77,133,91,103,105
Diethyl-pyrazine ***	11:42:6	121,136,107,80
trans-Anethole ***	13:20:5	148,147,117,77,133,91,103,105
p-Methoxy-acetophenone ***	16:05:4	135,77,150,43,92,107,119
p-Methoxy-cinnamaldehyde ***		162,161,147,91,65,77,133,131
2-(4-isopropyl-phenyl)propenal ***	17:17:0	147,105,91,69,163,133,176
p-Methoxy-phenyl acetone ***	17:48:8	121,43,164,77,122,91,65,107
Carvacrol ***	27:08:3	149,164,91,119,137,117
p-Methoxy-cinnamaldehyde ***	27:31:4	126,161,131,91,65,77,133,147
Octadecane ***	43:34:4	43,57,71,85,99,113,127,140,254
Ethyl Hexadecanoate ***	57:07:6	88,43,41,101,55,73,89,69
Hexadecanoic ***	52:56:4	43,41,60,73,59,69,129,254
Ethyl octadecadienoate ***	59:00:4	41,55,67,81,95,109,263,280
9,12-Octadecadienoic acid ***	1:00:06	41,43,67,55,81,95,60,109
Ethyl octadecenoate ***	1:00:28	41,43,55,69,83,97,111,282

cis-9-octadecenoic acid ***		73,59,45,87,129, 101,115,282
Ethyl octadecanoate ***	1:01:12	43,57,71,85,284,113, 127,312
Tricosane ***	1:10:12	43,57,71,85,99,113, 127,141,324
Pentacosane ***	1:14:00	43,57,71,85,99,113, 155
Heptacosane ***	1:21:35	43,57,71,85,99, 113,141,380
Squalene ***	1:24:52	69,41,81,95,55, 121,137,341
Nonacosane ***	1:28:34	43,57,71,85,99, 113,127,142,155
Cholesterol *	1:31:28	43,389,55,81,95, 69,275,107
Stigmasterol *	1:37:57	43,414,55,329,81, 93,107,396

----

* Tentative identification from mass spectra data.
*** Positive identification from mass spestrum and retention time which agree with authentic compound.

REFERENCES

1. D.M.Collyer, Bakers Digest (1964), 43-54.
2. M.P.De Figueiredo, Bakers Digest (1964), 48-51.
3. E.J.Mulders, H.Maarse, C.Weurman. Z.Lebensm. Unters. -Forsch. 150, (1972), 6874.
4. E.J.Mulders, J.H.Dhond. Ibid. 150, (1972) 228-32.
5. E.J.Mulders, M.C.Ten Noever de Brauw, S.Van Straten. Ibid. 150, (1973) 306-10.
6. E.J.Mulders. Ibid. 151, (1973) 310-17.
7. M.C.Nago, Contribution a l etude de l aroma de pain francaise, Doctora de 3 cycle, Paris, 1977.

8. E.Voudouris, M.E.Komaitis, V.Pattakou, in: G.Charalambous (ed) Flavour of Food and Beverage Chemistry and Technology Academic Press N.Y.-San Francisco-London, 1978, p.p. 57-64.
9. R.Schierlebe and W.Grosch. Topics in Flavour Research, (1985) 161-85.
10. R.Schierlebe, W.Grosch. J. Agr. Food Chem. 35(2), (1987) 252-57.
11. D.J.Folkes, J.W.Gramshaw. J.Food Technol. 12, (1972) 1-8.
12. J.M.Ames, G.Macleod. J.Food Sci. 50, (1985) 125-131.
13. K.Hunter, A.H.Rose, In: A.H. Rose (ed) "The yeast, Vol.2, Physiology and Biochemistry of Yeast" and Harrison, J.S. Academic Press, New York. (1971).

DEFINING ROASTED PEANUT FLAVOR QUALITY. PART 1. CORRELATION OF GC VOLATILES WITH ROAST COLOR AS AN ESTIMATE OF QUALITY

J.R. Vercellotti,[1] K.L. Crippen,[1] N.V. Lovegren,[1] and T.H. Sanders[2]

[1] Southern Regional Research Center, U.S. Department of Agriculture, Agricultural Research Service, 1100 Robert E. Lee Blvd., New Orleans, LA 70124

[2] National Peanut Research Laboratory, U.S. Department of Agriculture, Agricultural Research Service, 1011 Forrester Dr., S.E., Dawson, GA 31742

SUMMARY

A technique was developed for reproducible analysis of peanut butter volatile principles by direct gas chromatography at two purge temperatures (60° and 127° C) with flame ionization or sulfur specific flame photometric detection. Quality of peanut volatiles as well as degree of roast (e.g., several roasts of the same peanut lot with Hunter L values ranging from 60 to 40) can be measured using a uniform film of peanut butter on the wall of a glass cartridge. Examples are reported for Florunner medium (two crop years, 1985 and 1988) and Florunner #1 (1987 crop) commercial sized peanuts. All three crop year samples also had been defined for flavor quality by descriptive sensory panel analysis. Statistical correlation was made with quantities of key GC marker peaks and Hunter L–values as color indicators of degree of roast. Balanced peanut roast characteristics are present in Florunner peanuts roasted to a Hunter colorimeter L–value of 49 to 50, at which color quantities of volatile roasted peanut marker compounds are found in a rather narrow range of intensities.

1. INTRODUCTION

Fisher et al. (1), Lovegren et al. (2), Dupuy et al. (3), and St. Angelo et al. (4) developed procedures for determining volatiles in raw peanuts and legumes which can be used as indicators of inherent quality on any product that can be weighed into the glass tube used for direct gas chromatography. Fore et al. (5), (6), (7), (8) devised methods for quantitating peanut butter flavor volatiles, used this data to correlate GC profiles with sensory scores, and were able to employ the technique to assess shelf life stability of peanut butters.

These methods have been extended to many other foods such as vegetable oils, meat, chocolate, and fish as well as proven to be applicable to higher resolution gas chromatography on capillary columns (9), (10), (11), (12). Buckholz et al. (13), (14) have considered the effect of roasting time, commercial size, and peanut variety on the quality of flavor volatiles produced. Pattee and Singleton (15) reviewed the significance of volatile flavor compounds to peanut quality and included many references from their own work going back to 1965 as well as results from other laboratories through the 1960's and 1970's. Pattee et al. (16) also considered the effects of peanut size and time in storage for varieties of Virginia peanuts with respect to changes in flavor. How (17) described effects of variety, availability of precursors, roasting, and modified storage atmosphere on the chemical composition, headspace volatiles, and sensory flavor profiles of peanuts. Sanders et al. (18), (19) reported the influence of peanut maturity and curing conditions on the flavor character notes of peanuts. Young and Hovis (20) reported a headspace method for rapid analysis of volatiles in raw and roasted peanuts. Of the peaks produced from headspace analysis, eight were related to specific flavor characteristics of peanuts involved in objectionable flavor defects resulting from improper postharvest treatment.

The present paper reports gas chromatographic delineation of degree of peanut roast using volatiles analysis from samples purged at two different temperatures and using two detector types. These measurements of volatiles which are consistently highest in quantity permit correlation of peanut roast color with quantities of characteristic profile peaks. Targeting reproducible peanut roast characteristics through quantitative measurement of volatiles should considerably reinforce the time proven color card or reflectance colorimeter values (21) used by the industry. Determining roast quality in peanut butters by consistently reproducible gas chromatography has extensive economic ramifications. The homogenized roasted peanuts in peanut butter are more representative of an entire lot of peanuts than individual peanuts themselves. Also, peanut butter is a value–added product intended for the consumer which should represent the final production stage of this commodity.

2. MATERIALS AND METHODS

Three Florunner peanut lots, a 1985 crop Florunner medium grade size; a 1987 Florunner number one (#1) grade size; and a 1988 Florunner medium grade size, each from a single field source, were used in these studies. Medium grade sized kernel samples are retained on a 7.14 mm by 19.05 mm slotted screen (pass an 8.3 mm screen) and #1's, on a 6.4 mm by 19.05 mm slotted screen (pass a 7.1 mm screen). Five different roasts each of the 1988 crop medium and 1987 crop #1 Florunner peanuts were made at 162° C and 175 cubic feet per minute forced air flow in a carefully regulated drier (Surface Combustion, Inc., Maumee, OH 43537) using times varying from 7.5 minutes to 15 minutes. The screened sample baskets hold from 0.1 to 10 kg of peanut seed, and air flow is directed 50% of the duration of roast from the top surface of the peanut sample and 50% from the bottom. Three roast times were used for the 1985 crop medium peanut. Peanut paste samples were prepared with blanched peanuts by methods reported in Johnsen et al. (22) and Sanders et al. (18), (19) Hunter L values (HunterLab, D25–PC2, Reston, VA) for the peanut pastes from such samples ranged from 60 to 40. The U.S.D.A. plastic color guides (as described by Woodruff (23); Magnuson Engineers, Inc., 1010 Timothy Drive, San Jose, CA 95133) had the following L values referring to these roast colors: Guide #1, L = 55.4; Guide #2, L = 51.5; Guide #3, L = 49.3; Guide #4, L = 44.3. A raw paste of the medium and #1 size peanuts were used as an unroasted treatment and had Hunter L-values greater than 60.

2.1 Preparation of the Sample Tube for Direct Gas Chromatography

A folded plug of fine glass wool (50 to 55 mg) (8 micron, Pyrex Fiber Glass, Corning #3950) was placed about 5 mm above the base of an 84 x 9 mm O.D. glass cartridge used as a sample tube for direct gas chromatography of peanut butter volatiles (8). Approximately 2 grams of peanut butter at room temperature was placed in a 3 cc Luer lock disposable plastic syringe (Plastipak, Becton–Dickinson, East Rutherford, N.J., Catalog BD 5585) with a small weighing spatula. The plunger was inserted part way and the syringe was tapped on the table top on the hand end of the plunger to remove air in the sample. A 15 gauge stainless steel syringe needle, 10 cm long with 90° flat end and Luer lock hub (Unimetrics, Box 863, Joliet, Illinois) was attached to the syringe. Peanut butter (0.5000 to 0.5050 g total weight) is deposited above the glass wool plug on the inside wall of the direct gas chromatography sample tube in 2 to 3 strips about 3 mm wide, 1–2 mm thick, and 3.5 cm long using a short side to side motion as the needle is drawn up the tube. A 14 gauge or larger bore needle can be used for coarser peanut butters if necessary. Additional peanut butter sample was added with the syringe or removed with a small spatula to obtain closely reproducible weights. Each syringe will hold sufficient peanut butter to prepare two sample tubes. Blockages of the needle by small pieces of coarse peanut in the peanut butter were removed from the needle hub with a micro spatula. Uniformly ground peanut butters do not usually have this problem. Upon washing the needle and syringe with non–aromatic detergent, after rinsing thoroughly, a suitably sized wire was used to push small pieces of tissue paper through the needle to dry it for immediate reuse.

2.2 Direct Gas Chromatography Procedure at Higher Temperature (127° C)

The peanut butter sample tube prepared as above for direct gas chromatography was placed, with the glass wool plug at the bottom, in the injection port inlet of a 7.12/Tracor 222 gas chromatograph (10) or external closed inlet device (ECID, Scientific Instrumentation Service, River Ridge, LA) for direct gas chromatography (24), (3).

The carrier gas is swept over the strips of peanut butter in the glass cartridge and through the glass wool before entering the column. At a maximum inlet temperature of 127° C (Tracor) the sample was purged with nitrogen for 28 minutes at 20 ml/min carrier gas flow onto the top of a Tenax GC–8% polymetaphenylether column (8 feet x 1/8 inch; Ni 200). (When employing the ECID a block temperature of 132°C was applied to achieve 127°C inside the sample cartridge.) The Tenax column was cooled to about 20°C with a wet towel during volatiles concentration to allow at least 28 minutes of stripping time and still keep the first peak (methanol) on the column.

The sample cartridge was removed from the injection port after completion of volatiles stripping. To separate the concentrated flavor compounds the column was temperature programmed first to 50° C, held for 2 minutes, increased at 3°C/minute to 225° C, and then held for a total run time of about 85 minutes. Data collection and analysis was accomplished with a Hewlett–Packard 3357 Laboratory Automation System computer. Base lines on computer reconstruction analysis of curves were used which followed the lower valleys of the profile. Each sample was run gas chromatographically in duplicate and means of peak areas used in tabulating results after checking standard deviations.

2.3 Analysis of Peanut Butter Volatiles by Low Temperature (60°C) Dynamic Purge and Trap Gas Chromatography

Purge and trap analyses of peanut butter volatiles were carried out by dynamic purge and trap gas chromatography with a combination flame photometric and flame ionization detector using principles described by Brown et al. (25) for egg volatiles. An adaptation of the Tekmar volatiles impinger assembly (**Figure 1**) was substituted for the Tekmar semiautomatic purge and trap concentrator (Model LSC–3) as a generally applicable method. Peanut butter volatiles were sparged at 60°C for 28 minutes from a 25 ml Tekmar ALS needle impinger assembly containing 1.25 ± 0.1 g of peanut butter spread in a thin film on the walls with a flow rate of 20 cc/min of nitrogen carrier gas (Tekmar Co., Cincinnati, OH 45222–1856; component parts assembled as in diagramatic illustration #14–2258–000). The volatiles were concentrated on a packed Tenax GC/8% polymetaphenyl ether column (10 ft x 1/8") at ambient temperature after passing through a heated transfer line and six port 1/16" Valco valve (VICI Valco Instruments, Houston, TX 77255; part #C–6–T). The Tenax column was cooled to about 20° C with a wet towel during volatiles concentration. Chromatographic separation conditions were the same as for the high temperature (127°C) FID method above. The sample tube was removed from the injection port after completion of volatiles stripping and replaced with a tube containing a few milliliters of water to effect steam distillation. The six port valve permitted switching to a valve purge position that allowed the valve and transfer lines to be cleaned between runs by steam distillation from an impinger tube containing water alone.

2.4b Calibration of Flame Ionization and Flame Photometric Detectors

The flame ionization detectors on both the gas chromatographs were calibrated by injecting several concentrations of each of the peaks identified and obtaining response factors which were linear within the FID response ranges (1 to 50 ppm) found for the peanut butters. Unknowns as well as total volatiles were quantitated by using the response factor for pentane (1 to 50 ppm) as external standard of comparison. Concentrations of peaks for the flame ionization detectors are recorded as parts per million (micrograms of volatile per gram of the original sample weight of peanut butter). Responses for each of the flame ionization detectors were similar, and permitted closely matched degrees of sensitivity for the two systems. Calibration of the flame photometric detector with standards of sulfur containing compounds was carried out as in Brown et al. (25) with standards in the range of 1 to 500 parts per billion (ppb; ng per gram of peanut butter sample spiked). Recovery spikes of 42 ng of dimethyl sulfide were used to check system efficiency and FPD detection of 25 to 38 ng of recovered sulfide were found (61 – 89%) with this system. Concentrations of unknowns and total volatiles were quantitated by comparison with the FPD response factor for dimethyl sulfide as an external standard. Mass spectral identification of peaks was carried out as in Fore et al. (8) using either the packed column with fritted membrane separator for GC/MS or preconcentration of the peanut butter volatiles on a cartridge of Tenax GC followed by thermal desorption for three minutes at 200° C in the Legendre–Fisher–Dupuy external inlet with cryofocusing onto the capillary column (24), (3), (9), (12). A Finnegan 4500 mass spectrometer and Incos data system were used to identify peaks using a source potential of 70 eV. Gas chromatographic data are reported both in tables of quantities of each peak (parts per million or parts per billion with respect to original samples size) in order of GC elution as well as with three dimensional block diagrams in figures which attempt to enhance visualization of differences in the roasting process.

3. RESULTS AND DISCUSSION

3.1 FID analysis of peanut butter volatiles purged at 127° C

A medium florunner peanut butter (1985 crop) with roast color, L=51.2, was analyzed three times to determine the reproducibility of the volatiles profile. These analyses were all carried out under similar conditions, and comparison of peaks as well as means and standard deviations are listed in **Table 1**. The three analyses on the same medium roast sample (Analyses 1, 2, and 3 in **Table 1**) can be essentially superimposed, especially from 16 to 54 minutes retention time. Near the end of the analysis they deviate slightly from each other. Means and standard deviations in **Table 1** are diagnostic of the reproducibility of this gas chromatographic peanut butter profile of volatile flavor compounds. To see whether additional roasting time continued to accumulate volatiles, a fourth sample of this medium roast peanut butter was analyzed as the other samples in **Table 1** except that the sample was heated in the inlet an extra four minutes for a total stripping time of 32 minutes. The results of extended heating time are compared in Analysis 4 with the mean and standard deviations of **Table 1**. Total integrator counts in Analysis 4 are only slightly larger than the others in total volatiles as well as individual key peaks. This result may be attributed to the additional four minutes of purging used in the sample's volatiles concentration.

TABLE 1

REPLICATION OF VOLATILES PROFILES OF PEANUT BUTTER CONTROL 1985 FLORUNNER MEDIUM PEANUTS

PEAK NUMBER	COMPOUND (a)	RET TIME* MIN	1 PPM	2 PPM	3 PPM	MEAN PPM	STD DEV PPM	ANAL 4 + 4 MIN PPM
1	Free Methanol	6.7	4.1	4.0	3.8	3.9	0.15	4.2
2	Produced Methanol	8.4	3.2	2.8	2.6	2.9	0.30	3.3
3	Pentane	19.5-21.6	0.5	0.4	0.4	0.4	0.02	0.5
4	Methyl acetate	23.5	0.0	0.1	0.1	0.1	0.01	0.1
5	Methylpropanal	24.8	1.4	1.4	1.5	1.4	0.03	1.6
6	Unknown 1	27.5	0.2	0.2	0.2	0.2	0.01	0.2
7	Methylbutanal	31.1	1.9	1.9	1.9	1.9	0.02	2.0
8	Pentanal	33.2	0.1	0.2	0.2	0.2	0.02	0.2
9	Methylbutanol	34.3	0.2	0.3	0.3	0.3	0.03	0.3
10	N-Methylpyrrole	36.0	0.6	0.7	0.7	0.7	0.03	0.8
11	Hexanal	38.2	0.3	0.3	0.3	0.3	0.01	0.3
12	Unknown 2	39.6	0.1	0.1	0.2	0.1	0.01	0.2
13	Hexanol/Methylpyrazine	40.9	0.4	0.6	0.6	0.5	0.06	0.6
14	Dimethylpyrazine	44.5	3.1	3.3	3.3	3.2	0.09	3.4
15	Methylethylpyrazine	48.1	2.1	2.2	2.2	2.2	0.03	2.3
16	Tetrasubstituted pyrazines**	49.8-51.9	2.1	2.1	2.1	2.1	0.03	2.3
17	Vinylphenol	57.1	2.5	3.0	3.2	2.9	0.29	3.8
18	Unknown 3	60.0	0.8	0.8	0.8	0.8	0.02	1.0
19	Unknown 4	62.9	0.2	0.2	0.2	0.2	0.02	0.3
	SUM VOLATILE PEAKS (b)	12.6	13.4	13.4	13.1	0.36	14.7	
	INTEGRATOR TOTALS (c)	16.6	16.3	18.1	17.0	0.80	21.6	

(a) Medium roast 1985 Florunner with Hunter color of 51.2.
(b) Sum volatile peaks is a peak to valley integration (baseline connects lower valleys) calculated with respect to the response factor for pentane.
(c) Total volatiles two is an integration with a perpendicular drop to baseline (a flatter baseline including nearly all of the volatiles) calculated with respect to the response factor of pentane.
*Retention time is from the start of the GC run.
**Includes benzaldehyde.

Similar results are obtained with the Dupuy–Legendre–Fisher external closed inlet system (24) (3). The packed Tenax GC–8% polymetaphenyl ether column used in the current work can be replaced with a wide bore (0.75 mm o.d.) capillary column coated with phenylmethylsilicone. However, as reported by Ang et al. (26) concerning analysis of similar volatiles from ground meat, while the capillary column offered increased sensitivity for a particular compound, the packed column appeared to be more practical when changes in volatile profiles of the sample were to be measured. The present study reinforces these observations by Ang concerning the capillary versus packed column's utility in comparing volatiles from sample to sample.

Peak identification is essentially that listed by Fore et al. (8) for compound retention times on the Tenax GC–polymetaphenylether column. The GC retention time data for these compounds have been confirmed by GC–mass spectroscopy a number of times. Peak 2 in the paper by Fore et al. (8) was later found by mass spectroscopy to be mostly methanol with acetaldehyde near the beginning of the peak and methanethiol near the end (when it is present). In this work, the first peak with 6 minute retention time is essentially free methanol and is stripped off the sample initially. The second peak with 8.4 minute retention time is methanol that is produced by a hydrolytic chemical reaction in the sample during heating and is deposited later on the GC column than the free methanol. The intensity of this peak with 8.4 minute retention time is partially dependent on the amount of water in the sample if other conditions are the same. In addition, the

TABLE 2

1985 Florunner Mediums Direct Gas Chromatography, 127°C, FID

Hunter L value (a)	RET TIME MIN	56.7 lt.rst. PPM	51.2 med.rst. PPM	44.6 dk.rst. PPM	R-Squared
COMPOUND					
Free Methanol	6.7	15.6	4.1	1.9	0.83
Produced Methanol	8.4	3.2	3.2	4.4	0.82
Pentane/Acetone	19.5-21.6	0.4	0.4	0.3	0.85
Methyl acetate	23.5	0.0	0.0	0.1	0.90
Methylpropanal	24.8	0.8	1.6	2.9	0.99
Unknown 1	27.5	0.2	0.2	0.2	0.79
Methylbutanal	31.1	0.8	1.3	2.7	0.96
Pentanal	33.2	0.1	0.1	0.2	0.94
Methylbutanol	34.3	0.2	0.3	0.3	0.99
N-Methylpyrrole	36.0	1.4	1.2	1.8	0.42
Hexanal	38.2	0.5	0.6	0.3	0.66
Hexanol/Methylpyrazine	40.9	0.2	0.5	1.4	0.96
Dimethylpyrazine	44.5	1.0	2.9	5.2	1.00
Methylethylpyrazine	48.1	0.8	1.9	3.1	1.00
Tetrasubstituted pyrazines*	49.8-51.9	1.3	2.4	2.0	0.40
Vinylphenol	57.1	1.1	4.7	6.3	0.93
2,4-Decadienal	58.3	0.1	3.0	0.1	0.00
Unknown 2	60.0	0.5	0.9	1.2	0.94
Unknown 3	62.9	0.1	0.2	0.3	0.99
SUM VOLATILE PEAKS		28.1	29.6	34.6	0.93

(a) lt.rst., light roast; med.rst., medium roast; dk.rst., dark roast. Retention times and integration program as in Table 1.
* Includes benzeneacetaldehyde.

small peak with retention time 23.5 minutes is tentatively identified as methyl acetate. If hexanol is present it elutes as a shoulder on the front of the methylpyrazine peak about 2.3 minutes after the hexanal peak. The small peak with retention time of 34.3 minutes is methylbutanol. In the subsequent **Tables** only the major component in each peak is listed. Although a larger number of peaks identified as well as a broader base of total volatiles is accounted for in this work compared to that of Young and Hovis (20), all of the peaks reported by them are also included in these tabulations. Relative quantities of each peak in the Young and Hovis paper (20) cannot be compared to those reported here, however, because of lack of data.

TABLE 3

1988 FLORUNNER MEDIUM PEANUTS. DIRECT GAS CHROMATOGRAPHY (127°C).

Peak No.	Chemical Peaks	Retention Time* MIN	Hunter L Value (a) 62.0 (raw) PPM	60.7 (vltrst) PPM	52.4 (ltrst) PPM	50.5 (medrst) PPM	45.7 (dkrst) PPM	41.3 (vdkrst) PPM	R-Squared
1	Free Methanol	6.7	28.33	21.85	0.00	0.00	0.00	0.00	0.77
2	Produced Methanol	8.4	0.34	0.06	0.00	0.00	0.00	0.00	0.48
3	Ethanol	15.5	0.13	0.00	0.00	0.00	0.00	0.00	0.35
4	Pentane/acetone	19.5-21.6	0.39	10.42	6.53	4.70	1.61	0.65	0.19
5	Unknown 1	23.5	0.00	0.00	0.00	0.01	0.03	0.05	0.81
6	Methylpropanal	24.8	0.38	0.61	0.94	1.56	1.58	1.85	0.92
7	Methylbutanal	31.1	0.22	0.61	0.97	1.60	1.40	1.85	0.88
8	Pentanal	33.2	0.04	0.12	0.11	0.13	0.10	0.12	0.29
9	Methylbutanol	34.3	0.00	0.00	0.05	0.07	0.08	0.08	0.91
10	N-Methylpyrrole	36.0	0.98	1.94	1.34	1.59	1.94	2.53	0.50
11	Hexanal	38.2	0.27	0.62	0.32	0.50	0.26	0.19	0.30
12	Unknown 4	39.6	0.00	0.19	0.03	0.06	0.08	0.08	0.00
13	Hexanol/methylpyrazine	40.9	0.28	0.34	0.22	0.40	0.78	1.31	0.68
14	Dimethylpyrazine/ 2-pentylfuran	44.5-45.6	0.02	0.67	1.94	3.22	4.97	6.63	0.96
15	Unknown 5	46.2	0.25	1.20	0.57	0.24	0.16	0.19	0.34
16	Methylethylpyrazine	48.1	0.25	1.13	1.58	2.08	3.05	3.70	0.95
17	Tetrasubstituted pyrazines**	49.8-51.9	1.00	1.53	1.97	2.89	4.21	4.92	0.93
18	Unknown 6	54.1-55.9	0.07	0.37	0.04	0.02	0.17	0.27	0.00
19	Vinyl phenol	57.1	0.00	3.61	1.77	2.36	5.16	9.28	0.64
20	Decadienal	57.8	0.53	0.00	3.02	2.99	2.26	0.00	0.05
21	Unknown 7	60.0	0.12	0.30	0.58	0.79	1.09	1.30	0.98
	SUM VOLATILE PEAKS		33.61	45.58	21.97	25.21	28.94	34.99	0.14
	Total volatiles one (b)		3.62	19.85	17.00	18.36	19.48	23.00	0.47
	Total volatiles two (c)		7.32	24.73	21.88	20.64	26.60	31.78	0.57

(a) Peanut butters; vltrst, very light roast; ltrst, light roast; medrst, medium roast; dkrst, dark roast; vdkrst, very dark roast.
(b) Total volatiles one is a peak to valley integration calculated with respect to the response factor for pentane.
(c) Total volatiles two is an integration with a perpendicular drop to baseline calculated with respect to the response factor of pentane.
*Retention time is from the start of the GC temperature program.
**Includes benzeneacetaldehyde.

Three variable roasts from the 1985 medium florunner peanut are plotted in **Table 2**. Methylpropanal (24.8 minutes retention time), methylbutanal (31.1 minutes), methylbutanol (34.3 minutes), methylpyrazine (40.9 minutes), dimethylpyrazine (44.5 minutes), methylethylpyrazine (48.1 minutes), vinylphenol (57.1 minutes), unknown (60.0 minutes), and an unknown (62.9 minutes) all vary with the degree of roast. Free methanol decreased with increased roast time. Benzeneacetaldehyde (51.2 minutes) is recorded as a peak with the tetrasubstituted pyrazines but does not appear to increase with degree of roast whereas the smaller peaks around it do increase.

This GC technique for analyzing peanut butter can be used to show differences in the samples that may also be easily differentiated through sensory analysis. Flavor characteristics of the samples used in this study were assessed by the SRRC peanut flavor descriptive sensory analysis panel (The Spectrum Method of descriptive sensory analysis, (27)). The trained panel rated intensities for character notes presumably related to degree of roast (e.g., roasted peanutty, sweet aromatic, dark roast, raw beany, bitter (22). Intensities of character notes were found to be comparable to values in previously published studies (18), (19). With the present methodology we are working to correlate descriptive sensory intensity scores with regions or groups of peaks (18), (19), (22), (28), (29), (30). Off-flavored peanut butters have large peaks in their volatile profile not present in the good samples or peaks much larger than normally present in the good samples. Samples with non-volatile, off-flavor components would not be detected by this method. Also, samples containing compounds in GC peaks with little concentration or low detector response would not be recorded in these chromatograms. On the other hand, thresholds of sensory perception (31), (32) for some of these same compounds may be quite low and their impact quite great in the total flavor of the peanut butter while not being detectable at all on the gas chromatographic trace (compare **Tables 9** and **10**). Improved preconcentration and separation by highly efficient capillary columns should permit better delineation of some of these low threshold peaks.

All of these roasted peanut samples were analyzed in duplicate by low temperature volatiles concentration (60° sweep) with both flame ionization and flame photometric detection in addition to higher temperature direct gas chromatography (127°) with flame ionization detection only. Standard deviations from all these analyses were similar to those in **Table 1** for the 1985 crop medium peanuts. The higher temperature sweep (127°) was not suitable for flame photometric detection because excessive amounts of sulfur compounds were concentrated that tended to overload the FPD detector. The high temperature sweep (127°) FID data for roasts of both commercial grade sizes of the 1988 crop (mediums) and 1987 crop (#1's) is listed in **Tables 3** and **4**, respectively, as well as **Figures 2a and 2b**. Although not tabulated in this report very similar quantitative GC relationships were obtained using the high temperature method for medium Florunner peanuts roasted approximately to Hunter L-values of 50 and analyzed by descriptive sensory analysis in all crop years from 1984 through 1989.

Lovegren and St. Angelo (33) analyzed the volatiles produced by heating ground raw peanuts at various temperatures in the same direct GC inlet used in the present report to effect roasting under inert gas sweep. This work supports the present use of using a sweep temperature no higher than 130° C for a period of a half hour to avoid producing additional peanut volatiles under heating conditions, but to obtain a representative quantity of each peak. Thus, in a series of 79 raw peanut samples examined, nine component volatiles so produced comprised over 80% of the total component volatiles. Of these nine components of the profile, five were produced in steadily increasing concentrations at temperatures ranging from 104° C to 172° C: methanol, acetaldehyde, 3–methylbutanal, $\underline{N}$–methylpyrrole, and trimethylpyrazine. At temperatures above 145° C, 2–methylpropanal also followed a trend of steady increase with temperature. Only above 154° C, the temperature at which physical browning of the raw peanut sample began, did dimethylpyrazine, dimethylethylpyrazine, and benzeneacetaldehyde form in increasingly larger quantity with temperature. Other volatile compounds tabulated in the present work did not increase with temperature of the inlet or were masked by the large quanitity of neighboring peaks. These results have been confirmed in the present study and have served as a guide for inlet sweep temperature settings.

There are many subtle Maillard reaction products in the peanut volatiles mixture. Roasted peanut Maillard products have been extensively studied by Mason et al. (34), (35); Walradt et al. (36); Waller et al. (37); Buckholz et al. (13), (14); and Ho et al. (38). The many heterocyclic nitrogen compounds such as pyrazines, thiazoles, thiophenes, and other aromatics or sulfides suggest a role in the total flavor impact. Ahmed and Young (39), Mason and Waller (34), and Newell et al. (40) have reviewed the role of precursors as well as enumerated the collective heteroatomic compounds produced in peanut flavor. In comparing relative quantities of volatiles produced by roasting medium and #1 Florunner peanuts, it should be considered that proximate compositional analysis and precursor concentrations differ between these sizes (39).

3.2 Low Temperature (60° C) Purge and Trap Volatiles Identified by FID

As described earlier the low temperature purge was employed for several reasons. First, the total volatiles in the head space at this lower temperature will more reasonably approach the olfactory perception of a subject perceiving the aroma. Secondly, the lower temperature will prevent formation of new volatiles in the mixture either by Maillard reactions or through cracking of hydroperoxides previously formed (41). Selke and

Frankel (41) showed that in soybean oils at 60° C the volatiles of lipid oxidation were much less than in oils heated over 120° C.

TABLE 4

1987 FLORUNNER NUMBER ONE PEANUTS. DIRECT GAS CHROMATOGRAPHY (127°C) FID

Peak No.	Chemical Peaks	Retention Time*	Hunter L Value (a) 63.2 (raw) PPM	59.4 (vltrst) PPM	54.5 (ltrst) PPM	50.0 (medrst) PPM	44.9 (dkrst) PPM	41.1 (vdkrst) PPM	R-Squared
1	Free Methanol	6.7	14.63	25.41	16.41	9.63	5.96	2.15	0.70
2	Produced Methanol	8.4	0.38	0.14	0.00	0.00	0.00	0.00	0.63
3	Ethanol	15.5	0.06	0.05	0.00	0.00	0.00	0.00	0.71
4	Pentane/acetone	19.5-21.6	0.27	0.63	0.52	0.30	0.21	0.32	0.19
5	Unknown 1	23.5	0.00	0.02	0.03	0.04	0.09	0.47	0.56
6	Methylpropanal	24.8	0.73	2.19	3.15	3.90	5.89	5.35	0.94
7	Methylbutanal	31.1	0.42	1.45	2.75	3.16	4.99	4.92	0.97
8	Pentanal	33.2	0.00	0.08	0.12	0.10	0.11	0.08	0.34
9	Methylbutanol	34.3	0.25	0.31	0.44	0.41	0.42	0.37	0.41
10	N-Methylpyrrole	36.0	1.13	2.14	2.09	1.79	2.05	2.25	0.40
11	Hexanal	38.2	1.64	2.60	2.64	2.13	1.39	1.45	0.26
12	Unknown 4	39.6	0.00	0.00	0.00	0.00	0.43	0.52	0.72
13	Hexanol/methylpyrazine	40.9	0.53	0.41	0.50	0.68	1.22	2.04	0.74
14	Dimethylpyrazine/ 2-pentylfuran	44.5-45.6	1.55	1.69	3.97	5.48	9.81	13.75	0.92
15	Unknown 5	46.2	0.33	0.47	0.24	0.27	0.41	0.49	0.10
16	Methylethylpyrazine	48.1	0.49	1.42	2.63	3.61	6.05	8.37	0.96
17	Tetrasubstituted pyrazines**	49.8-51.9	2.30	3.85	5.13	6.46	10.10	12.87	0.96
18	Unknown 6	54.1-56.9	0.11	0.11	0.34	0.49	1.00	1.34	0.92
19	Vinyl phenol	57.1	0.00	0.92	3.40	5.13	9.89	14.11	0.95
20	Decadienal	58.3	0.61	1.26	0.00	0.00	0.00	0.00	0.51
21	Unknown 7	60.0	0.23	0.59	0.94	1.20	1.91	2.41	0.98
	SUM VOLATILE PEAKS		25.66	45.74	45.32	44.77	61.92	73.26	0.86
	Total volatiles one (b)		7.16	14.37	19.96	23.61	36.89	45.96	0.97
	Total volatiles two (c)		12.48	25.37	32.90	35.79	54.33	70.69	0.95

(a) Peanut butters: vltrst, very light roast; ltrst, light roast; medrst, medium roast; dkrst, dark roast; vdkrst, very dark roast.
(b) Total volatiles one is a peak to valley integration calculated with respect to the response factor for pentane.
(c) Total volatiles two is an integration with a perpendicular drop to baseline calculated with respect to the response
*Retention time is from the beginning of the GC temperature program.
**Includes benzeneacetaldehyde.

A combined flame ionization (FID) and flame photometric detector (FPD) permitted simultaneous detection of typical FID active flavor volatiles (as in the Dupuy et al. method (3)) and the FPD active sulfur containing compounds (Brown et al. (25)). The low temperature FID volatiles (60° C) purge data for the above roasts (1988 Florunner mediums and number ones) are listed in **Tables 5** and **6** as well as **Figures 3a and 3b**.

Some 18 FID active compounds (alcohols, lipid oxidation products, Strecker aldehydes, pyrazines, etc.) were identifiable as markers for this low temperature (60° C purge and trap) degree of roast study. The FID active compounds purged at 60° have all been previously reported by Fore et al. (8) with the exception that at this lower temperature the last identifiable peak is benzeneacetaldehyde. This mixture of peanut butter flavor volatiles differs somewhat from those purged at 127°, both qualitatively and quantitatively, while the complete set reported by Fore et al. (8) are present in the higher temperature purge (i.e., peaks extend beyond vinyl phenol and the decadienals).

The fact that more pyrazines are collected on concentration of the sparged volatiles at the lower temperature than the higher indicates that there are head space and sample heating differences between the two methods (see **Figure 1**). Koehler and Odell (42) following earlier work by Koehler et al. (43) demonstrated that below 100° C little formation of pyrazines occurs in peanuts or model systems of sugars and amino acids. However, above 115° C thermal decomposition of certain pyrazines becomes significant and loss of these flavor principles is quite probable. The work of Koehler is at least supportive of using the lower temperature to sparge volatiles from peanut butter. Whether these differences are reflected in the cross section of volatile stimuli presented to a subject perceiving the peanut flavor aromas under the two sampling conditions is not known from this study.

TABLE 5

1988 Florunner Mediums Purge and Trap, 60°C, FID

Peak Number	Chemical Peaks	Retention Time* MIN	Hunter L-Value 62.0 PPM	60.7 PPM	52.4 PPM	50.5 PPM	45.7 PPM	41.3 PPM	R-Squared
1	Free Methanol	21.8	0.00	10.29	14.69	45.94	47.08	50.94	0.84
2	Produced Methanol	31.9	0.00	2.66	0.00	12.46	16.66	11.66	0.61
3	Ethanol	40.0	0.09	0.00	8.32	0.00	0.00	0.86	0.00
4	Pentane/Acetone	43.4	0.12	1.99	0.80	2.55	1.36	2.07	0.20
5	Unknown 1	45.8	0.00	0.00	0.00	0.25	0.27	0.55	0.80
6	Methylpropanal	47.5	0.00	0.66	1.99	5.44	5.72	6.84	0.90
7	Unknown 2	50.1	0.00	0.28	0.45	0.61	0.42	0.77	0.75
8	Methylbutanal	53.8	0.03	0.72	2.63	4.71	4.88	5.84	0.94
9	Unknown 3	55.8	0.00	0.32	0.49	0.58	0.42	0.68	0.68
10	N-Methylpyrrole	58.6	0.25	2.44	3.41	6.67	6.81	8.70	0.90
11	Hexanal	60.9	0.11	0.80	0.86	1.44	0.89	0.88	0.29
12	Unknown 4	62.4	0.00	0.12	0.18	0.80	0.27	0.44	0.33
13	Hexanol/Methylpyrazine	63.6	0.16	0.32	0.51	1.23	0.99	1.60	0.84
14	Dimepyr/2-Pentylfuran	67.4	0.15	0.54	4.42	9.86	9.39	20.23	0.88
15	Methylethylpyrazine	71.1	0.52	0.42	2.48	5.51	3.57	8.57	0.81
16	Unknown 5	72.5	0.00	0.31	0.50	0.77	0.50	0.58	0.55
17	Benzeneacetaldehyde	73.5	0.00	0.00	2.24	0.84	1.62	2.95	0.76
18	Tetrasubstituted pyrazines	74.9	0.20	0.00	0.00	1.39	0.00	2.83	0.42
	SUM VOLATILE PEAKS		1.63	21.90	43.97	101.05	100.84	126.97	0.91

*Retention time is measured from the beginning of the GC temperature program. Total trapping time: 30 minutes.

Indication of the relative impact of each of these compounds in the low and high temperature elution method is given in the table of threshold values for volatiles in aqueous medium (**Table 9**). For most of the high temperature (127° C) FID-active compounds, the thresholds are above the level monitored with the detector. Methylpropanal, methylbutanal, N-methylpyrrole, hexanal, hexanol, 2-pentylfuran, vinyl phenol, and decadienal all have thresholds below concentrations monitored by the FID detector. We have used these FID and FPD markers throughout this work to track our roast studies. Since in this work our major concern is to correlate very accurately sensory intensity data with the presence of volatiles in the GC, these markers have been very useful to perform statistical comparisons (30).

In **Table 5** degree of roast is often related to Peaks 6, methylpropanal, and 8, methylbutanal, along with N–methylpyrrole (Peak 10) and the pyrazines ranging from Peaks 13 through 17 (17). Sanders and Green (44) demonstrated that methylpropanal is higher in less mature peanuts, which is confirmed here with respect to the smaller commercial sized #1's. Methylpyrazine (Peak 13), dimethylpyrazine (Peak 14), methylethylpyrazine (Peak 15), and the tetrasubstituted pyrazines (Peak 16) all continue rising in total concentration with degree of roast. Possibly the increasingly large quanitities of alkaloidal pyrazine compounds in the very dark roasts might be responsible for some of the bitter and dark roast off–flavors involved (45), (30).

TABLE 6

1987 Florunner Number Ones Purge and Trap, 60°C, FID

Peak Number	Chemical Peaks	Retention Time* MIN	Hunter L-Value 63.20 PPM	59.40 PPM	54.50 PPM	50.00 PPM	44.90 PPM	41.10 PPM	R-Squared
1	Free Methanol	21.8	0.00	15.57	9.02	23.62	42.15	14.43	0.40
2	Produced Methanol	31.9	0.06	2.60	2.41	6.50	11.17	6.24	0.69
3	Ethanol	40.0	0.00	0.00	0.00	0.00	0.00	0.00	0.00
4	Pentane/Acetone	43.4	0.14	0.76	0.47	0.94	1.61	1.19	0.73
5	Unknown 1	45.8	0.00	0.00	0.00	0.10	0.22	0.21	0.85
6	Methylpropanal	47.5	0.05	1.37	2.32	4.45	10.41	8.18	0.86
7	Unknown 2	50.1	0.05	0.31	0.30	0.48	0.70	0.53	0.81
8	Methylbutanal	53.8	0.08	2.25	3.89	7.44	15.34	13.21	0.91
9	Unknown 3	55.8	0.00	0.29	0.27	0.46	0.77	0.62	0.85
10	N-Methylpyrrole	58.6	0.89	4.14	2.94	4.13	6.58	6.08	0.78
11	Hexanal	60.9	0.00	1.81	1.30	1.71	2.14	1.51	0.40
12	Unknown 4	62.4	1.82	2.64	2.19	2.52	1.20	1.09	0.41
13	Hexanol/ Methylpyrazine	63.6	2.25	3.93	3.13	3.16	2.91	1.53	0.19
14	Dimethylpyrazine/ 2-Pentylfuran	67.4	8.09	11.28	11.04	12.88	28.11	28.58	0.82
15	Methylethylpyrazine	71.1	5.24	6.48	9.28	5.96	10.82	14.13	0.71
16	Unknown 5	72.5	0.00	0.83	2.05	0.79	0.78	0.74	0.03
17	Benzeneacetaldehyde	73.5	1.10	1.32	2.00	4.24	5.10	7.12	0.94
18	Tetrasubstituted pyrazines	74.9	0.00	2.04	4.41	0.00	0.00	3.37	0.02
	SUM VOLATILE PEAKS		19.77	57.63	57.03	79.39	140.02	108.77	0.82

* Retention time is measured from the beginning of the GC temperature program. Total trapping time: 30 minutes.

Benzeneacetaldehyde (shoulder on Peak 17) may contribute to the sweet aroma that occurs in peanut flavor volatiles. Buckholz et al. (13) demonstrated a high correlation between the intensity of benzeneacetaldehyde and desirable flavor in roasted peanuts.

In the present study the relative quantity of benzeneacetaldehyde is highest at medium roast (Hunter L = 50.5) before declining. Vinyl phenol (Peak 19; p–hydroxystyrene) possesses a strong chemical plastic odor reminiscent of coal gas and disinfectant. In **Tables 2, 3, and 4** vinyl phenol increases in quantity throughout the darkest roasts. Lovegren et al. (10) defined relative concentrations of each of the above gas chromatographic peaks in parts per million using response factors from external standards.

3.3 Sulfur Containing Compounds Detected by the FPD in Medium Florunners

Many off–flavor compounds produced by Maillard reactions of sulfur amino acids and carbohydrates have intense sulfide or sulfur heterocyclic off–flavors. Some fourteen sulfur–containing, FPD active peaks (mercaptans, mono– and disulfides, hydrogen sulfide, and carbonyl sulfide) were routinely monitored using this low temperature concentration system. Sulfur–containing compounds were detected from the 60° purge sample with simultaneous FPD detection and are listed for florunner medium and number one peanuts in **Tables 7** and **8**.

Although many of these compounds have undesirable character in themselves, in proper proportion they add considerable to the positive blend of desirable flavors (46). Most of these compounds have aromatic thresholds of perception that are less than 1 ppb in water. Thresholds of perception of the sulfur containing compounds identified by FPD detection are also listed in **Table 10**. Therefore, because the impact of sulfur compounds is so subtle in peanut roasts, the sulfur containing compounds are of great import to establish a balance of peanut flavor.

Of the sulfur compounds listed in **Tables 7, 8,** and **10**, the simplest degradation product of cysteine is hydrogen sulfide and has the off–flavor "rotten eggs". Methyl sulfide has the off–flavor of "sickening sulfide, extremely diffusive, repulsive reminiscent of sharp green or burnt cabbage". Methyl sulfide is found in cooked corn or freeze damaged vegetables and legumes such as navy beans and peanuts. The higher sulfides such as dibutyl sulfide are reminiscent of off–flavors in rotten onion or scorched rubber. Dimethyl disulfide is intensely onion–like, very diffusive with a sickening cooked cabbage off–flavor. Dimethyl trisulfide is sulfurous, burnt cabbage or onion off–flavor. The allyl sulfides are similar to these latter but with more of a garlic–like overtone. These Maillard off–flavors are generated under a variety of circumstances included microbial degradation of metabolites that form these sulfides. Although not yet identified in the present work but possibly among the unknowns listed, the Strecker degradation product of methionine, methional, imparts a powerful, diffusive onion or meat like aroma that is present in coffee or the "cooked beef brothy" blend of beef flavor, but which turns into a burnt sweet corn or vulcanized rubber pungency when in too high a concentration (32).

TABLE 7

1988 Florunner Mediums, Purge and Trap, 60°C, FPD

Peak Number	Chemical Peaks	Retention Time* MIN	Hunter L-Value 62.0 PPB	60.7 PPB	52.4 PPB	50.5 PPB	45.7 PPB	41.3 PPB	R-Squared
1	Hydrogen sulfide/COS	10.0-26.5	0.0	0.0	5.5	321.2	83.3	3473.9	0.46
2	Unknown eight	31.8	0.0	4.3	52.1	58.5	129.9	201.9	0.92
3	Methanethiol	34.5	0.0	9.4	19.7	1331.9	1833.5	3752.9	0.79
4	Dimethyl sulfide	43.8	0.0	7.1	1.5	597.0	858.3	312.5	0.43
5	Carbon disulfide	46.8	0.0	0.0	1.5	35.7	55.2	42.4	0.73
6	Unknown ten	51.6	0.0	0.0	0.4	2.7	6.8	2.8	0.53
7	Propanethiol	54.3	0.0	0.0	1.3	7.0	16.7	29.4	0.81
8	Diethyl sulfide	56.1	0.0	0.0	0.3	3.0	8.0	9.8	0.83
9	Dimethyl disulfide	58.5	0.0	15.3	14.5	1113.4	1146.3	759.1	0.56
10	Unknown eleven	64.3	0.0	0.0	0.0	1.7	1.6	1.7	0.71
11	Unknown twelve	65.4	0.0	0.0	0.0	3.2	3.8	8.7	0.77
12	Unknown thirteen	66.7	0.0	0.0	0.0	2.8	2.9	4.4	0.80
13	Unknown fourteen	68.7	0.0	0.0	0.0	6.0	16.4	49.0	0.67
14	Unknown fifteen	70.3	0.0	0.0	7.8	41.5	39.5	79.7	0.84
15	Unknown sixteen	73.0	0.0	0.0	3.3	4.0	0.0	22.5	0.48
16	Unknown seventeen	75.4	0.0	0.0	0.0	0.6	0.0	7.2	0.44
	SUM VOLATILE PEAKS		0.0	36.1	107.9	3530.2	4202.3	8757.8	0.80

* Retention time is measured from the beginning of the GC temperature program. Total trapping time: 30 minutes.

The sulfur containing compounds detectable by this system are quite intense immediately after roasting. Considering that the flame ionization detector is able to detect in the parts <u>per million range</u>, on the FPD chromatogram the peaks are in the <u>parts per billion</u> range. For the present study we have identified and used hydrogen sulfide, carbonyl sulfide, methanethiol, dimethyl sulfide, carbon disulfide, propanethiol, diethyl sulfide, and dimethyl-disulfide as peanut volatile marker compounds. Nine unknown sulfur compounds are also present. A study of sulfur containing peanut flavor volatiles has been completed by Watkins (47) and Watkins and Young (48) using a different method of sampling the volatiles. Watkins listed most of the same FPD active sulfur compounds and several others from peanut butter which are also similar to the /compounds reported here. In comparison to the work of Watkins the present low temperature (60° C) purge and trap method not only permits sulfur compound analysis of peanut butter (as contrasted to raw peanuts roasted at 150° C <u>in situ</u>) at a mild temperature but also simultaneously provides detection of the volatile profile of FID active compounds. Thresholds listed for the sulfur containing compounds in **Table 10** are also all below the quantities found by low temperature purging and FPD analysis in the present peanut roast study. Although one would have expected dimethyltrisulfide in the peanut volatiles we were unable to identify this compound, whose retention time is near that of Peak 14. The other unknown sulfur compounds were quite regular and reproducible and served as useful references in the roast studies.

3.4 FID and FPD Active Compounds in Commercial Size #1 Peanuts

In general, in the present experiment the #1 peanuts were observed to have elevated peak intensities when compared to the medium peanuts (compare **Tables 4, 6,** and **8**). As has been demonstrated in other studies of immature peanuts, methylpropanal is also higher in these roasted #1 peanuts than in the medium Florunners (44). Likewise methylbutanal is higher in these peanuts. In the #1 peanuts the pyrazines are higher in darker roasts than in the mediums, and the floral aromatic, benzeneacetaldehyde, also increases more in the #1's.

TABLE 8

1988 Florunner Number Ones, Purge and Trap, 60°C, FPD

Peak Number	Chemical Peaks	Retention Time MIN	Hunter L-value 63.2 PPB	59.4 PPB	54.4 PPB	50.0 PPB	44.9 PPB	41.1 PPB	R-Squared
1	Hydrogen sulfide/COS	10.0-26.5	0.8	62.4	0.0	0.0	191.1	63.3	0.27
2	Unknown eight	31.8	0.0	87.9	7.0	15.5	103.0	80.5	0.27
3	Methanethiol	34.5	0.5	41.4	28.1	77.6	665.9	152.3	0.35
4	Dimethyl sulfide	43.8	6.0	51.9	22.3	27.8	73.4	30.9	0.19
5	Carbon disulfide	46.8	0.9	4.0	4.6	4.9	42.2	27.8	0.65
6	Unknown ten	51.6	0.0	1.0	0.0	1.2	1.1	3.5	0.61
7	Propanethiol	54.3	0.0	0.4	0.5	1.4	10.3	10.8	0.78
8	Diethyl sulfide	56.1	0.0	0.0	0.0	0.0	3.5	3.0	0.67
9	Dimethyl disulfide	58.5	3.7	4.1	13.4	63.8	470.2	563.8	0.78
10	Unknown eleven	64.3	0.0	0.0	0.0	1.9	0.5	1.7	0.48
11	Unknown twelve	65.4	0.0	0.0	0.0	0.0	1.0	3.8	0.58
12	Unknown thirteen	66.7	0.0	0.0	0.0	0.0	1.1	4.0	0.60
13	Unknown fourteen	68.7	0.0	0.0	0.0	3.6	18.0	38.9	0.73
14	Unknown fifteen	70.3	0.0	0.7	3.4	9.7	47.3	89.2	0.76
15	Unknown sixteen	73.0	0.0	0.0	0.0	0.0	0.7	18.1	0.44
16	Unknown seventeen	75.4	0.0	0.0	0.0	3.4	0.7	11.4	0.52
	SUM VOLATILE PEAKS		11.8	253.7	79.4	210.9	1630.0	1103.0	

* Retention time is measured from the beginning of the GC temperature program. Total trapping time: 30 minutes.

Although the Florunner medium and #1 peanuts contain qualitatively the same key sulfur compounds, the quantity of all the sulfur compounds in the medium peanuts is 5 to 10 times greater than in the #1's roasted to the same color. In the light of literature on the development of proteins during peanut maturation (39), methionine- and cysteine-containing precursors are probably implicated in these differences in sulfur roast yields between medium and #1 florunners.

The unknown sulfur compounds in the FPD chromatograms shown in **Tables 7 and 8** are in some cases of greater quantity for the #1's than for mediums. Relative quantities of these unknowns were calculated with reference to dimethyl sulfide as external standard. These could well be contributing to burnt rubber or scorched corn off-flavors in the darker roasted #1's. Many of the other sulfur containing Maillard reaction compounds, too numerous to give all their off-flavor descriptors and molecular formulas, impart off-flavors (13), (14). These are thiophenes, thiazoles, thiolanes, and thioesters which are present almost universally in baked or roasted cereal products, roasted coffee, cocoa, as well as in peanuts. The sulfur containing heterocycles such as benzothiazole (intense burnt rubber or scorched milk off-flavor) have a peculiar place in off-flavor chemistry (32). Such off-flavors are familiar in sensory analysis of roasted coffee, cocoa, peanuts, and baked cereal products.

TABLE 9

THRESHOLDS FOR FID COMPOUNDS, FLORUNNER MEDIUM AND NUMBER ONE PEANUTS

Peak No.	Chemical Peaks	Retention time* MIN	Threshhold of perception** (PPM)
1	Free Methanol	6.7	200.0
2	Produced Methanol	8.4	200.0
3	Ethanol	15.5	10.0
4	Pentane/acetone	19.5-26.6	340/200
5	Unknown 1	23.5	unk
6	Methylpropanal	24.8	0.9
7	Methylbutanal	31.1	0.2
8	Pentanal	33.2	0.3
9	Methylbutanol	34.2	4.0
10	N-Methylpyrrole	36.0	less than 0.1
11	Hexanal	38.2	0.2
12	Unknown 4	39.7	unk
13	Hexanol/ methylpyrazine	40.9	0.5/110
14	Dimethylpyrazine/ 2-pentylfuran	44.5-45.5	50/1
15	Unknown 5	46.4	unk
16	Methylethylpyrazine	48.1	7.0
17	Tetrasubstituted pyrazines*	49.8-51.9	>100
18	Unknown 6	54.1-58.9	unk
19	Vinyl phenol	57.1	0.1
20	Decadienal	58.3	0.1
21	Unknown 7	60.0	unk

* Retention time is measured from the time that the temperature program begins.
**References: Stahl, 1973 and Fors, 1983.

3.5 Regression analyses of GC peak intensities with respect to Hunter L-values for roast color

The high temperature FID data is the mean of two repeated measures on each sample. Low temperature FID and FPD data are tabulated as means of three repeated measures, respectively. Standard deviations for these means were within 5% and are not listed in the tables. Regression analyses were carried out by plotting GC peak quantities (in ppm) as tabulated above versus Hunter L-values for respective roast colors. R-squared values for these correlations are included in each of **Tables 2** through **8**. Notable differences in the volatile patterns of samples roasted to various degrees are made in the summarizing remarks of subsequent paragraphs.

3.6 Correlation of GC peaks intensities with color for high temperature GC method (127° C) for medium and #1 peanuts with FID

– In **Tables 3** and **4** for high temperature sweep (127° C) volatiles on 1988 crop medium and 1987 crop #1 peanuts, methylpropanal (peak 6), methylbutanal (peak 7), dimethylpyrazine (peak 14), methylethylpyrazine (peak 16), tetracarbon–substituted pyrazine (peak 17) have correlation coefficients that are greater than 0.9 and correlate well with degree of roast.

– Total volatiles at this sweep temperature (with adjusted baseline) were better correlated with roasting for the #1 peanuts than for the mediums, and the medium peanuts in **Table 3** show little correlation of total volatiles with degree of roast.

TABLE 10

THRESHOLDS FOR FPD COMPOUNDS, FLORUNNER MEDIUM AND NUMBER ONE PEANUTS. PURGE AND TRAP GC.

Peak Number	Chemical Peaks	Retention Time* MIN	Threshold of perception**
1	Hydrogen sulfide/COS	10.0–26.5	0.47 ppb
2	Unknown eight	31.8	unk
3	Methanethiol	34.5	2 ppb
4	Dimethyl sulfide	43.8	1 ppb
5	Carbon disulfide	46.8	0.2 ppm
6	Unknown ten	51.6	unk
7	Propanethiol	54.3	0.06 ppb
8	Diethyl sulfide	56.1	0.4 ppb
9	Dimethyl disulfide	58.5	1.2 ppb

* Retention time is measured from the beginning of the GC temperature program. Total trapping time: 30 minutes.
**References: Stahl, 1973 and Fors, 1983.

– Free and produced methanol (peak 1 and 2) as well as ethanol (peak 3) decreased with roasting time (decreased Hunter L–value) probably because more was evaporated during longer roasting times.

– In medium peanuts unknown 1 (peak 5) and methylbutanal (peak 7) increased with roasting time, but both these peaks were more intense in the #1's at this higher temperature for volatiles concentration than were the mediums.

– In the #1's unknown 4 (peak 12), hexanol/methylpyrazine (peak 13), unknown 6 (peak 18), vinyl phenol (peak 19) and total volatiles–2 increased with an increase in roasting time. Methylbutanol (peak 9) in the #1 peanut sample was the only peak with maximum area at Hunter L–value ca. 50 (medium roast).

– In **Table 2** many of the same relationships hold for the 1985 medium florunner sample as for the 1987 #1's and 1988 mediums. However, with only three degrees of roast to correlate for the 1985 crop year, peak size and degree of roast in **Table 2** is much more regular than in the other two crop year samples (much higher R-squared values overall).

3.7 Correlation of GC peaks with roast color for low temperature GC method using purge and trap at 60° C with FID

The yield of volatiles and kinds of compounds dominant in the low temperature sweep of peanut butters differ from the higher temperature concentration method. Correlation of these with roast color is nonetheless important since as mentioned above the mixture of volatiles at 60° C more closely approximates the sensory subject's impression.

– From **Tables 5** and **6** Unknown 1 (peak 5), methylpropanal (peak 6), unknown 2 (peak 7), $\underline{N}$–methylpyrrole (peak 10), dimethylpyrazine (peak 14), methylethylpyrazine (peak 15), and benzeneacetaldehyde (peak 17) were highly correlated with roasting. All increased as peanuts were roasted for longer periods (Hunter L–values decreased). No peaks decreased as roasting time was lengthened. Unknown 4 (peak 12) was maximum at a medium roast with Hunter L–value of 50.

– Hexanol/methylpyrazine (peak 13) in the #1's and unknown 5 (peak 16) in the #1's tended to be maximized at a medium roast (Hunter L–value, ca. 50), but this was not so in the medium sized peanuts. Hexanol/methylpyrazine (peak 13) was highly correlated with roast in the mediums but not in the #1's. This is probably due to the fact that 2 compounds make up the same peak.

– Pentane (peak 4) was highly correlated with roast in the #1's but not as high for the mediums. (Pentane correlation with roast color was opposite in the high temperature method (correlates well with roast in mediums)). Unknown 3 (peak 9) correlates highly with roast in the #1's but not in mediums at low temperature purging. (Unknown 3 was not monitored in the high temperature method).

3.8 Low temperature (60° C) purge and trap for GC volatiles with FPD

In **Tables 7** and **8** are listed sulfur compounds detected with FPD for medium and #1 florunner peanuts. Correlation of sulfur containing peaks with degree of roast is interesting because so many of the overtones of balanced peanut flavor contain sulfury notes.

– Carbondisulfide (peak 5), propanethiol (peak 7), diethyl sulfide (peak 8), unknown 13 (peak 12), unknown 14 (peak 13) and unknown 15 (peak 14) increased with increases in roast with high correlation coefficients ($r^2 > 0.60$).

— In the mediums, unknown 8 (peak 2), methanethiol (peak 3), unknown 11 (peak 10), and unknown 12 (peak 11) increased with increases in roasting time (with $r^2 > 0.60$), but not in #1's.

— In the #1's dimethyldisulfide (peak 9) and unknown 10 (peak 6) increased with increases in roasting time, but did not increase as much in the mediums.

— No sulfur peaks reached their maximum at the medium roast with L = 50, nor did any peaks decrease with increased roasting time. Overall the florunner mediums had higher sulfur volatiles than the #1 peanuts. Total volatiles also had a higher correlation with degree of roast for the mediums than for the #1's.

3.9 Overview of applying direct gas chromatographic analysis to roasted peanut volatiles

Both the higher (127° C) and lower temperature sweep (60° C) methods described herein are purge and trap volatile concentrations (3), (9), (25). They are both direct gas chromatography methods because the system is closed and the same packed column is used to concentrate the samples that is subsequently used to separate the component volatiles. Neither thermal desorption nor solvent elution is necessary to effect chromatography. In fact, it would appear that some separation is effected on the packed column at ambient temperature before the actual temperature ramp rates are begun. Heating and sample size are uniform in both these methods so that flame ionization and photometric detection can be applied quantitatively. There are more than 300 flavor compounds now identified in roast peanuts using a variety of concentration and gas chromatographic techniques (13), (14), (38). From these total peanut volatiles the packed column of Tenax GC coated with 8% polymetaphenylether separates only 35 or 40 significant peaks that are dealt with in this paper. However, this separation is very consistent and measures a cross section of the volatiles in peanut aroma. It is useful in measuring differences in raw or roasted peanuts to apply in defining flavor quality of commercial lots or defining degree of roast as was done here. Current work in progress in these laboratories is developing methodology to effect separation of many more compounds with capillary gas chromatography using the principles described in this paper. Nonetheless, the simplicity and reproducibility of the present technique recommends the volatiles analysis described here for application to solving research and industrial problems.

4. **SUMMARY AND CONCLUSIONS**

1. Degree of roast was assessed gas chromatographically on florunner medium and #1 commercial sized peanuts roasted to five Hunter L values ranging from 60 to 40.

2. A descriptive sensory panel identified flavor character notes and their intensities that typify changes in degree of roast (e.g., roasted peanutty, sweet aromatic, dark roast, raw beany, bitter) to authenticate roast quality (correlations of GC and sensory flavor analysis to be reported in a separate accompanying paper (30)).

3. A sparging device designed for this application is reported which concentrates roasted peanut volatiles of peanut butters by dynamic headspace technique onto a packed gas chromatographic column (Tenax GC–8% PMPE) at moderate sample temperatures (60° C).

4. A combined flame ionization (FID) and flame photometric detector (FPD) permitted simultaneous detection of 18 typical FID active flavor volatiles and 14 sulfur containing compounds. Roasted peanut volatiles were also run by direct gas chromatography in a sample injection port at 127° C using FID.

5. A simple technique has been developed for depositing thin layers of peanut butter on the inside of glass sample tube cartridges or purge and trap impinger tubes for the purpose of uniformly sweeping off the flavor volatiles from the paste surface on samples of similar weight. Reproducible volatile profiles were used as indicators of relative quality depending on concentrations of specific marker flavor compounds in the peanut butter.

6. Quantitative gas chromatographic data so generated was statistically compared with roast color intensities. Optimization of roast as determined by gas chromatographic correlation with roast color permitted establishment of a reference framework of GC marker peak quantities to define comparative degrees of peanut roast.

REFERENCES

1. G.S. Fisher, M.G. Legendre, N.V. Lovegren, W.H. Schuller, and J.A. Wells, J. Agric. Food Chem. 27 (1979) 7–11.
2. N.V. Lovegren, C.H. Vinnett, and A.J. St. Angelo, Peanut Sci. 9 (1982) 93–96.
3. H.P. Dupuy, M. Brown, G.S. Fisher, N.V. Lovegren, and A.J. St. Angelo, APRES Peanut Quality Methods Manual. Method QM 1. Amer. Peanut Res. and Educ. Soc., Stillwater, OK, 1983.
4. A.J. St. Angelo, N.V. Lovegren, and C.H. Vinnett, Peanut Sci. 11 (1984) 36–40.
5. S.P. Fore, L.A. Goldblatt, and H.P. Dupuy, J. Am. Peanut Res. Educ. Assoc. 4(1) (1972) 177–185.
6. S.P. Fore, H.P. Dupuy, J.I. Wadsworth, and L.A. Goldblatt, J. Am. Peanut Res. Educ. Assoc. 5(1) (1973) 59–65.

7. S.P. Fore, H.P. Dupuy, and J.I. Wadsworth, Peanut Sci. 3(2) (1976) 86–89.

8. S.P. Fore, G.S. Fisher, M.G Legendre, and J.I. Wadsworth, Peanut Sci. 6 (1979) 58–61.

9. H.P. Dupuy, G.H. Flick, Jr., M.E. Bailey, A.J. St. Angelo, M.G. Legendre, and G. Sumrell, J.Am. Oil Chem. Soc. 62 (1985) 1690–1693.

10. N.V. Lovegren, H.P. Dupuy, J.R. Vercellotti, and T.H. Sanders, Proc. Amer. Peanut Res. and Educ. Soc., 19 (1987) 43.

11. J.R. Vercellotti, N.V. Lovegren, T.H. Sanders, and G.V. Civille, Abstr. 194th Meeting Amer. Chem. Soc. 8 (1987) AGFD 42.

12. J.R. Vercellotti, A.J. St. Angelo, M.G. Legendre, G. Sumrell, H.P.Dupuy, and G.J. Flick, Jr., J. Food Comp. Anal. 1(3) (1988) 239–249.

13. L.L. Buckholz, Jr., H. Daun, E. Stier, and R. Trout, J. Food Sci. 45 (1980) 547–554.

14. L.L. Buckholz, Jr., and H. Daun, in: R. Teranishi and H. Barrera–Benitez (Eds) Quality of Selected Fruits and Vegetables of North America. ACS Symposium Series No. 170. American Chemical Society, Washington, D.C., 1981, pp. 163–181.

15. H. E. Patee and J.A. Singleton, in: R. Teranishi and H. Barrera–Benitez (Eds), Quality of Selected Fruits and Vegetables of North America. ACS Symposium Series No. 170. American Chemical Society, Washington, D.C., 1981 pp. 147–161.

16. H.E. Pattee, J.L. Pearson, C.T. Young, and F.G. Giesbrecht, J. Food Sci. 47 (1982) 455–460.

17. J.S.L. How, Effects of variety, roasting, modified atmosphere packaging, and storage on the chemical composition, headspace volatiles, and flavor profiles of peanuts. Ph.D. North Carolina State University, Raleigh, 1984.

18. T.H. Sanders, J.R. Vercellotti, K.L. Crippen, and G.V. Civille, J. Food Sci. 54 (1989) 475–477.

19. T.H. Sanders, J.R. Vercellotti, P.D. Blankenship, K.L. Crippen, and G.V.Civille, 54 (1989) 1066–1069.

20. C.T. Young and A.R. Hovis, J. Food Sci. 55 (1990) 279–280.

21. J.G. Woodruff, Peanuts. Production, Processing, Products. Third edition. AVIPublishing Co., Westport, CT. (1983) pp. 394–395.

22. P.B. Johnsen, G.V. Civille, J.R. Vercellotti, T.H. Sanders, and C.A. Dus, J. Sensory Studies 3(1) (1988) 9–18.

23. J.G. Woodruff, Peanuts. Production, Processing, Products. Third edition. AVIPublishing Co., Westport, CT. (1983) pp. 394–395.

24. M.G. Legendre, G.S. Fisher, W.H. Schuller, H.P. Dupuy, and E.T. Rayner, J. Am. Oil Chem. Soc. 56 (1979) 552–555.

25. M.L. Brown, D.M. Holbrook, E.F. Hoerning, M.G. Legendre, and A.J. St. Angelo, Poultry Science, 65 (1986) 1925–1233.

26. C.Y.W. Ang and L.L. Young, J. Assoc. Off. Anal. Chem., 72(2) (1989) 277–281.

27. M. Meilgaard, G.V. Civille, and B.T. Carr, Sensory Evaluation Techniques, Vols. I and II. CRC Press, Inc., Boca Raton, FL, 1987.

28. T.H. Sanders, J.R Vercellotti, P.D. Blankenship, and G.V. Civille, Abstr. 194th Meeting Amer. Chem. Soc., AGFD 41 (1987).

29. T.H. Sanders, J.R. Vercellotti, and G.V. Civille, Proc. Amer. Peanut Res. Educ. Soc. 19 (1987) 42.

30. K.L. Crippen, J.R Vercellotti, N.V. Lovegren, and T.H. Sanders, Elsevier, This volume, 1991.

31. W.H. Stahl (Ed.), Odor and taste threshold values data. American Society for Testing and Materials. Data Series 48. Philadelphia, PA., 1973, 250 pp.

32. S. Fors, in: G.R. Waller and M.S. Feather (Eds), The Maillard Reaction in Foods and Nutrition. ACS Symposium Series 215. American Chemical Society, Washington, D.C., 1983, pp. 185–286.

33. N.V. Lovegren, and A.J. St. Angelo, Proc. Amer. Peanut Res. and Educ. Soc. 13 (1981) 102.

34. M.E. Mason, and G.R. Waller, Agr. Food Chem. 12 (1964) 274–278.

35. M.E. Mason, B. Johnson, and M. Hamming, J. Agric. Food Chem. 14 (1966) 454–460.

36. J.P. Walradt, A.O. Pittet, T.E. Kinlin, R. Muralidhara, and R.Sanderson, J. Agric. Food Chem. 19 (1971) 972–979.

37. G.R. Waller, A. Khettry, and C.T. Young, Proc. Amer. Peanut Res. and Educ. Soc. 11 (1979) 16.

38. C.-T. Ho, M.-H. Lee, and S.S. Chang, J. Food Sci. 47(1) (1982) 127–133.

39. E.M. Ahmed and C.T. Young, in: H.E. Pattee and C.T. Young, (Eds), Peanut Science and Technology, American Peanut Research and Education Soc., Yoakum, TX, 1982, p. 655–688.

40. J. A. Newell, M.E. Mason, and R.S Matlock, J. Agric. Food Chem. 15 (1967) 767–772.

41. E. Selke and E.N. Frankel, J. Am. Oil Chem. Soc. 64 (1987) 749–753.

42. P.E. Koehler and G.V. Odell, J. Agric. Food Chem. 18 (1970) 895–898.

43. P.E. Koehler, M.E. Mason, and J.A Newell, J. Agric. Food Chem. 17 (1969) 393–396.

44. T.H. Sanders, and R.L. Green, J. Am. Oil Chem. Soc. 66 (1989) 576–580.

45. H.-D. Belitz and H. Wieser, Food Reviews International, 1 (2) (1985) 271–354.

46. R. Teranishi, R.G. Buttery, and D.G.Guadagni, Annals of the New York Academy of Sciences. 237 (1974) 209–216.

47. R.H. Watkins, "Characterization of Major Sulfur Compounds in Peanut Headspace by Gas Chromatography", M.S. thesis, North Carolina State University (1987), Raleigh, NC

48. R.H. Watkins and C.T. Young, Proceedings of the Am. Peanut Res. and Educ.Soc., 19 (1987) 45.

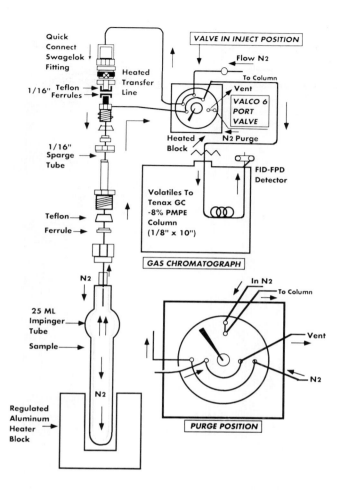

Figure 1. Purge and trap assembly for gas chromatography of flavors.

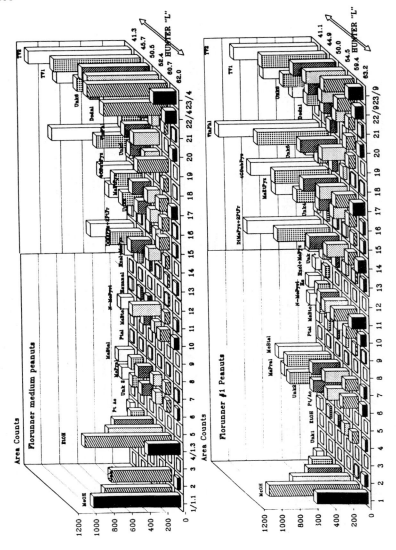

Figures 2a and 2b. Graph of area counts for direct GC peaks with FID at higher temperature (127°C): Degree of roast for medium and #1 Florunner peanuts.

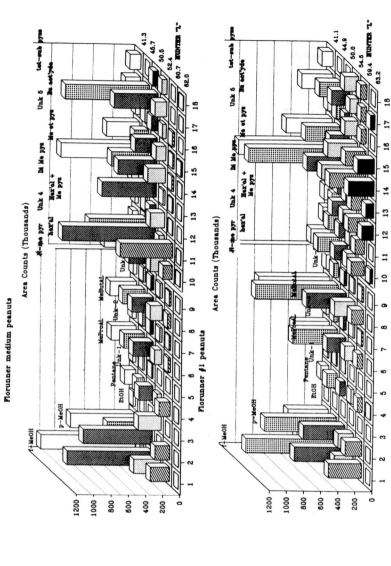

Figures 3a and 3b. Graph of area counts for purge and trap GC with FID at lower temperature (60°C): Degree of roast for medium and #1 Florunner peanuts.

G. Charalambous (Ed.), Food Science and Human Nutrition
1992 Elsevier Science Publishers B.V.

DEFINING ROASTED PEANUT FLAVOR QUALITY. PART 2. CORRELATION OF GC VOLATILES AND SENSORY FLAVOR ATTRIBUTES

K.L. Crippen[1], J.R. Vercellotti[1], N.V. Lovegren[1], and T.H. Sanders[2]

[1]Southern Regional Research Center, USDA, ARS, P.O. Box 19687, New Orleans, LA 70179 (USA)

[2]National Peanut Research Laboratory, USDA, ARS, 1011 Forrester Dr., Dawson, GA 31742 (USA)

SUMMARY

Two lots of florunner peanuts were prepared to varying degrees ranging from raw to very dark roasted (Hunter L values ranging from 60 to 40). Peanut flavor was evaluated using a descriptive flavor analysis panel. First, volatile compounds were monitored using dynamic headspace technique with a packed gas chromatographic column. Volatiles were purged at 60°C and trapped on a room temperature column. Combined flame ionization and flame photometric detectors were used to monitor peaks. Second, peanut volatiles were monitored by direct gas chromatography with a 127°C sample injection port. Several peaks related ($R \geq |0.84|$) with dark roasted and the woody/hulls/skins flavor. No peaks monitored linearly related with the roasted peanutty flavor.

1. INTRODUCTION

As with most food systems, roasted peanut flavor is very complex. Many aspects of production and processing, such as peanut maturity and post-harvest curing conditions (1), (2) can affect peanut flavor quality. Freeze damage to windrow peanuts has a detrimental effect on flavor (3). A sensory panel can perceive these flavors and evaluate the intensities, but it is difficult to make precise instrumental measurements of flavor quality. Research has demonstrated that high concentrations of volatiles indicate poor peanut quality (4), (5), (6), (7).

Some research has been done to relate specific chemical compounds to peanut flavors or off-flavor development processes. Pattee et al. (8) have related hexanal and pentane to raw peanut flavor. Brown et al. (9) indicated that volatile components such as ethanol, pentane, pentanal, and hexanal are associated with lipid oxidation. Clark and Nursten (10) reported the sensory characteristics of 2-nonenal to be peanutty and 2-ethyl-3-methylpyrazine was described as nutty/roasted. Fischer and Grosch (11) identified the legume-like flavor with a combination of γ-butyrolactone, benzaldehyde, indene, 2–methoxy–3–isopropylpyrazine, nonanal, benzyl alcohol, and alkyl–substituted benzenes. If the compounds that contribute to a flavor can be identified, then the precursor compounds and the path of development may potentially be identified.

Research relating descriptive sensory flavor characteristics of peanuts to chemical compounds is limited. Buckholz et al. (12) correlated GC volatiles of peanuts with hedonic ratings. It was found that the peak identified as pentanal had a negative correlation coefficient (R) with flavor preference. The peak identified as 2–ethyl–6–methylpyrazine correlated positively with flavor preference. The sensory methods utilized yielded little information about the flavor characteristics of roasted peanuts. Therefore, the conclusions from the correlations can not readily be interpreted.

The present investigation utilizes descriptive sensory flavor data from peanuts roasted to varying degrees and relates individual flavor characteristics to gas chromatographic peanut volatile peaks.

2. MATERIALS AND METHODS

2.1 Peanut samples

Two different lots of peanuts were used for this experiment. One was medium grade size ($\geq$ 7.15mm < 8.3mm diameter) florunner peanuts from a field in southwestern Georgia and the other was # 1 grade size ($\geq$ 5.95mm < 7.14mm diameter) florunner peanuts from a separate Southwestern Georgia field.

The peanuts were roasted in a surface combustion roaster as described by Johnsen et al. (13). Peanut paste was prepared according to Sanders et al. (2). Roast color was measured on peanut pastes with a Hunter Lab Color meter and only the L value was used. The range was from raw (L value=62) to very dark roasted (L value=45). Six different roast levels were made from each lot of peanuts.

2.2 Color Measurement

Peanut paste samples were placed on a 25 x 75 mm microscope slide using as a form a 6 x 25 mm o.d. polyethylene ring, made by cutting out the center of a plastic snap cap from a sample vial. The diameter of the ring on the microscope slide made a circular exposure of peanut paste to the colorimeter source with adequate width to cover the light aperture and register intensiity. After standardizing and reading the black and white color plates with the Hunterlab D 25–PC2A colorimeter according to operating procedures, the peanut paste was measured five times for the L, a, and b color values. Five L value readings were then averaged. Each of the raw and roasted peanut paste samples were similarly treated and the data used as a measure of roast color.

2.3 Sensory Methods

Descriptive flavor analysis methods were used to quantify the intensities of defined peanut flavor terms (1) (13). The 12 panelists were trained in descriptive flavor analysis according to Meilgaard et al., (14). The flavor characteristics evaluated by the panel were roasted peanutty (RPT), sweet aromatic (SAC), raw/beany (RBN), astringent (AST), sweet (SWT), woody/hulls/skins (WHS), dark roasted (DRT) and bitter (BTR). Intensity of peanut flavor characteristics were evaluated using a 15–point universal intensity scale (14). The samples were presented to panelists in plastic 1 oz. cups labeled with 3–digit random numbers. Red lighting was utilized in the evaluation room to mask the peanut paste color. Samples were presented in random order and all degrees of roast within a commercial size were presented at one session to facilitate comparison between roasts. Two repeated measures (presentation) of each sample were presented to the panel alternating sessions between the two lots of peanuts.

2.4 Gas Chromatographic Methods

Two different gas chromatographic methods as described below were used to measure peanut volatiles. One method utilized low temperature sparging (60°C) with flame ionization and flame photometric detectors. The other GC method purged volatiles at 127°C and was equipped with a flame ionization detector.

TABLE 1

Peaks (compounds) and retention times monitored with the low temperature GC method and the FID detector.

Peak No.	Compound	Retention Time[1]
1	free methanol[2]	21.8
2	produced methanol[3]	31.9
3	ethanol	40.0
4	pentane	43.4
5	unknown 1	45.8
6	methylpropanal	47.5
7	unknown 2	50.1
8	methylbutanal	53.8
9	unknown 3	55.8
10	N-methylpyrrole	58.6
11	hexanal	60.9
12	unknown 4	62.4
13	hexanol/methylpyrazine	63.6
14	dimethylpyrazine	67.4
15	methylethylpyrazine	71.1
16	unknown 5	72.5
17	benzeneacetaldehyde	73.5
18	4-C substituted pyrazine	74.9

[1] retention time is from the start of collection of volatiles at ambient temperature
[2] methanol that is inherent in the peanut
[3] methanol produced in the sample by drying in the inlet and is related to moisture content

2.4.1 Low Temperature FID and FPD GC. Peanut paste (1.25 g) on the walls of a screw-top conical test tube placed within a regulated heating block was purged for 30 min at 60°C with nitrogen carrier gas. A closed loop device with an injection valve was made to concentrate the peanut volatiles at moderate temperatures (15) (16). Volatiles were concentrated at ambient temperature onto a Tenax GC-8% polymetaphenylether (PMPE) column. After temperature programming, a combined flame ionization detector (FID) and flame photometric detector (FPD) permitted simultaneous detection of typical FID active volatiles and the FPD, sulfur containing compounds. Eighteen FID active compounds and sixteen FPD active compounds were routinely monitored (16). Low volatilization temperatures were used to simulate volatile compound release similar to occurrences in the mouth. The peaks monitored are found in **Table 1** and **2** in the order of shortest to longest retention times.

TABLE 2

Peaks (compounds) and retention times monitored with the low temperature GC method and the FPD detector.

Peak No.	Compound	Retention time[1]
1	hydrogen sulfide	10.0-26.5
2	unknown 8	31.8
3	methanethiol	34.5
4	dimethylsulfide	43.9
5	carbondisulfide/unknown 9	46.8
6	unknown 10	51.6
7	propanethiol	54.3
8	diethylsulfide	56.1
9	dimethyldisulfide	58.5
10	unknown 11	64.3
11	unknown 12	65.4
12	unknown 13	66.7
13	unknown 14	68.7
14	unknown 15	70.3
15	unknown 16	73.0
16	unknown 17	75.4

[1]Retention time is from the start of collection of volatiles at ambient temperatures

2.4.2 High Temperature FID GC. The volatiles were eluted from 0.50 g of peanut paste distributed on the walls of a sample tube in the injection port at 127°C and absorbed at ambient temperature onto a Tenax GC-8% PMPE column for 28 min. After sample collection, the column was temperature programmed according to Lovegren et al. (7) for chromatographic analysis. This higher temperature method results in increased volatilization of compounds and higher peak area counts (6), (17), (18). The identification of volatile compounds monitored in this experiment was accomplished by Fore et al. (19). Peak compound names are found in **Table 3**. Only the major compound was listed in the tables for each GC peak.

2.4.3 Gas Chromatographic Sample Preparation.

Peanut paste was placed in a disposable plastic syringe fitted with a 15 gauge stainless steel syringe needle, 10 cm long with 90 degree flat end (16). For the two GC methods the peanut paste was deposited on the inside wall of a sample tube or conical test tube. Respectively, these tubes were placed in the GC inlet in the high temperature method and in a heating block in the low temperature method (16).

2.5 Analysis of Data

The intensities of individual flavor attributes and the area counts of individual peaks were plotted against the roast color (L value) (20). Correlation coefficients (R) and the linear equations were determined. The FPD or sulfur data were plotted on a log to log scale because of the nonlinearity of the detector. All of the peaks, and all the flavor attributes were sorted based on the shape and direction of the curve. For example when the plot was a straight line with a negative slope it was grouped with plots with similar equations. Peaks of a certain curve shape and direction were regressed on the flavor attributes with similar direction and curve. For sulfur compounds the flavor intensity was regressed on log (peak areas). Only those correlations with $R \geq |0.84|$ were included in this report.

TABLE 3

Peaks (compounds) and retention times monitored with the high temperature GC method and the FID detector[1].

Peak No.	Compound	Retention Time[2]
1	free methanol[3]	6.7
2	produced methanol[4]	8.4
3	ethanol	15.5
4	pentane/acetone	19.5-21.6
5	unknown 1	23.5
6	methylpropanal	24.8
7	methylbutanal	31.1
8	pentanal	33.2
9	methylbutanol	34.3
10	N-methylpyrrole	36.0
11	hexanal	38.2
12	unknown 4	39.6
13	hexanol/methylpyrazine	40.9
14	dimethylpyrazine	44.5
15	2-pentylfuran	45.6
16	methylethylpyrazine	48.1
17	4-C substituted pyrazine	49.8-51.9
18	unknown 6	54.1-55.9
19	vinylphenol	57.1
20	decadienal	57.8
21	unknown 7	60.0

[1]Adapted from Fore et al., 1979
[2]retention time is from the start of the temperature program
[3]methanol that is inherent in the peanut
[4]methanol produced in the sample by drying in the inlet and is related to moisture content

3. RESULTS

3.1 Flavor vs. Roast

Raw/beany and dark roasted flavors had strong linear correlations with roast color in both the medium and the #1 size peanuts. As degree of roast increased (L value decreased), intensity of dark roasted flavor increased and raw/beany flavor intensity decreased (**Fig. 1a** and **1b**). Roasted peanutty flavor and sweet aromatic flavor had non-linear trends with maximum intensities in medium roasted peanuts (L value~50), and lower intensities in under roasted and over roasted peanuts. **Figure 2** displays this trend for roasted peanutty. The mediums displayed a higher intensity roasted peanutty flavor than the #1's. Sweet taste showed the same trend as roasted peanutty and sweet aromatic flavor. Darker roasted peanuts tended to have more intense bitter taste. The increase was linear in the #1 size peanuts; however, in the medium size peanuts, low correlation coefficients (R) indicated a lack of linearity. In both lots very dark roasted peanuts had more intense bitter flavor than did the raw and under roasted samples.

3.2 FID Detector Peak Compounds vs. Dark Roasted Flavor

Methylpropanal, methylbutanal, dimethylpyrazine and methylethylpyrazine linearly related with dark roasted flavor ($R \geq |0.84|$) in both the medium and #1 size peanuts using both GC methods (**Table 4**). Slopes and intercepts varied with peanut source and GC method. Differences in slopes denote that for the same change in area counts of the peak, the change in specific flavor intensity was higher in samples with steeper slopes (i.e., higher number). In the high temperature method, medium size peanuts had steeper slopes for these compounds than #1's. Intercepts for methylpropanal, methylbutanal and methylethylpyrazine were higher for #1's than mediums (**Table 4**). For dimethylpyrazine in the high temperature method, the medium and #1 size peanuts had similar intercepts, but different slopes. In the low temperature method methylbutanal and methylethylpyrazine had higher intercepts and steeper slopes for the medium size peanuts than for the #1 size peanuts. The intercept represents the intensity of dark roasted flavor at the GC's 0 area counts level. The high temperature data for these compounds fit dark roasted flavor intensity consistently better (R) than the low temperature data. This is probably due to higher concentrations being driven off at higher purging temperatures which reduces the amount of fluctuations of the monitoring of these compounds. Methylpropanal results for the low temperature method had similar slopes and intercept patterns as in the high temperature GC method (**Table 4**). Methylpyrazine/hexanal peak (both mediums and #1's) measured by the high temperature method linearly related with dark roasted flavor, and had slope and intercept trends similar to dimethylpyrazine (**Table 4**). Using the low temperature method the medium size peanuts correlated well, but the #1's did not. The noncorrelation of the #1's with dark roasted flavor was probably due to interference from the rich mixture of hexanal, methylpyrazine, and perhaps other unseparated compounds that occur in this peak. Taking out possible outliers did not cause this line to conform to the linear patterns of the mediums or high temperature #1's.

TABLE 4

Correlation between flavor and FID active chemical compounds in GC peaks.

Flavor	Compound	GC Method	Peanut Source	|R|	Intercept	Slope
DRT[1]	methylpropanal	low temp	medium	0.94	0.49	1.1×10^{-5}**
DRT	methylpropanal	low temp	#1's	0.89	0.88	7.1×10^{-6}*
DRT	methylpropanal	high temp	medium	0.95	-0.72	1.3×10^{-4}**
DRT	methylpropanal	high temp	#1's	0.94	-0.31	3.9×10^{-5}**
DRT	methylbutanal	low temp	medium	0.95	0.26	1.0×10^{-5}*
DRT	methylbutanal	low temp	#1's	0.92	0.76	3.9×10^{-6}**
DRT	methylbutanal	high temp	medium	0.93	-0.41	9.9×10^{-5}**
DRT	methylbutanal	high temp	#1's	0.96	-0.04	3.4×10^{-5}
DRT	methylpyrazine/hex-al	low temp	medium	0.91	0.19	6.2×10^{-5}*
DRT	methylpyrazine/hex-al	low temp	#1's	0.41	4.76	-1.9×10^{-5}
DRT	methylpyrazine/hex-al	high temp	medium	0.85	0.46	2.0×10^{-4}*
DRT	methylpyrazine/hex-al	high temp	#1's	0.88	0.44	1.3×10^{-4}*
DRT	dimethylpyrazine	low temp	medium	0.93	0.81	5.4×10^{-6}**
DRT	dimethylpyrazine	low temp	#1's	0.92	-0.24	4.3×10^{-6}*
DRT	dimethylpyrazine	high temp	medium	0.98	0.47	4.2×10^{-5}**
DRT	dimethylpyrazine	high temp	#1's	0.96	0.54	2.1×10^{-5}**
DRT	methylethylpyrazine	low temp	medium	0.88	0.70	1.2×10^{-5}*
DRT	methylethylpyrazine	low temp	#1's	0.91	-1.26	1.1×10^{-5}*
DRT	methylethylpyrazine	high temp	medium	0.99	-0.22	8.6×10^{-5}**
DRT	methylethylpyrazine	high temp	#1's	0.98	0.46	3.6×10^{-5}**
DRT	4-C sub. pyrazine	low temp	medium	0.64	1.64	2.4×10^{-5}
DRT	4-C sub. pyrazine	low temp	#1's	0.30	2.06	6.6×10^{-6}
DRT	4-C sub. pyrazine	high temp	medium	0.97	-0.53	6.9×10^{-5}**
DRT	4-C sub. pyrazine	high temp	#1's	0.98	-0.23	2.7×10^{-5}**
DRT	N-methylpyrrole	low temp	medium	0.95	-0.77×10^{-3}	1.3×10^{-5}**
DRT	N-methylpyrrole	low temp	#1's	0.90	-0.43	1.9×10^{-5}*
DRT	N-methylpyrrole	high temp	medium	0.78	-1.78	1.6×10^{-4}
DRT	N-methylpyrrole	high temp	#1's	0.74	-3.11	1.9×10^{-4}
DRT	benzeneacetaldehyde	low temp	medium	0.86	0.82	2.4×10^{-5}*
DRT	benzeneacetaldehyde	low temp	#1's	0.94	0.27	1.3×10^{-5}**
DRT	benzeneacetaldehyde	high temp	medium	--	--	--
DRT	benzeneacetaldehyde	high temp	#1's	--	--	--
DRT	vinylphenol	low temp	medium	--	--	--
DRT	vinylphenol	low temp	#1's	--	--	--
DRT	vinylphenol	high temp	medium	0.86	0.71	2.2×10^{-5}*
DRT	vinylphenol	high temp	#1's	0.97	0.87*	1.4×10^{-5}**
DRT	unknown 1	low temp	medium	0.89	1.10	8.9×10^{-5}*
DRT	unknown 1	low temp	#1's	0.88	1.20	1.9×10^{-4}*
DRT	unknown 1	high temp	medium	0.92	1.16**	2.7×10^{-3}*
DRT	unknown 1	high temp	#1's	0.81	1.69*	2.4×10^{-4}*
DRT	unknown 2	low temp	medium	0.87	0.02	7.2×10^{-5}*
DRT	unknown 2	low temp	#1's	0.87	0.01	8.1×10^{-5}*
DRT	unknown 2	high temp	medium	--	--	--
DRT	unknown 2	high temp	#1's	--	--	--
DRT	unknown 3	low temp	medium	0.84	-0.13	7.9×10^{-5}*
DRT	unknown 3	low temp	#1's	0.90	0.33	7.1×10^{-5}*
DRT	unknown 3	high temp	medium	--	--	--
DRT	unknown 3	high temp	#1's	--	--	--
DRT	unknown 7	low temp	medium	--	--	--
DRT	unknown 7	low temp	#1's	--	--	--
DRT	unknown 7	high temp	medium	0.99	-0.19	1.2×10^{-4}**
DRT	unknown 7	high temp	#1's	0.99	0.10	6.5×10^{-5}**

[1]DRT = dark roasted flavor

TABLE 4 (continued)

Correlation between flavor and FID active chemical compounds in GC peaks.

Flavor	Compound	GC Method	Peanut Source	$|R|$	Intercept	Slope
WHS[2]	methylbutanal	low temp	medium	0.85	1.49**	2.5×10^{-6}*
WHS	methylbutanal	low temp	#1's	0.71	1.63	7.4×10^{-7}**
WHS	methylbutanal	high temp	medium	0.85	1.32**	2.3×10^{-5}*
WHS	methylbutanal	high temp	#1's	0.79	0.62	6.9×10^{-6}*
WHS	unknown 3	low temp	medium	0.84	1.33**	2.1×10^{-5}*
WHS	unknown 3	low temp	#1's	0.84	1.46	1.6×10^{-5}*
WHS	unknown 3	high temp	medium	--	--	--
WHS	unknown 3	high temp	#1's	--	--	--
WHS	unknown 2	low temp	medium	0.82	0.62**	4.9×10^{-6}*
WHS	unknown 2	low temp	#1's	0.87	1.34**	2.1×10^{-5}*
WHS	unknown 2	high temp	medium	--	--	--
WHS	unknown 2	high temp	#1's	--	--	--
WHS	methylpropanal	low temp	medium	0.82	1.55**	2.4×10^{-6}*
WHS	methylpropanal	low temp	#1's	0.69	1.65**	1.4×10^{-6}
WHS	methylpropanal	high temp	medium	0.85	1.25**	3.1×10^{-5}*
WHS	methylpropanal	high temp	#1's	0.82	1.35**	8.5×10^{-6}
WHS	methylethylpyrazine	low temp	medium	0.71	1.63**	2.6×10^{-6}
WHS	methylethylpyrazine	low temp	#1's	0.57	1.38*	1.8×10^{-6}
WHS	methylethylpyrazine	high temp	medium	0.95	1.34**	2.1×10^{-5}**
WHS	methylethylpyrazine	high temp	#1's	0.65	1.62**	5.8×10^{-6}
WHS	4-C sub. pyrazine	low temp	medium	0.46	1.85*	4.5×10^{-6}
WHS	4-C sub. pyrazine	low temp	#1's	0.28	1.86*	1.5×10^{-6}
WHS	4-C sub. pyrazine	high temp	medium	0.89	1.29**	1.7×10^{-5}*
WHS	4-C sub. pyrazine	high temp	#1's	0.66	1.50**	4.4×10^{-6}
WHS	N-methylpyrrole	low temp	medium	0.88	1.41**	3.2×10^{-6}*
WHS	N-methylpyrrole	low temp	#1's	0.88	1.26**	4.5×10^{-6}*
WHS	N-methylpyrrole	high temp	medium	0.84	0.82	4.4×10^{-5}*
WHS	N-methylpyrrole	high temp	#1's	0.91	0.27	5.9×10^{-5}*
WHS	vinylphenol	low temp	medium	--	--	--
WHS	vinylphenol	low temp	#1's	--	--	--
WHS	vinylphenol	high temp	medium	0.85	1.55**	5.7×10^{-6}*
WHS	vinylphenol	high temp	#1's	0.62	1.70**	2.2×10^{-6}
WHS	unknown 7	low temp	medium	--	--	--
WHS	unknown 7	low temp	#1's	--	--	--
WHS	unknown 7	high temp	medium	0.92	1.36**	2.9×10^{-5}**
WHS	unknown 7	high temp	#1's	0.70	1.54**	1.1×10^{-5}
WHS	dimethyldisulfide	FPD	medium	0.87	0.69	0.24*
WHS	dimethyldisulfide	FPD	#1's	0.65	0.59	0.27
RBN	free methanol	low temp	medium	0.62	3.52**	-1.6×10^{-6}
RBN	free methanol	low temp	#1's	0.66	3.88*	-2.8×10^{-6}
RBN	free methanol	high temp	medium	0.93	1.80**	-1.0×10^{-5}**
RBN	free methanol	high temp	#1's	0.67	1.15	-1.2×10^{-5}
RBN	produced methanol	low temp	medium	0.75	3.78**	-2.6×10^{-6}
RBN	produced methanol	low temp	#1's	0.81	4.16**	-4.1×10^{-6}*
RBN	produced methanol	high temp	medium	0.79	2.11*	-2.8×10^{-4}
RBN	produced methanol	high temp	#1's	0.90	1.90**	-3.0×10^{-4}*
RBN	ethanol	low temp	medium	0.10	2.72*	-7.4×10^{-7}
RBN	ethanol	low temp	#1's	0.00	2.66	-0.0
RBN	ethanol	high temp	medium	0.69	2.25*	-1.2×10^{-3}
RBN	ethanol	high temp	#1's	0.87	1.82*	-3.0×10^{-3}*

*, ** parameter was significantly different than zero at $\alpha \leq 0.05$ and 0.01, respectively based on t-test.
[2]WHS = woody/hulls/skins flavor, RBN = raw/beany flavor

The compounds included in the 4-C substituted pyrazines peak correlated well with dark roasted flavor when the high temperature GC method was used but not with the low temperature method (**Table 4**). In the high temperature GC/flavor data correlations the intercept was greater in the #1's and the slope was steeper in the mediums. Further separation of this peak into its component compounds may yield better relationships and enhance understanding of flavor compound formation and influence on roasted flavor.

The GC data collected at the high temperature for N–methylpyrrole did not correlate as well with dark roasted flavor as the low temperature method (**Table 4**). The trend in both low and high temperature data sets was an increase in dark roasted flavor with an increase in N–methylpyrrole.

Benzeneacetaldehyde was not monitored with the high temperature GC method, but had good correlations with dark roasted flavor in the low temperature method (**Table 4**). The mediums had a higher intercept and steeper slope than the #1's. The #1's had a higher correlation coefficient than the mediums due to one GC point in the medium peanut data being out of sequence. Benzeneacetaldehyde has a sweet aroma, and it's contribution to dark roasted flavor is still under investigation.

Vinylphenol, monitored in the high temperature GC data only, correlated well with dark roasted flavor (**Table 4**). The mediums had a lower intercept and a steeper slope than the #1's. The mediums also had a higher correlation coefficient than the #1's. Vinylphenol has a characteristic phenolic/plastic aroma and its actual contribution to dark roasted flavor is not known.

Unknown 1 correlated highly (R > |0.84|) with dark roasted flavor in both GC methods (**Table 4**). In the low temperature method unknown 1 was not detected by the GC detector until the peanuts reached a medium roast (L value≈50). In the high temperature method there was a slight increase in peak area counts between the raw and the under roasted samples, but the increase between medium roasted and over roasted was much greater. Concurrently the sensory panel intensity scores for dark roasted flavor increased from raw peanuts to very over roasted peanuts. In the correlation between the flavor and GC data the slope was steeper and the intercept was higher in the #1 size peanuts than the medium size peanuts for both GC methods. The high temperature method resulted in higher intercepts and steeper slopes than the low temperature method. This is probably due to variations between methods in sample weight and purging temperature. Unknown 2 was monitored in the low temperature GC method only (**Table 4**). It correlated well with dark roasted flavor for both the medium and #1 size peanuts. The intercept was not different between the two peanut sizes and the slope was steeper in the #1's. Unknown 3 was monitored in the low temperature GC method only (**Table 4**). The intercept was higher in the #1's and the slopes in both size peanuts were not different. Unknown 7 was monitored in the high temperature method only (**Table 4**). The correlations with dark roasted flavor were very high for both the mediums and the #1's (i.e., R=0.99). The intercept was lower and the slope was steeper in the medium size peanuts. More work is needed to determine the chemical makeup of these peaks and their relationship to dark roasted flavor.

3.3 FPD Detector Peak Compounds vs. Dark Roasted Flavor

Methanethiol, carbondisulfide/unknown 9, propanethiol, diethylsulfide, dimethyldisulfide and unknowns 12, 13, 14, and 15 correlated highly with dark roasted flavor in both #1's and mediums (**Table 5**). None of these compounds have aromas that resemble dark roasted flavor based on sniffer port work done at SRRC, New Orleans, LA (21). They may be only by–products of reactions that take place during roasting and thus have high correlations with degree of roast (22), (23), (24), (25), (26).

Two unknowns, 8 and 10 correlate highly with dark roasted flavor in the medium size peanuts, but not with #1 size peanuts (**Table 5**). Unknown 16 correlated highly with dark roasted flavor in the #1 size peanuts but not in the mediums. Even though high correlations exist, in some cases it is likely that these compounds are not contributors to roasted flavors.

TABLE 5

Correlation between flavor and FPD active chemical compounds in GC peaks.

Flavor	Compound	GC Method	Peanut Source	$|R|$	Intercept	Slope
DRT[1]	methanethiol	FPD	medium	0.92	-2.46	0.88*
DRT	methanethiol	FPD	#1's	0.84	-4.08	1.3*
DRT	carbondisulfide/unk 9	FPD	medium	0.90	-2.64	1.2*
DRT	carbondisulfide/unk 9	FPD	#1's	0.94	-8.35*	2.5**
DRT	propanethiol	FPD	medium	0.96	-3.75*	1.6**
DRT	propanethiol	FPD	#1's	0.96	-4.83*	2.0**
DRT	diethylsulfide	FPD	medium	0.93	-4.08*	1.8**
DRT	diethylsulfide	FPD	#1's	0.85	-3.82	2.0*
DRT	dimethyldisulfide	FPD	medium	0.85	-2.49	0.9*
DRT	dimethyldisulfide	FPD	#1's	0.93	-5.45*	1.5**
DRT	unknown 12	FPD	medium	0.87	-3.64	1.7*
DRT	unknown 12	FPD	#1's	0.88	-4.84	2.4*
DRT	unknown 13	FPD	medium	0.85	-4.09	1.9*
DRT	unknown 13	FPD	#1's	0.88	-4.68	2.3*
DRT	unknown 14	FPD	medium	0.89	-2.43	1.3
DRT	unknown 14	FPD	#1's	0.89	-2.26	1.3*
DRT	unknown 15	FPD	medium	0.92	-2.83	1.2*
DRT	unknown 15	FPD	#1's	0.97	-3.73**	1.5**
DRT	unknown 8	FPD	medium	0.91	-3.80	1.3**
DRT	unknown 8	FPD	#1's	0.75	-2.81	1.1
DRT	unknown 10	FPD	medium	0.87	-4.55	2.0*
DRT	unknown 10	FPD	#1's	0.78	-5.27	2.3
DRT	unknown 16	FPD	medium	0.62	-1.52	1.1
DRT	unknown 16	FPD	#1's	0.84	-2.67	1.6*
WHS	methanethiol	FPD	medium	0.90	0.75	0.22*
WHS	methanethiol	FPD	#1's	0.97	0.86	0.36**
WHS	unknown 8	FPD	medium	0.94	0.31	0.34**
WHS	unknown 8	FPD	#1's	0.94	0.32	0.35**
WHS	dimethylsulfide	FPD	medium	0.79	0.89	0.22
WHS	dimethylsulfide	FPD	#1's	0.93	-2.93*	0.98**
WHS	propanethiol	FPD	medium	0.85	0.57	0.36*
WHS	propanethiol	FPD	#1's	0.73	0.59	0.38

*, ** parameter was significantly different than zero at $\alpha \leq 0.05$ and 0.01, respectively based on t-test.

[1]DRT = dark roasted flavor, WHS = woody/hulls/skins flavor, RBN = raw/beany flavor

3.4 FID Detector Peak Compounds vs. Woody/Hulls/Skins

N–methylpyrrole correlated well with woody/hulls/skins flavor in both the mediums and the #1's using both the high and low temperature GC methods (**Table 4**). N–methylpyrrole does not smell like wood, hulls, or skins, so the significance of the relationship is not obvious.

Methylbutanal correlated highly with woody/hulls/skins in the mediums using both GC methods, but did not correlate well in the #1's (**Table 4**). This indicated that methylbutanal was not a major individual contributing compound to woody/hulls/skins.

Unknown 3 correlated highly with woody/hulls/skins in both mediums and #1's for the low temperature GC method (**Table 4**). It was not monitored in the high temperature method. Unknown 2 correlated well with woody/hulls/skins in the #1's but in the mediums the correlation coefficient was 0.82 or below the 0.84 cutoff (**Table 4**). It was not monitored in the low temperature GC method. The compounds correlating with woody/hulls/skins flavor also correlated with dark roasted flavor. Further investigations are needed to differentiate between the compounds contributing to woody/hulls/skins and dark roasted flavors.

3.5 FPD Detector Peak Compounds vs. Woody/Hulls/Skins

Woody/hulls/skins correlated well with methanethiol and unknown 8 in both sizes of peanuts (**Table 5**). Neither of these compounds smell like wood, hulls or skins. Dimethylsulfide correlated with woody/hulls/skins in the #1 size peanuts but not in the mediums (**Table 5**). Propanethiol and dimethyldisulfide correlate well with woody/hulls/skins in the mediums, but not in the #1's (**Table 5**).

3.6 FID Detector Peak Compounds vs. Raw/Beany

Raw/beany correlates well with (free) methanol in the mediums but not in the #1's (**Table 4**). Methanol (produced by drying the peanut sample in the inlet) and ethanol correlate well with raw/beany in the #1's, but not in the mediums (**Table 4**). No monitored sulfur containing compounds correlated with raw/beany.

4. DISCUSSION

Roasted peanutty and sweet aromatic flavors did not correlate with any of the peaks monitored. GC techniques, instruments and detectors have limits and many compounds go undetected even in application of current technology. The peanutty and sweet aromatic flavors probably involve combinations of compounds and probably involve coupounds not detected by the methods employed in this investigation. These flavors are complex and single volatiles do not necessarily define sensory flavor characteristics.

These GC methods utilize packed columns, which are appropriate for quality comparison purposes on raw peanuts or roasted peanuts, and have been quite useful for identifying peanuts with flavor problems. They are particularly useful in identifying lipid oxidation compounds (hexanal, hexanol, pentane), fermentation products due to freeze damage or improper drying procedures (excess ethanol, acetaldehyde) and deviations from normal volatile profiles (excess total volatiles or an abundance of certain individual peaks in good volatile profiles) for raw peanuts or peanut butter which indicate problems (5),(16), (27). These packed column procedures fail to detect or separate the many minor peaks found with various capillary column procedures. Minor compounds or combinations of minor compounds may be major contributors to some flavors.

This experiment utilized discriptive sensory flavor analysis to identify intensities of the two distinct flavors, roasted peanutty, and dark roasted. This helped us understand that many compounds previously related to roasted flavor were really related to dark roasted flavor and not roasted peanutty flavor. Roasted peanutty flavor is still a mystery.

5. CONCLUSIONS

The pyrazines and some other compounds, such as methylbutanal and methylpropanal correlate highly with dark roasted flavor. Woody/hulls/skins correlated highly with N-methlypyrrole. Several sulfur compounds related to dark roasted flavor, but their characteristic aromas were not reminiscent of dark roasted peanuts.

Roasted peanutty and sweet aromatic (two desirable flavors in peanuts) did not correlate with peaks obtained as markers in these gas chromatographic methods. These flavors are very complicated, and observation of relationships among them and the 34 peaks detected was likely complicated by the lack of detection of compounds critical to flavor expression, or the combinations of compounds that produce specific flavors.

ACKNOWLEDGEMENTS

The authors thank Peter Johnsen, Bryan Vinyard, Brenda Lyon and James How for their reviewer comments and suggestions to improved the manuscript. They extend appreciation to Bryan Vinyard for statistical consultation.

REFERENCES

1 T.H. Sanders, J.R. Vercellotti, K.L. Crippen, and G.V. Civille, J. Food Sci., 54 (1989) 475–477.

2 T.H. Sanders, J.R. Vercellotti, P.D. Blankenship, K.L. Crippen, and G.V.Civille, J. Food Sci., 54 (1989) 1066–1069.

3 K.L. Crippen, J.R. Vercellotti, J.L. Butler, E.J. Williams, E.S. Wright, and D.M. Porter, Unpublished data. U.S.D.A.–A.R.S., Southern Regional Research Center, New Orleans, LA (1989).

4 H.E. Pattee, E.O. Beasley, and J.A. Singleton, J. Food Sci., 30 (1965) 388–392.

5 C.T. Young and A.R. Hovis, J.Food Sci. 55(1990) 279–280.

6 A.J. St. Angelo, N.V. Lovegren, and C.H. Vinnett, Peanut Sci., 11 (1984) 36–40.

7 N.V. Lovegren, C.H. Vinnett, and A.J. St. Angelo, Peanut Sci., 9 (1982) 93–96.

8 H.E. Pattee, J.A. Singleton, and W.Y. Cobb, J. Food Sci., 34 (1969) 625–627.

9 M.L. Brown, J.I. Wadsworth, H.P. Dupuy, and R.W. Mozingo, Peanut Sci., 4 (1977) 54–56.

10 R.G. Clark and H.E. Nursten, IFFA, 8 (1977) 197–201.

11 K.H. Fischer and W. Grosch, in: P. Schreier (Ed.), Flavour '81, Weurman Symposium, 3rd edition, Walter de Gruyter, New York, NY (1981) p. 195–201.

12 L.L. Buckholz, Jr., H. Daun, E. Stier, and R. Trout, J. Food Sci., 45 (1980) 547–554.

13 P.B. Johnsen, G.V. Civille, J.R. Vercellotti, T.H. Sanders, and C.A. Dus, J. Sensory Studies, 3 (1988) 9–18.

14 M. Meilgaard, G.V. Civille, and B.T. Carr, Sensory Evaluation Techniques, Vols. I and II. CRC Press, Inc., Boca Raton, FL, 1987.

15 M.L. Brown, M. Holbrook, E.F. Hoerning, M.G. Legendre, and A.J. St. Angelo, Poultry Sci. 65 (1986) 1925–1933.

16 J.R. Vercellotti, K.L. Crippen, N.V. Lovegren, and T.H. Sanders, Elsevier, This volume, 1991.

17 H.P. Dupuy, M.L. Brown, G.S. Fisher, N.V. Lovegren, and A.J. St. Angelo, "Quality Methods", C.T. Young (Ed.), Amer. Peanut Res. Educ. Soc., Inc. Stillwater, OK, QM 1 (1983).

18 N.V. Lovegren, H.P. Dupuy, and J.R. Vercellotti, Proc. Amer. Peanut Res. Educ. Soc., 19 (1987) 43.

19 S.P. Fore, G.S. Fisher, M.G. Legendre, and J.I. Wadsworth, Peanut Sci., 6 (1979) 58–61.

20 SAS/STAT User's Guide. SAS Institute, Inc., Cary, NC, 1988.

21 K.L. Crippen and J.R. Vercellotti, Unpublished data on correlation of sensory peanut flavor and G.C. data. U.S.D.A.–A.R.S., Southern Regional Research Center, New Orleans, LA (1990).

22 C.T. Young and K.T. Holley. "Comparison of peanut varieties in storage and roasting", Ga. Agric. Expt. Station, Bull. No. 41 (1965) p. 7.

23 J.P. Walradt, A.O. Pittet, T.E. Kinlin, R. Muralidhara, and R. Sanderson, J. Agric. Food Chem., 19 (1971) 972–979.

24 M.H. Lee, C.T. Ho, and S.S. Chang, J. Agric. Food Chem., 29 (1981) 684–686.

25 C.T. Ho and Q.Z. Jin, Lebensm.–Wiss. U. –Technol., 15 (1982) 366–367.

26 R.H. Watkins, "Characterization of Major Sulfur Compounds in Peanut Headspace by Gas Chromatography", M.S. thesis, North Carolina State University (1987), Raleigh, NC.

27 J.A. Singleton and H.E. Pattee, J. Food Sci., 52 (1987) 242–244.

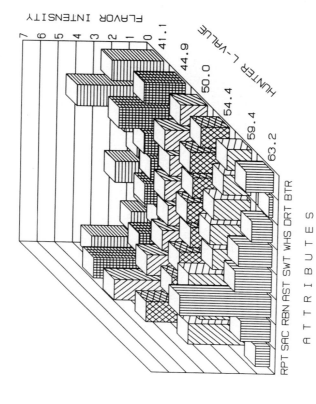

Figure 1a. Mean flavor intensity across the degrees of roast for the medium size peanuts.

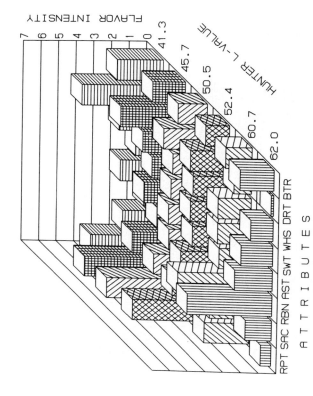

Figure 1b. Mean flavor intensity across the degrees of roast for the #1 size peanuts.

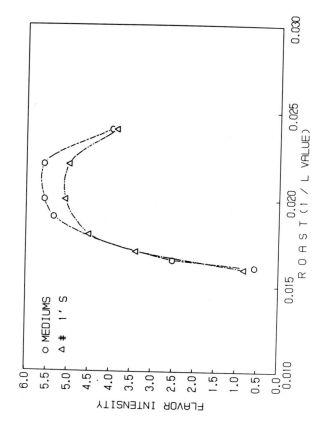

Figure 2. Mean roated peanutty flavor intensity for medium and #1 size peanuts.

GROWTH RESPONSE OF THE MUSHROOM AGARICUS CAMPESTRIS TO NITROGEN SOURCES WHEN CULTIVATED IN SUBMERGED FERMENTATION.

A.M. MARTIN

Food Science Program, Department of Biochemistry, Memorial University of Newfoundland, St. John's, Newfoundland, Canada, A1B 3X9

SUMMARY

Several sources of nitrogen were employed to study the mycelial growth of the edible mushroom Agaricus campestris. The organic nitrogen sources tested were peptone, urea and yeast extract. The inorganic sources were ammonium citrate, ammonium nitrate, ammonium phosphate dibasic and potassium nitrate. The concentrations of the different sources of nitrogen were calculated to provide 0.5 g/L to a peat extract medium used as substrate. Different concentrations of yeast extract, which was the best nitrogen source added, were studied for their effects on growth and on the nitrogen content of the mycelial biomass.

1. INTRODUCTION

The first commercially-oriented research on submerged culture production of mushrooms was conducted in 1948 (1). Since then, several researchers have attempted to improve the process of biomass production in submerged fermentation by higher fungi. Sugihara and Humfeld (2) reported the growth in submerged culture of several mushroom species. Eddy (3) studied the growth of 20 species of mushrooms in synthetic culture. In a series of patents, Szuecs (4), Humfeld (5) and Cirillo (6) disclosed methods for producing mushroom mycelium in submerged culture. Reviews of the work done in submerged culture of mushroom mycelium have been presented by Litchfield (7,8) and Worgan (9). The cultivation of basidiomycetes in fermenters has been used in physiological studies in order to determine single parameters for biomass production, to produce special enzymes or as a screening program for antibiotics (10).

Mushroom mycelium grown in submerged culture has been reported to be capable of producing materials with good nutritive value (11,12), and has a potential use as a food, food additive or food supplement (6,8,13). Litchfield (14) has stated that a pleasant-flavoured protein supplement from mushroom could be of particular interest to developing countries where chronic protein shortages exist.

Mushrooms are used as a flavouring agent in soups, sauces and gravy mixes, besides their direct consumption (15,3). If the mycelium produced by submerged culture were to have the characteristic mushroom flavour, it could then be expected that consumer acceptance could be found for such a product. Dijkstra and Wikén (16) and Litchfield (17) have reported that the flavour of mushroom mycelium was dependent on the substrate and the organism's strain.

Agaricus campestris, a mushroom species commonly eaten in several countries, has received much of the attention given to the study of the nutrition and development of mushroom flavour in submerged cultivation (18). Peat extracts have been employed as the only nutrient source in the growth of Agaricus campestris mycelium (19). The composition of the mushroom mycelium produced is influenced by the chemical composition of the peat extract substrate. Peat extracts have been found deficient in nitrogen and phosphorus for the best growth of microorganisms (20).

When the yeast Candida utilis was grown in supplemented peat extracts, its protein and amino acid composition was close to that of the commercial Fleischmann's yeast. The growth of an unidentified acidophilic fungus on supplemented peat extracts produced only about one-half of the protein content of the Fleischmann's yeast (21). Lower protein content is expected in fungi as compared to yeast. However, the protein content reported for A. campestris, both for the sporophore (22) and for the mycelium produced in submerged fermentation (23) is comparable to the range of 45.5 - 58.0% protein content reported for fodder yeast cultivated in peat extract media (21).

When cane molasses medium was utilized in the submerged growth of A. campestris, addition of yeast extract had a promoting effect on the biomass yield. It was also reported that the carbohydrate to nitrogen balance of the medium is an important factor in the growth of A. campestris mycelium (18).

The objective of the present work has been to test several supplemented peat extract media in the submerged fermentation of Agaricus campestris and to evaluate the nitrogen and protein contents and the amino acid composition of the mushroom mycelium produced.

2. Materials and Methods

2.1 Peat extracts

Ground *Sphagnum* peat moss from Sundew Peat Bog, Newfoundland, Canada, was mixed with 1.5% (v/v) H_2SO_4 (33g dry peat / 100g solution) and autoclaved at 15 psig (121°C) for two hours. The extracts were obtained by pressing the autoclaved product followed by filtration through Whatman No. 1 filter paper. Peat extracts with approximately 30 g/L total carbohydrate concentration were supplemented with different sources of nitrogen in different fermentations.

2.2 Organism

Agaricus campestris NRRL 2334 (American Type Culture Collection), previously adapted to growth in peat extracts (24).

2.3 Culture conditions

Agaricus campestris was aseptically inoculated into 100 mL of sterile culture media in 250 mL shake flasks and incubated in a Gyrotory water bath shaker (Model G76, New Brunswick Scientific Co., Inc.) at the previously found optimum conditions for growth (19). The initial pH was adjusted before inoculation by adding 15 N NaOH.

2.4 Nitrogen supplementation of the culture media

The effect of different sources of nitrogen (ammonium citrate, ammonium phosphate dibasic, ammonium sulfate, ammonium nitrate, potassium nitrate, urea, yeast extract and peptone) were studied to determine the possibility of supplementing the low nitrogen content in the peat extract. Different concentrations of yeast extract (1.0, 3.0, 5.0, 8.0, and 10.0 g/L) which was the best nitrogen source, were added to the peat extract medium to study their effects on growth and on crude protein production. The concentrations of the different sources of nitrogen used were calculated to provide 0.5 g/L of nitrogen to the culture media. This was the most suitable concentration found in previous experiments on the cultivation of mushroom mycelium in peat extract media (25).

2.5 Total carbohydrates (TCH)

Total carbohydrates in the culture media before and after fermentation were determined by the anthrone reagent method without correction factor for color interference (26).

2.6 Mycelial dry weight

The culture medium, after fermentation, was filtered through oven dried (105°C to constant weight), Whatman No.1 filter paper. The filter paper with mycelium was oven dried (105°C) and the mycelial weight determined.

2.7 Nitrogen content

The nitrogen content of the mycelium was calculated by the Kjeldahl method in a Kjeltec System (Tecator, Höganäs, Sweden).

2.8 Amino acid composition

The mushroom mycelium was hydrolysed under vacuum with 6 N HCl for 24 hours. The samples were reconstituted with 0.2 N lithium citrate buffer and analyzed on a Beckman 121 MB amino acid analyzer (Beckman Instruments, Palo Alto, California) using a single column method.

All results are average values from three different experiments.

3. RESULTS AND DISCUSSION

The final biomass concentration and the nitrogen content of $\underline{A}$. campestris mycelium grown in nitrogen-supplemented peat extracts is shown in Table 1. It can be seen that the nutrients added to the basic peat extract medium increased both the concentration and the nitrogen content of the mycelium in all cases. The effect of the nitrogen supplementation depended on the nitrogen source. Maximal growth values were obtained with yeast extract as the nutrient source, ammonium phosphate producing the second best growth, which confirms previous findings concerning the effect of those nutrient supplements on the growth of mushroom mycelium, as discussed by Manu-Tawiah and Martin (27).

Because yeast extract enhanced the dry biomass produced and its nitrogen content to a greater extent than ammonium phosphate, it is suggested that besides nitrogen and phosphorus, other growth factors available in the yeast extracts are required to improve the growth of $\underline{A}$. campestris in a peat extract medium.

Table 2 shows that the protein content for $\underline{A}$. campestris grown in a nitrogen-supplemented peat extract medium compares well with the protein content of yeast grown in peat extract basal medium.

Table 1. Effect of different sources of nitrogen on the growth of A. campestris in a peat extract medium.*

Nitrogen source (0.5 g/L N)	Dry biomass concentration (g/L)	Nitrogen content of the biomass, % (w/w dry basis)
None	1.8±0.3	3.5±1.1
Ammonium citrate	2.1±0.2	5.2±0.9
Ammonium nitrate	2.2±0.1	5.5±1.5
Ammonium phosphate, dibasic	2.8±0.3	5.7±0.8
Ammonium sulfate	2.5±0.5	5.4±1.1
Peptone	2.5±0.3	5.4±1.1
Potassium nitrate	2.1±0.2	5.5±1.4
Urea	2.5±0.2	5.3±0.8
Yeast extract	3.5±0.4	6.0±1.0

* Mean values ± standard deviations.

The concentration of individual amino acids from mycelial biomass of A. campestris cultivated in nitrogen-supplemented peat extracts was superior, in all cases, to the concentration of the mycelium when no supplementation was done (data not presented in this work). The amino acid composition of A. campestris cultivated in the peat extract supplemented with yeast extract is compared with that of the yeast Candida utilis biomass also grown in a peat extract-based medium, with the Food and Agricultural Organization (FAO) standards for amino acid composition and with the reported value for the sporocarp of A. campestris mushroom cultivated in solid medium (Table 3). Although the concentrations for the individual amino acids for A. campestris were, in general, lower than the amino acids concentrations for the yeast, A. campestris mycelium biomass showed higher concentrations than C. utilis for the amino acids Glycine and Methionine. Regarding the FAO standards, A. campestris mycelium biomass has higher concentrations of Cystine, Lysine and Threonine. It is important to note that although the information for the amino acid composition for the A.

Table 2. Protein content of microbial biomass cultivated in peat extracts[a].

Organisms	Protein content (% of dry weight)	References
Active dry yeast (Fleischmann)	41.4	LeDuy, 1981 (30)
Candida utilis	48.1	LeDuy, 1981 (30)
Acidophilus fungus	24.3	Boa and LeDuy, 1983 (31)
Morchella esculenta	26.0	Martin, 1983 (32)
Scytalidium acidophilum	42.1	Martin and White, 1985 (33)
Agaricus campestris	44.4[b]	Martin and Bailey, 1985 (25)
	37.5[c]	This work
Pleurotus ostreatus	40	Manu-Tawiah and Martin, 1987 (34)

[a] % Protein = % Nitrogen x 6.25
[b] Experiments in a 1L aerated and agitated fermenter
[c] Experiments in shake flasks

campestris mycelium cultivated in this work is presented as the means of three determinations plus and minus the standard deviations, no statistical analysis was conducted with the rest of the information reported in Table 3; therefore, the preceding discussion does not consider the statistical value of the differences noted. It is also of interest to note that the biomass concentration and the concentrations of amino acids for A. campestris mycelium cultivated in peat extract in an agitated and aerated fermenter, as reported by Martin and Bailey (25), were higher than those obtained in this work, in which the experiments were conducted in shake flasks. Although it is to be expected that growth conditions should affect the biomass growth, it was found in this work that those conditions, in addition to media composition, also affected the composition of A. campestris mycelium in submerged culture.

The concentration of yeast extract in the medium influenced both the final mycelial biomass concentration produced and its nitrogen content. A concentration of 5 g/L of yeast extract produced the maximal growth of the biomass and the highest biomass nitrogen content, the values not presenting a significant difference ($P>0.05$) from their corresponding values when higher values of yeast extract concentrations were tested (Figure 1). Manu-Tawiah and Martin (27) reported similar results for Pleurotus ostreatus grown in peat extracts. Other researchers have presented similar conclusions in regards to the effect of increasing nitrogen concentration in their culture medium (7,12,14,23,28,29).

Table 3. Comparison of the amino acid composition (g/100 g protein) of Agaricus campestris with other microbial biomass.

	FAO standard (35)	Candida utilis	Agaricus campestris	
		yeast grown in peat extracts (36)	Sporo-carp (22)	Mycelium grown in peat extracts[a]
Alanine		10.7		8.5±0.8
Arginine		6.6		2.1±0.5
Aspartic acid		12.2		10.7±3.1
Cystine	2.0			5.1±1.8
Glutamic acid		15.2		12.0±2.0
Glycine		4.7		7.8±1.5
Histidine		2.6		
Isoleucine	4.2	3.6	2.6	1.8±0.4
Leucine	4.8	7.0	4.3	2.7±0.9
Lysine	4.2	12.2	4.8	6.0±1.3
Methionine	2.2	0.9	1.0	1.5±0.3
Phenylalanine	2.8	2.1	2.6	1.8±0.5
Proline		6.3		5.7±1.0
Serine		6.0		5.3±0.9
Threonine	2.8	5.6		4.8±0.7
Tryptophan	1.4	[b]	3.1	[b]
Tyrosine	2.8	3.1		2.1±0.4
Valine	4.2	4.6	3.2	3.9±0.7

[a] This work, medium supplemented with 5 g/L yeast extract
[b] Not determined due to destruction of protein biomass due to acid hydrolysis.

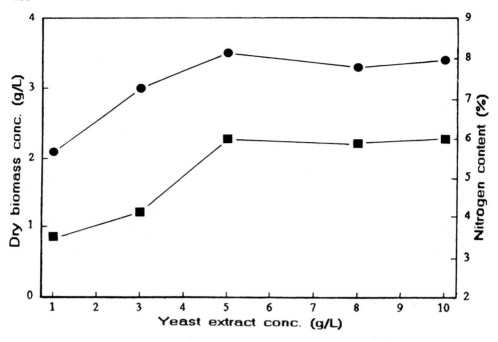

Figure 1: Effect of different concentrations of yeast extract on the growth and nitrogen content of A. campestris mycelium grown in peat extracts. Dry biomass concentration: (●); nitrogen content (■).

4. CONCLUSIONS

In general, it can be concluded that in the growth of A. campestris mushroom mycelium in submerged culture, nitrogen supplementation of the medium enhanced the growth, and the nitrogen and amino acid contents of the biomass. The effect of the nitrogen sources utilized were affected by the kind of supplement utilized. The fact that the best nutrient supplement, yeast extract, is a source of other nutrients besides nitrogen, indicates that other nutrients will also have the potential to enhance the growth of the mushroom mycelium.

REFERENCES

1. H. Humfeld, Science, 107 (1948) 373.
2. T.F. Sugihara, and H. Humfeld, Appl. Microbiol., 2 (1954) 170-172.
3. B.P. Eddy, J. Sci. Food Agric., 9 (1958) 644-649.
4. J. Szuecs, (1958). U.S. Patent 2,850,841.
5. H. Humfeld, (1954). U.S. Patent 2,693,665.
6. V. Cirillo, (1960). U.S. Patent 2,928,210.
7. J.H. Litchfield, in: H.J. Peppler (Ed.), Microbial Technology, Reinhold, New York, 1967, pp. 107-144.
8. J.H. Litchfield, in: R.I. Mateles and S.R. Tannebaum (Eds.), Single Cell Protein, MIT Press, Cambridge Mass. and London, 1968, pp. 309-329.
9. J.T. Worgan, in: D.J.D. Hockenhull (Ed.), Progress in Industrial Microbiology, vol. 8, J. and A. Churchill, London 1968, pp. 72-139.
10. F. Zadrazil and K. Grabbe, in: H. Dellweg (Ed.), Biotechnology, Vol. 3, Verlag Chemie, Weinheim, 1983, pp.145-187.
11. S.S. Block, G. Tsao and L. Han, J. Agric. Food Chem., 6 (1958) 923-965.
12. F.J. Reusser, F.T. Spencer and H.R. Sallans, Appl. Microbiol., 6 (1958) 1-4.
13. K.K. Janardhanan, T.N. Kaul and A. Husain, J. Food Sci. Technol., 7 (1970) 197.
14. J.H. Litchfield, in: M.P. Starr (Ed.), Global Impact of Applied Microbiology, John Wiley and Sons, Inc., New York, N.Y. (1963), pp. 327-337.
15. S.T. Chang, Bioscience, 30(6) (1980) 399-401.
16. F.I. Dijkstra and T.O. Wikén., Z. Lebensm. Unters.-Forsch. 160 (1976) 255-262.
17. J.H. Litchfield, Biotechnol. Bioeng., 9 (1967) 289-304.
18. A.M. Moustafa, Appl. Microbiol., 8 (1960) 63-67.
19. A.M. Martin, J. Food Sci., 48 (1983) 206-207.
20. P. Quierzy, N. Therien and A. LeDuy, Biotechnol. Bioeng., 21 (1979) 1175-1190.
21. A. LeDuy, in: C.H. Fuchsman and S.A. Spigarelli (Eds.), Proceedings of the International Symposium on Peat Utilization, Bemidji State University, Bemidji, Minn., 1981, pp. 89-115.
22. N. Kosaric, A. LeDuy and J.E. Zajic, Can. J. Chem. Eng., 51 (1973) 186-190.
23. H. Humfeld and T.F. Sugihara, Mycologia, 44 (1952) 605-620.
24. A.M. Martin, Can. J. Microbiol., 29 (1983) 108-110.
25. A.M. Martin and V.I. Bailey, Can. Inst. Food Sci. Technol. J., 18 (1985) 185-188.
26. A. LeDuy, N. Kosaric and J.E. Zajic, in: T.C. Hutchinson (Ed.), Proceedings of the 10th Canadian Water Pollution Research Symposium, University of Toronto, Toronto, Ontario, Canada, 1975, pp. 126-131.
27. W. Manu-Tawiah and A.M. Martin, Can. Inst. Food Sci. Technol. J., 21 (1988) 194-199.
28. H. Falanghe, Appl. Microbiol., 10 (1962) 572-576.
29. H.C. Srivastava and Z. Bano, Appl. Microbiol., 19 (1970) 166-169.
30. A. LeDuy, in: Proceedings of the peat as an energy alternative symposium, The Institute of Gas Technology, pp. 479-493.

31 M.J. Boa and A. LeDuy, Can. J. Chem. Eng., 60 (1982) 532-537.
32 A.M.Martin, Can. Inst. Food Sci. Technol. J., 16 (1983) 215-217.
33 A.M. Martin and M.D. White, J. Food Sci., 50 (1985) 197-200.
34 W. Manu-Tawiah and A.M. Martin, Food Microbiol., 4 (1987) 303-310.
35 FAO/WHO, WHO Tech. Rep. Ser. No. 522, Geneva, Switzerland, 1973.
36 A. LeDuy, Paper Presented at the International Peat Symposium, Bemidji State Univ., Bemidji, Minn., Oct. 21-23, 1981.

G. Charalambous (Ed.), Food Science and Human Nutrition
© 1992 Elsevier Science Publishers B.V. All rights reserved.

STUDY OF THE GROWTH AND BIOMASS COMPOSITION OF THE EDIBLE MUSHROOM PLEUROTUS OSTREATUS.

A. M. Martin

Food Science Program, Department of Biochemistry, Memorial University of Newfoundland, St. John's, Newfoundland, Canada, A1B 3X9.

SUMMARY

The edible mushroom Pleurotus ostreatus, also known as the oyster mushroom, was cultivated in liquid and solid media using peat as the main substrate source. Amino acids, fat, fibre, moisture, nitrogen, and protein contents were determined for the mushroom biomass produced.

The protein contents of the mushrooms cultivated on liquid and solid media were approximately 40% and 36%, respectively, calculated on a dry weight basis. These are promising values, when compared to those reported with the use of other substrates. In addition, the amino acid profile of the mushroom biomass showed that the essential amino acids were present in fairly good concentrations.

1. INTRODUCTION

Edible mushrooms have been increasingly recognized by the Food Industry worldwide as nutritious and popular foods (1). In recent years, the consumption of mushrooms has attained an approximately 10% growth rate per year in industrialized Western countries (2,3), including Canada (4), where this interest has resulted in mushrooms becoming the second most valuable vegetable crop, with 51,400 tonnes valued at 136 million dollars produced in 1985 (5).

Mushrooms are mostly used as flavoring agents rather than as food staples. Only one-third of the world's annual crop is sold fresh, while the remaining two-thirds are processed into flavoring agents or canned (6).

Only a few of the edible mushroom species are commercially cultivated. The five most important cultivated mushrooms are: the white mushroom/button mushroom (Agaricus bisporus), the black forest mushroom/shiitake (Lentinus edodes), the winter mushroom (Flammulina velutipes), the straw mushroom (Volvariella volvacea) and the oyster mushroom (Pleurotus ostreatus) (3,7). Agaricus is cultivated in seventy-four countries but is commonly consumed mainly in Europe and North America. <u>Lentinus</u> and <u>Flammulina</u> are commonly grown in China and Japan. China is the main producer of <u>Volvariella</u>, but it is familiar to all Southeast Asians, and Pleurotus is gaining popularity in Europe and Asia.

Mushroom protein contains all the essential amino acids (8) in high concentrations. In addition to proteins, mushrooms are a good source of the B vitamins (9), are low in calories, and are valued as flavoring agents in foods (3,6). There are more than 2,000 edible fungi in the world but so far only about 25 species are widely accepted for human consumption (10).

<u>Pleurotus ostreatus</u>, more commonly known as the oyster mushroom, has been gaining favor among mushroom lovers due to its delicate flavor (8). <u>P. ostreatus</u> may be grown on wastepaper (11) and other cullulose sources such as straw, corn cobs and sawdust (5), and in peat (12, 13).

<u>Pleurotus</u> species have a relatively simple growth requirement. It is reported that for both mycelium growth and fruiting body development, lignin-cellulose materials are sufficient (14). Cultivation of <u>Pleurotus</u> species does not require composting. In some cases, pasteurization or sterilization of the substrate is not necessary either. Comprehensive literature on the cultivation of <u>Pleurotus</u> species has been presented (15). It has been reported that supplementing the substrate with some organic and/or inorganic sources of nitrogen could increase yield and total nitrogen contents of <u>Pleurotus</u>. The possibilities of nitrogen fixation by <u>Pleurotus</u> have been comprehensively reviewed by Kurtzman (16). <u>Pleurotus</u> species can be cultivated over wide ranges of temperature (21 to 33°C) and relative humidity (67 to 72%) (17).

The production of mushroom mycelium in submerged culture for use as a food or in food products is relatively recent, compared with the traditional technique of producing mushroom fruiting bodies (or sporophores) in manure or in compost beds. Experience gained since World War II in antibiotic fermentation processes led to the idea of growing mushroom mycelium in agitated and aerated fermenters. In this way, a mushroom-flavored product could be produced throughout the year. In addition, low-cost materials, such as food industry wastes, can be utilized as substrate sources for mushroom production and at the same time reduce the biochemical oxygen demand of the wastes. The flavored mushroom mycelium should be suitable for use in formulated foods, such as instant soups, sauces, etc. (6). Commercial production of morel mushroom mycelium was initiated in 1963 by a company in the United States using the Szuecs process. The production was discontinued because apparently the market was not yet prepared for the acceptance of such a product.

The process of extracting nutrients from peat to be employed in submerged fermentations for the growth of various microorganisms with potential commercial value has been studied for a long time (18). A review of the literature shows that the fermentation of peat extracts or peat hydrolysates has been conducted extensively in the Soviet Union and on a lesser scale in Ireland, the United States and Canada. The bulk of the research in these countries has been done utilizing acid hydrolysates from peat as the basic media in the submerged culture of microorganisms, mainly yeast species (18-20) and fungi (21-25).

This work reviews the activities which have been conducted at the Department of Biochemistry, Memorial University of Newfoundland, Canada, in the cultivation of P. ostreatus mushroom in liquid and solid media utilizing peat as the main nutrient source (12, 13).

2. MATERIALS AND METHODS

2.1 Organism

Pleurotus ostreatus No. 152 (Department of Plant Sciences, University of Western Ontario, London, Canada).

2.2 Peat hydrolysates

The work reported here utilized a high-moor Sphagnum peat moss, of a relatively low degree of decomposition, taken from a bog near the city of St. John's. The initial moisture content of this peat was approximately 80%, but there was some variation between samples, and peat also tends to lose moisture in storage. Before the preparation of the hydrolysates, the peat was dried in a laboratory oven (Blue M Electric Co.) to obtain a standard moisture content of approximately 10%.

The results reported in this work correspond to the process using ground peat of 18 to 60 mesh particle size, 1.5% (v/v) H_2SO_4, a dry-peat: H_2SO_4 solution ratio of 1:6 (w/w), and autoclaving at 15 psig (121°C) for two hours. Before autoclaving, the peat and H_2SO_4 solution are mixed together thoroughly.

The hydrolysates were obtained by pressing the autoclaved product in a modified laboratory press (Model C, F.S. Carver, Inc.), followed by vacuum filtration through Whatman #1 filter paper. The hydrolysates have been tested without additional nutrients (non-supplemented), and with the addition of various concentrations of several inorganic salts and organic nutrient sources, alone or in combinations. The aim has been to rely as much as possible on the nutrients in the peat hydrolysate itself, minimizing the addition of supplements and choosing the cheapest ones, although better growth could be achieved with more expensive media formulations. The pH of the hydrolysates was adjusted by 15N NaOH or with concentrated NH_4OH solutions. NaOH was utilized when the effect of the nitrogen concentrations in the peat extract or in other nitrogen supplements was being tested.

2.3 Culture conditions

The sterile growth media (100 mL in 250 mL shake flasks) were aseptically inoculated with blended pure culture mycelia and incubated in a Gyrotory water bath shaker (Model G76, New Brunswick Sci. Co., Inc.). Fermentations have also been conducted in a 1-litre aerated and agitated fermenter (Bioflo, New Brunswick Sci. Co., Inc.). Various values of inoculum ratio, temperature, initial pH, fermentation time and agitation speed have been tested to optimize the growth conditions of the microbial species (13, 24, 25).

2.4 Spawn preparation

Wheat grain, raw peat and calcium carbonate were used for the preparation of the spawn. The wheat grain was first immersed in water and then autoclaved for 20 minutes at 15 psig (121°C). Excess water was removed and the grain was mixed with 10% raw peat and 1% $CaCO_3$, based on the boiled grain weight. Glass bottles containing 200g of the mixture were sterilized for 20 minutes at 15 psig (121°C), cooled to room temperature (approximately 25°C) and inoculated aseptically with the growth of one slant culture of P. ostreatus. The inoculated mixture was incubated at room temperature for 14 days and used as spawn to inoculate the solid culture substrate.

2.5 Substrate for fruiting body production

Sphagnum peat moss was used as the substrate source and support for the P. ostreatus fruiting body development. The pre-treatment involved only addition of sufficient water to the raw peat to obtain an initial substrate moisture content of 75-80%, and addition of $CaCO_3$ to raise the pH to near neutral values. The substrate was supplemented with 5% (by weight of dry peat) wheat bran, and sterilized by autoclaving for 20 minutes at 15 psig (121°C). After the substrate was cooled to room temperature, spawn was added at the rate of 7% of the sterilized substrate weight. About 300g of the spawned substrate was aseptically packed into sterile aluminum trays (22 x 15 x 2.5 cm) and covered with a sterile polythene film. Six holes of approximately 1.5 mm diameter each were made in the polythene cover to allow gas exchange with the environment. The covered containers were incubated at $27 \pm 2°C$ in the absence of light for 14 days, and then exposed to light from a tungsten source. Thereafter, the colonized substrate was watered twice a day. The air in the cultivation chamber was constantly humidified. The first flush of mushrooms appeared between 10 and 14 days, and the fruiting bodies were harvested when they were considered to have attained their maximum growth.

2.6 Analytical methods

The total carbohydrate concentrations in the peat hydrolysates and in the fermented media were determined by the anthrone reagent method (26). The moisture content was determined by oven drying, nitrogen by the AOAC 47.003 micro-Kjeldahl method, and crude protein by multiplying the % nitrogen by 6.25. Fat was determined gravimetrically after ether extraction, ash was determined by combustion at 600°C, and crude fibre by the AOAC 7.061 method (27). For the amino acid analyses, freeze-dried samples were hydrolysed with 6N HCl under vacuum for 24 hours at 110°C. The samples were reconstituted with 0.2N lithium citrate buffer and analysed with a Beckman 121 MB amino acid analyser using a single column method. All the results are average values from at least three different determinations.

3. RESULTS AND DISCUSSION

3.1 Composition of substrates

Table 1 shows the composition of the peat extracts utilized in the submerged cultivation of Pleurotus ostreatus mushroom mycelium, and of the solid peat utilized for the growth of fruiting bodies.

TABLE 1

Basic composition of the peat hydrolysates and solid peat substrates.[a]

Component	Peat hydrolysates (29)	Peat (12)
Total carbohydrate	32.75 ± 1.23 g/L	b
Moisture	b	77.5 ± 3.5%
Nitrogen	0.60 ± 0.01 g/L	1.3 ± 0.1%

[a]Means of three determinations ± standard deviations.
[b]Not determined.

3.2 Growth parameters in submerged cultivation

The production of mushroom mycelium was optimized by varying the growth parameters. The conditions resulting in the best growth are presented in Table 2. In addition to the total dry mycelium concentration produced, the value for the biomass yield (grams of dry mycelium produced per gram of total carbohydrate consumed) was calculated. As it may be seen, the yield obtained, approximately 60%, was relatively high in comparison to other fermentation processes for the production of microbial biomass.

TABLE 2

Growth parameters for the mushroom Pleurotus ostreatus produced in submerged cultivation in peat hydrolysates (13).

Parameter	Value
Agitation (rpm)	150
Inoculum ratio % (v/v)	5
pH	5
Temperature (°C)	28
Final biomass concentration (g/L)	5
Biomass yield (%)	60

3.3 Composition of the mycelium and fruiting bodies of P. ostreatus mushroom cultivated in peat substrates

The concentration of the main components for both the mycelial biomass and the fruiting bodies of P. ostreatus is reported in Table 3. The most significant characteristic is the protein content, which was higher than those reported for the same mushroom species grown in other substrates. In the case of the fruiting bodies, it has been reported (14) that the higher nitrogen concentration in the peat substrates, as compared with other cellulosic substrates generally employed in the solid cultivation of P. ostreatus, contributed to the higher protein content of the fungus grown.

Finally, Table 4 shows the essential amino acid composition of P. ostreatus mycelium grown in submerged culture and of the fruiting bodies grown in solid medium. It shows that all essential amino acids were present in satisfactory amounts. In general, the mycelium presented higher values than the fruiting bodies for the crude protein content and for the individual essential amino acids. These findings could highlight the potential of the mushroom mycelium as a protein supplement for foods.

TABLE 3

Composition of the mycelium and fruiting bodies of P. ostreatus mushroom cultivated in peat substrates.[a]

Component (%)	Mycelium (30)	Fruiting bodies (12)
Ash	6.5 ± 0.5	8.6 ± 0.5
Crude Protein	40.1 ± 1.8	36.0 ± 4.9
Fat	2.6 ± 0.2	1.9 ± 0.1
Fibre	5.9 ± 0.4	6.5 ± 0.3
Moisture	78.2 ± 2.5	89.6 ± 0.6

[a]Means of three determinations ± standard deviations. With the exception of the % moisture content, all values are reported on a dry weight basis.

TABLE 4

Essential amino acid composition of P. ostreatus grown in peat hydrolysates (g/100g protein).[a]

Amino Acid	Mycelium (31)	Fruiting bodies (12)
Isoleucine	3.5 ± 0.2	2.1 ± 0.3
Leucine	6.1 ± 0.3	3.5 ± 0.2
Lysine	5.7 ± 0.4	3.4 ± 0.4
Methionine	1.0 ± 0.1	1.0 ± 0.1
Phenylalanine	3.4 ± 0.3	2.2 ± 0.1
Threonine	4.9 ± 0.3	2.7 ± 0.2
Tryptophan	1.2 ± 0.1	[b]
Valine	3.9 ± 0.2	1.8 ± 0.1

[a]Means of three determinations ± standard deviations.
[b]Not reported.

3.4 Production of mycelial pellets

Generally, the main objective in the production of mushroom mycelium is to obtain, consistently, a safe, flavoured, marketable product. In the cultivation of mushrooms in submerged fermentation, the production of mycelial pellets is reportedly important for flavour development, probably because of autolysis in the center of the pellets (28). In addition, a pellet suspension decreases the viscosity of the medium, enhancing mixing, mass transfer and the separation of the biomass from the rest of the medium. The study of the production of mycelial pellets of Agaricus campestris (bisporus) has been reported (22).

4. CONCLUSIONS

The edible mushroom P. ostreatus, also known as the oyster mushroom, was adapted and cultivated in both solid and liquid media for the first time using peat and peat hydrolysates as the only or main substrate source.

Peat, which is often used as casing soil in the production of Agaricus bisporus, the well-known button mushroom, can be also employed as a source of nutrients in the submerged growth of mushroom mycelial biomass, with the objective of producing, under controlled conditions a mushroom-flavoured product for the food industry.

REFERENCES

1. F. Zadrazil and K. Grabbe, in: H. Dellweg (Ed), Biotechnology. Volume 3, Verlag Chemie, Weinheim, F.R. Germany, 1983, pp. 147-187.
2. W. A. Hayes and N. G. Nair, in: J. E. Smith and D. R. Barry (Eds), The Filamentous Fungi. Volume 1: Industrial Mycology, Edward Arnold Ltd., London, England, 1975, pp. 212-248.
3. M. C. Tseng and J. H. Loung, Annual Reports of Fermentation Processes, 7 (1984) 45-79.
4. Anonymous. Can. Inst. Food Sci. Technol. J., 14 (1981) 358.
5. J. K. Scott, Reader's Digest, 130 No. 780 (1987) 13-18.
6. J. H. Litchfield, Food Technol., 21 No. 159 (1967) 55.
7. S. T. Chang and P. G. Miles, in: S. T. Chang and T. H. Quimio (Eds), Tropical Mushrooms. Chinese University Press, Hong Kong, 1982, pp. 3-10.
8. S. T. Chang, O. W. Lau, K. Y. Cho, Europ. J. Appl. Microbiol. Biotechnol., 12 (1981) 58-62.
9. E. V. Crisan and A. Sands, in: S. T. Chang and W. A. Hayes (Eds), The Biology and Cultivation of Edible Mushrooms. Academic Press, New York, N.Y. (1978) pp. 137-168.
10. E. A. Bessey, Morphology and Taxonomy of Fungi, Hafner Publishing Co., New York, N.Y. (1961).
11. K. H. Steinkraus and R. E. Cullen, New York's Food and Life Sciences, 11 No. 4 (1978) 5-7.
12. W. Manu-Tawiah and A. M. Martin, J. Sci. Food Agric., 37 (1986) 833-838.
13. W. Manu-Tawiah and A. M. Martin, Appl. Biochem. Biotechnol., 14 (1987) 221-229.
14. S. S. Block, Appl. Microbiol., 13 (1965) 5-9.
15. F. Zadrazil and R. H. Kurtzman, in: S. T. Chang and T. H. Quimio (Eds), Tropical Mushrooms. Chinese University Press, Hong Kong, 1982, pp. 277-298.
16. R. H. Kurtzman and F. Zadrazil, in: S. T. Chang and T. H. Quimio (Eds), Tropical Mushrooms. Chinese University Press, Hong Kong, 1982, pp. 299-348.
17. Z. Bano, H. C. Srinivasan and H. C. Srivastava, Appl. Microbiol., 11 (1963) 184-187.
18. A. LeDuy, Process Biochem., 15 (1979) 5-7.
19. C. H. Fuchsman, Peat, Industrial Chemistry and Technology, Academic Press, New York, N.Y., 1980, pp. 119-134.
20. P. Quierzy, N. Therien and A. LeDuy, Biotechnol. Bioeng., 21 (1979) 1175-1190.
21. J. M. Boa and A. LeDuy, Can. J. Chem. Eng., 60 (1982) 532-537.
22. A. M. Martin and V. I. Bailey, Appl. Environ. Microbiol., 49 (1985) 1502-1506.
23. A. M. Martin and M. D. White, Appl. Microbiol. Biotechnol., 24 (1986) 84-88.
24. A. M. Martin, J. Food Sci., 48 (1983) 206-207.
25. A. M. Martin, Can. Inst. Food Sci. Technol. J., 16 (1983) 215-217.
26. A. LeDuy, N. Kosaric and J. E. Zajic, in: T. C. Hutchinson (Ed), Correction Factor for Anthrone Carbohydrate in Coloured Wastewater Samples. Proceedings of the 10th Canadian Symposium on Water Pollution Research, Toronto, Canada, University of Toronto, 1975, pp. 126-131.
27. A.O.A.C., Official Methods of Analysis, 13th Edition, Association of Official Analytical Chemists, Washington, D.C., 1980.

28. J. C. Suijdam, N.W.F. Kassan and P. G. Paul, Europ. J. Appl. Microbiol. Biotechnol., 10 (1980) 211-221.
29. W. Manu-Tawiah and A. M. Martin, in: K. Grabbe and O. Hilber (Eds), Uses of Nitrogen - Supplemented Peat Extracts for the Cultivation of _Pleurotus_ _ostreatus_ Mushroom Mycelium. Mushroom Science XII (Part II), Proceedings of the Twelfth International Congress on the Science and Cultivation of Edible Fungi, Braunschweig, F. R. Germany, September 1987, International Society for Mushroom Science, Berlin, 1989. pp. 157-167.
30. A. M. Martin and W. Manu-Tawiah, in: E. D. Primo Yufera and P. Fito Maupoey (Eds), Biomass Composition of the Edible Mushroom _Pleurotus_ _ostreatus_. Advances in Food Technology, Vol. 1. Proceedings of the Second World Congress of Food Technology, Barcelona, Spain, 3-6 March, 1987, PROSEMA, Valencia, 1989, pp. 667-676.
31. W. Manu-Tawiah and A. M. Martin, Food Microbiol., 4 (1987) 303-310.

G. Charalambous (Ed.), Food Science and Human Nutrition
© 1992 Elsevier Science Publishers B.V. All rights reserved.

IMPROVED RETENTION OF MUSHROOM FLAVOUR IN MICROWAVE-HOT AIR DRYING

L.F. DI CESARE[1], M. RIVA[2] and A.SCHIRALDI[2]

[1] I.V.T.P.A., Via Venezian 26, 20133 Milano (Italy)
[2] DI.S.T.A.M., Sez. Tecnologie Alimentari, Universita' di Milano, Via Celoria 2, 20133 Milano (Italy)

SUMMARY

The most relevant quality index of mushrooms is their flavour. This mainly depends on the redox balance between 1-octen-3 ol and 1-octen-3 one. Drying treatments can modify the natural balance by increasing the ketone fraction, which induces a metallic note in the flavour. Microwave heating combined with hot air flow allows shortening of the drying time and improves the retention of the mushroom like flavour. A simple kinetic model is suggested to justify the above behaviour.

1. INTRODUCTION

Aroma of mushrooms comes from more than 150 volatiles (1), the most important of which are 1-octen-3 ol and its oxidation derivative 1-octen-3 one, since they induce the fresh mushroom flavour (2, 3).

Systematic odour evaluations have been reported (3, 4) which allow correlation between concentration of either compound and flavour note of fresh mushrooms.

Results concerning Agaricus bisporus studied by Cronin and Ward (3) allowed to assess two different odour tresholds, viz., 0.1 and 0.01 ppm for the alcohol and ketone, respectively. At concentration of 1 ppm, the flavour note of the alcohol is weak mushroom-like, while that of the ketone includes an extra weak metallic component. At 10 ppm, the alcohol produces the full raw mushroom like aroma, and the ketone a sickly fungal smell with strong metallic note.

The alcohol comes from a chemical reaction catalyzed by an enzymic pool of lipoxygenase and hydroperoxide lyase in the presence of oxygen (5). The reaction rate increases just after slicing or finely cutting the fresh mushrooms (6). Once formed, the alcohol is oxidized to ketone with an increase of the flavour pungency.

These considerations may justify the typical aroma of dried mushrooms, which undergo slicing and prolonged exposure to the air in the course of the drying process.

Since the flavour is the only quality parameter which justifies the commercial value of this product, a special care is required to retain it as much as possible in any preservation process.

To this respect drying, i.e. the usual preservation treatment, must be carefully designed. This is traditionally achieved with adequate drying temperature, previous blanching of the product, and monitoring the colour changes in the course of the treatment.

While a general agreement exists about the choice of temperature and final humidity of the product, the literature reports different opinions about the necessity of the blanching (6-9).

In a previous paper (10) the comparison between drying procedures, viz., with hot air flow (HA) and microwave + hot air flow (MW + HA), allowed to prefer the latter for a better preservation of the original quality of raw mushrooms.

As a matter of fact, the combined treatment required a shorter drying time with limited thermal injury of the diced samples; the rehydratability of the samples was comparable in the two cases, but the flavour retention was quite better in (MW + HA) dried product.

It was recognized that the improvements found in the combined treatment could be mainly explained with the larger water diffusivity and the smoother thermal gradient within the samples.

In the present work we present a more detailed discussion about the retention of aroma compounds observed in the previously reported different drying techniques.

2. MATERIALS AND METHODS

Commercial mushrooms (Agaricus bisporus) previously stored at 5° C were selected according to the size of the carpophores (from 2.5 to 3.5 cm.) and cut into slices of 5.1 ($\mp$ 0.1) mm.

Drying experiments were carried out in an especially

deviced equipment (ALM 1600, SFAMO, Plombieres Les Bains, France) which allowed either HA or MW + HA treatment in the conditions reported elsewhere (10).

Optical fiber thermocouples (Fiber Optic Sensor KZ1, ASEA, France) allowed temperature monitoring with a ∓ 0.2°C accuracy of both hot air and sample core in the course of the experiment.

A feed-back control was acting on the preheated air flow.

In MW + HA treatments this control allowed to keep constant the temperature of the air flow and simultaneously tune the microwave power so that sample core too could remain at the same preplanned temperature.

The water loss was gravimetrically determined at various times; the relevant moisture content was referred to the residual humidity in the final products (evaluated after eight hour annealing at 100°C).

The change of the thickness of the slices during the treatments was determined at the microscope, and empirically fit vs drying time (10).

Flavour compounds (1-octen-3 ol and 1-octen-3 one) were analyzed in three 5 kg lots of mushrooms, two of which were examined after HA and MW + HA drying at 60°C. The third lot was examined as fresh product.

The sample were homogenized with 22 l of distilled water after a previous freezing at -20°C which induced breaking of cellular walls on rewarming.

A glass climbing film evaporator adequately designed (11) was employed to strip the flavour compounds at 40 - 45°C and 799 Pa.

They were then flushed through a glass column (40 cm length, 2 cm int. diam.) packed with 60 ml of KS112 (Dow Chemical, Italia) apolar resin, and eluted with 100 - 120 ml of pure ethyl ether after drainage of the solution.

After dehydration with anhydrous Na_2SO_4 the solutions were distilled until complete evaporation of the solvent.

The final analysis was carried out with a gascromatograph (DANI 8400 FID) equipped with a Carbowax 20 M wide bore (25 m lenght, 0.55 mm internal diameter, 10 µm fill tickness).

0.05 µl of the extracts were injected. The following operating conditions were employed. Gas flow: H_2 30 ml/min, air 300 ml/min and He (carrier) 30 ml/min; temperature: injector

180°C, detector 221°C; column programme: from 70 to 190°C in 25 min at 2°C/min.

Recognition of 1-octen-3 ol and 1-octen-3 one was carried out by comparison of the retention times of standards. The two-point calibration curve method was used for quantitative analysis.

Figure 1 reports three typical aromagrams from fresh, HA and MW + HA dried mushromms, respectively. The signals of the two characteristic flavour compounds are indicated. The pattern obtained presents a large number of peaks, which confirms the results reported in literature (1, 3, 4).

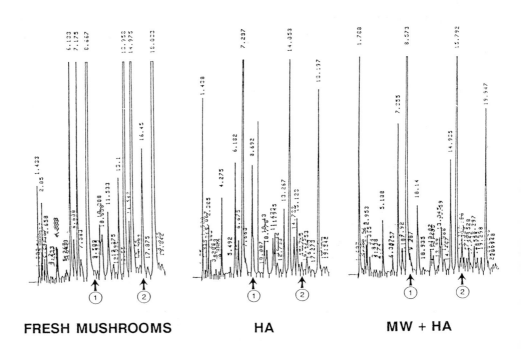

Fig. 1. Aromagrams obtained from distilled ether extracts of fresh, HA and MW + HA dried Agaricus bisporus mushrooms. Peaks numbered with 1 and 2 correspond to 1-octen-3 one and 1-octen-3 ol, respectively.

3. **RESULTS AND DISCUSSION**

Since flavour loss is correlated with water release during dehydration, it seemed reasonable to previously assess the drying kinetics in either treatment considered, at a given temperature of the hot air flow. Fig. 2 reports the results obtained at 60° C.

These allowed, via a fickian approach, evaluation of the average water diffusivity, viz., 2.77 10^{-7} and 5.77 10^{-7} cm^2 s^{-1} for HA and MW+HA treatment, respectively.

These results were consistent with a more rapid dehydration in the MW + HA treatment and suggested that the residue would have a lower concentration of the alcohol in samples dried with HA than with MW + HA technique. The activation energies of water diffusivity were found to be rather close to each other (10) for either treatment; the water release was therefore assumed to occur with the same mechanism. Accordingly, the larger water diffusion would depend on the retention of a better porosity in MW+HA treated samples.

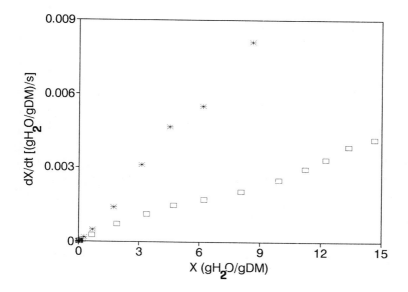

Fig. 2. Drying rate vs absolute humidity of the samples at 60° C. □ HA, * MW+HA drying technique.

Since part of the alcohol undergoes oxidation to ketone, the decrease of its concentration would be even larger than expected for the liquid-vapour equilibrium.

Table 1 reports the concentrations of either aroma compound observed after HA and MW+HA treatment for comparable sample humidity (about 0.05 kg H_2O/kg DM) at 60° C.

TABLE 1
Retention of aroma compounds after drying

Aroma Compound	CONTENT (µg/kg raw mushrooms)		
	RAW	HA	MW + HA
1-octen-3 ol	212 ∓ 8.06	31 ∓ 0.37	60 ∓ 1.25
1-octen-3 one	4 ∓ 0.25	48 ∓ 1.85	6 ∓ 0.78

These data showed that, in spite of the expected larger volatility of the ketone, this compound tends to accumulate within the samples: the reason could be the longer drying time required in the HA treatment which implies a larger amount of ketone and, therefore, justifies the more pronounced metallic flavour note of mushrooms dried with this technique.

These data were worked out according to a simple model which takes into account both the kinetic and the diffusivity contribution to the change of concentration:

$$\begin{cases} \frac{dA}{dt} = \chi_o - \chi A - D_A \cdot \nabla A \cdot S \cdot \rho \\ \frac{dK}{dt} = \chi A - D_K \cdot \nabla K \cdot S \cdot \rho \end{cases} \quad [1]$$

where A and K are the residual concentrations (µg/kg raw mushroom) of alcohol and ketone, respectively, in the dried mushrooms, t is the time (s), χ_o is kinetic constant (µg/kg s^{-1}) of the enzymic formation of A from its precursor, χ is the kinetic constant (s^{-1}), D's are the diffusivities (cm^2/s), S is the actual surface of aroma release (cm^2) and ρ is the density of raw mushrooms (kg/cm^3).

The concentration gradients, ∇A and ∇K, can be reliably represented with the ratio between concentration and half thickness of the mushroom slice, A/(L/2) and K/(L/2).

Since dK/dt is positive, one can argue that the formation rate of the ketone is larger than its escape from the mushroom. Either contribution conversely acts to reduce the concentration of the alcohol.

Summation of the second equation from the first leads to:

$$\frac{dA}{dt} + \frac{dK}{dt} = \chi_o - \frac{2S \cdot \rho \cdot (D_A A - D_K K)}{L} \quad [2]$$

Figure 3 reports the data of the table 1 vs the corresponding drying time. The descending trend of alcohol concentration implies a first severe decrease followed by a moderate reduction in the final steps. An opposite behaviour is observed for the ketone concentration.

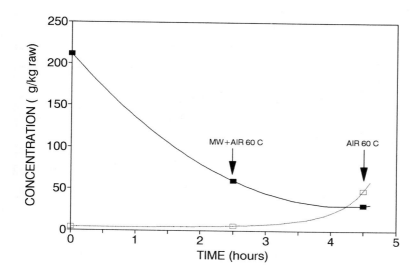

Fig. 3. Change of the 1-octen-3 ol (■) and 1-octen-3 one (□) concentration with drying time in HA and MW+HA treated samples.

A polynomial fitting of the experimental trends reported in Fig. 3 allowed evaluation of the corresponding derivatives appearing in [2]. This could be therefore rewritten as

$$x_o - \frac{2S \cdot \rho \cdot (D_A A - D_K K)}{L} = -97.3 + 29.72\ t \qquad [3]$$

When t = 0 this reduces to:

$$x_o = \frac{2S \cdot \rho \cdot (D_A A_o)}{L_o} - 97.3 \qquad [4]$$

where the terms relevant to the ketone have been neglected, since they are much smaller than those relevant to the alcohol.

[4] allows a rough evaluation of D_A which is almost two orders of magnitude larger than D_{H_2O}.

If the change of ketone concentration is assumed to mainly depend on its formation from the alcohol, then one can roughly estimate the kinetic constant, χ, which is about $4 \cdot 10^{-4}$ s^{-1}.

4 CONCLUSIONS

This result confirms that any lengthening of the heat treatment will favour accumulation of the ketone and reduction of the alcohol pool which should be adequately large to allow release of flavour when mushrooms undergo cooking.

The last consideration is in favour of a short drying treatment, like that allowed by use of microwaves.

This work brings new information about the opportunities offered by the use of microwaves in food treatments, especially for preservation of subtle properties like aroma.

In the case of mushrooms, combined microwave and hot air drying allows to shorten the process; this leads to limited thermal injury, easier water diffusion and larger aroma retention with an almost complete preservation of the original ratio between the volatiles responsible of the mushroom like flavour.

REFERENCES

1. S.Van Straten and H.Maarse, Volatile Compounds in Food. Zeist: Division for Nutrition and Food Research, TNO, 1983
2. W.Freytag and K.H.Ney, Europ.J.Biochem., 4 (1968), 315-318
3. D.A.Cronin and M.K.Ward, J.Sci.Food Agric., 22 (1971), 477-479.
4. K.H.Fischer and W.Grosch, Lebensm.Wiss.u.Technol., 20 (1987), 233-236
5. M.Wurzenberger and W.Grosch, Biochim. Biophys. Acta, 795 (1984), 163-165.
6. M.Komanowsky, Food Technol., 24 (9) (1970), 80-84
7. W.M.Crues and E.M.Mrak, Fruit Product J., 21 (1942), 302
8. F.J.McArdle and D.Curven, Mushroom Science, 5 (1962), 547
9. G.B.Bartholomai, Rev.Agronomica y Tecnologia de Alimentos, 14 (3) (1974), 429-438
10. M.Riva, A.Schiraldi and L.F.Di Cesare, Lebensm. Wiss. u.Technol., in press (1991)
11. L.F.Di Cesare, R.Nani and G.Bertolo, Imbottigliamento, 2 (1982), 42

G. Charalambous (Ed.), Food Science and Human Nutrition
© 1992 Elsevier Science Publishers B.V. All rights reserved.

STUDY OF THE INTERACTION BETWEEN POLYVINYL CHLORIDE AND VINYL CHLORIDE MONOMER USING INVERSE GAS CHROMATOGRAPHY - THERMODYNAMIC AND STRUCTURAL CONSIDERATIONS.

DIMITRIOS APOSTOLOPOULOS

Kraft General Foods, General Foods USA, Packaging Evaluation Center South Broadway, Tarrytown, NY 10591, USA.

SUMMARY

The interaction between residual vinyl chloride monomer (VCM) and polyvinyl chloride (PVC), a polymer of major use in packaging, was evaluated by using inverse gas chromatography (IGC). The polymer constituted the stationary phase and pulses of monomer were introduced into mobile phase. The specific retention volume, V_g^o, as well as, the thermodynamic parameters of the PVC-VCM interaction were calculated from chromatographic data. The results showed that the polymer-monomer interaction increased as the monomer concentration and temperature decreased. Also it was found that the number of binding active sites present in the polymeric matrix, an inherent part of the polymer structure, had an effect on the polymer-monomer interaction. Those findings suggest that the migration of VCM from PVC packaging materials with very low concentrations of residual monomer should be practically nil at ambient temperature.

INTRODUCTION

Due to incomplete polymerization unreacted vinylchloride monomer (VCM) remains physically trapped among the interstices of the polymeric chains in polyvinylchloride (PVC) based polymers. Residual VCM may migrate to commercial mouthwashes, alcoholic liquors, water, vegetable oil or other foods packaged in PVC bottles, food wrappings and other plastic articles with as little as 1-2 PPM of monomer (1-6).

Considerable attention was focused on the migration of residual VCM after it was realized that the latter is a potential carcinogen and can constitute a serious health hazard to the public (7).

The migration of VCM from a polymer to a contacting phase can be considered as a function of the polymer-monomer interaction and diffusion. The thermodynamics of the interaction determine the equilibrium distribution of the migrant and diffusion affects the rate of attaining the equilibrium (8).

One way to asses the propensity for migration of residual VCM in a PVC polymeric package is by studying the interaction between the polymer and monomer. The stronger the interaction between the two species the less is the chance that migration will occur (9). Because of the analytical difficulties involved there is only limited information available on the PVC-VCM interaction at lower VCM concentration ranges. Classical partition equilibria methods do not provide adequate sensitivity and in addition, they are time consuming. These limitations can be overcome by using Inverse Gas Chromatography (IGC). Numerous researchers have previously used IGC for studying polymer-monomer interactions (10-12). However, the absence of a contacting liquid phase does limit the usefulness of IGC somewhat, as the affect of solvent (food) penetration upon the polymer is not accounted for.

The present work was undertaken with the objective to study the PVC-VCM interaction at various temperatures and low VCM concentrations. In order to elucidate also the effect of PVC structure, PVC resin was treated with iodine (Wijs) solution to modify the polymer structure. Both treated and untreated resins were used in the study.

MATERIALS AND METHODS
Materials.

Unplasticized PVC resin with a density of 1.41g/ml, designated as VC47BE-1, supplied by Borden Chemical Company, North Andover, MA; Vinyl chloride monomer (VCM) of chromatographic grade and high purity (1066 PPM), supplied by Matheson Gas Products Co., East Rutherford, N.J.; Glacial acetic acid (99%); and Iodine (Wijs) solution, approximately 0.2N, containing glacial acetic acid, iodine and chrorine, supplied by Fisher Scientific Co., Fair Lawn, N.J.

Preparation of Monomer "Free" PVC Resin.

Prior to use PVC resin was sieved and the 100/150 mesh fraction collected. Sieved resin was further stripped of its residual monomer by heating at $60°-65°C$ in a vacuum oven under vacuum of 28 in. mercury for 24 hours. The removal of residual VCM was confirmed by using gas chromatography in combination with the hot jar technique as modified by Gilbert (13), sensitive to approximately 2×10^{-9}g VCM/g PVC.

Treatment of PVC Resin With Iodine Solution.

Monomer free PVC resin samples of 20g were placed in 250 ml Erlenmeyer flasks with 25ml iodine solution to soak for 24 hours at room temperature ($23°C$) and $60°C$. Afterwards samples were filtered, washed with excess of distilled water, methanol and again distilled water and dried in a vacuum oven at $60°C$ under vacuum of 28 in mercury for 24 hours.

Determination of Swelling For Iodine Treated PVC Resin.

Samples of monomer free PVC resin were treated with glacial acetic acid (99%) at $60°C$, in a manner similar to that previously described for the samples of PVC resin treated with iodine solution. This was necessary in order to differenciate between the effects of iodine and glacial acetic acid, both present in Wijs solution, on the swelling of polymer. Four (4) g of dry treated and untreated resins were placed separately into 20 ml glass test tubes and shaken to settle. The height (cm) of each resin inside the test tube was measured using a ruler and the occupied volume calculated. The volume difference observed between the untreated and treated resins was used to calculate percent of swelling for treated resins.

Preparation of Chromatographic Columns.

Monomer free untreated and iodine treated PVC resins were packed in 6'x 1/4" aluminum chromatographic grade columns. The packing was done with the aid of a vacuum pump and a mechanical vibrator to assure adequate settling of the polymeric resin. The amount of the polymer packed in the column was determined by weighing the column before and after packing. The amounts of PVC resin packed in the columns used with this study ranged from 19g to 21g. All columns were conditioned before use by purging overnight with nitrogen.

Preparation of VCM Standards.

Known volumes of VCM were introduced directly into glass serum vials, which had been tightly sealed and pre-flushed with pure nitrogen. One-half milliliter (0.5 ml) aliquots of VCM standards within the concentration range of 2 to 1066 PPM (V/V) were injected into G.C.

Measurement of Retention Time for VCM Probe/Apparatus.

A Hewlett Packard gas chromatograph, model 5990A, equipped with a dual flame ionization detector was used for measuring the retention time of VCM. Constant oven temperature was maintained to within $\pm$ 1°C by means of circulating air. A uniform temperature was assured throughout the chromatographic column by placing insulated spacers on column ends to prevent overheating from contact with injection port and detector. Nitrogen was used as the carrier gas. Its flow rate was measured at room temperature (25°C) by a soap bubble flow meter attached to the column outlet in combination with a stopwatch. The inlet pressure was measured on a mercury manometer with a range up to 100 cm Hg. The gas chromatograph operation conditions were as follows: column temperatures 30°C, 60°C; injection port temperatures 30°C, 60°C; detector temperature 215°C; carrier gas flow rate 60cc/min.

Determination of Specific Retention Volume (V_g^o).

As mentioned earlier IGC required packing of a chromatographic column with the polymeric resin under study and injection of small amounts of monomer in the mobile phase. The chromatographic system was assumed to attain true equilibrium instantaneously since small amounts of monomer were injected. After equilibration of the system the monomer was partitioned between stationary and mobile phase.

The volume of a carrier gas per unit weight of polymer necessary to elute the sorbed monomer from the polymer is defined as specific retention volume, V_g^o when corrected to 0°C. The latter which is absolutely characteristic of the under study polymer-monomer system was calculated using the following equation:

$$V_g^o = JF_m(t_r - t_a)((P_o - P_{f1})/P_o) \frac{273}{T_r} \frac{1}{W_s} \qquad (1)$$

where t_r is the retention time of the monomer; t_a is the retention time of an unsorbed species (air); F_m is the measured flow rate; P_o is the column outlet pressure; P_{f1} is the pressure inside a soap bubble flow meter; T_r is the room temperature; W_s is the polymer weight; and J is the James and Martin (14) compressibility factor accounting for pressure drop along the column which is calculated from equation:

$$J = \frac{3}{2} \left(\frac{(P_i/P_o)^2 - 1}{(P_i/P_o)^3 - 1} \right) \qquad (2)$$

where P_i is the column inlet pressure.

Determination of Thermodynamic Parameters.

Since the chromatographic system was assumed to attain instantaneous local equilibrium, the V_g^o was considered to be strictly dependent on the thermodynamic equilibrium of the polymer-monomer interaction unaffected by any operational parameters. Thus, the V_g^o values at infinite dilution were used to calculate the thermodynamic parameters of the interaction between the polymer and the monomer using equations:

$$-\frac{\Delta H_s^o}{R} = \frac{\partial \ln V_g^o}{\partial \frac{1}{T_{col}}} \qquad (3)$$

$$\Delta G_s^o = -RT_{col} \ln K_p \qquad (4)$$

$$K_p = \frac{V_g^o d \, T_{col}}{273} \qquad (5)$$

$$\Delta S_s^o = \frac{\Delta H_s^o - \Delta G_s^o}{T_{col}} \qquad (6)$$

where ΔH_s^o, ΔG_s^o and ΔS_s^o are the enthalpy, Gibb's free energy and entropy of sorption, respectively; R is the universal gas constant: K_p is the partition coefficient of monomer in the polymer/mobile phase; d is the density of the polymer (15,16).

RESULTS AND DISCUSSION.

Evaluation of the Specific Retention Volumes, V_g^o, and Thermodynamic Parameters.

1. Specific Retention Volumes, V_g^o.

The specific retention volumes, V_g^o, obtained for the interaction between VCM and untreated and iodine treated PVC at 30°C and 60°C are the average of replicate experiments, involving three determinations per experiment. For better illustration V_g^o values were plotted as a function of the amount injected and temperature (See Figs.1-3). Fig. 1 shows the effect of the amount of VCM injected and temperature on the V_g^o of untreated PVC resin.

The observed concentration dependence of V_g^o, clearly suggests a nonlinear distribution of the monomer in favor of the polymer phase. This nonlinearity of the partition coefficient as a function of the size of the injected VCM sample was rationalized in terms of the dual-mode sorption model (17,18). According to this model, the mechanism which controlled the monomer concentration in the polymer involved two distinctly different modes and the monomer present in the polymer existed in two thermodynamically distinct molecular species;

(i) molecules that following ordinary solution chemistry and obeying Henry's law were dissolved in the amorphous polymer matrix

(ii) molecules that following an activated sorption mechanism and obeying a Langmuirian law were physicochemically bound onto submicroscopic structural irregularities referred to as "active binding sites". Active binding sites represent regions of localized lower density, frozen into polymer matrix as a result of incomplete volume relaxation during quenching of the polymer from the rubbery to the glassy state. The total concentration of VCM in the polymer (C_T) can be expressed analytically as follows:

$$C_T = C_D + C_H \tag{7}$$

where C_D and C_H refer to the dissolved and Langmuirian concentrations, respectively.

The equilibrium distribution of VCM is given by equation:

$$K_p = K_{p_o} (1 + (C_H/C_D)) \tag{8}$$

where K_p is the experimentally derived partition coefficient, difined as the total concentration of VCM in the polymer (C_T) over the concentration of VCM in the mobile phase (C_m) at equilibrium:

$$K_p = \frac{C_T}{C_m} \tag{9}$$

and K_{p_o} is the ideal distribution law coefficient, defined as the concentration of VCM dissolved in the amorphous region of the polymer matrix (C_D) over the concentration of VCM in the mobile phase (C_m) at equilibrium:

$$K_p = \frac{C_D}{C_m} \tag{10}$$

Assuming that there is a finite number of active sites in the polymer matrix, two limiting cases can be discerned:

<u>Case I.</u> Where the amount of injected VCM was very low or the number of active sites were significant with respect to the concentration of VCM in the mobile phase. The rate constant for VCM sorption on active sites (K_H) was greater than the rate constant for dissolution in the amorphous polymer matrix (K_D), $K_H \geqslant K_D$ and the equilibrium $C_D \rightleftharpoons C_H$ was such that the concentration of VCM in the bound state (C_H) was equal to or exceeded that of the unbound (dissolved) species (C_D), $C_H \geqslant C_D$. The partition coefficient (K_p) became a function of C_H/C_D, and V_g^o which is another form of partition coefficient increased as the amount of injected monomer

decreased to a very low level.

Case II. Where the amount of injected VCM was very high or the number of active sites were insignificant with respect to the concentration of VCM in the mobile phase.

With a large amount of injected VCM the active sites were saturated, the concentration of monomer dissolved in the amprphous polymer matrix (C_D) became much greater than the concentration of bound species (C_H), $C_D \gg C_H$, the ratio C_H/C_D approached zero, the partition coefficient (K_p) became equivalant to K_{p_o}, $K_p \simeq K_{p_o}$ and V_g^o became concentration independent.

Besides the amount of injected VCM also the temperature had an effect on V_g^o. The temperature effect was twofold. As temperature increased V_g^o decreased and also became concentration independent at a lower VCM concentration as shown in Fig. 1. Apparently at an increased temperature the $C_D \rightleftharpoons C_m$ equilibrium shifted to the right, the ratio $-\dfrac{C_D}{C_m}-$ and the product of $K_{p_o}(1+ (C_H/C_D))$ decreased and as it becomes obvious from Equation 8 and 10, K_p also decreased. Consequently, as the monomer distribution equilibrium favored the mobile phase, V_g^o decreased. Also at higher temperature, the higher kinetic energy and increased perturbation acquired by VCM molecules bound onto active binding sites allowed them to overcome the sorption energy barrier, desorb and bounce back into mobile phase. Therefore, C_H decreased and C_m increased. This means that the number of active sites with high enough binding energy for monomer sorption became very small or insignificant with respect to the concentration of VCM in the mobile phase (C_m). The active sites of such a limited number were saturated at very low VCM concentration where C_H/C_D approached zero, Equation 8 was reduced to $K_p \simeq K_{p_o}$ and V_g^o became concentration independent.

Another parameter that affected also the specific volume, V_g^o was the type of resin. Significant V_g^o differences were observed amongst the various resins included in this study. PVC resin treated with iodine solution at 60°C exhibited the highest V_g^o values, followed by the resin treated with the same reagent at 23°C. Untreated PVC resin showed the lowest V_g^o values (See Figs. 1-3). Those V_g^o differences were thought to reflect structural changes induced by the treatment of PVC resin with the iodine solution and were interpreted in terms of the number of active binding sites present in the polymer matrix. As it might been expected treatment of the PVC resin with iodine solution resulted in sorption of bulky iodine molecules mainly and to a lesser extend of glacial acetic acid, both present in Wijs solution, which induced swelling and created stress-strain effects within the polymer's matrix, opened up the network of polymeric chains and uncovered new active sites. Application of heat with the resin treated at 60°C, facilitated penetration of additional sorbent into polymer which consequently caused more swelling.

As a result, there were more active sites uncovered and readily available for sorption of monomer molecules. The concentration of bound VCM (C_H), the ratio C_H/C_D, K_p and subsequently the V_g^o values increased. This explains why PVC resin treated with Wijs solution at 60°C exhibited greater V_g^o values than its treated at 23°C and untreated counterparts.

2. Gibb's Free Energy (ΔG_s^o).

The free energy changes (ΔG_s^o) for all studied resins are shown in Figs 4-6. ΔG_s^o was plotted as a function of the amount of injected VCM and temperature. As it is apparent, ΔG_s^o values followed the trend of V_g^o values. This supported the presence of active sites in the PVC matrix and signified their importance on the free energy of the PVC/VCM system.

The more negative or less positive ΔG_s^o values obtained at

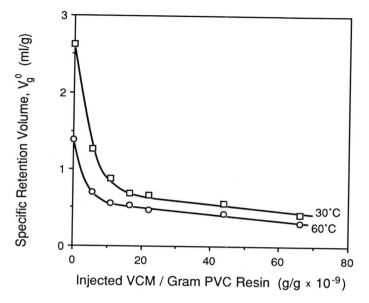

Figure 1. Specific retention volume (V_g^0) for untreated PVC resin as a function of VCM concentration and temperature

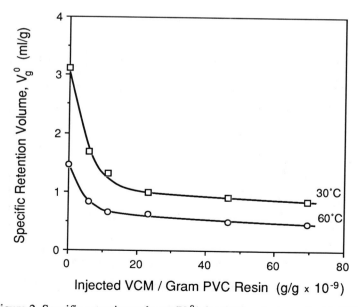

Figure 2. Specific retention volume (V_g^0) for PVC resin treated with Wijs solution at 23°C as a function of VCM concentration and temperature

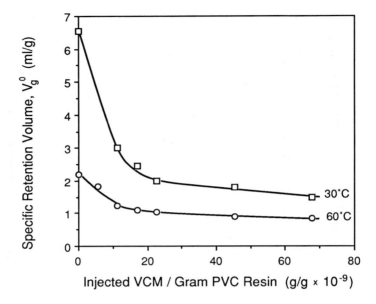

Figure 3. Specific retention volume (V_g^0) for PVC resin treated with Wijs solution at 60°C as a function of VCM concentration and temperature

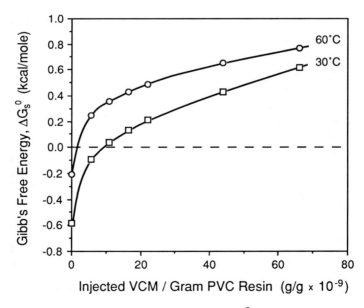

Figure 4. Gibb's free energy of sorption (ΔG_s^0) for untreated PVC resin as a function of VCM concentration and temperature

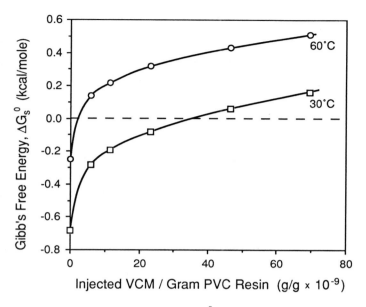

Figure 5. Gibb's free energy of sorption (ΔG_s^0) for PVC resin treated with Wijs solution at 23°C as a function of VCM concentration and temperature

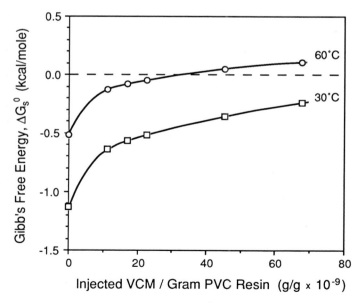

Figure 6. Gibb's free energy of sorption (ΔG_s^0) for PVC resin treated with Wijs solution at 60°C as a function of VCM concentration and temperature

lower temperature shows that binding of VCM was favored at lower temperatures. Also, $\triangle G_S^O$ became more rapidly concentration independent at higher temperatures. This provides evidence that less active site binding or greater matrix penetration occurred at higher temperatures. Therefore, it is easier for residual VCM to desorb and migrate from a PVC matrix at higher, rather than at lower temperatures. Resin treated with Wijs solution at 60^OC showed the more negative $\triangle G_S^O$ values. All the other resins had $\triangle G_S^O$ values that were less negative or even positive with the untreated resin more so. This indicates that the iodine treated resin at 60^OC was the most reactive due to the greater number of active sites available for sorption of VCM. The untreated resin with positive $\triangle G_S^O$ values was the least reactive. As a matter of fact the positive $\triangle G_S^O$ values obtained for PVC resins treated with iodine solution at 23^OC and untreated resin violate the second law of thermodynamics and indicate that the PVC/VCM system reached no equilibrium. This is probably due to the convoluted structure of VC47BE-1 PVC resin which did not allow VCM molecules to penetrate readily the PVC matrix, reach and interact with the active sites. The problem was further intensified with the relatively high carrier gas flow rates employed.

However, in studies of this type, it may be possible to generate retention and thermodynamic data corresponding to equilibrium conditions by optimization of flow rate, temperature and resin particle size (Courval and Gray 19).

3. Enthalpy ($\triangle H_S^O$).

The enthalping changes ($\triangle H_S^O$) as a function of VCM concentration are shown in Fig. 7. The concentration dependence of the $\triangle H_S^O$ values observed at the lower VCM concentrations indicates a relation between the enthalpy of the PVC-VCM system and the polymer structure. Apparently, the latter affected the number and binding capacity of the active sites present in the PVC matrix. Those active sites ultimately were involved in the rise of ΔH_s^o at lower VCM concentrations. PVC resin treated with Wijs solution at 60°C had the most negative ΔH_s^o values followed by the resin treated with Wijs solution at 23°C. Untreated resin had the least negative ΔH_s^o of the PVC resin treated with Wijs solution at 60°C when compared to other resins and especially to untreated resin, indicate that the former exhibited strongest total binding forces. This apparently resulted from the greater number of active sites exposed in this kind of resin.

4. Entropy of Sorption (ΔS_s^o).

Figs 8-10, show the effect of VCM concentration and temperature on ΔS_s^o values of untreated and treated PVC resins.

The differences in ΔS_s^o values and patterns of concentration shown by the studied resins indicate the existence of structural differences amongst those resins. The PVC resin treated with Wijs solution at 60°C exhibited the most negative ΔS_s^o values followed by the resin treated with Wijs solution at 23°C. The untreated resin had the least negative ΔS_s^o values. Such ΔS_s^o values clearly suggest that the VCM molecules sorbed onto resin treated with Wijs solution at 60°C assumed a more ordered arrangement as compared to VCM molecules sorbed by the untreated resin which appeared to be the most disordered. The order/disorder magnitude of the PVC-VCM system for the resin treated with Wijs solution at 23°C was in between. The greater order of VCM molecules sorbed onto resin treated with Wijs solution at 60°C was attributed to the structural changes that occurred within the polymer matrix during the treatment. The latter induced swelling of the polymer matrix and stress-strain effects that initiated some orientation

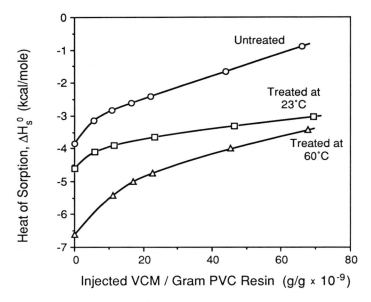

Figure 7. Heat of sorption (ΔH_s^0) for untreated and treated resins with Wijs solution as a function of VCM concentration

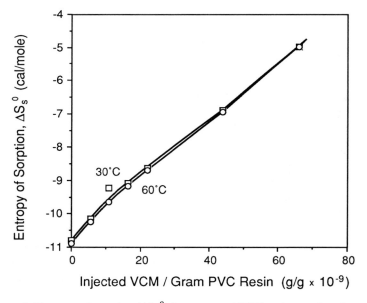

Figure 8. Entropy of sorption (ΔS_s^0) for untreated PVC resin as a function of VCM concentration and temperature

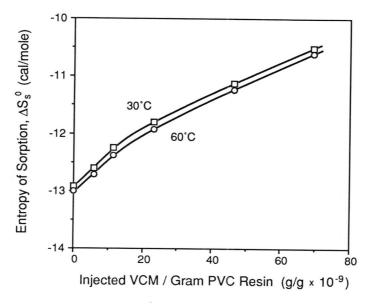

Figure 9. Entropy of sorption (ΔS_s^0) for PVC resin treated with Wijs solution at 23°C as a function of VCM concentration and temperature

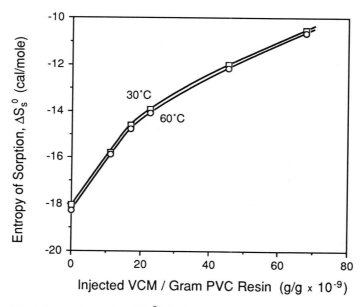

Figure 10. Entropy of sorption (ΔS_s^0) for PVC resin treated with Wijs solution at 60°C as a function of VCM concentration and temperature

of the polymer chains and simultaneously uncovered more binding active sites. The more ordered structure of the polymer matrix achieved through the chain orientation and the presence of more active sites allowed a more ordered accomodation of the sorbed VCM molecules. As a result the PVC-VCM system appeared to exhibit more order. Swelling of the polymer matrix was the result of the combined effect of heat and sorption of the bulky iodine molecules. The separate effects of those two factors on the structure of the polymer are manifested by the differences in ΔS_s^o values between the resin treated with Wijs solution at $60^{\circ}C$ and $23^{\circ}C$. The former exhibited more negative ΔS_s^o values than the latter. This indicates that heat must had a more significant effect on the change of the physical structure of the polymer than the Wijs solution itself. Furthermore, the change of the physical structure of the PVC resin upon treatment with Wijs solution, was evidenced by comparison of the specific gravity the untreated versus the treated resins. Treated resins and specifically the one of $60^{\circ}C$ showed a significant increase in volume upon the treatment (See Table 1).

TABLE 1

Swelling for Treated PVC Resins

Resin Treatment	Swelling(%)
PVC resin treated with Wijs solution at $23^{\circ}C$.	3.21
PVC resin treated with Wijs solution at $60^{\circ}C$.	76.50
PVC resin treated with glacial acetic acid at $60^{\circ}C$.	13.21

The concentration dependence of ΔS_s^o values at low VCM concentrations, observed particularly on the resins treated with Wijs solution, is one more manifestation of the active sites existence. As indicated by the small differences of ΔS_s^o values obtained at 30°C and 60°C where the polymer-monomer interaction was measured, temperature did not have as much of an impact on the order/disorder of the sorbed VCM molecules, as the polymer structure did.

The slightly more negative ΔS_s^o values at the lower temperature indicate a more ordered structure for the PVC-VCM system as compared to that at higher temperatures. This can be directly related to the kinetic energy of VCM molecules. The VCM molecules at the lower temperature did not have enough energy to overcome the sorption energy barrier and remained strongly bound on the active sites contributing to the overall order of the system. At the higher temperature the VCM molecules acquired excessive energy and perturbation that allowed them to overcome the sorption energy barrier of active sites and bounce back in the gaseous phase, creating instability and disorder amongst the sorbed VCM molecules.

CONCLUSIONS

Inverse gas chromatography (IGC) was used successfully to generate data that revealed very useful information about the nature of the interaction between VCM and PVC, a polymer of wide use in packaging. The momomer-polymer interaction increased with the decrease in temperature and the amount of VCM injected into the gas chromatograph. This is in agreement with findings by other investigators and supports point of view, that at ambient temperature and low enough residual VCM concentrations the monomer-polymer interaction may become so strong that residual monomer will likely possess a limited potential for migration into package contents.

ACKNOWLEDGEMENT

This work was done at Rutgers, The State University of New Jersey, in partial fulfilment of the requirements for the degree of Master of Science/Graduate Program in Food Science.

REFERENCES

1. K. Figge, Food Cosmet. Tox., (1972) 10, 815.
2. Federal Register, Food and Drug Administration (21 CFR Part 121) (1975) 40 (171), 40529.
3. G.A. Daniels and D.E. Proctor, Modern Packaging (1975) 48 (4), 45.
4. C.V. Breder, J.L. Dennison and M.E. Brown, J. Assoc. Off. Anal. Chem. (1975) 58 (6), 1214.
5. M.E. Kashtock, J,R. Giacin and S.G. Gilbert, J.Food Sci.(1980) 45, 1008-1011.
6. P. Kinigakis, J. Miltz and S.G. Gilbert, J. Food Process Preserv. (1987) 11, 247.
7. C. Maltoni and G. LeFemine, Annals of the New York Academy of Science (1975) 246, 195.
8. J.R. Morano, J.R. Giacin and S. G. Gilbert, J. Food Sci (1977) 42, 230-233.
9. S.G.Gilbert, J. Miltz and J.R. Giacin, J. Food Process Preserv. (1980) 4, 27.
10. J.M. Braun and J.E. Guillet, Macromolecules (1976) 9, 340.
11. M.A. Llorente, C. Meduina and A.Horta, J. Polym. Sci (1979) 24(1), 230.
12. P.G. Demertzis and M.G. Kontominas, Lebensm-Wiss + Technol. (1986) 19,249.
13. ASTM: F 151, Annual Book of ASTM Standards (1972) 42, 367.
14. A.T. James and A.J.P. Martin, Biochem. J.(1952) 50, 679.
15. J.L. Varsano and S.G.Gilbert, J. Pharm. Sci (1973) 62(1),87-91.
16. V.Rebar, E.R. Fischbach and D.Apostolopoulos, Biotech and Bioengineer (1984) XXVI, 513.
17. W.R. Vieth and K.J.Sladek, J. Colloid Sci (1965)20, 1014.
18. W.J. Koros and H.B. Hopfenberg, Food Technl. (1979) 33 (4),56.

INVERSE GAS CHROMATOGRAPHIC STUDY OF MOISTURE SORPTION BY WHEAT AND SOY FLOUR AND THE EFFECT OF SPECIFIC HEAT TREATMENT ON THEIR SORPTION BEHAVIOR.

K.A. RIGANAKOS, P.G. DEMERTZIS and M.G. KONTOMINAS

Lab.of Food Chemistry, Dept. of Chemistry, Univ. of Ioannina, 451 10 - Ioannina, Greece.

SUMMARY

Moisture sorption by wheat and soy flours was studied at 35 and 45°C using Inverse Gas Chromatography. Wheat flour showed a higher moisture uptake than soy flour. This was attributed to the higher percentage of hydrophilic starch in wheat flour as compared to soy flour. Both flours were subsequently heated at 150°C for 1 hr to investigate possible structural modifications of starch and/or protein, induced by the heat treatment. Sorption isotherms of the treated flours were then constructed at 35 and 45°C. Results showed no significant differences between untreated and heat treated samples. It seems that under present experimental conditions (low RH, short heating times) no significant phase transitions in the starch or denaturation in the proteins occured. Experimental data were successfully fitted to the BET equation and the monolayer value (V_m), sorption constant (C), specific surface area of the flours and the heat of adsorption of water were determined.

INTRODUCTION

Knowledge of the water sorption characteristics of flour based food products can aid: (a) in the development of formulations by showing the direction of moisture transfer of components in a mixture and (b) in the selection of proper packaging materials to optimize storage stability.

Wheat and soy flours are products rich in starch and protein respectively. Gluten is the main protein of wheat flour while glycinin is the main protein of soy flour. Both starch and proteins, due to their amorphous nature are known to adsorb water strongly, especially at low water activity values. It is apparent that water sorption directly affects the keeping quality of flours.

A factor which is expected to affect the sorption behavior of flours is heat treatment, since such a treatment is responsible for phase transitions in starch and denaturation in proteins as reported in the literature (ref.1). Heat treatment is a process that almost all dough containing mixtures undergo for the production of various commercial products (i.e. bread, cakes, cookies etc.).

Sorption of water by flour has been studied previously (refs. 2,3). However there has been very little attempt to account for the adsorptive capacity of flour on the basis of its chemical structure. The flour-water interaction has been studied by a number of techniques (ref.4-6). Among these, inverse gas chromatography is a rapid and efficient well established method for the study of moisture sorption of a variety of substrates (refs. 6-12).

The specific objectives of this paper were: (a) to study the effect of heating on moisture sorption by wheat and soy flour using inverse gas chromatography and X-ray diffraction spectroscopy, (b) to attempt to fit the experimental data to the BET equation model and (c) to determine the specific area and the heat of adsorption of water for both substrates.

MATERIALS AND METHODS

Wheat flour of 70% extraction rate was donated by "Mills of Saint George" Co., Athens, Greece, and soy flour by "Fytro Foods" Co., Athens, Greece. Proximate analysis of the two flours in accordance with AOAC methods (ref.13) is given in Table 1. Heat treatment consisted of heating the samples for 1 hr at 150°C in a vacuum oven. These time/temperature conditions were selected as representing those during commercial preparation of products such as bread, cakes, pies etc. All the samples were dried in a vacuum oven at 40°C for 24 hrs before use. Wheat and soy flours were sieved and fractions of particle size 60-80 Mesh were collected. Each sample then was mixed with inert support, chromosorb (W-Acid Washed DMCS-treated 60-80 Mesh, SERVA, W.Germany) in a ratio of 1% (w/w) and was used to pack a stainless steel column of dimensions 0,90 m x 0,64 cm (1/4 in o.d.). The amount of the flour in the column was kept at a minimum amount in order to minimize diffusion effects within the column which would result in broadening of the chromatographic peaks.

TABLE 1. Proximate analysis of wheat and soy flour

Type of flour	Moisture (%)	Starch (%)	Protein (%)	Fat (%)	Ash,Fibers (%)
Wheat flour of 70% extraction rate	12	70	13	2	3
Soy flour	10.5	30.5	48.5	1.5	6

The column was then connected to a VARIAN 3700 gas chromatograph equipped with a thermal conductivity detector and conditioned for 24 hrs using helium as the carrier gas. In all the experiments distilled water was injected into the column via a microsyringe in volumes ranging from 0,1μl to 10μl. All experiments were carried out in triplicate at 35 and 45°C. Peak and peak areas were recorded on a VARIAN 9176 recorder. Gas chromatographic operational conditions were as follows: Carrier gas flow rate: 30ml/min; injection port temperature: 155°C; detector temperature: 170°C; filament current: 150mA. Moisture-free helium was used as the carrier gas.

X-ray diffraction spectra of all the samples were recorded using a Siemens D-500 X-ray diffractometer. The operational conditions were: 30mA, 40kV; diffraction angle was 3-60°; scanning rate was 1°/min; X-ray source was Copper-K_a with a graphite monochromator. Prior to recording X-ray diffraction spectra, the samples were dried for 24 hrs in a vacuum oven at 40°C.

RESULTS AND DISCUSSION

Details on the use of inverse gas chromatography to calculate water uptake (a) by substrates are given elsewhere (refs. 8,14-15).

Sorption isotherms of wheat and soy flour at 35 and 45°C are shown in figures 1 and 2, as moisture uptake (a) versus partial vapour pressure (P). Sorption isotherms are of sigmoid shape (BET type II) which is typical of most food products (ref.16). The shape of the

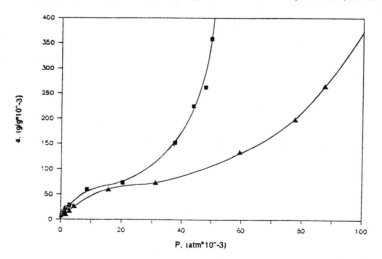

Fig. 1: Water sorption isotherms for wheat flour at 35°C (■) and 45°C (▲).

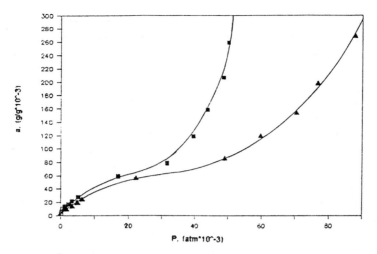

Fig. 2: Water sorption isotherms for wheat soy flour at 35°C (■) and 45°C (▲).

isotherms can be explained in terms of the three-step moisture sorption process for starch and proteins given in previous work (refs. 6,12).

In figure 3 the sorption isotherms of wheat and soy flour at 35°C are given for comparison purposes. It is clear that wheat flour adsorbs a larger amount of water at a

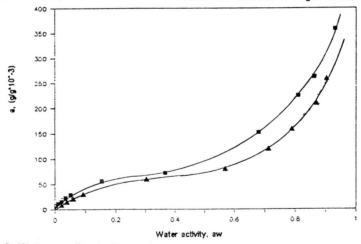

Fig. 3: Water sorption isotherms for wheat flour (■) and soy flour (▲) at 35°C.

given water activity value than soy flour. This can be related to the higher sorptive capacity of the hydrophilic starch (wheat flour is rich in starch) possessing more active sites (OH$^-$ groups) than the less hydrophilic protein (soy flour is reach in protein) possessing fewer active sites (>C=O, COO$^-$, NH$_4^+$). (ref.2).

Sorption isotherms of untreated and heat treated wheat and soy flour are shown in figures 4 and 5 at two different temperatures. Figures 4 and 5 show a rather insignificant effect of heat treatment for both flours, especially at low water activity values.

It seems that present heat treatment conditions had no effect on protein structure (denaturation). Similar findings have been reported by Labuza (1968). (ref.1). According to Altman and Benson (1959) (ref.17) denaturation of egg albumin does not occur at a measurable rate until the relative huminity exceeds 0.60. Present heat treatment conditions correspond to relative humidity values significantly lower than 0.60 since the flours were heated in the absence of water. Bushuk and Winkler (ref. 2) reported a 20% reduction in wheat flours sorptive capacity for water after a heat treatment at 100°C for 24 hrs. In these experiments the flour was heated in the absence of water. Reduction of sorptive capacity of the flours for water after 4 and even 8 hrs of heating under same conditions was insignificant.

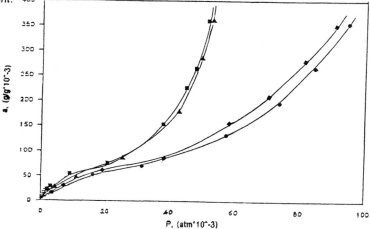

Fig. 4: Water sorption isotherms for untreated and heat-treated wheat flour at 35°C [untreated (■), heat-treated (▲)] and 45°C [untreated (♦), heat-treated (●)].

The effect of heat treatment on starch is also insignificant with the possible exception of wheat flour rich in starch, at high relative humidity values. It is possible that at the higher

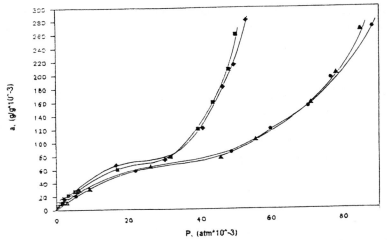

Fig. 5: Water sorption isotherms for untreated and heat-treated wheat flour at 35°C [untreated (♦), heat-treated (■)] and 45°C [untreated (▲), heat-treated (●)].

temperature (45°C) and relative humidity values (>0.50) the amount of crystalline. water impenetrable starch increases slightly at the expense of the amorphous starch (ref.1).

Above results are supported by X-ray diffraction spectra (figure 6). Any phase transition

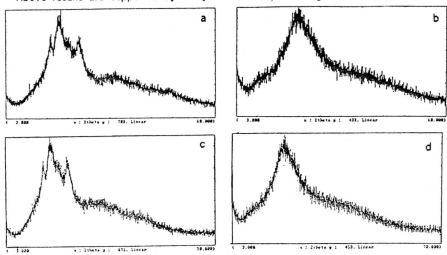

Fig. 6: X-ray diffraction spectra of: a) untreated wheat flour, b) untreated soy flour, c) heat-treated wheat flour and d) heat-treated soy flour

(amorphous ⟶ crystalline) affecting the sorption behavior of the flour would have shown up in the X-ray spectra. Figure 6a is identical to fig.6c and fig.,6b is identical to fig.6d evident of no significant structural modifications of the flours during heat treatment (ref.18).

BET Isotherm

The isotherm model most widely used in food systems is that of Brunauer et al (BET) (19) which is expressed by the equation (1):

$$\frac{a_w}{(1-a_w)V} = \frac{1}{V_m C} + \frac{a_w(C-1)}{V_m C} \tag{1}$$

where V is the amount sorbed, V_m is the monolayer value, a_w is the water activity, C is a sorption constant equal to:

$$C = Ke^{Q_s/RT} \tag{2}$$

where Q_s is the heat of sorption, K is a factor $\cong 1$, R is the universal gas constant and T is the absolute temperature.

A plot of $a_w/(1-a_w)V$ vs a_w gives a straight line, from the slope and intercept of which the monolayer value, (V_m) and the sorption constant (C) can be calculated (Tables 2 and 3). V_m can be considered as equivalent to the amount of water held adsorbed on specific sites of the adsorbent. It has been suggested (refs. 20,21) that the BET water monolayer value corresponds to optimum storage stability of dehydrated foods because of the protective effect of water against oxygen adsorption and/or interaction of adjacent polar groups.

TABLE 2. BET constants (V_m, C), BET surface area (S_o) and heat of sorption (Q_S, Q_T) for untreated and heat-treated wheat flour.

Material	Temperature (°C)	Vm (g/gx10⁻³)	C	S_o (m²/g)	Q_S (Kcal/mol)	Q_T (Kcal/mol)
Untreated	35	0.061	31.09	213.5	-2.10	-12.54
	45	0.061	30.62	213.5	-2.16	-12.60
Heat-treated	35	0.058	29.76	203.0	-2.08	-12.52
	45	0.057	28.61	199.5	-2.12	-12.56

TABLE 3. BET constants (V_m, C), BET surface area (S_o) and heat of sorption (Q_S, Q_T) for untreated and heat-treated soy flour.

Material	Temperature (°C)	V_m (g/g×10⁻³)	C	S_o (m³/g)	Q_S (Kcal/mol)	Q_T (Kcal/mol)
Untreated	35	0.053	23.50	185.5	-1.93	-12.37
	45	0.052	22.56	182.0	-1.97	-12.41
Heat-treated	35	0.050	24.20	175.0	-1.95	-12.39
	45	0.049	20.93	171.5	-1.92	-12.36

Application of sorption data to the BET equation gave a very good correlation (R^2=0.97-0.99).

V_m and C values for untreated and heat treated flour samples are very similar (tables 2 and 3).

The most significant factor for the success of the BET theory is that it provides a means of evaluating the specific surface area of the adsorbent (determined from V_m) and the heat of adsorption for the first layer (determined from C).

The specific surface area (S_o) in given by the equation (3) (ref.1,22):

$$S_o = \frac{1}{M_{H_2O}} N_o A_{H_2O} \cdot V_m \quad (m^2/gr \text{ solid}) \qquad (3)$$

Where: M_{H_2O} is the relative molecular mass of water (=18 gr/mole), N_o is Avogadro's number (6.023×10²³ molecules/mole) and A_{H_2O} is the apparent surface area of one water molecule (10.6×10⁻²⁰ m²). Specific surface area values are given in Tables 2 and 3. Our specific surface area value for untreated wheat flour (213.5 m²/g) is in good agreement with that of Bushuk and Winkler (235 m²/g) (ref. 2).

The heat of sorption Q_S is the heat required for partial or total dehydration of food. According to the assumptions of the BET isotherm model, the total heat of sorption Q_T for the first layer is equal to the ΔH_v (heat of vaporization =-10.44 kcal/mol) plus the heat of sorption (due to site interaction) Q_S and for all layers above the monolayer Q_T is equal to ΔH_v. Q_S and Q_T values are given in tables 2 and 3. The value of Q_T for wheat flour (approximately, -12.50kcal/mol) correlates very well with that of Bushuk and Winkler (12.60 kcal/mol) (ref. 2).

In conclusion, it should be stressed that heat treatment of the flour samples under conditions of low RH and short heating times has no significant effect on the moisture sorption profile of these food products. Investigation of moisture sorption of flours under various heat treatment conditions (% RH, time, temperature) will be the objective of a forthcoming paper.

REFERENCES
1. T.P.Labuza, Sorption phenomena in foods, Food Technol., 22 (1968) 263-271.
2. W.Bushuk and C.A.Winkler, Sorption of water vapor on wheat flour, starch and gluten. Cereal Chem., 34 (1957) 73-84.
3. J.Hlynka and A.D.Robinson, Moisture and its measurement In : J.A.Anderson and A.W.Alcock, (eds.) Storage of cereal grains and their products, Am. Assoc. Cereal Chemists, St. Paul, Minnesota (1954).
4. K.F.Finney and W.T.Yamazari, Water retention capacity as an index of the loaf volume potentialities and protein quality of hard red winter wheats, Cereal Chem., 23 (1946) 416-427.
5. J.D.Geerdes and R.H.Harris, Characterizations of hard red spring and durum wheat proteins by some physico-chemical properties, Cereal Chem., 29(1952), 132-141.
6. K.A.Riganakos, P.G.Demertzis and M.G.Kontominas, Gas Chromatographic Study of Water sorption by wheat flour, J.Cereal Science, 9 (1989), 261-271.
7. D.G.Gray and J.E.Guillet, A gas chromatographic method for the study of sorption on polymers, Macromolecules, 5(3) (1972) 316-321.
8. U.Coelho, J.Miltz and S.G.Gilbert, Water binding on collagen by inverse phase gas chromatography: Thermodynamic considerations, Macromolecules, 12 (1979) 284-287.
9. D.S.Smith, C.H.Mannheim and S.G.Gilbert, Water sorption isotherms of sucrose and glucose by inverse gas chromatography, J.Food Sci., 46 (1981) 1051-1053.
10. H.J.Helen and S.G.Gilbert, Moisture sorption of dry bakery products by inverse gas chromatography, J.Food Sci., 50(1985) 454-458.
11. D.Apostolopoulos and S.G.Gilbert, Frontal inverse gas chromatography as used in studying water sorption of coffee solubles, J.Food Sci., 53 (1988) 882-884.
12. P.G.Demertzis and M.G.Kontominas, Study of water sorption of egg powders by inverse gas chromatography, Z.Lebensm.Unters.Forsch., 186 (1988) 213-217.
13. AOAC, Official methods of analysis, 12th edn., Washington DC (1975).
14. A.V.Kiselev and Y.I.Yashin, "Gas Adsorption Chromatography", Plenum Press, New York (1969).

15 P.G.Demertzis, M.G.Kontominas and S.G.Gilbert, Gas Chromatographic determination of sorption isotherms of vinylidene chloride on vinylidene chloride copolymers, J.Food Science, 52 (1978) 747-750.
16 N.W.Desrosier, Elements of Food Technology, AVI Dubl. Co., Westport (1977).
17 R.L.Altman and S.W.Benson, The effect of water upon the rate of heat denaturation of egg albumin, J.Am.Chem.Soc., 82(1960), 3852-3857.
18 W.T.Astbury and R.Lomax, An x-ray study of the hydration and denaturation of proteins, J.Chem.Soc. (1935) 846-851.
19 J.Brunauer, P.H.Emmett and E.Teller, Adsorption of gases in multimolecular layers, J.Amer.Chem.Soc., 60(1938) 309-319.
20 H.Salwin, Moisture levels required for stability in dehydrated foods, Food Technol., 174(1963) 34-41.
21 A.T.Aguerre, C.Suarez and P.E.Viollaz, Some aspects derived from BET theory and their relation with food conservation, Lebensm.-Wiss u.Technol., 19 (1986) 328-330.
22 P.G.Demertzis, K.A.Riganakos and M.G.Kontominas, Water sorption isotherms of crystalline raffinose by inverse gas chromatography, Inter. J. Food Sci. Technol., 24 (1989), 629-636.

APPLICATION OF A MODIFIED I.G.C. METHOD IN THE STUDY OF THE WATER SORPTIONAL BEHAVIOR OF SELECTED PROTEINS I. LYSOZYME-WATER INTERACTIONS.

P.G. DEMERTZIS[1], S.G. GILBERT[2] AND H. DAUN[2]

[1]University of Ioannina, Department of Chemistry, Laboratory of Food Science, P.O. Box 1186, 45110-Ioannina, Greece.

[2]Department of Food Science and the Center for Advanced Food Technology, Cook College, Rutgers University, P.O. Box 231, New Brunswick, N.J. 08903.

SUMMARY

The water sorptional bahavior of a hydrophilic protein (purified lysozyme) as affected by sample pretreatment (slow freezing, fast freezing, glycosylation and predrying) was studied using a modified pulse inverse gas chromatographic method. Fast-frozen lysozyme showed a slightly higher water adsorption than slow-frozen one, where glycosylated lysozyme adsorbed less compared to the unglycosylated sample. On the other hand, predrying of the substrates caused a relatively significant diminishing on their sorptional behavior because of structural changes (restructuring) occuring during predrying. Data were succesfully fitted to the Guggenheim, Anderson and De Boer (G.A.B.) equation and analysed according to the Zimm-Lundberg cluster theory. Results showed enhanced cluster formation tendency for predried materials as well as for glycosylated lysozyme.

INTRODUCTION

In recent years, protein-water interactions have received increasing attention as these interactions play an important role in determining the three dimentional structure of the protein molecules as well as many of the functional properties of proteins in foods (refs 1-3). Water molecules are linked to the active site of the substrate changing the individual structures to more cohesive and thus affecting the physical properties of fabricated foodstuffs. The amount of water absorbed depends on the type of protein, the degree of bioactivity (native or denaturated) and the conformational (spacial) structure of protein (ref. 4).

Lysozyme is a well-known protein with approximate molecular weight of 14,400. Each molecule consists of a single polypeptide chain with 129 aminoacids, the main of them being arginine (8.5%), aspartic acid (16%), threonine (8%), glycine and alanine (ref. 5). The protein exhibits high hydrophilicity and is stable to heat up to 55°C. Thus lysozyme serves as a good substrate for investigating protein-water interactions involving polar binding sites (refs 6-8)).

Numerous methods have been used to study water binding by proteins or, generally, the properties of protein-water interaction. The simplest and most accepted technique used to study these properties is sorption-desorption isotherm, e.g. graph of water activity (a_w) versus moisture content at constant temperature. Water sorption isotherms of protein systems can give the necessary knowledge to understand the mechanism of water sorption and the role of water in some reactions critical for the performance of commercial foods such as Maillard reactiosn etc (refs 4,9,10).

Water sorption isotherms can be analysed with theoretical models derived from physicochemical calculations. Specifically, this analysis can provide values for monolayer coverage of the substrate, specific active sites and clustering levels at variable coverage.

The use of the method of inverse gas chromatography (IGC) for the determination of sorption isotherms is especially advantageous when there is a need for rapid water sorption determination and limited amounts of substrates are available (ref. 11). The rapidity of the method has been further inhanced by using a recently developed modified pulse technique which produces a sorption isotherm from a single chromatographic elution peak (ref.12). Moreover, the method does not require that moisture equilibrium be attained during data collection. Based on mass balances and equations well described elsewhere (ref. 9,12,13) the evaluation of water uptake, water content and water activity are based on the following mathematical relations:

$$W_U = \frac{k_t t_i - k_a A_i}{m_s} \quad (1)$$

where W_U is the water uptake (g/g); m_s is the amount of stationary phase (g); t_i is the time (s); A_i is the area under the elution peak at time t_i; k_t is time constant; and k_a is area constant,

$$a_w = \frac{V_{t_i}}{V_{max}} \quad (2)$$

where V_{t_i} is the voltage at time t_i; and V_{max} is the maximum peak voltage in an empty (calibration) column under the same conditions.

The objectives of the present study were:
a) To use the new modified IGC technique for determination of water sorption isotherms of various lysozyme samples.
(b) To study the effect of pretreatment (fast freezing, slow freezing and predrying) on the water sorptional behaviour of purified lysozyme.

(c) To gain new insight on posible water-water and water-protein interactions by using model equations (G.A.B) and Zimm-Lundberg cluster analysis.

MATERIALS AND METHODS

MATERIALS

Purified slow-frozen and fast-frozen samples were prepared as follows: A preweighed amount of lysozyme (Sigma Chem. Co., cat. #6876) was dissolved in deionized water and filtered through 0.45 micron cellulose acetate filter (Millipore, type HV). The sample was dialyzed against deionized water using a preconditioned dialysis tubing (boiled six times in deionized water using a preconditioned dialysis tybing (boiled six times in deionized water) of molecular weight cut-off (MWCO) 3,500, for 4 days at 4°C, changing water 1-2 times per day. A portion of the sample was slow-freezed and freeze-dried for 48 hours at lowest vacuum (slow-frozen lysozyme). Another portion of the sample was immersed in a dry-ice bath for a few seconds (fast-frozen lysozyme).

Glycosylated slow-frozen lysozyme was prepared as follows: 1g purified slow-frozen lysozyme and 3000mg anhydrous D-glucose (Analytical grade) were dissolved in 15 ml of deionized water, slow-freezed (overnight in freezer) and freeze-dried for 48 hours at lowest vacuum. Lyophilized material was placed into chamber under controlled atmosphere equilibrated at 65% R.H. and 50°C for 15 days. After this, 15 ml of water were added to the reaction vial and the sample was dialyzed using dialysis tubing of (a) MWCO = 1,000 for 8 hours, (b) MWCO = 3,500 for 8 hours and (c) MWCO = 10,000 for 8 hours. Aliquots were collected each two hours and the disappearance of glucose was measured using a spectrophotometric test (Methods in Enzymology, 1984, Vol.116, 77-87). The sample was finaly slow freezed and freeze-dried for 48 yours at lowest vacuum.

The predried materials for each of the above samples were prepared by packing an appropriate amount of them into a GC column which was placed into the GC oven at 55°C and subjected to 1 hour drying under inert gas flow adjusted at 40ml N_2/min to a presumed constant weight since water vapor pressure of sample was below the sensitivity of the thermal conductivity detector.

METHODS

1. IGC instrumentation and procedure

A schematic diagram of the setup equipment used in the present study is shown in Figure 1. The gas chromatogram was a Varian 3700 equipped with a thermal conductivity detector and a liquid carbon dioxide cryogenic system. The analog to digital (A/D) converter, model Dash-8 (12 bit resulution) and the analog input submultiplexer expansion, model EXP-16, were purchased from Metrabyte Co (Tannton, MA, USA). The personal computer was an IBM-XT (International Business Machines Corp.). The Labtech Notebook software (Laboratory Technologies Corp., Cambridge, MA) version 4.1, was used for the data acquisition, while for the data analysis the Lotus 1-2-3- program, version 2.01 was used.

The GC columns were pure-sample and short lenght. A swagelok reducer fitting was used as column loaded with approximately 50 mg of sample with the aid of a vacuum pump and a mechanical vibrator. A relatively large amount of solute e.g. 25-30 μl water) was injected using an empty (calibration) column first and then using a loaded one. The analog response from the GC was digitized while displayed in real-time mode on the monitor screen and simultaneously was stored in a real ASCII file on the computer's hard disk. Further analysis of data to obtain water sorption isotherms was performed using a BASIC language program.

Model equation analysis was carried out using the Labtech's Notebook curve-fit (non-linear regression analysis) program.

2. Density measurements

True density measurements (for cluster analysis) were carried out using a gas pycnometer (Quantachrome, model SPY-2 stereopycnometer) which utilized helium gas (20 psig) to measure the true volume of a preweighed aliquot of the sample).

RESULTS AND DISCUSSION

1. Water Sorption isotherms

Figures 2-4 show the GC profiles of "as is" and "predried" materials studied (fast-frozen lysozyme, slow-frozen lysozyme and glycosylated lysozyme at 25ºC. The corresponding water sorption isotherms for the above materials at 25ºC are given in fugures 5-7. Figures for fast-frozen lysozyme samples show the high sorption capacity of highly amorphous lysozyme as well as the transition occuring at abour 65% R.H. when water organizes in clusters. This restructuring effect is more pronounced in case of "as is" sample and depends on the extent of exposure time to permit water cluster formation into the matrix of the substrate and also on temperature. In case of slow-frozen lysozyme (Figs 2 and 5), the observed transitions were much less pronounced. This can be attributed to the significantly less matestable structure obtained by the slow-freeze procedure. Similarly, transitions have not been observed in case of glycosylated lysozyme (Figs 3 and 6) indicating more stable structure. Above results are in general accordance with previous experimental results on similar substrates (refs 9,13) and

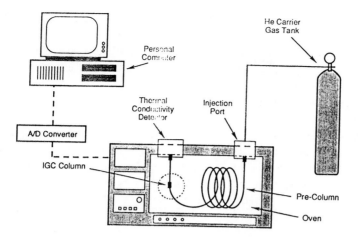

Figure 1: Schematic diagram of the I.G.C. setup equipment

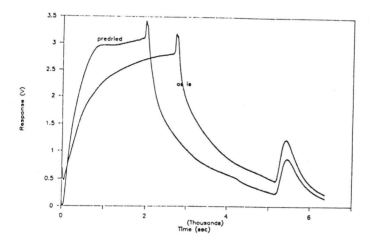

Figure 2: Chromatograms of "as is" and "predried" fast-frozen purified lysozyme samples at 25°C.

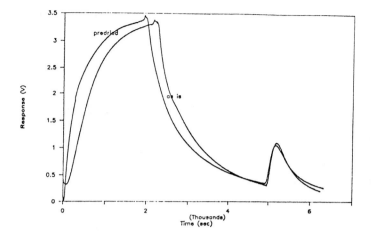

Figure 3: Chromatograms of "as is" and "predried" slow-frozen purified lysozyme samples at 25°C.

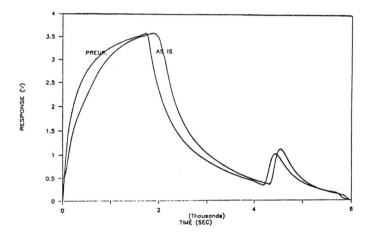

Figure 4: Chromatograms of "as is" and "predried" glycosylated slow-frozen lysozyme samples at 25°C.

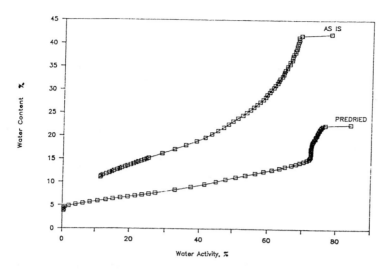

Figure 5: Water sorption isothrems of "as is" and "predried" fast-frozen purified lysozyme samples at 25°C.

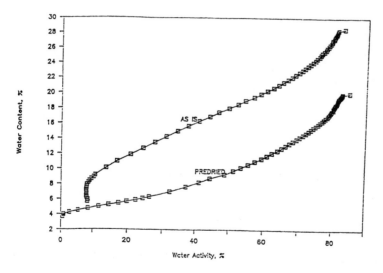

Figure 6: Water sorption isothrems of "as is" and "predried" slow-frozen purified lysozyme samples at 25°C.

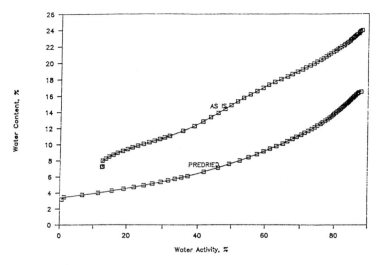

Figure 7: Water sorption isothrems of "as is" and "predried" glycosylated slow-frozen lysozyme samples at 25°C.

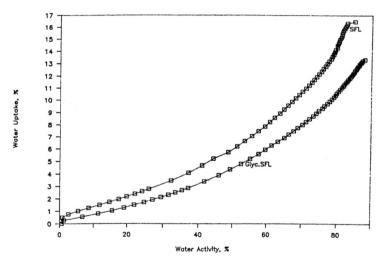

Figure 8: Comparison between water sorption isotherms of "predried" slow-frozen lysozyme and glycosylated lysozyme samples at 25°C.

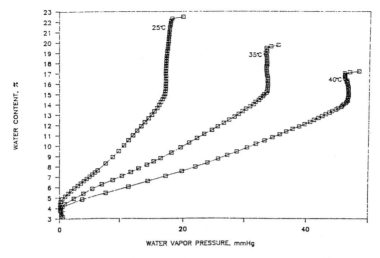

Figure 9: Water sorption isotherms of fast-frozen purified lysozyme at different temperatures.

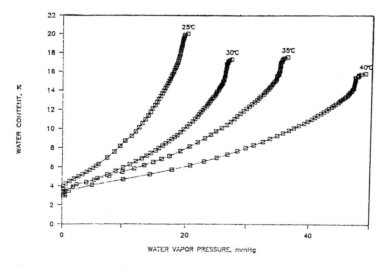

Figure 10: Water sorption isotherms of slow-frozen purified lysozyme at different temperatures.

indicate, once again, the potential of IGC in elucidating the eccect of water on restructuring of food systems.

The effect of glycosylation on water sorptional behavior of lysozyme is clearly shown in Figure 8. This figure shows that glycosylated lysozyme absorbs less than the unglycosylated one, under the same conditions. This finding can be attributed to the partial coverage of lysozyme high hydrophilicity amino groups as they react with glucose, as well as to possible structural changes occuring during glycosylation process.

Sorption isotherms of the majority of the substrates were of sigmoid type (BET type II) which is typical of most food constituents. Only in case of "predried" glycosylated lysozyme sample "sugar-like" (BET type III) isotherm was obtained indicating less hydrophilicity for this substrate.

The effect of temperature on water sorption isotherm of the three substrates is shown in Figs 9-11. Temperature shifts can have important effects on chemical and microbiological reactivity related to quality deterioration of preserved foods. It is also well known that temperature affects the mobility of water molecules and the dynamic equilibrium between the vapor and adsorbed phase. As can be seen from Figs 9-11, under constant vapor pressure (or a_w), increase in temperature causes a decrease in the amount of sorbed water. This is observed in most foods and indicates that substrate becomes less hygroscopic with increasing temperature. This is neccesitated by the thermodynamic relationship,

$$\Delta G = \Delta H - T\Delta S \qquad (3)$$

Since $\Delta G<0$ (spontaneous process) and $\Delta S<0$ (sorbed water has less freedom), $\Delta H<0$. Therefore, an increase of temperature represents unfavorable condition to the sorption process.

2. Model equation analysis - Application of G.A.B. equation

Equations for fitting water sorption isotherms are of special interest in many aspects of food preservation (shelf-life prediction of dried packaged products, prediction of drying times, prediction of equilibrium conditions for mixtures of products with various water activities). They are also needed for evaluating the thermodynamic parameters of the water sorbed in foods.

There are a great number of theoretical and empirical equations in the literature, which have been proposed for correlating equilibrium moisture content in food systems.

The G.A.B. equation (for Guggenheim-Anderson-De Boer) has been recognized as the best theoretical model for foods (refs 14,15). It is a three parameter equation recently favored by the majority of European Food Research Laboratories. The G.A.B. equation is in the form:

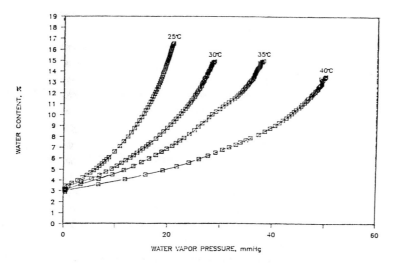

Figure 11: Water sorption isotherms of glycosylated slow-frozen lysozyme at different temperatures.

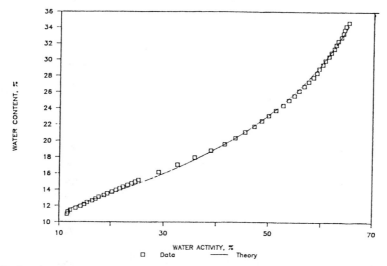

Figure 12: Least square fitting of the G.A.B. equation on "as is" fast-frozen purified lysozyme at 25 °C.

$$\frac{W}{W_m} = \frac{Cka_w}{(1-ka_w)(1-ka_w + Cka_w)} \tag{4}$$

where:

W is % water content on dry basis

W_m is % water content corresponding to saturation of all primary adsorption sites by one water molecule (formerly called B.E.T. monolayer value).

a_w is water activity

C is the Guggenheim constant $= c' \exp[(H_i - H_m) / RT]$

k is a factor correcting properties of the multilayer molecules with respect to the bulk liquid: $k = k' \exp[(H_i - H_q) / RT]$

H_i is heat of condensation of pure water vapor

H_q is total heat of sorption of the multilayer water molecules.

G.A.B. model can be considered as an extention of the B.E.T. model taking into account the modified properties of the sorbate in the multilayer region.

The G.A.B. model was fitted to our data using non-linear regression analysis. Figure 12 shows a depicted example of the data together with the fitted theory. The G.A.B. model gave a very good fit either for the whole water activity range or for the a_w range from 10 to 65% in the case of fast- and slow-frozen lysozyme samples. The estimated coefficients from G.A.B. equation are given in table **1**. Of special interest are the W_m values of various substrates as they give the amount of water corresponding to the monolayer coverage. Results in table 1 indicate that there is a significant difference in W_m values between "as is" and "predried" samples. More specifically, for the same substrate, the "as is" sample exhibits greater W_m value compared to the "predried" sample. These differences can be attributed to structural changes occuring during predrying (retrogradation) which reduce the water sorptive capacity of the material.

3. Zimm-Lundberg cluster analysis

Zimm and Lundberg (ref. 16) proposed a "cluster theory" in order to explain the sorption of vapors by high polymers, which can be used to study the water sorption behavior of biopolymer/solute systems. The theory defines a function (cluster function) that measures the tendency of the adsorbed molecules to cluster. This approach includes a direct measurment of nonrandom mixing in a two-component system without using any preconceived model and thus provides a means of interpreting the sorption data in molecular terms. The clustering function (G_{11}/V_1) is the mean number of water molecules in the vicinity of similar molecule in ecess of the number that might be anticipated in the vicinity if the distribution were solely a consequence of random mixing, and is equal to:

$$G_{11}/V_1 = \varphi_2 \, [\, (a_w/\varphi_1) \, / \, a_w]_{P,T} - 1 \tag{5}$$

where G_{11} = the cluster integral,
V_1 = partial molar volume of component 1 (water),
φ_1 = volume fraction of component 1,
$\varphi_2 = (1-\varphi_1)$ = volume fraction of component 2 (sorption substrate).

In terms of molar concentration, the cluster function is given by:

$$\varphi_1 \, G_{11} \, / \, V_1 \, = \, C_1 G_{11} \tag{6}$$

where C_1 = molar concentration of component 1.

The average number of molecules existing in a cluster (average cluster size) is then given by:

$$\varphi_1 G_{11}/V_1 + 1 \text{ or } C_1 G_{11} + 1 \tag{7}$$

Negative cluster values, especially smaller than -1, indicate no cluster formation and also that sorbate molecules are widely dispersed in the system and are probably attached to specific sites sorption. A positive cluster value means that the average solute molecule has more neighbors of its own nature than would be present in a random distribution. Furthermore, cluster formation leads to a matrix expansion and thus new active sites may be exposed. In an ideal solution the clustering function, in terms of average cluster size, is equal to +1, i.e. type 1 molecule excludes its own volume to other molecules.

Cluster analysis was applied to fast- and slow-frozen lysozyme ("as is" and "predried" samples), and average cluster size functions vs water activity were plotted at 25°C (figures 13 and 14). From these figures some interesting results can be arisen:
(a) There is a significant difference in the tendency to cluster formation between the "as is" and the corresponding "predried" sample. For instance, in the case of slow-frozen lysozyme the "as is" sample starts to exhibit clustering conditions at a_w=0.90 while the "predried" sample starts to exhibit clustering conditions at significantly lower a_w(=0.63). The same behavior is also observed for fast-frozen sample. The explanation is the same as that already given for the W_m values. It seems that the tendency for adsorbed water to form clusters is mainly related to the hydrophobicity of the system, e.g., the more hydrophobic the system the greater the

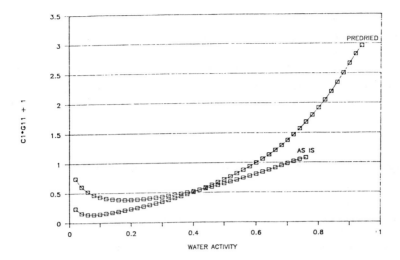

Figure 13: Cluster function (average cluster size) vs. water activity for "as is" and "predried" fast-frozen purified lysozyme at 25 °C.

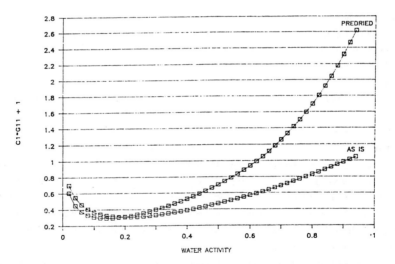

Figure 14: Cluster function (average cluster size) vs. water activity for "as is" and "predried" slow-frozen purified lysozyme at 25 °C.

tendency of sorbed water to form clusters. In other words, at a given a_w value, water/water interactions are favored in case of a hydrophobic system while substrate/water interactions are favored in case of a hydrophilic one, as expected.

(b) The initial shape of curves in Figs 14 and 15 can be rationalized as follows: A fraction of the initially adsorbed water molecules are penetrated the protein matrix causing partial swelling which in turn exposes additional active sites for water binding, resulting in decrease in clustering.

Table 1: Calculated G.A.B. constants from experimental water sorption isotherm data at 25°C

Substrate	Wm(x102)	C	k
As is fast-fr. lysozyme	13.7±0.1	17.5±4.1	0.94±0.02
Predr.fast-fr. lysozyme	5.8±0.1	176.8±34.4	0.91±0.01
As is slow-fr. lysozyme	12.3±0.2	27.6±1.7	0.70±0.01
Predr.slow-fr. lysozyme	5.6±0.1	37.8±4.8	0.87±0.00
As is glycosyl. lysozyme	11.8±0.2	16.4±0.9	0.61±0.01
Predr. glycosyl. lysozyme	4.9±0.1	21.6±2.1	0.81±0.00

CONCLUSIONS

(a) Present results demonstrate again the potential of the IGC method in evaluating restructuring phenomena in metastable food systems. The transitions in the structure and composition of food substrates are reflected in the changes of water vapor pressure measured by the TCD detector. These structural changes produced by swelling and shrinkage during sorption measurements may be great enough to make invalid any hydration process model which neglects these effects.

(b) G.A.B. model and Zimm-Lundberg cluster analysis were succesfully applied in an effort to gain insight into the mechanism of water build up in the protein substrates as affected by sample treatment (drying, fast- and slow-freezing and glycosylation). Results showed that drying process results in a considerable reduce in water sorption capacity of substrates because of structural changes occuring during this process.

REFERENCES
1. M.Schnerf, Protein-water interactions, in: T.M.Hardman (Ed.), Water and Food Quality, Elsewier, Amsterdam, 1989, p.135.
2. W.Kausmann, Some factors in the interpretation of protein denaturation. Adv.Prot.Chem., 14(195) 1-63.
3. L.Slade, H.Levine and J.W.Finley, Protein-water interactions: Water as a plasticizer of fluten and other protein polymers, in: R.D.Phillips and J.W.Finley (Eds), Protein quality and the effects of processing, Marcel Dekker, N.York, 1989, pp.9-124.
4. J.A.Rupley, P.H.Yang and G.Tollin, Thermodynamic and related studies of water interacting with proteins, in: S.P.Rowland (Ed.,) Water in Polymers, A.C.S, Washington D.C., 1980, pp.111-132.
5. D.C.Phillips, The three dimensional structure of an enzyme molecule, Sci.Amer. 215(6) (1966), 78.
6. P.Cerruti, S.L.Resnik, A.Seldes and C.Ferro-Fontan, Kinetics of deteriorative reactiosn in model food systems of high water activity, J.Food Sci 50(1985), 627.
7. J.D.Kuntz and W.Kauzmann, Hydration of Proteins and polypeptides, Adv.Prot.Chem., 28 (1974), 239.
8. J.D.Leeder and L.C.Watt, Stoichiometry of water sorption by proteins, J.Colloid Interf.Sci. 48(2) (1974), 339.
9. P.N.Giannakakos, Water Relations in the Lysozyme-Glucose System, Ph.D.Thesis, Rutgers Univ.New Brunswick, New Jersey (1990).
10. J.N.Morozov, T.Y.Morozova, G.S.Kachaloca and E.T.Myacin, Interpretation of water desorption isotherms of lysozyme, Int.J.Biol.Macromol., 10 (1988), 329-336.
11. S.G.Gilbert, Inverse Gas Chromatography in: J.C.Giddings, E.Grusha, J.Gazes and P.R.Brown (Eds), Advances in Chromatography, Vol.23, Marcel Dekker, N.York, 1984.
12. S.G.Gilbert, A modified frontal chromatrographic method for water sorption isotherms of biological macromolecules, in: D.R.Lloyd, T.C.Ward and H.P.Schreiber (Eds), Inverse Gas Chromatography, ACS Symp. ser.391, ACS, Washington, D.C., 1988, pp.306-317.
13. O.Ramon, H.Daun, C.Frenkel and S.G.Gilbert, Characteristics of hydrophilic water related hysteresis in food systems by IGC, in: G.Charalmbous (ed.) Flavors and Off-flavors 89, Elsevier, Amsterdam (1989), pp.419-437.
14. C.Van den Berg, Description of water activity of foods for engineering purposes by means of the G.A.B. model of sorption, in: B.M. Mc Kenna (ed.), Engineering and Food Vol 1, Elsevier, London, 1984, pp. 311-320.
15. W. Schar and M. Ruegg, The evaluation of G.A.B. constants for water vapor sorption data, Lebensm. Wiss. u.-Technol., 18 (1985) 225-229.
16. B.H. Zimm and J.L. Lundberg, Sorption of vapors by high polymerrs, J. Phys. Chem., 60 (1956) 425-428.

G. Charalambous (Ed.), Food Science and Human Nutrition
© 1992 Elsevier Science Publishers B.V. All rights reserved.

APPLICATION OF A MODIFIED IGC METHOD IN THE STUDY OF THE WATER SORPTIONAL BEHAVIOR OF SELECTED PROTEINS. II. GLIADIN-WATER INTERACTIONS.

P.G. DEMERTZIS[1], S.G. GILBERT[2] and H. DAUN[2]

[1]University of Ioannina, Department of Chemistry, Laboratory of Food Science, P.O. Box 1186, 45110-Ioannina, Greece.

[2]Department of Food Science and the Center for Advanced Food Technology, Rutgers University, P.O. Box 231, New Brunswick, N.J. 08903.

SUMMARY

A modified pulse inverse gas chromatographic method was applied to the study of water sorptional behavior of hydrophobic protein (purified slow-frozen gliadin) as affected by sample pretreatment (predrying and glycosylation). The water sorption isotherms obtained showed lower water adsorption capacity for gliadin compared to the hydrophilic lysozyme samples studied in our previous paper. On the other hand, predrying of the sample diminshed its sorptional ability due to structural changes occuring during predrying. Glycosylation of the sample caused a slight increase in its corptional capacity, possibly due to the attachment of more hydrophilic groups on the protein molecule. Analysis of sorption data according to Zimm-Lundberg cluster theory also showed an enhanced cluster formation tendency for gliadin compared to the lysozyme samples.

INTRODUCTION

Water is one of the most widespread chemical substrances in the environment and in biological terms is perhaps the most important constituent of living tissues. Water is present in tissues of animal or plant origin with high moisture content as well as in substrates with restricted moisture content (low moisture level).

In practice, most of food products do not contain a continuous liquid phase, but only adsorbed water in equilibrium with the surrounding vapor phase. The speed and intensity of chemical reactions (e.g. oxidation, Maillard reactions) occuring in food systems as well as the growth of microorganisms and the modification of their physical properties are controlled by the thermodynamic activity of this type of water.

Protein-water interactions in various food systems have received increasing attention in recent years. The majority of proteins exhibit regions which are more or less ordered and which interact with adsorbed water. Considering that a significant amount of the amino acids that constitute the side chains of proteins have no affinity for water, it is clear that the so called "hydrophobic interactions" must play an important role in proteinic structure as well as in denaturation processes. Hydrophobic interactions are possibly in part responsible for the globular conformation of many proteins (ref. 1).

Gliadin and glutenin are the two major proteins of gluten. They are located in the wheat endosperm and serve as storage protein as they are rapidly broken down to amino acids and peptides upon germination of the seed, thus providing a source of nitrogen for the protein being synthesized for use by the embryo. The storage proteins are characterized by high contents of glutamine and of proline (ref. 2).

Gliadin is a mixture of proteins (α-, β-, γ- and ω- gliadins) having similar amino acid composition. All gliadin components contain extremely high glutamic acid and proline contents. Glutamic acid, which is present mainly as glutamine, promotes hydrogen bonding, while proline is known to interrupt ordered secondary structures such as α- helices and β- structures, thus preventing the peptide chains of gliadin from assuming extended ordered secondary structures and facilitating the folding of the polypeptide chains into globular conformations.

The structure of the protein can influence the affinity for water and mainly the accessibility of polar sites to water. Two different types of accessible polar sites can be interpreted: (a) The polar sites of amino acid chains. Each of them is able to bind 6 water molecules (refs 3,4), (b) According to other investigators (refs 5,6) the major adsorption sites are in the polypeptide backbone (...-CO-NH-CH$_2$-...). The two types of hydration most probably exist simultaneously. In addition, interchain bridges between peptide bonds can be formed in the basis of a hexagonal network of water molecules linking the hydrophilic surfaces of the peptide bonds (ref. 6).

The structure and properties of gluten depend on the state of aggregation of its components, i.e., on the interactions that are related with the conformation of protein molecules and their ability to associate through hydrogen and ionic linkages, disulfide fridges and hydrophobic interactrions. The role of hydrophobic interactions in the structure of proteins has been studied by many investigators (refs 7-11). The high content of gluten in non-polar amino acids indicates the importance of hydrophobic interactions in determining its properties. Studies of Greene and Kasarda (ref. 7) on α-gliadin showed that apolar areas exist on the surface of the molecules and that hydrobicity relies upon conformatinal changes. Popineau and Godon (ref. 10) studied the surface hydrophobicity of gliadin components. Their results confirmed that the hydrophobicity of gliadins is generally high and that surface hydrophobicity of gliadins influences their surfactant properties.

In a previous paper (ref. 12) we studied the water sorptional behavior of lysozyme samples using a recently established modified pulse IGC technique. In the present work we used this modified IGC technique with the aims:

a) To further apply and test the modified IGC method for constructing water sorption isotherms of various gliadin samples.
b) To study the effect of sample pretreatment (predrying and glycosylation) on water/gliadin interactions using model equation analysis and Zimm-Lundberg cluster theory.

MATERIALS AND METHODS
MATERIALS

Purified slow-frozen gliadin was isolated by a Ponca hard red winter wheat flour grown and milled at the University of Kansas, U.S.A.. This was 100% pure in terms of both the variety and treatment after harvest. The flour was extracted with 0.5 N sodiium chloride solution firtst and then with 70% (v/v) aqueous ethanol. The ethanol extract was subjected to ultrafiltration and freeze drying.

Glycosylated gliadin was prepared as follows: A mixture of purified gliadin and glucose (10:1 w/w) was dissolved in a 0.1 N acetic acid solution (pH=4.0) and freeze-dried for 48 hours. The freeze-dried sample was incubated at 50°C and 65% R.H. for 15 days.

METHODS

The whole experimental methodology followed in this study concerning IGC instrumentation and procedure as well as true density measurments has been described in details elsewhere (refs. 12-14)

RESULTS AND DISCUSSION

GC profiles and water sorption isotherms obtained for both "as is" and "predried" materials (slow-frozed gliadin, glycosylated slow-frozen gliadin) at 25°C, are shown in Figs 1-4. As can be seen from these figures, no transitions have been observed in case of gliadin samples (both unglycosylated and glycosylated), compared to significant transitions observed in case of unglycosylated lysozyme samples (ref. 12). This finding is indicative of more stable or less metastable structures in case of gliadin samples.

On the other hand, "predried" samples adsorb less water than corresponding "as is" materials. This indicates that predrying process may influence the structure and the mechanical properties of biopolymers and therefore their sorption behavior. This is a main disadvandage of the conventional static method for sorption isotherm determination, which usually requires predrying of the sorbent samples previous to the characterization of their sorption behavior.

A comparison between sorption isotherm of "as is" fast- and slow-frozen lysozyme (studied previously) and gliadin samples is shown in Fig. 5. It is observed that, under the same conditions, gliadin adsorbs considerably less than lysozyme. This is mainly attributed to the hydrophobic nature of the gliadin itself.

Fig. 6. shows the effect of glycosylation on water sorptional behavior of slow-frozen gliadin. It is observed that the glycosylated gliadin adsorbs a little more than the unglycosylated one. This fact can be attributed to the attachment of more hydrophilic (glucose) molecules on the hydrophobic gliadin molecules..

Furthermore, the sorption isotherms obtained for gliadin samples were rather "sugar like" (BET type III) than sigmoid (BET type II), indicating reduced hydrophilicity for theses substrates.

The G.A.B. equation (ref. 12) was also applied to our data of both gliadin samples and gave good fit for the whole water activity range. The estimated coefficients for G.A.B. equation are tabulated in table 1. It is obsreved that, for the same substrate, the "as is" sample exhibits greater W_m value compared to the "predried" sample. These differences, although less prenounced compared to those of hydrophilic (lysozyme) substrates (ref.12), can be attributed to restructuring phenomena occuring during predrying. The W_m values for gliadin samples are also significantly lower than the corresponding values for both fast- and slow-frozen lysozyme samples (table 1, ref. 12). This is expected because of the hydrophobic structure of gliadin.

Table 1. Estimated coefficients for the G.A.B equation from experimental sorption isotherm data at 25°C.

Substrate	W_m (x10^2)	C	K
Slow-frozen gliadin (as is)	6.4 ± 0.2	485.7 ± 860.1	0.82 ± 0.02
Slow-frozen gliadin (predried)	3.6 ± 0.0	602.1 ± 499.5	0.99 ± 0.00
glycosylated gliadin (as is)	6.6 ± 0.4	742.3 ± 879.6	0.74 ± 0.03
glycosylated gliadin (predried)	4.0 ± 0.1	19.9 ± 6.1	0.94 ± 0.01

Zimm-Lundberg cluster analysis (ref. 12) was also applied to gliadin samples. Fig.7 shows a plot of average cluster size vs. a_w for "as is" and "predried" gliadin samples. It is observed that the "predired" sample exhibits greater tendency to cluster formation than the "as is" sample The same behavior was, observed for lysozyme samples (ref.12). Furthermore, in case of gliadin samples, the tendency for adsorbed water to form clusters is considerably higher

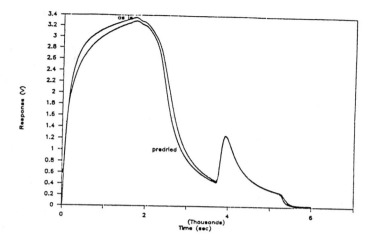

Figure 1: GC profiles of "as is" and predried slow-frozen purified gliadin at 25°C.

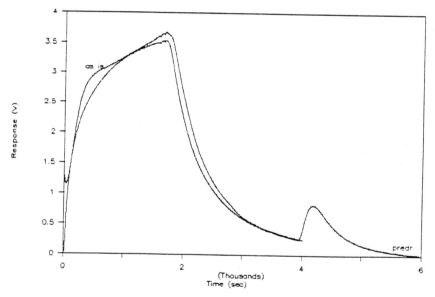

Figure 2: GC profiles of "as is" and predried glycosylated slow-frozen purified gliadin at 25°C.

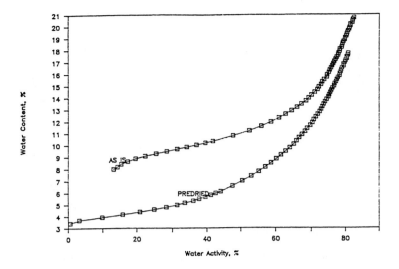

Figure 3: Water sorption isotherms of "as is" and "predried" slow-frozen purified gliadin at 25°C.

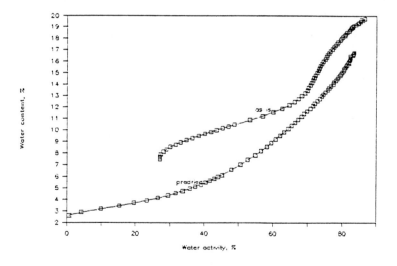

Figure 4: Water sorption isotherms of "as is" and "predried" glycosylated slow-frozen purified gliadin at 25°C.

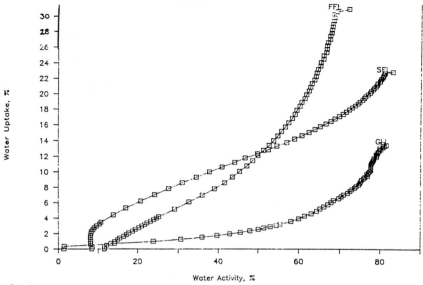

Figure 5: Comparison between water sorption isotherms of "as is" fast- and slow-frozen lysozyme and gliadin samples at 25°C.

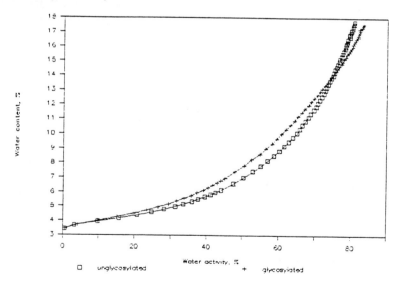

Figure 6: Comparison between water sorption isotherms of glycosylated and unglycosylated slow-frozen gliadin.

compared to that of the corresponding lysozyme samples. The explanation is the same as that already given for the W_m values.

In conclusion, present work again demonstrates the significance of IGC measurments of sorption characteristics of biopolymers, since IGC is a dynamic method that measures continuously the sorption behavior in contrast to the time averaging representation of the static method and may therefore reveal transitions and changes that are time and moisrure dependent and have been almost impossible to be detected by the traditional static or long-tme period techniques.

REFERENCES
1. J.L.Multon, Interactions berween water and the constituents of grains, seeds and by-products in: J.L.Multon (Ed.), Preservation and Storage of Grains, seeds and their by-products, Lavoisier Publ., Paris, 1988, pp.89-129.
2. D.D.Kasarda, C.C.Nimmo and G.O.Kohler, Proteins an the amino acid composition of wheat fractions, in: Y.Pomeranz (Ed.), Wheat Chemistry and Technology, AACC, St.Paul, Minnesota, 1978, pp. 227-299.
3. L.Pauling, Chimie generale, 2nd Ed., Dunod, Paris, 1960.
4. A.McLaren and J.Rowen, Sorption of water by proteins and polymers: A review, J.Polym.Sci. 7(2-3) (1951), 289-324.
5. R.Duckworth and G.Smith, The environment for chemical change in dried and frozen foods. Proc.Nutr.Soc., 22 (1963), 182-189.
6. D.T.Warner, Theoretical studes of water on Carbohydrates and Proteins, in: L.B.Rockland and G.F.Stewart (Eds), Water activity: Influences on food quality, Academic Press, N.York, 1981, pp.435-465.
7F.C.Greene and D.D. Kasarda, Apolar interaction of a-gliadin, Cereal Chem. 48(1971), 601.
8. B.Codon and Y.Popineau, Difference d'hydrophobicite de surface des gliadines de deux bles durs de bonne et de mauvais qualite. Agronomie, 1(1981), 77.
9. K.Kahn and W.Bushuk, Glutenin structure and functionality in breadmaking, Bakers Dig. 52 (1978), 2.
10. Y.Popineau and B.Godon, Surface hydrophobicity of gliadin components, Cereal Chem., 59(1) (1982), 55-62.
11. R.S.Spolar, J.-H.Ha and M.T.Record, JR., Hydrophobic effect in protein folding and other moncovalent processes involving proteins, Proc.Natl.Acad.USA, 86 (1989), 8382-85.
12. P.G.Demertzis, S.G.Gilbert and H.Daun, Application of a modified IGC method in the Study of the water sorptional behaviour of selected proteins. I.Lysozyme-water interactions. 7th International Conference "Recent Developments in Food Science and Nutrition, Samos-Greece (1991), Proceedings in Press.
13. S.G.Gilbert, A Modified Frontal Chromatographic Method for Water Sorption Isotherms of Biological Macromolecules, in: D.R.Lloyd, T.C.Ward and H.P.Schreiber (Eds), I.G.C. Characterization of Polymers and Other Materials, A.C.S, Washington, D.C., 1989, pp.306-317.
14. O.Ramon, H.Daun, C.Frenkel and S.G.Gilbert, Characterization of hydrophilic water related hysteresis in food systems by IGC, in: G.Charalambous (Ed.) Flavors and Off-flavors '89, Elsevier, Amsterdam, 1990, pp. 419-437.

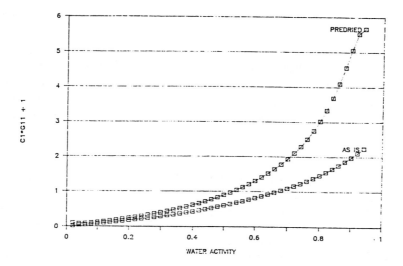

Figure 7: Average cluster size vs. water activity for "as is" and "predried" slow frozen purified gliadin at 25°C.

WATER SORPTION HYSTERESIS IN POTATO STARCH AND EGG ALBUMIN

M. LAGOUDAKI and P.G. DEMERTZIS

Lab. of Food Chemistry, Dept. of Chemistry, University of Ioannina, 45110 Ioannina, Greece

SUMMARY

Moisture adsorption and desorption isotherms at 30°C for potato starch and egg albumin over the water activity (a_w) range 0.07-0.97 were determined gravimetrically, by exposing the samples to atmospheres of known relative humidities. Both materials exhibited the hysteresis phenomenon, which was more pronounced in the case of potato starch. The Brunauer, Emmett and Teller (B.E.T.), Guggenheim, Anderson and De Boer (G.A.B.) and Freundlich equations were successfully applied to the sorption data and the monolayer as well as the sorptive capacity values were calculated.

INTRODUCTION

The importance of water to the stability and acceptability of foods has been known for many years. To predict stability of foods a knowledge of the function and state of water is necessary. The interaction between water and food components can be studied by several techniques (refs. 1, 2). The majority of the studies in that area have been done by a thermodynamic method, the water sorption isotherms. According to this technique the degree of hydration of a material is measured as a function of water activity at constant temperature. The objective of this work was to determine the water adsorption and desorption isotherms for potato starch and egg albumine.

MATERIALS AND METHODS

Both potato starch and egg albumin were purchased from Sigma Chemical Co., U.S.A. They were dried under vacuum at 45°C for 24h and kept in a desiccator for 48h before they were used. The samples were placed in aluminium foil cups and were equilibrated against nine saturated salt solutions ranging in a_w from 0.07 to 0.97 in equilibration chambers. The samples were equilibrated at 30 ± 0.5°C in a constant temperature desiccator. Triplicate determinations were done and the averages are presented. To obtain the desorption isotherms the sample equilibrated at the highest humidity atmosphere was successively exposed to each of the lower constant humidity atmospheres.

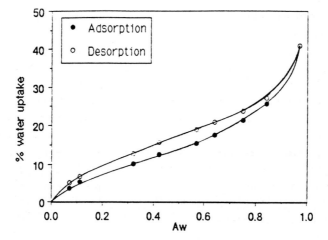

Figure 1. Sorption isotherms of potato starch at 30°C

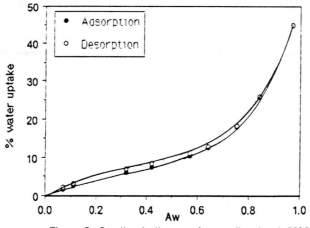

Figure 2. Sorption isotherms of egg albumin at 30°C

RESULTS AND DISCUSSION
Water Sorption Hysteresis

The adsorption and desorption isotherms for potato starch and egg albumin at 30°C are given in Figs. 1 and 2 respectively. Both adsorption and desorption branches were of sigmoid shape (BET type II) which is typical of most food products.

Moisture sorption hysteresis is the phenomenon in which different paths exist for adsorption and desorption isotherms and it has important theoritical and practical implications in foods. The theoretical implications range from general considerations of the irreversibility of the sorption process to the question of validity of thermodynamic functions derived therefrom. The practical implications deal with ease of drying, change in surface structure of the adsorbent by dehydration and the effects of hysteresis on chemical and microbiological deterioration (refs. 3, 4). The several causes of sorption hysteresis are impurities on the surface of the adsorbent, the presence of some irreversible water phase change, irreversible swelling of the adsorbent and a capillary condensation-evaporation process in small pores. In nature, hysteresis may be considered as a built-in protective mechanism against extremities such as loss of water due to a dry atmosphere, frost damage and freezer burn. Figure 3 shows four types of hysteresis according to the classification of Everett (ref. 5). In type A the loop occurs over a limited range of relative pressures. In type B the loop extends from the saturation vapor pressure down to a well-defined closure point, which is characteristic mainly of the kind of the vapor adsorbed. In type C the loop extends over the entire range of vapor pressure. In type D, which is a mixture of types B and C, the desorption curve follows the pattern of type B loop but before meeting the adsorption curve it bends away downward to the zero vapor pressure as in type C.

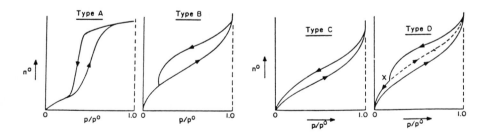

Fig. 3. Main types of Sorption Hysteresis

In general, the type of changes encountered upon adsorption and desorption will depend on a) the initial state of the sorbent (amorphous versus crystalline), b) the transitions taking place during adsorption, c) the final a_w adsorption point and d) the speed of desorption. With regard to (c) and (d), if the saturation point has been reached and the material has gone into solution, rapid desorption may preserve the amorphous state due to supersaturation.

In our experiments a reproducible hysteresis loop between the adsorption and desorption isotherms was obtained for both materials. In potato starch a relatively large hysteresis loop occured with a maximum at about $a_w=0.6$ which is within the capillary condensation region. In egg albumin, a small total hysteresis was observed which began in the capillary condensation region at about $a_w=0.75$ and extended over the rest of the isotherm. Results obtained are in accordance with those reported for starchy and high-protein foods (refs. 6, 7).

The moisture sorption hysteresis may be interpreted either by the capillary condensation theory, according to which a vapor condenses to a liquid in pores, or by conformational changes, intermolecular phase annealing, incomplete phase change and swelling effects induced by water sorption. According to experiments carried out by certain investigators (refs. 7-9) neither starch nor albumin are porous substrates and therefore capillary condensation can't play a significant role in water binding, although, according to other investigators (ref. 4), the hysteresis loops obtained for starchy foods were attributed to capillary condensation as well as to the reasons mentioned before.

Sorption Models

B.E.T. Isotherm

It is the most widely used model in food systems. It is expressed by equation (1).

$$a_w / (1-a_w) \cdot V = 1/V_m \cdot C + a_w \cdot (C-1) / V_m \cdot C \qquad (1)$$

where V: water uptake, (g/g)
 V_m: monolayer value, (g/g)
 a_w: water activity
 C: sorption constant

Application of sorption data to the B.E.T. equation gave a very good fit ($R^2=0.98-0.99$) for a_w between 0.07-0.60. The values of the B.E.T. constants are given in Table 1. A number of investigators (refs. 10, 11) noticed that knowledge of water uptake at the monolayer value is of great importance because it is the level of moisture content at which dehydrated foods have optimum storage stability because of the protective effect of water against oxygen adsorption and interactions of adjacent polar groups.

TABLE 1. B.E.T. isotherm constants for water sorption by potato starch and egg albumin at 30°C.

	V_m	C
Potato starch	0.07	21.01
Egg albumin	0.05	7.56

G.A.B. Isotherm

This model can be considered as an extension of the B.E.T. multimolecular localised homogeneous adsorption model. It is reported as giving a remarkable fit over a wide range of water activity (up to 0.9) and a very good evaluation for the amount of water tightly bound by the primary adsorption sites (refs. 12-14). The G.A.B. model is expressed by equation (2).

$$W / W_m = C \cdot K \cdot a_w / (1-Ka_w) \cdot (1-Ka_w+CKa_w) \qquad (2)$$

where W: water uptake, (g/g)

W_m: water uptake corresponding to monolayer value. (g/g)

a_w: water activity

C: Guggenheim's constant

K: correction factor

Equation (2) can be transformed into equation (3).

$$a_w / W = A \cdot a_w^2 + B \cdot a_w + \Gamma \qquad (3)$$

where $A = K(1-C) / W_m \cdot C$, (4) $B = (C-2) / W_m \cdot C$, (5) and $\Gamma = 1 / W_m \cdot C \cdot K$ (6)
A plot of a_w/W vs a_w gives a parabolic curve. Using equations (4), (5), (6) parameters W_m, C and K can be calculated (Table 2).

TABLE 2. G.A.B. isotherm constants for water sorption by potato starch and egg albumin at 30°C.

	Wm	C	K
Potato starch	0.09	10.52	0.78
Egg albumin	0.06	6.02	0.93

Statistical treatment of sorption data gave a very good fit (R^2=0.97-0.98) to the G.A.B. equation for a_w between 0.07-0.85.

Freundliich Isotherm

This model is important for explaining the sorption behaviour of heterogeneous surfaces such as those of most foods. It has also been successfully applied to various foodstuffs (refs. 15, 16). It is expressed by equation (7).

$$V = k \cdot a_w^{1/n} \qquad (7)$$
$$\text{or} \qquad \log V = \log k + 1/n \cdot \log a_w \qquad (8)$$

where V: water uptake, (g/g)
a_w: water activity
k, n: constants related to the sorptive efficiency of the sorbent

Constant k is known as the sorptive capacity of the material. Plot of logV vs loga_w permits the calculation of k and n (Table 3).

TABLE 3. Freundlich isotherm constants for water sorption by potato starch and egg albumin at 30°C.

	k	n
Potato starch	0.215	1.032
Egg albumin	0.253	1.372

Statistical analysis of sorption data for a_w between 0.07-0.80 gave a good fit (R^2=0.96-0.98) to the Freundlich equation.

REFERENCES

1 A.G. Gurme, J.S. Schmidt and P.M. Steinberg, Mobility and Activity of Water in Casein Model Systems as Determined by ^{2}H NMR and Sorption Isotherms, J. Food Sci., 55 (1990) 430-433.
2 I.D. Kuntz and W. Kauzmann, Hydration of Proteins and Polypeptides, Adv. in Protein Chem., 28 (1974) 239-345.
3 J.G. Kapsalis, Moisture sorption hysteresis, in: L.B. Rockland and G.F. Stewart (Eds), Water Activity: Influences on Food Quality, Academic Press, New York, 1981, pp. 143-178.
4 K. Boki and S. Ohno, Moisture Sorption Hysteresis in Kudzu Starch and Sweet Potato Starch, J. Food Sci., 56(1) (1991) 125-127.
5 D.H. Everett, Adsorption hysteresis, in: E.A. Flood (Ed.), The Solid-Gas Interface, Marcel Dekker Inc., New York, 1967, pp. 1055.
6 J.G. Kapsalis, Influences of Hysteresis and Temperature on Moisture Sorption Isotherms, in: L.B. Rockland and L.R. Beuchat, (Eds), Water Activity: Theory and Applications to Food, Marcell Dekker Inc., New York, 1987, pp. 173-214.
7 C. Van Den Berg, S.F. Kapel, G.A.J. Welbring and J. Wolters, Water Binding by Potato Starch, J. Food Technol., 10 (1975) 589-602.

8 F.E. Mellon and R.S. Hoover, Hygroscopicity of Amino Acids and Its Relationship to the Vapor Phase Water Absorption of Proteins, J. Amer. Chem. Soc., 73 (1951) 3879-3882.
9 W.P. Bryan, Thermodynamic Models for Water-Protein Sorption Hysteresis, Biopolymers, 26 (1987) 1705-1716.
10 H. Salwin, Moisture Levels Required for Stability in Dehydrated Foods, Food Technology, 17 (1963) 34-41.
11 J.R. Aguerre, C. Suarez and E.P. Viollaz, Some Aspects Derived from BET Theory and their Relation with Food Conservation, Lebensm. Wiss u. - Technol., 19 (1986) 328-330.
12 C. Van Den Berg, Description of water activity of foods for engineering purposes by means of the G.A.B. model of sorption, in: B.M. Mc Kenna, (Ed.), Engineering and Food Vol. 1, Elsevier Appl. Sci. Publ., London, 1984, pp. 311-320.
13 M. Wolf, W.E.L. Spiess and G. Jung, Standarization of isotherm measurements, in: D. Simatos and J.L. Multon (Eds), Properties of water in Foods, Martinus Nijhoff Publ., Dordrecht, 1985, pp. 661-667.
14 W. Schar and M. Ruegg, The Evaluation of G.A.B. Constants from Water Vapor Sorption Data, Lebensm. Wiss. u. - Technol., 18 (1985) 225-229.
15 D.S. Smith, C.H. Mannheim and S.G. Gilbert, Water Sorption Isotherms of Sucrose and Glucose by Inverse Gas Chromatography, J. Food Sci., 46 (1981) 1051-1053.
16 P.G. Demertzis and M.G. Kontominas, Study of water sorption of egg powders by Inverse Gas Chromatography, Zeitsch. Lebensm. Unters. Forsch., 186 (1988) 213-217.

STUDY OF WATER VAPOR DIFFUSION THROUGH PLASTICS PACKAGING MATERIALS USING INVERSE GAS CHROMATOGRAPHY

P.J. KALAOUZIS and P.G. DEMERTZIS

Lab. of Food Chemistry, Dept. of Chemistry, University of Ioannina, 45110 Ioannina, Greece

SUMMARY

In this work the diffusion of water through plasticized and unplasticized food-grade PVC was studied in the temperature range 25-50ºC. By an appropriate choice of conditions, Van Deemter equation was used for the calculation of diffusion coefficients from the variation in peak width with carrier gas linear velocity. Furthermore, the Arrhenious plots of diffusion coefficients in the PVC-plasticizer mixtures were constructed and the activation energies for diffusion were computed. Diffusion coefficients increase with increasing temperature and plasticizer content, while activation energies for diffusion decrease with increasing plasticizer content. The Inverse Gas Chromatographic method for studing diffusion of water through polymers was found to be a simple, fast and accurate one.

INTRODUCTION

Polyvilylchloride films have found wide applications, over the past several years, in the packaging of a large variety of foodstuffs such as fresh meat, fruits and vegetables, cheeses etc (refs. 1-3). These films contain a number of plastics additives added to improve the physical and mainly the mechanical properties of the films. One of the most important category of additives are plasticizers. Plasticizers are low-volatility solvents for plastics while plasticize or soften the plastic. PVC is a stiff and brittle polymer when unplasticized. The plasticizer is incorporated into polymer to increase workability, flexibility, or extensibility.

In recent years, inverse gas chromatography, (I.G.C), was found to be very effective in measuring sorption tendency and diffusion coefficients of gases and volatile liquids in molten polymers (refs. 4-9). In this work the diffusion of water vapors through plasticized and unplasticized low M.W. PVC was studied using inverse gas chromatography.

DATA TREATMENT

Van Deemter et al. related peak broadening in a gas chromatographic column to column properties through equation 1:

$$H = A + B/u + Cu \qquad (1)$$

where H is the theoretical plate height, u is the linear velocity of the carrier gas, and A, B, C are constants independent of u. Whereas A and B are related to instrument perfomance and gas phase spreading, C depends on a number of factors, including the diffusion coefficient of the probe molecule in the stationary phase. The constant C has been related to the diffusion coefficient (D_p) by means of the relationship:

$$C = (8/\pi^2) (d_f^2/D_p) [k/(1+k)^2] \qquad (2)$$

where d_f is the thickness of the stationary phase and k the partition ratio, given by

$$k = (t_r-t_f)/t_f \qquad (3)$$

where t_r and t_f are, respectively, the retention times of solvent and unadsorbed indicator, such as air. Millen and Hawkes (ref. 10), following Giddings (ref. 11), claimed that a value of 2/3 should be used as the constant in equation 2 instead of $8/\pi^2$. In order to make use of equation 1 it is necessary to evaluate both H and u. The plate height H, can be obtained from the eluted peaks displayed on a chart recorder by using the following equation:

$$H = (L/5.54) (W_{1/2}/t_r)^2 \qquad (4)$$

where L is the column length and $W_{1/2}$ is the peak width at half the peak height. The linear velocity of the carrier gas u, is calculated from the expresion

$$u = j \, LT_c / t_r T_r \qquad (5)$$

where j is the James and Martin compressibility factor, accounting for pressure drop along the chromatographic column, T_c is the temperature of the column, T_r is the temperature of the enviroment. The thickness of the stationary phase is given by

$$d_f = (1/3) \, W \, (\rho_s/\rho_p) \, r_s \qquad (6)$$

where W is the % loading of the polymer, ρ_s is the density of inert support, ρ_p is the density of polymer and r_s is the radius of inert support particles.

In accordance with the theory of activated diffusion, a plot of log (D_p) versus 1/T should produce a straight line of slope $-E_a/2.303 \, R$

$$D_p = D_o^{-E_a/RT} \qquad (7)$$

where D_o is a constant, E_a the activation energy for diffusion, and R is the gas constant.

MATERIALS AND METHODS

The polymer investigated in the present work supplied by Polyscience, Inc. (U.S.A). It was Polyvinylchloride (PVC), having low molecular weight (M.W.=48000). As plasticizer was used a polyadipic ester (Santicizer 409A) supplied by Monsanto (U.S.A). The G.C equipment was a Shimatzu 8A, equipped with TCD. The chromatographic parameters were as follows:

flow rate (ml/min): 30-500
carrier gas : helium, high purity
temperature (°C) : injection port - 130
:column - 25-50
:detector - 130

The column packing material were prepared as follows. The 3 polymers were dissolved in tetrahydrofuran and coated onto the inert support by slow evaporation of the solvent with gentle stirring and heating. After vacuum drying for approximately 24h at 60°C, the chromatographic supports were packed into 1/4" O.D. aluminum columns with the aid of a mechanical vibrator.

The column parameters are described in Table 1.

TABLE 1. Stationary phase and column parameters

Polymer type	loading (%)	polymer mass (g)	column dimensions (length O.D. cm)	
A: PVC 92%-plasticizer 8%	9.34	0.4656	100	0.63
B: PVC 85%-plasticizer 15%	8.42	0.4221	100	0.63
Γ: PVC 75%-plasticizer 25%	10.96	0.5543	100	0.63

RESULTS AND DISCUSSION

The Van Deemter equation plots of plate heigh (H) versus linear velocity (u) were constructed at 25, 32, 40 and 50°C. The results obtained are shown in figures 1-3. It is observed that at higher flow rates linear plots were obtained whose slopes were then equal to the coefficient C in equation 1. The values of diffusion coefficients were calculated using equation 2 and are listed in table 2. The values of activation energy for diffusion of the three polymeric mixtures in studied were calculated from the slope of figure 4 and are also listed in table 2.

Diffusion coefficients increase with increasing temperature. This fact can be attributed to the increasing flexibility of polymer chains.

Diffusion coefficients are also increasing with increasing the amount of plasticizer in polymer and this increase is accompanied by a decrease in activation energy. The addition of a plasticizer to a polymer decreases the cohesive forces between the chains resulting in an increase in segmental mobility. It is clear that this should result in an increased rate of diffusion and a lower activation energy.

TABLE 2. Diffusion coefficients and activation energies for water diffusion in the three polymeric mixtures between 25 and 50°C

Polymer	Temperature (°C)	D_p (cm^2 s^{-1}/10^8)	E_a (Kcal/mole)
A	25 32 40 50	0.95 1.18 1.99 3.74	9.19
B	25 32 40 50	1.92 3.78 4.71 6.62	8.00
Γ	25 32 40 50	4.44 6.20 9.07 13.4	7.31

The values of diffusion coefficients of water in low M.W. PVC (plasticized and unplasticized) compared to those obtained for high M.W. PVC/plasticizer systems (ref. 12) are of the same order of magnitude. This confirms the fact that the diffusion coefficient of solvents in polymers are independent of the M.W. of polymers. This result seems reasonable as the diffusion process of the solvent is a jump of the solvent molecule from one chain unit to another and therefore should not be affected by the length of the entire chain (ref. 13).

REFERENCES

1 D. Messady and J.M. Vergnaud, Quick indentification and analysis of plasticizers in PVC by programmed-temperature gas chromatography using the best stationary phases. J. Appl. Polym. Sci., 24 (1979) 1215-1225.
2 J.L. Taverdet and J.M. Vergnaud, Study of transfer procces of liquid into and plasticizer out of plasticized PVC by using short tests, J. Appl. Polym. Sci., 29 (1984) 3391-3400.
3 J.K. Sears, N.W. Touchette and J.R. Darby, Plasticizers, in: R.W. Tess and G.W. Poehleim (Eds), Applied Polymer Science, 2nd Ed., ACS, Washington, DC. (1985), pp. 611-641.

4 D.G. Gray and G.E. Guillet, Studies of diffusion in polymers by gas chromatography. *Macromolecules*, **6** (1973) 223-227.
5 J.M. Braun, S. Poos and J.E. Guillet, Determination of diffusion coefficients of antioxidants in polyethylene by gas chromatography., *J. Polym. Sci., Polym. Let. Ed.* **14** (1976) 257-261.
6 J.M. Kong and S.L. Hawkes, Diffusion in silicone stationary phases, *J. Chromatogr. Sci.*, **14** (1976) 279-283.
7 P.J. Tait and A.M. Abushihada, The use of gas chromatographic technique for study of diffusion coefficients, *J. Chromatogr. Sci.*, **17** (1979) 219-223.
8 D.S. Hu, C.D. Han and L.I. Stiel, Gas chromatographic measurments of infite dilution diffusion coefficients of volatile liquids in amorphous polymer at elevated temperatures, *J. Appl. Polym. Sci.*, **33** (1987) 551-576.
9 P.G. Demertzis and M.G. Kontominas, Thermodynamic study of water sorption and water vapor diffusion in Poly(vinylidene chloride) copolymers, in D.C. Lloyd, T.C. Ward and H.P. Schreiber (Eds), *Inverse Gas Chromatography*, ACS, Washington, DC. (1989) pp. 77-86.
10 W. Millen and S.J. Hawkes, Determination of diffusion coefficient in polyethylene by gas chromatography, *J. Polym. Sci., Polym. Let. Ed.*, **15** (1977) 463-465.
11 S.J. Hawkes, Modernization of the Van Deemter equation for chromatographic zone dispersion, *J. Chem. Educ.*, **60** (1983) 393-398.
12 P.J. Kalaouzis, P.G. Demertzis and M.G. Kontominas, Gas chromatographic study of water diffusion in food containers from PVC according to the including plasticizer, 3rd Panhellenic Conference on Food Science and Technology, Proceedings under Publ., Athens - Greece (1990).
13 K. Ueberreiter, The solution process, in: J. Crank and G.S. Park, (Eds) *Diffusion in Polymers*, Academic Press, London, (1968), pp. 220-256.

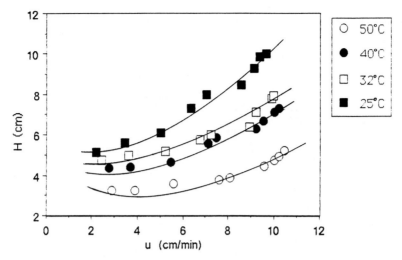

Fig. 1. Van Deemter curves for PVC 92%-Polymeric plasticizer 8%

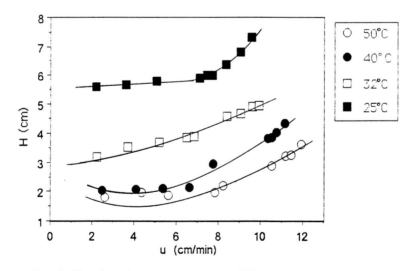

Fig. 2. Van Deemter curves for PVC 85%-Polymeric plasticizer 15%

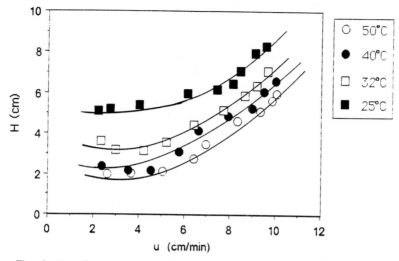

Fig. 3. Van Deemter curves for PVC 75%-Polymeric plasticizer 25%

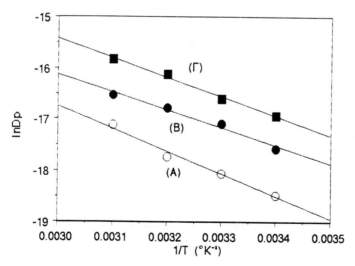

Fig. 4. Arrhenius plots of diffusion coefficients of water for the 3 polymers

DIFFUSION OF WATER IN STARCH MATERIALS

G.D. SARAVACOS[1], V.T. KARATHANOS[1] and S.N. MAROUSIS[2]

[1]Food Science Department and Center for Advanced Food Technology, Rutgers University, New Brunswick, NJ 08903 (USA)
[2]Central Engineering, Procter and Gamble Co, Cincinnati OH 45232 (USA)

SUMMARY

The diffusion of water in starch materials is a fundamental mass transport process, which is important in the processing and storage of various starch-based foods. The effective diffusivity of water in heterogeneous starch systems is a complex function of the moisture content, the temperature and the pressure. The water diffusivity, estimated from the drying data or moisture-distribution curves, depends strongly on the physical structure (bulk porosity) of the material. Mechanical compression, air pressure, gelatinization or addition of sugars reduced substantially the water diffusivity. Water may be transported by liquid or vapor diffusion, depending on the physical structure of the starch system. The diffusion of water is involved in various physical and chemical processes applied to foods, such as cooking, baking, dehydration and extrusion cooking.

INTRODUCTION

The diffusion (transport at molecular level) of water in food systems is of fundamental importance in various food processes, such as dehydration, packaging and storage. Molecular diffusion is the principal mechanism of mass transfer, involved in several food processes (ref. 1). The effective or apparent water diffusivity is a useful overall transport property of water in food materials, which includes transport by molecular diffusion (liquid or vapor), surface diffusion and hydrodynamic flow (ref. 2).

Reliable values of the transport properties of water and other small molecules are required in computations and simulation/optimization of food processing and quality retention of food products. Starch materials are the basic carbohydrate polymers of many food products and they can be used as model food materials in investigations of the mechanism of physicochemical processes such as sorption and diffusion (ref. 3).

The diffusivity of water in food materials varies widely, due to their different physical and chemical structure. Fish (ref. 4), using the sorption technique, found that the water diffusivity in potato starch gels decreased considerably at low moisture contents. Saravacos and Raouzeos (ref. 5), using the drying technique, observed a maximum of water diffusivity in corn starch gels at intermediate moisture contents. Marousis et al. (ref. 6), using the drying technique, found that water-soluble carbohydrates (sugars) reduced significantly the water diffusivity in hydrated granular starches. This reduction was related to the decrease of bulk porosity of the dried material, caused by the precipitation of sugars in the intergranular spaces.

Leslie et al. (ref. 3) reported that the water diffusivity in starch systems depends in a complex way on the moisture content, the temperature, the physical structure of the material and the method of determination. Higher diffusivities were obtained by the drying method than the sorption technique, evidently due to the porous structure developed during drying. Incorporation of inert particles (silica, carbon black) in the granular starch increased the water diffusivity due to the higher bulk porosity. The water diffusivity was found to decrease sharply when the starch materials are gelatinized by heat (ref. 7). This reduction in water diffusivity has been related to the decrease of the porosity of the starch samples, caused by the gelatinization process.

MATERIALS AND METHODS
Materials

Two native corn starches were used in granular or gelatinized form, Hylon 7 (63% amylose) and Amioca (98% amylopectin). Granular starch samples were at moisture contents 0 to 1 kg water/kg dry solids, by mixing the starch powder with distilled water and equilibrating at room temperature for 24 hours. Gelatinized samples were prepared by heating mixtures of Amioca starch/water (1/1) at

100°C or Hylon 7 starch/water (1/2) at 120°C for 15 min. Mixtures of 75% starch and 25% sugar (glucose, sucrose or dextrin) were prepared in granular or gelatinized form (ref. 6).

Compressed starch samples were prepared using a laboratory compression Instron, model TM. The starch material, equilibrated at fixed moisture contents, was compressed at pressures 1-40 atm in an aluminum ring 33 mm diameter and 3.5 mm thick.

Extrusion-cooked starches were prepared at moisture contents 0.15-0.35 kg water/kg dry solids, using a laboratory single-screw extruder (Brabender) operated at 50-250 RPM and temperatures 100°-180°C.

Density/Porosity

The particle density (ρ_p) of the granular starches at various moisture contents was determined with a helium gas stereopycnometer (model SPY-2, Quantachrome Corp.). The bulk density (ρ_b) of the starch materials was estimated from the weight and the volume of the samples (spheres, cylinders or slabs). The bulk porosity (ϵ) of the starch samples was estimated from the equation:

$$\epsilon = 1 - \rho_b/\rho_p \tag{1}$$

Diffusivity from Drying Data

The effective diffusivity of water in starch materials was estimated by applying the unsteady-state diffusion equation to the drying data of starch samples (refs. 8, 9). Samples of starch (spheres, 2 cm diameter or slabs, 3.5 mm thick) were dried in a pilot-plant air dryer (Sargent Corp.), operated at 2 m/s air velocity and 10% relative humidity (ref. 9). The moisture content (X) of the samples was determined gravimetrically at various drying times (t) and the water diffusivity (D) was estimated at various moisture contents (X) from the following equations for the slab and the sphere respectively:

$$\frac{X-X_e}{X_o-X_e} = \frac{8}{\pi^2} \sum_{n=1}^{\infty} \frac{1}{(2n-1)^2} \exp\left[-\frac{(2n-1)^2 \cdot \pi^2 \cdot D \cdot t}{4 \cdot L^2}\right] \tag{2}$$

$$\frac{X-X_e}{X_o-X_e} = \frac{6}{\pi^2} \sum_{n=1}^{\infty} \frac{1}{n^2} \exp\left[-\frac{n^2 \cdot \pi^2 \cdot D \cdot t}{r_o^2}\right] \tag{3}$$

where, X_o=initial moisture content, X_e=equilibrium moisture content (dry basis), L=thickness of slab drying from one side, r_o=radius of spherical sample.

The shrinkage of the starch samples during drying was taken into consideration by measuring their dimensions (L, r_o) at various drying times.

Diffusivity from Moisture Distribution

The water diffusivity at pressures higher than atmospheric was determined using the moisture distribution method in cylindrical starch samples (ref. 10). Two cylinders of starch samples at different moisture contents, 13 mm diameter and 100 mm long, were joined at one end and put in a pressure reactor (Parr Instruments), which was maintained at the desired air pressure 1-40 atm and temperature 25°-140°C. After a specified time the cylinders were removed from the reactor and the moisture distribution was determined by slicing the cylinders and determining gravimetrically the moisture content of the starch slices. The water diffusivities in the two cylinders (D_1 and D_2) were estimated from the solution of the Fick diffusion equation for the experimental system under consideration (refs. 8, 10):

$$\frac{c_1(\infty) - c_1(z_{1i})}{c_1(\infty) - c_1(0)} = \mathrm{erfc}\left(\frac{z_{1i}}{2(D_1 t)^{0.5}}\right) \qquad (4)$$

$$\frac{c_2(-\infty) - c_2(z_{2i})}{c_2(-\infty) - c_2(0)} = 1 + \mathrm{erf}\left(\frac{z_{2i}}{2(D_2 t)^{0.5}}\right) \qquad (5)$$

Two effective water diffusivities (D_1 and D_2) were obtained, reflecting the different moisture content and different physical structures of the two cylindrical samples.

RESULTS AND DISCUSSION
Diffusion in Granular Starch

The transport of water through a heterogeneous medium, such as granular starch, is a complex process of diffusion through the starch particles and the air-filled pores. Experimental data from drying experiments indicate that the water diffusivity is a complicated function of the moisture contents the main transport mechanism might be liquid diffusion, which is affected positively by the temperature (Arrhenius-type relationship). As the drying progressed, the water diffusivity increased, indicating a vapor-type diffusion through the porous material (Fig. 1). At moisture contents less than 10% the water diffusivity decreased sharply, possibly due to the reduced mobility of adsorbed water molecules. Similar results were obtained with the two types of starches used, i.e. Hylon 7 (linear amylose molecules) and Amioca (branched

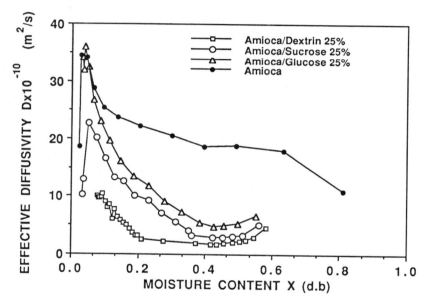

Fig. 1. Effective water diffusivity in granular hydrated Amioca and mixtures of Amioca with water-soluble carbohydrates.

amylopectin molecules), suggesting that the transport of water is affected mainly by the macroscopic structure of the material.

Incorporation of water-soluble carbohydrates in granular starches reduced significantly the water diffusivity (Fig. 1). This reduction appeared to be proportional to the size of the carbohydrate molecule, with dextrin 15 DE (15 dextrose equivalent) having the strongest effect. Measurements of the bulk porosity showed that the water-soluble carbohydrate reduced significantly the bulk porosity (ϵ) of the dried starch material, e.g. from $\epsilon=0.45$ (granular Amioca) to $\epsilon=0.30$ (granular Amioca 75%/dextrin 25%). The reduction of bulk porosity can be explained by the precipitation of the water-soluble carbohydrates in the intergranular spaces (pores) of the material during the drying process. This effect was proportional to the sugar concentration (0-25%) in the starch mixture (ref. 6). The filling of the pores and intergranular channels by the precipitated sugars was confirmed by microscopic observations (ref. 11). The reduction of water diffusivity by sugars and dextrins can be utilized in forming moisture barriers in dehydrated or intermediate moisture foods for improved quality.

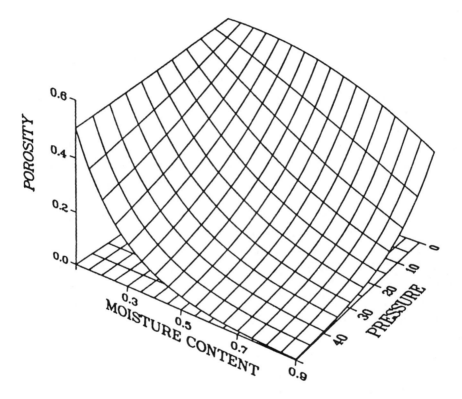

Fig. 2. Effect of mechanical pressure and moisture content on the bulk porosity of granular Amioca.

Mechanical compression of granular starches reduced significantly the bulk porosity and the water diffusivity. The effect of pressure was stronger in wet starches than in dry materials (Fig. 2). Regression analysis of the experimental bulk porosity (ϵ) versus pressure (P, atm) and moisture content (X, dry basis) yielded the following equation for granular Amioca (ref. 12):

$$\epsilon = (0.600 + 0.0643 \cdot X - 0.370 \cdot X^2) \cdot \exp(0.0077 - 0.1113 \cdot X \cdot P) \qquad (6)$$

The water diffusivity D (m²/s) in granular starch (Amioca) was found to be a complex function of bulk porosity (ϵ) temperature T (K) and moisture content (X, dry basis):

$$D = 10^{-10} \cdot \{4842 + 0.5735 \cdot X^{-4.34} + 3412 \cdot [\frac{\epsilon^3}{(1-\epsilon)^2}]\} \cdot \exp(-\frac{4.5}{R \cdot T}) \qquad (7)$$

The energy of activation for diffusion of water in granular starch was relatively low (4.5 kcal/mol), but it increased significantly when water-soluble carbohydrates were added, or when starch was gelatinized.

Diffusion in Gelatinized Starch

Gelatinization of starch reduced in general the water diffusivity (ref. 7). The physicochemical changes brought about to starch materials by heat and water absorption resulted in rupture of starch granules and formation of a gel structure (ref. 13), in which the diffusion of water molecules was slower. Fig. 3 shows the effect of gelatinization on the water diffusivity in Amioca starch. The reduced water diffusivity was related to the lower porosity of the gelatinized starch materials (ref. 7). The samples of gelatinized Amioca (high-amylopectin) starch experienced more shrinkage during drying, resulting in lower porosity and reduced water diffusivity than the gelatinized samples of Hylon 7 (high-amylose) starch. The Hylon 7 gels were more rigid than the Amioca gels, and they formed more cracks and pores during drying, which increased considerably the effective water diffusivity.

The changes in water diffusivity due to gelatinization are important in the thermal processing of starch-based food, e.g. cooking, baking, sterilization and dehydration.

Diffusion at High Pressures

The diffusivity of water vapor in gases is inversely proportional to the total pressure, according to the kinetic theory of gases (ref. 14). Thus, the water diffusivity in porous freeze-dried starch at low pressures (vacuum) was found much higher than at atmospheric pressure (ref. 15).

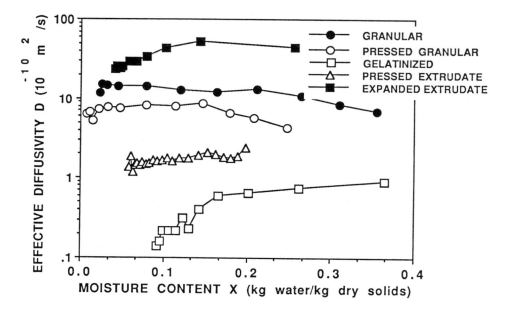

Fig. 3. Effective water diffusivity in granular, gelatinized and extruded Amioca starch.

Experimental measurements, using the moisture distribution method, showed that the water diffusivity in both granular and gelatinized starches decreased from 1 to 40 atm (ref. 10). Temperature had a positive Arrhenius-type effect in the range of 25°-140°C (Figs. 4 and 5). The effect of air pressure was more pronounced in granular (Fig. 4) than in gelatinized (Fig. 5) Amioca starch, evidently due to the higher porosity of the particulate material. The higher air pressures reduced the mobility of water vapor in the gas phase (pores) of the porous material. Air pressure had also a significant negative effect on the water diffusivity in gelatinized starch, possibly due to a reduction of the free volume of the polymer system.

Regression analysis of the experimental data in granular and gelatinized starch (Amioca) yielded the following empirical equations (8) and (9) respectively:

$$D(\text{x}10^{-10} \text{ m}^2/\text{s}) = \frac{[D_o \cdot \exp(-E_a/RT + k_2 \cdot X)]}{P^{k_1}} \qquad (8)$$

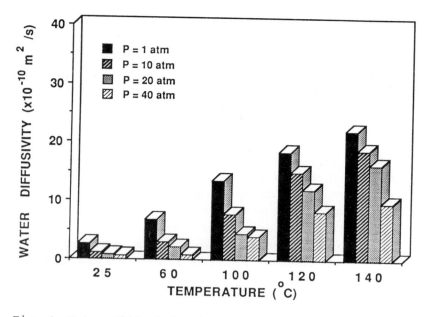

Fig. 4. Water diffusivity in granular Amioca at high pressures and temperatures.

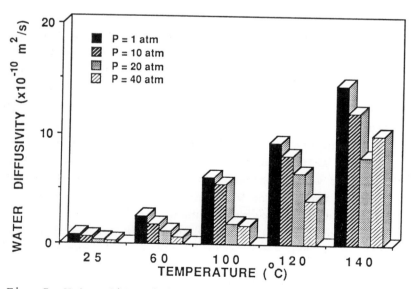

Fig. 5. Water diffusivity in gelatinized Amioca at high pressures and temperatures.

where R=gas constant, R=1.987 kcal/mol·K.
D_o (x10^{-10} m^2/s) = exp(10.882) E_a=5.66 kcal/mol
k_1=0.3122 k_2=-1.5111 (kg water/kg dry starch)
X=moisture content, dry basis.

$$D = D_o \cdot \exp(-E_a/RT - k_1 P) \tag{9}$$

D_o(x10^{-10} m^2/s) = exp(10.848) E_a = 6.66 kcal/mol
k_1 = 0.02717 atm^{-1}

The energy of activation for diffusion of water (E_a) was 5.66 kcal/mol in the granular starch and 6.66 kcal/mol in the gelatinized samples, indicating stronger interactions of the starch/water system in the gelatinized material (ref. 10).

The diffusion of water at high pressures is of importance to food processes such as pressure cooking, pasta extrusion and drying (ref. 16) and extrusion cooking.

Diffusion in Extrusion Cooking

The diffusion of water in starch materials is of fundamental importance in the extrusion cooking of various starch-based foods. In an extrusion cooker, the granular (powder) food material is mixed with water, compressed mechanically up to 50 atm, partially gelatinized (or melted) at temperatures up to 150°C and finally expanded through a die to atmospheric pressure (ref. 17).

Diffusion of water is fast in the mixing section of the extruder due to the high porosity of the granular (particulate) material. Compression of the food particles reduces significantly the water diffusivity, e.g. from 15x10^{-10} to 8x10^{-10}m^2/s (Fig. 3). Gelatinization of the starch granules reduced sharply the water diffusivity to about 1x10^{-10}m^2/s. The water diffusivity in expanded starch extrudates was very high (about 40x10^{-10}m^2/s) due to the high bulk porosity (about ϵ=0.7). The water diffusivity is important in the drying of expanded extrudates. When the extruded starch material was compressed to low porosity the water diffusivity was reduced drastically to the level of the gelatinized starch (Fig. 3).

Conversion of granular to gelatinized starch can be accomplished at low moistures by the combining action of high temperature and mechanical shear. Under these conditions, the long starch molecules may be broken down to small fragments, such as dextrins, which can affect adversely the water diffusivity. The production of extruded food products of desirable quality may be affected by the diffusion of water during and after the extrusion process.

ACKNOWLEDGEMENTS

New Jersey Agricultural Experiment Station publication No. F-10535-1-91 supported in part by the Center for Advanced Food Technology, Rutgers University and the New Jersey Agricultural Experiment Station. The Center for Advanced Food Technology is a N.J. Commission on Science and Technology Center.

REFERENCES

1. G.D. Saravacos. Mass transfer properties of foods, in M.A. Rao and S.S.H. Rizvi (Eds.) Engineering Properties of Foods, Marcel Dekker, New York, 1986, pp. 89-132.
2. M.A. Roques. Diffusion in foods. The work of COST 90bis sub-group, in R. Jowitt, F. Escher, M. Kent, B. McKenna and M. Roques (Eds.), Physical Properties of Foods-2, Elsevier Applied Science Publ., London, 1987, pp. 13-25.
3. R.B. Leslie, P.J. Carillo, T.Y. Chung, S.G. Gilbert, K. Hayakawa, S.N. Marousis, G.D. Saravacos and M. Solberg, in H. Levine and L. Slade (Eds.), Water Relationships in Food, Plenum Press, New York, 1991, in press.
4. B.P. Fish, 1958, Diffusion and thermodynamic properties of water in potato starch gels, in Fundamental Aspects of Dehydration of Foodstuffs, Society of Chemical Industry, London, 1958, pp. 148.
5. G.D. Saravacos and G.S. Raouzeos, Diffusivity of moisture during air drying of starch gels, in B.M. McKenna (Ed.) Engineering and Food, Vol.1, Elsevier Applied Science Publ., London, pp. 499-507.
6. S.N. Marousis, V.T. Karathanos and G.D. Saravacos, Effect of sugars on the water diffusivity in hydrated granular starches, J. Food Sci. 54 (1989), 1496-1500.
7. G.D. Saravacos, V.T. Karathanos, S.N. Marousis, A.E. Drouzas and Z.B. Maroulis, Effect of gelatinization on the heat and mass transport properties of starch materials, in W.E.L. Spiess and H. Schubert (Eds.) Engineering and Food Vol. 1-Physical Properties and Process Control, Elsevier Applied Science Publ., New York, 1990, pp. 390-398.
8. J. Crank, The Mathematics of Diffusion. 2nd ed., Pergamon

Press, Oxford, 1975.
9. V.T. Karathanos, G. Villalobos and G.D. Saravacos, Comparison of two methods of estimation of effective moisture diffusivity from drying data, J. Food Sci. 55 (1990), 218-223.
10. V.T. Karathanos, G.K. Vagenas and G.D. Saravacos, Water diffusivity in starches at high temperatures and pressures, Biotechnol. Prog. 7 (1991) 178-184.
11. S.N. Marousis and G.D. Saravacos, Density and porosity of drying starch materials. J. Food Sci. 55 (1990) 1367-1372.
12. S.N. Marousis, V.T. Karathanos and G.D. Saravacos, Effect of physical structure of starch materials on water diffusivity, J. Food Proc. and Pres. 15 (1991), in press.
13. C.G. Biliaderis, C.M. Page, T.J. Maurice and B.O. Juliano, Thermal characterization of rice starches: A polymeric approach to phase transitions of granular starch, J. Agric. Food Chem. 34 (1986) 6-14.
14. R.C. Reid, J.M. Prausnitz and B.E. Poling. The Properties of Gases and Liquids, 4th ed., McGraw-Hill, New York, 1987.
15. G.D. Saravacos and R.M. Stinchfield, Effect of temperature and pressure on sorption of water vapor by freeze dried food materials, J. Food Sci. 30 (1965) 779-786.
16. J. Andrieu and A. Stamatopoulos, Moisture and heat transfer modeling during durum wheat pasta drying, in A. Mujumdar (Ed.), Drying '86, Hemisphere Publ., New York, 1986, pp. 492-497.
17. V.T. Karathanos and G.D. Saravacos, Water diffusivity in extrusion cooking of starch materials, in J.L. Kokini, C.T. Ho and M. Karwe (Eds.), Applied Food Extrusion Science, Marcel Dekker, New York, 1991, in press.

SOLUBLE COFFEE'S NEW BIOTECHNOLOGY

RALPH L. COLTON

BRAMCAFE INTERNATIONAL LTD., Lansdale, PA 18446 - U.S.A.

This report is on a recently developed method for producing liquid coffee extract which could revolutionize the manufacture of soluble coffee. Liquid coffee extract is the intermediate stage between roasted coffee and the final dehydrated product.

Freeze-dry, spray-dry (regular instant) and liquid coffee concentrate are all classed as "soluble coffee." Together, they make up almost 25 percent of the coffee consumption in the industrialized nations. This varies widely by country with the U.K. and Australia being the highest with 80 percent and 70 percent respectively. Japan, now the fourth largest coffee consuming nation, drinks 50 percent as soluble. The U.S. uses about 30 percent soluble.

This new method is exciting for three major reasons:

a) It provides a substantially higher yield of soluble solids with a massive reduction in the cost of manufacturing.

b) It provides greater consumer satisfaction since it obtains much more of the coffee flavor fraction from the roasted bean and hence produces a "coffier" soluble coffee.

c) It is more environmentally benign, a truly "green" soluble coffee, with considerably less atmospheric pollution.

First, a brief background of soluble coffee:

Before World War II, little powdered or instant coffee was sold. And during the War all production was purchased by the Armed Forces as an essential ingredient of the Army Field Ration.

After WWII, returning soldiers and a changing life-style demanding more convenience foods created a ready market for instant coffee. Many manufacturers (General Foods, Standard Brands, Borden, Tenco etc.) joined Nestle in exploiting this burgeoning market. Nestle had supplied most of the instant coffee during the War and had the most advanced technology.

At this time, the product was sold with "50 percent Malto-dextrin added." Malto-dextrin is a bland-tasting corn sugar which was added to retard caking in the container, facilitate reconstitution to a beverage and to aid in dehydration.

Marketing pressure for a "100 percent Pure Instant Coffee"

sent process engineers in search of a way to solubilize part of the expended grounds as a replacement for malto-dextrin.

Three approaches were researched:

1. Acid hydrolysis, which gave high yields, was rejected for technical reasons and problems of removing precipitates following pH adjustment prior to dehydration.

2. Enzymatic hydrolysis, in spite of its many potential advantages, was abandoned because of disappointingly low yields.

3. Aqueous hydrolysis (industrial pressure-cooking), in spite of many manufacturing problems, more than doubled the total yield of soluble solids and, by 1950, was almost universally employed in the manufacture of instant coffee.

This latter system generally consists of a battery of 7 tall, stainless-steel columns interconnected by piping and valves. One column is generally off-stream for discharge and recharge with ground roasted coffee. It is operated counter-currently with superheated water at about 177°C. (350°F.) under steam-pressure of about 155-160 psi entering the most expended column and proceeding sequentially, at increasingly lower temperatures, through to the most recently charged column where it exits at about 85°C. (185°F). Upon exiting, the extract has a concentration of soluble coffee solids of about 20 percent.

The cycle time is 20-30 minutes for a total residence time of 2-3 hours.

The function of the freshly charged column is to concentrate the extract passing through by selective absorption of water and, at the same time, wetting the fresh ground coffee in preparation for the extraction of the coffee flavor fraction in the following column.

Most of the solubilization (hydrolysis) of the expended grounds from the second column occurs in the last column which receives the superheated water.

An excellent description of this process is in "Coffee Technology," Sivetz and Desrosier, AVI Publishing 1979. This is the text-book of the soluble coffee industry and explains in detail the process and its many problems.

And now to the story of this new biotechnological development and its manifold advantages:

Several years ago, this author, who had long experience of manufacturing soluble coffee (freeze-dry and liquid coffee concentrate) in the United States and Brazil, became intrigued by the possibility of making enzymatic hydrolysis viable.

He did not have much encouragement. Sivetz, in a paragraph entitled "Useless Techniques" states that "the use of enzymes to solubilize cellulose portions of roasted coffee is impractical." The co-discoverer of Trichoderma reesei, a mutant strain of T. viride, a fungus which produces the most potent cellulosic enzymes, told this author that they would be ineffectual with coffee as being "too fibrous." Two U.S. Patents issued in 1942 to William Kellogg include claims of "greatly enhanced yield of coffee solubles" using the enzyme diastases. Kellogg pressure-cooks his ground roasted coffee at 15 psi for one hour to "soften and loosen the fibers" before cooling the product and separating the extract.

Unfortunately, Kellogg provided no figures as to his "Greatly enhanced yield." Replication of his method, using much more powerful enzymes, gave only 1 percent more yield than with coffee which had not been pressure-cooked. Incidently, have you ever tasted coffee which has been pressure-cooked for one hour? No? Well, don't!

This author knew that, in order for enzymes (organic catalysts) to perform their function of cleaving large insoluble molecules into smaller, soluble ones, it is necessary to have adequate receptor contact (i.e. sufficient surface area).

Even the enzyme of T. reesei is relatively large (nominal dimension is 51 Angstrom units, about 15 times that of the water molecule) so it would not be able to penetrate most of the pores and laminae of ground roasted coffee.

The goal was to solubilize at least 35 percent of the expended grounds in order to approximate the yield of the standard method.

The first approach was to increase the surface area by finer and finer grinding. The yield did increase, as expected. However, even when the grounds were disc-milled almost to the consistency of face-powder, the yield using four different enzymes in conjunction, was only 18-20 percent. And this was with 24 hours of enzymatic activity. Very frustrating.

Then the idea of using steam-explosion came forward as a possible solution to the problem of increasing the surface area. It was hypothesized that the escaping steam would enlarge the pores and expand the laminae providing more receptor contact.

The first trial was an immediate success. In fact, the 35

percent goal was exceeded substantially by a yield of 55 percent. There was great elation and thinking became directed to the many potential advantages of enzymatic hydrolysis.

There, of course, is a great deal more technology involved that can be discussed in this short paper; the parameters of the steam-explosion, the pH, concentration and temperature of the slurry, organic and inorganic inhibitors, adjuvants and on and on. It is a very exciting field and enzymatic hydrolysis has manifold advantages over the conventional industrial pressure-cooking.

One interesting advantage is that of selectivity:

Whereas the conventional method is a "shot-gun" approach to solubilization, relying primarily on residence-time and temperature, enzymes are highly selective. Each class of enzyme can only bioconvert one constituent. For instance, the enzyme, cellulase converts cellulose into glucose and cellobiose which further reduces to glucose. It can only solubilize cellulose not starch, protein or any other material.

It was found that this selectivity factor could be used to great advantage in soluble coffee manufacture. For instance, roasted coffee contains 10-12 percent protein which, when solubilized becomes peptides and polypeptides which tend to be bitter. However, if the enzyme, protease is not used in the process, most of the protein remains in the final residue and the beverage is less bitter. Since some bitterness may be desired, this can be controlled by the amount of enzyme used or at which point in the process it is introduced.

In contrast to the above control and selectivity, the conventional method is a "shot-gun" approach relying on residence-time and temperature to effect solubilization.

This method, as explained by Sivetz, has about reached its yield limit since a 5 degree increase in temperature, in a short time, softens the grounds turning them into "a foul-smelling mass, destroying the extract."

Now an exciting revelation for you environmentalists.

The final residue of the conventional method is generally dewatered and burned to produce process-steam. It has been estimated that the soluble coffee industry, worldwide, pollutes the atmosphere with over 750 million tons of particulates and carbon dioxide each year.

However, the final residue of the new method is digestible to cattle and, if protease is not employed in the process, it would contain a nutritious 25 percent protein level.

There is much, much more but time is running out. However, we should touch on the following because it could be important for developing nations which want to create jobs and industrialize part of their coffee crop. This method is not only considerably lower in capital and operating costs than the conventional, but it has fewer operating and maintenance problems so requires fewer highly skilled workers.

Another point of interest. The final residue of soluble coffee manufacturing contains about 25 percent coffee oil. This is a high quality, largely poly-unsaturated, comestible vegetable oil. In using the new method, at least 80 percent of this coffee oil can be recovered vs. a claim of 50 percent in a 1985 U.S. patent assigned to General Foods.

Which coffee-producing, developing country does not need jobs, cattle-feed and a more healthful vegetable oil to replace the usual palm oil?

Finally, and perhaps most important, is the following:

PROBLEM: If the 20 percent higher total yield of soluble coffee solids were primarily in the non-coffee flavor fraction (the hydrolysate), there would be a substantially weaker coffee flavor in the final product.

SOLUTION: In spite of the higher total yield of solubles, the new method obtains much more of the coffee-flavor fraction. In fact it produces a considerably "coffier" soluble coffee.

EXPLANATION: It is well known (see Sivetz) that a yield of over 30 percent by weight of the roasted coffee can be obtained if it is pulverized. This is not practical in the conventional system which requires a very coarse grind and the yield of coffee-flavor solubles is generally 18-20 percent.

When combined with the second extraction (the hydrolysate), the ratio of flavor solubles to the filler is about 40/60.

In contrast, this <u>new method obtains the full 30 percent of coffee-flavor solubles obtainable</u> from roasted coffee.

So, even with a total yield of soluble solids some 20 percent more than the conventional method, the ratio of coffee-flavor solubles to the hydrolysate is about 50/50. As a result, it is a substantially "coffier" coffee extract. <u>(50/50 vs 40/60</u>

This means that the final product will contain a higher level of coffee flavor and provide greater consumer acceptance.

Finally, as we look to the future, the enzyme, ligninase will soon be commercially available to further increase the yield from roasted coffee. Even then, the "Colton Method" (U.S. Patent 4,983,408, January 8, 1991 with foreign filings in major coffee consuming countries) will obtain enough of the coffee-flavor fraction such that the ratio remains better than that of the conventional method. It will still be a "coffier" soluble coffee.

One last note: a process system has been engineered such that the conventional method can be modernized to use this new biotechnology for under US $5 per bag (60 kg) of operating capacity. The expected annual manufacturing cost-savings are estimated as being US $15-20 per bag processed.

And this cost-saving is in addition to being able to provide the consumer with a truly "coffier" soluble coffee which is, without doubt, the greatest value of the "Colton Process."

Thank you for your attention, I trust that you have found this report interesting.

AROMA OF CHINESE SCENTED GREEN TEA WITH Citrus aurantium var. arama

LUO S.-J., GUO W.-F. and FU H.-J.

Hangzhou Tea Processing Research Institute of Ministry of Commerce, Hangzhou, Zhejiang (People's Republic of China)

SUMMARY

The aroma concentrate of Chinese scented green tea with Citrus aurantium var. arama was prepared by simultaneous distillation and extraction method and then qualitatively analysed by GC-MS and quantitatively analysed by GC-FID. The main constituents and the percentages of the total aroma in this scented green tea were found as: linalool 63.1%, limonene 5.8%, β-pinene 2.5%, linalyl acetate 2.2%, α-terpineol 2.3%, nerolidol 3.1%, t,t-farnesol 2.4% and phytol 2.8%. These constituents contribute to make the attractive aroma characteristics of this scented green tea.

INTRODUCTION

The green tea scented with Citrus aurantium var. arama ("Daidai" in Chinese) is one of the Chinese traditional scented teas, which is well received by people for its strong flavor, the medical effect of helping digestion and being appetizing. And because the manufacturing season of Citrus aurantium scented tea is in April and May, earlier than other scented teas, it sells well on market. Here we report the analysis of the aroma composition of this scented green tea.

EXPERIMENTAL

1. Samples

The samples were made from basket-fired green tea and Citrus aurantium var. arama in Fuzhou Tea Factory.

2. Experimental methods

Experimental methods were the same as previously reported (1).

RESULTS AND DISCUSSION

The result of aroma composition of Citrus aurantium scented green tea is shown in Table 1 and Figure 1, in which 27 of the constituents were identified which make up 97.2% of the total aroma. The constituents of relative high concentration are: linalool, limonene, β-pinene, nerolidol and phytol, etc. Among the identified constituents, alcohols make up 79% of the aroma concentrate, and there are some esters (3.9%) and ketones (1.4%), etc. The aroma composition of Citrus aurantium scented green tea is similar to that of Citrus grandis scented green tea, which also mainly composes of alcohols (2). This may be because both the flowers are of Rutaceae family, citrus genus. Compared with other scented teas, there is small concentration of aldehydes and acids in the aroma of Citrus aurantium scented green tea (3-5). The concentration of aroma was about 0.08% of the scented tea, which was 15 times higher than that of the material green tea (6), and was the highest in scented teas except for jasmine tea. It is clearly because the quantity of flower used in scenting was higher than other scented teas.

It was reported that the main aroma constituents of Citrus aurantium were limonene, linalool, geraniol and citronellol, etc. (7). According to our analysis (6), before scenting the percentages of linalool, geraniol and nerolidol of the total aroma were 18.3, 0.16 and 0.84, respectively. So by scenting with Citrus aurantium, the concentrations of linalool, geraniol and nerolidol, etc. in the tea increased remarkably, and terpenes such as β-pinene and limonene also increased. Since the concentration of linalool in the aroma of Citrus aurantium is quite high (63.1%) with typical fragrance of Michelia alba or lily, combining with high concentrations of limonene (lemon-like), nerolidol (weak rose and apple-like), phytol and other compounds, it is suggested to make the strong fragrant characteristics of Citrus aurantium scented green tea.

Table 1
Aroma composition of Citrus aurantium scented green tea

Peak No	Constituent	Percent of total aroma
1	β-Pinene	2.49
2	Limonene	5.75
3	γ-Terpineol	0.18
4	cis-3,6-Linalooloxide	1.41
5	trans-3,6-Linalooloxide	0.69
6	Linalool	63.05
7	Linalyl acetate	2.23

Table 1 (Continued)

Peak No	Constituent	Percent of total aroma
8	4-Terpineol	0.70
9	α-Terpineol	2.29
10	cis-3,7-Linalooloxide	1.09
11	trans-3,7-Linalooloxide	1.11
12	Geranyl acetate	0.94
13	Nerol	0.13
14	Geraniol	1.62
15	Benzyl alcohol	0.73
16	Phenylethyl alcohol	0.59
17	β-Ionone	0.86
18	3,7-Dimethyl-1,5-octadien-3,7-diol	0.68
19	Nerolidol	3.11
20	Cedrol	0.10
21	3,7-Dimethyl-1,7-octadien-3,6-diol	1.00
22	Phytone	0.49
23	Dihydrobovolide	0.33
24	Methyl palmitate	0.06
25	Dihydroactinidiolide	0.35
26	t,t-Farnesol	2.42
27	Phytol	2.83

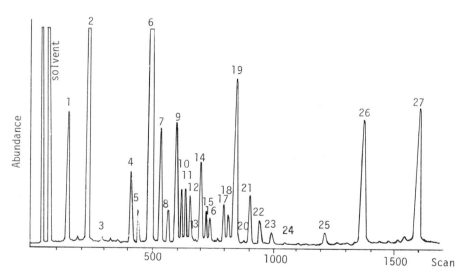

Fig. 1. TIC of aroma of <u>Citrus aurantium</u> scented green tea.

REFERENCES

1 Luo Shao-Jun, Guo Wen-Fei, Fu He-Juan and Tei Yamanishi, in: G. Charalambous (Ed.), Frontiers of Flavor. Proceedings of the 5th International Flavor Conference, Porto Karras, Chalkidiki, Greece, 1-3 July 1987, Elsevier, Amsterdam, 1988, pp. 191-199.

2   Luo Shao-Jun, Fu He-Juan and Guo Wen-Fei, Tea Science, (1990) 45-48.
3   Luo Shao-Jun et al., Fujian Tea, (1987.4.) 11-14.
4   Luo Shao-Jun et al., Fujian Tea, (1988.1.) 16-17.
5   Fu He-Juan et al., Fujian Tea, (1989.3.) 20-22.
6   Luo Shao-Jun et al., Fujian Tea, (1987.3.) 18-21.
7   Jiangsu New Medical College, Big Dictionary of Traditional Chinese Pharmacology, Vol.2, pp.1042, Shanghai People's Publishing House, Shanghai, 1977.

DESIGN AND APPLICATION OF A MULTIFUNCTIONAL COLUMN SWITCHING GC-MSD SYSTEM

K. MacNAMARA[1], P. BRUNERIE[2], S. KECK[1], A. HOFFMANN[3]
[1]Irish Distillers Group, Bow St. Smithfield, Dublin 7 (Irish Republic)
[2]Pernod-Ricard, 120 Av. du Marechal Foch, 94015 Creteil (France)
[3]Gerstel GmbH, Aktienstrasse 232-234, 4330 Muelheim a.d. Ruhr (Germany)

SUMMARY

A state-of-the-art double oven multidimensional gas chromatographic system is described which features electronic flow control and computer activated servo valves to achieve the pressure balancing necessary for pulseless switching in a multicolumn system configuration. A cold programmable injector is also an integral part of the system and its pneumatics, and permits solvent venting from large injections directly after the liner. Installation of selective detectors on the second oven or coupling to a mass selective detector results in a system with powerful applicability to trace analysis in complex matrices. Examples described will show the multifunctional nature of the system and its ability to offer solutions to complex problems in alcoholic beverage analysis.

INTRODUCTION

As our appreciation and knowledge of the complexity of natural mixtures increases it is becoming clear that the extra separating power of multidimensional separations will be required for routine analysis of the future. In this paper the concept of multidimensionality is as defined by Himberg (1) i.e. the sample flow of two or more GC columns are connected in such a way that selected, partly separated fractions of the sample eluting from the first column can be transferred to the second for further separation. The same author refers to this technique as two-stage gas chromatography or GC-GC. Bertsch (2) extends this definition to also include a sample that is analysed simultaneously on two columns of different selectivity for retention data correlation of the sample components.

Schomburg's group were among the earliest workers in this field, both in improving instrumental design and in application (3). Goekeler (4) used a multidimensional double-oven GC for separation and analysis of the antioxidant 2,6-ditertiarybutylphenol in aviation jet fuel. Gordon et al. (5) compared three commercially available capillary to capillary switching systems in terms of activity and the analysis of a complex sample and recommended the practical benefits of dual oven instruments for independent temperature control of each column. Bertsch (2,6) has published comprehensive reviews of multidimensional GC and rightly emphasises the need for powerful hyphenated systems comprising GC-GC with selective detectors including MS and IR. In the alcoholic beverage field Bicchi et al. (7) used multidimensional GC for the enrichment of minor components in an essential oil. In this application repeated cuts from the pre-column were stored in an intermediate cold trap in order to achieve sufficient enrichment to obtain clear mass spectra on transfer to the same polarity second column. Herraiz et al. (8) evaluated the aroma compounds of Chilean Pisco with a dual oven multidimensional GC using pre and main columns of opposing polarities. This system was also linked to a mass spectrometer and allowed reliable identification of many compounds by removing the overlapping that can be prevalent in one dimensional GC. In this regard Giddings (9) has calculated that 500 million theoretical plates would be required for 0.99 separation probability of a 100 component mixture, thus vividly illustrating the limitations of one dimensional chromatography. Van Ingen et al. (10) determined the restricted compound ethyl carbamate in alcoholic beverages by extraction followed by two dimensional GC and FID detection.

Multidimensional technology has traditionally not been used as a routine technique but rather has remained in the domain of a specialised technique for particularly difficult separations. This is in spite of the fact that commercial instrumentation has been available for some years either as complete stand-alone or add-on units. The problem seems to lie in the degree of manual input and customisation required for individual separation problems. Most commercial systems are based on the classic Deans design (11) wich used pneumatic flow switching requiring careful balancing of gas pressures. The Deans design was developed for packed columns where the high carrier gas flows did not put too strenuous demands on the required gas equilibrations.

However as Mueller (12) points out use of low flow narrow bore capillary columns in a Deans configuration places much greater demands on the pneumatic switching system.
Mueller (12) also lists the following requirements for a suitable capillary column coupling system:
- No deterioration of separation efficiency and peak symmetry by eluate transfer.
- Coupling of a monitor detector for the preseparation without creating a time lag between the cut region and the detector.
- Absence of adsorptive surfaces and movable valve parts.
- Intermediate trapping should not be necessary.

One commercial system for use with capillary columns (13) modifies the Deans concept and incorporates valveless "live switching" which uses the pressure drop across a coupling piece instead of the gas flows for column switching. In this paper we describe a system which allows multidimensional capillary GC according to the Deans design but also incorporates optimal coupling pieces and computer control and monitoring of mass flows and pressures for the critical required pressure balancing.

Using the same principles a further option of venting after the liner is incorporated into the system through use of a programmable cold injector as an integral part of the system. All the requirements recommended by Mueller above are satisfied and examples will be shown using the most stringent configuration of two narrow bore capillary columns. A software controlled preparative unit, again using the same technology can be fitted and an example is outlined of an automated separation of two closely eluting isomers.

The system used in this work was also fitted with a Mass Selective Detector after the second oven and a Chemiluminescent Sulfur Detector which was movable between FID's installed on both ovens.

SYSTEM DESIGN

The Gerstel-MCS (Multi Column Switching) Gas Chromatographic System (Gerstel GmbH, Muelheim a.d. Ruhr, Germany) is based on a Hewlett-Packard 5890 GC with pneumatic modification to allow installation of three electronic mass flow controllers (MFC) for carrier gas flow and pneumatic switching at both the inlet switching device (ISD) after the cold injection system (CIS) and at the column switching device (CSD).

Fig.1 shows the pneumatic diagram of the system. Switching occurs in two newly developed low dead volume switching devices and all connections in the system are with graphpack technology. All pneumatic and GC functions are controlled by a PC through an MCS power unit. An FID on this GC acts as a monitor detector for cutting from the precolumn to the main column.

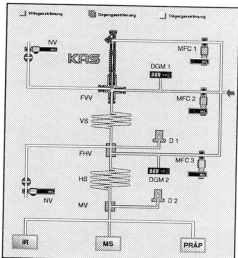

Fig. 1 : Pneumatics diagram, zero condition

The above unit is connected by a heated interface to another 5890 GC which houses the second column and allows independent temperature control of the chromatography of components cut and transferred to this column. This second GC is itself part of a Hewlett-Packard 5971A Mass Selective Detector controlled by its own workstation. Both GC's are linked by remote start cables to allow an MCS start command on the first GC to start the MS run on the second GC. The run delay on the GC/MS is then the pre-programmed time to switching and transfer on the first GC. Preparative applications are carried out simply by exchanging the MSD for the preparative unit with all preparative software control executed from the MCS workstation.

In **Fig. 1** the pneumatic configuration describes the condition in which the sample is transferred from the injector to the precolumn and to the main column without any switching. MFC1 provides this flow and MFC2 and MFC3 are closed. This uninterrupted carrier gas flow through the liner and both columns is defined as the zero condition.

Fig. 2 describes the pneumatic condition in which part of the injected sample is vented from the liner at some suitable intermediate temperature to the venting trap PC1. In this case MFC2 opens and provides a countercurrent venting flow exiting at PC1, which must be greater than the carrier gas flow. This flow serves both to vent the unwanted components and to maintain the previous carrier gas flow through the two capillary columns.

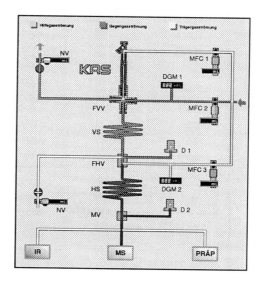

Fig. 2 : Solvent venting

Fig. 3 describes the pneumatic condition in which the sample exiting the precolumn is vented at PC2. In this case MFC3 is open and provides a countercurrent venting flow again greater than the carrier gas flow. The system operates under continous venting (non-zero condition) at the column switching device until a transfer or heart-cut from the first to the second column is desired. For this time period the system reverts to the zero condition at the column switching device i.e. MFC3 closed with uninterrupted flow from the first to the second column. After the desired transfer MFC3 is time programmed to open again so that all unwanted components from the precolumn are vented.

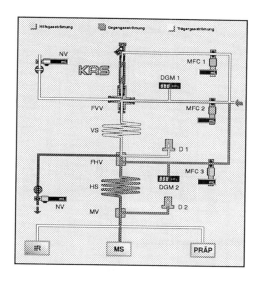

Fig. 3 : Continous venting

The utility and user friendliness of this system result from the automatic computer control and monitoring of mass flows and pressures, which in turn allow rapid equilibration and pressure balancing within the switching devices. The principles of switching and equilibration can be understood by reference to **Figs. 4** and **5**. The independent venting flows which prevent components of no interest from reaching either the first column or later the second column are produced by a rapid establishment of a countercurrent flow supplied through a mass flow controller (MFC2, MFC3) and a simultaneous opening of the corresponding outlet through a magnetic valve (MV1, MV2). To make a cut and transfer components of interest through the switching devices these venting flows are stopped for the required period, with the system returning to the zero condition. Both carrier and countercurrent flows within a switching device must be balanced so that carrier gas flow before and after switching remains the same for reproducible retention times. This is achieved by simulating a vent at the appropriate temperature and the computer either opens or closes electronic servo valves (NV) until that pressure which existed in the zero condition is re-established. Pressures at the switching devices are continually monitored by the bypass digital pressure gauges (DPG1, DPG2) and continuously displayed. These servo settings are stored by the computer so that during actual run switching the flows are precisely balanced giving fine tuned cuts and pulseless switching. In practice this means that the system can be set up for different applications in a very short time with all GC, GC-MS and pneumatic switching times stored in individual method aquisition files.

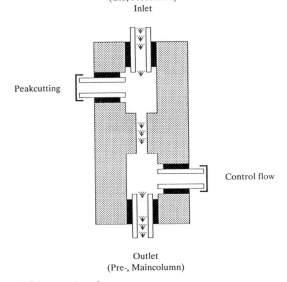

Fig. 4 : Principle of switching, no venting

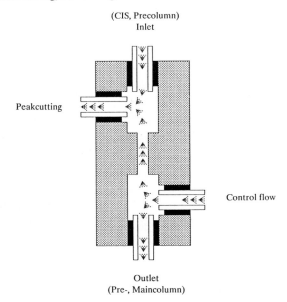

Fig. 5 : Principle of switching, venting

EXPERIMENTAL

The following columns and conditions were used for the analytical applications :

Precolumn in GC-1	:	Stabilwax-DA (Restec Corporation) 60 m x 0.25 mm ID x 0.25 µm df.
Oven Program	:	60°C, 3°C/min to 100°C, then 1.5°C/min to 220°C,
		and for the solvent venting ethyl carbamate analysis;
		100°C for 2 mins, then 2°C/min to 220°C.
Main Column in GC-2	:	Rtx-5 (Restec Corporation), 5% diphenylpolysiloxane, 50 m x 0.25 mm ID x 0.25 µm df.
Oven Program	:	30°C for the corresponding time to pneumatic switching in the first oven, then 5°C/min to 220°C.
Carrier Flow	:	1 ml/min Helium.

Large volume injections were made with a Hamilton 100 µl gas tight syringe fitted with a needle of outside diameter 0.65 mm for compatibility with the septum-less sampling head of the cold injection system. For the same application liners were packed with deactivated glass wool for temporary suspension of the solvent during its evaporation and removal from the liner.

The MSD was operated either in full scan or in selected ion monitoring (SIM) mode depending on the application. The following SIM ions were monitored :

Ethyl Carbamate	M/Z 62,74,89
Furaneol	M/Z 58,85,128

For the preparative application an FID was used in place of the mass selective detector :

Precolumn and Main Column	:	2.0 m, 4 mm ID glass column packed with 10% diglycerol on kieselgur.

Both columns were installed in the first oven which was kept at an isothermal 70°C.

Carrier Flow	:	10 mls/min Helium
Transferline to preparative device	:	130°C
Divider oven in Preparative device	:	150°C
Trap temperatures	:	-5°C with LN2
ALS Injection Volume	:	$3\mu l$/cycle
Number of cycles	:	230
Total volume injected	:	690 μl

APPLICATIONS

A.   DETECTION AND QUANTIFICATION OF FURANEOL IN WINE

Rapp et. al. (14) identified the compounds causing strawberry-like aroma in wine as 2,5-dimethyl-4-hydroxy-2,3-dihydro-3-furanone (furaneol) and 2,5-dimethyl-4-methoxy-2,3-dihydro-3-furanone (methoxyfuraneol). Since both compounds usually occur together detection of the major compound furaneol indicates a potential for strawberry-note properties. The sensory perception threshold of furaneol is 30 - 50 ppb and its analysis at and below this level is complicated by the fact that it is prone to coelution with other wine compounds. Even use of selected ion monitoring detection does not offer a complete solution as the major ions of furaneol (M/Z 57, 85 and 128) are not very specific.

Fig. 6 shows a 2 min heart-cut from the first polar column to the second non-polar column of a freon extract of a wine with ppm amounts of furaneol. For this transfer the venting flow at the column switching device was programmed to stop for the allotted time, allowing furaneol and co-eluting compounds to be transferred for separation on the second column. Peak shape of all components on the second column is excellent and a clean mass spectrum is obtained for furaneol eluting at 77.536 mins.

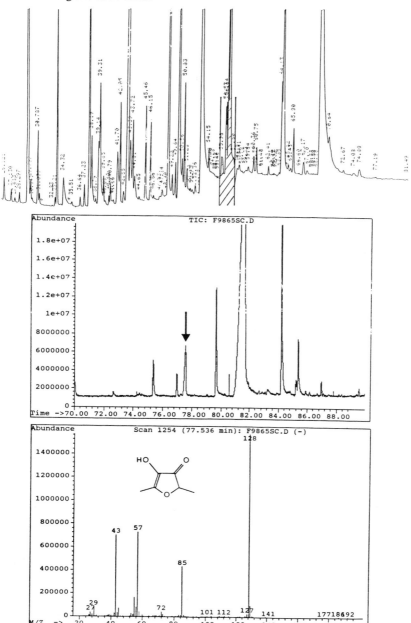

Fig. 6 : Heartcut of a freon extract of wine with ppm amounts of furaneol

Fig. 7 shows the same switching program applied to a wine with low ppb levels of furaneol but this time the MSD is operated in more sensitive SIM for M/Z 57, 85 and 128. Again furaneol is detected unambiguously and the common ions eluting after furaneol clearly demonstrate the need for a multidimensional input into the separation and detection of this compound.

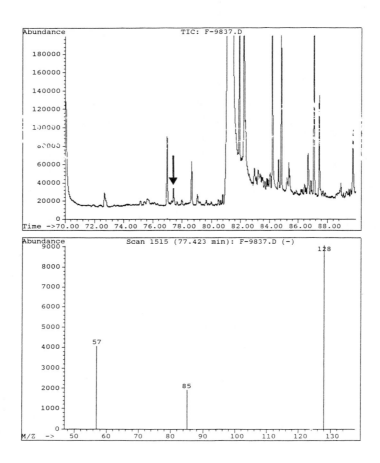

Fig. 7 : Heartcut of a freon extract of wine with ppb amounts of furaneol

B. USE OF A SPECIFIC SULFUR DETECTOR AND MS FOR DIASTOMERIC RATIOING AND CONFIRMATION OF A FLAVOUR COMPONENT

In this application the system capabilities are further extended by use of a highly sensitive Sulfur Chemiluminescence Detector (SCD Model 350, Sievers Research Inc. Colorado, U.S.A.) to locate sulfur isomers on the precolumn followed by transfer to the second column for clean mass spectral confirmation.

This detector has the following important advantages for trace sulfur compound analysis in complex matrices :

1. Sulfur compound detection is practically interference free as the detection mechanism is based on the selective chemiluminescent reaction of sulfur monoxide and ozone.

2. The detector uses an existing FID as the flame source and sulfur analytes are combusted to sulfur monoxide in a hydrogen-rich flame. A ceramic probe and vacuum system takes the sulfur monoxide formed to the detector cell where all other functions such as ozone generation, reaction and signal output occur automatically. In the 2-oven multidimensional system the ceramic probe can be easily moved between FID's of both ovens to investigate location of sulfur compounds in the complex precolumn run and after heart cutting to the second column.

P-methane-8-thiol-3-one is a component of Buchu Leaf Oil which is its sole natural source and is obtained in turn by steam distillation of the leaves of Barosma Betulina or Barosma Crenulata. This sulfur compound is used by the flavour industry because of its powerful fresh odour note; it exists in two diasteriomeric forms and the structures and configurations were assigned by Lamparsky and Schudel (15). The synthetic compound is generally obtained by chemical addition of hydrogen sulfide to pulegone and the diasteriomeric ratio is conveniently reversed depending on whether the source is synthetic or natural.

Fig. 8 shows an FID trace of a commercial peach-flavoured wine product, the corresponding chemiluminescent sulfur trace and the sulfur trace of diluted Buchu Leaf Oil. These sulfur traces immediately identify the synthetic p-methane-8-thiol-3-one diasteriomers in the flavour added to the wine product because of the inverted isomer ratio.

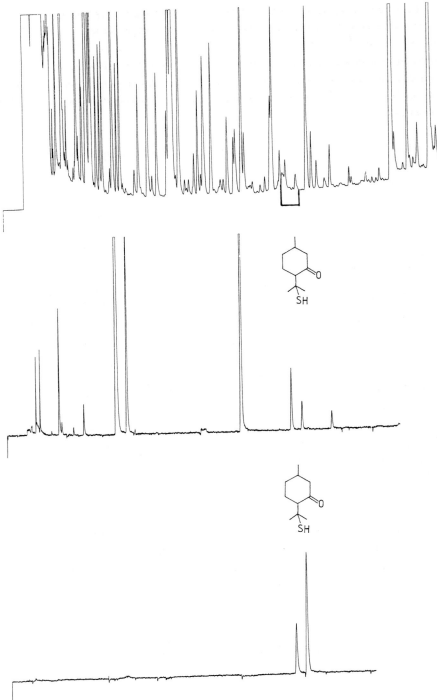

Fig. 8 : FID-Trace (TOP) of a wine product, SCD trace of a wine product and Buchu leaf oil

In **Fig. 8** the FID and SCD traces were taken from the monitor detector on the first oven of the MCS system. In a second experiment the switching system was programmed to transfer the two isomers in the wine product to the second coupled column into the MSD (based on their elution times from the sulfur trace). **Fig. 9** shows the resulting TIC trace where the isomers are now separated from other uninteresting matrix components and give high quality mass spectra. The excellent TIC peak shapes also testify to the integrity of the MCS switching technology and design.

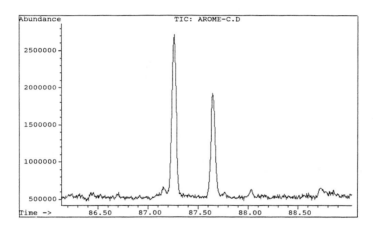

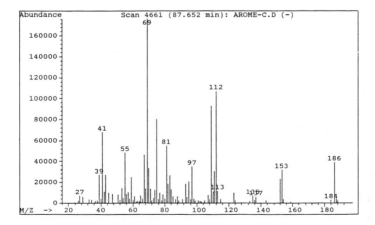

Fig. 9 : TIC and spectrum of p-methane-8-thiol-3-one

C. DIRECT LARGE VOLUME INJECTION OF ALCOHOLIC BEVERAGES FOR LOW PPB ETHYL CARBAMATE DETERMINATION WITH TARGET ION CONFIRMATION.

Ethyl Carbamate is a natural occurring carcinogen present in all fermented foods and beverages (16). Strict regulatory guidelines are in force with maximum allowable levels in the ppb range. Multi sample analysis of trace level ethyl carbamate involving sample preparation requires considerable resources and there are reported instances of pre-treatment operations involving heat leading to artifact formation. Even use of GC-MS in selected ion monitoring is not without difficulties as co-eluting ions from complex beverage matrix compounds can give interference.

Using both the inlet switching device and the column switching device in a single run we have been able to combine direct large volume injection and heart cutting of distilled spirits to allow low ppb quantification of ethyl carbamate with three ion confirmation of positives. Typically 25 μl of sample is injected into the packed liner of the cold injection system which is held at an intermediate temperature under venting to effect maximum solvent removal compatible with minimum solute loss. After this time period the system switches back to the zero condition (no venting) at the inlet switching device and the cold injector ramps to its final temperature to transfer the ethyl carbamate to the precolumn. Normal chromatography occurs on this column followed by heart cutting of the ethyl carbamate to the second column and the MSD in SIM detection.

	No Solvent Venting	Solvent venting
Injection Volume	1 μl	25 μl
Carrier Gas Flow	1 ml/min He	1 ml/min He
Liner Flow	1 ml/min He	10 mls/min He
Venting Flow	0	25 mls/min He
Venting Time	0	2 mins
Initial Temperature	100°C	100°C
Initial Time	0	2 mins
Injector Program Rate	10°C/sec	10°C/sec
Final Temperature	220°C	220°C
Final Time	3 mins	3 mins

Table 1 : Cold injector programmes

The cold injector programmes and inlet switching device pneumatic settings comparing the normal 1 μl and 25 μl injections are summarised in **Table 1**. A feature of this design is that in addition to the venting flow that removes the solvent, generation of much higher liner purging flow is possible at the same time. On reversion to the zero condition the venting flow stops and the liner flow reverts to the normal capillary flow of 1 ml/min. **Fig. 10** shows the enrichment effect that can be achieved by comparing on the monitor detector 1 μl injection of 200 ppm ethyl carbamate without solvent venting and 20 μl of 10 ppm ethyl carbamate with solvent venting. The recovery is typically greater than 85%. Using this enrichment technique it is possible to monitor M/Z 62, 74 and 89 from direct injection of low ppb levels of ethyl carbamate.

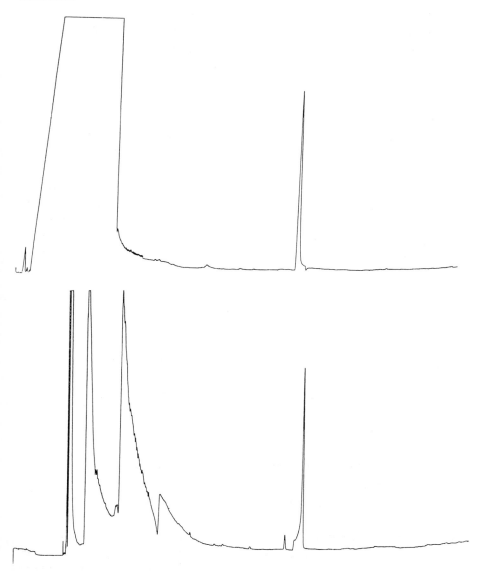

Fig. 10 : 1 μl of 200 ppm EC without solvent venting (Top) and 20 μl of 10 ppm EC with solvent venting

Use of M/Z 64 from isotopically labelled ethyl carbamate as internal standard assures good statistical accuracy. **Fig. 11** shows a target generated report of a whiskey with 35 ppb ethyl carbamate based on M/Z 62 for quantification and using M/Z 74 and 89 for qualifier ratio confirmation.

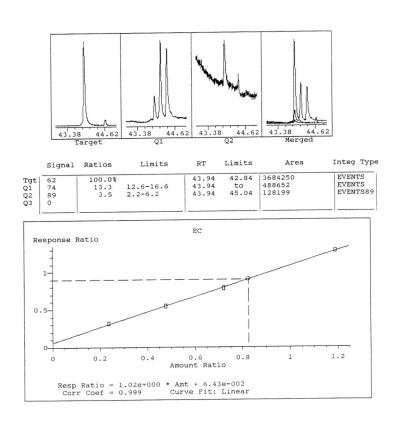

Fig. 11 : Target generated report of 35 ppb EC in a whiskey

D. PREPARATIVE SEPARATION OF TWO CLOSELY ELUTING ISOMERS

In this application the MSD is replaced by a preparative device which together with an automatic liquid sampler for repetitive injections is controlled from the MCS workstation. Both packed columns are mounted in the first oven and the second column is connected via an effluent splitting device to an FID so that each column has a monitor FID. In this way the preparative process can be monitored after each column and the final switching occurs in a preparative switching device via a heated transfer line from the effluent switching device.

The schematic drawing in **Fig. 12** outlines the configuration changes after the second column for this application.

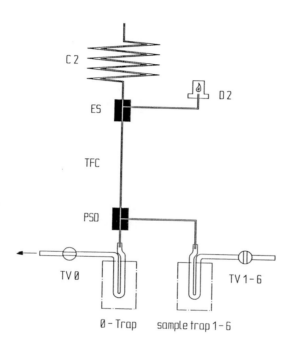

Fig. 12 : Preparative device (principle)

Fig. 13 shows monitor detector traces from both columns for one of 230 3 μl injections of a concentrated fusel oil in which the dominant components are natural 2- and 3-methyl-1-butanol. The 2-methyl isomer is 30% of the 3-methyl isomer and elutes first. The first column monitor detector trace (D1) shows practical coelution of the isomers. Therefore the first cut is programmed at the indicated tick marks on the D1 trace, i.e. from the base of the 2-methyl isomer to just after its apex. The second column monitor detector trace (D2) shows that the result of this cut is enrichment of the 2-methyl isomer but with some residual 3-methyl isomer. Therefore the second cut is made in the preparative switching device at the indicated D2 marks, i.e. near the base of the 2-methyl isomer and just at the end of the downslope.

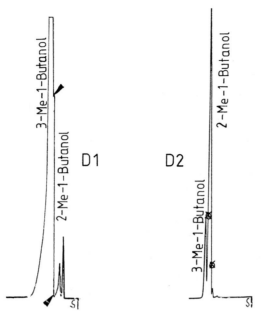

Fig. 13 : Cutting on pre-column and maincolumn (D1: pre-column, D2: maincolumn)
The above cutting parameters were software programmed and the liquid sampler delivered 230 3µl injections to the system under these conditions. The isolated purity of the 2-methyl-1-butanol was greater than 99%.

Fig. 14 shows the isomer components in the fusel oil (diluted 1/100 with ethanol) before and after the preparative operation.

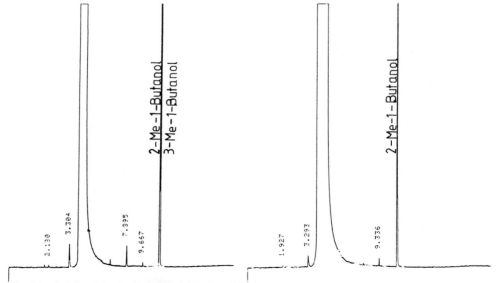

Fig. 14 : Original fusel oil (left) and isolated isomere from preparative trap

REFERENCES

1. K. Himberg et al., Journal of Microcolumn Separations Vol.1, No.6, 1989.

2. W.J. Bertsch, HRC & CC, 1, 85 (1978).

3. G. Schomburg and F. Weeke, Chromatographia 16, (1982).

4. U. Goekeler, American Laboratory, October 1984.

5. B.M. Gordon et al., Journal of Chromatographic Science Vol. 23, January 1985.

6. W.J. Bertsch in Multidimensional Chromatography, Techniques and Applications. Published by Marcel Dekker, New York.

7. C. Bicchi et al., Journal of High Resolution Chromatography Vol. 12, November 1989.

8. M. Herraiz et al., Journal Agric. Food Chem. 1990, 38

9. J.C. Giddings in Multidimensional Chromatography, Thechniques and Applications. Published by Marcel Dekker, New York.

10. R.M. van Ingen et al., HRC & CC, 19,151, 1987.

11. D.R. Deans, Chromatographia 1, 18 (1968).

12. F. Mueller and U. Goekeler, International Laboratory, June 1985.

13. F. Mueller, International Laboratory, July/August 1983.

14. A. Rapp and H. Mandery, Experimentia, Vol. 42 (8), 1986.

15. D. Lamparsky and P. Schudel, Tetrahedron Letters No. 36 (1971).

16. H. Connacher and B. Page, Proceedings of Euro Food Tox. 11, Zürich, 237, 1986.

G. Charalambous (Ed.), Food Science and Human Nutrition
© 1992 Elsevier Science Publishers B.V. All rights reserved.

SENSORY AND ANALYTICAL EVALUATION OF HOP OIL OXYGENATED FRACTIONS

Nora B. Sanchez[1], Cindy L. Lederer, Gail B. Nickerson[2], Leonard M. Libbey, Mina R. McDaniel[3]

Sensory Science Laboratory, Dept. of Food Science and Technology, Wiegand Hall, Oregon State University, Corvallis, OR 97331-6602

[1]CIATI - Bartolome Mitre y 20 de Junio (8336), Villa Regina-Rio Negro, Argentina Fax: 941-25377

[2]Agricultural Chemistry Department, Oregon State University 97331-6502

[3]Author to whom correspondence should be sent.

SUMMARY

Oxygenated fractions of Hallertauer Mittelfrüh, U.S.D.A. 21455 (Mt. Hood), and U.S.D.A. 21459 were evaluated for aroma by a descriptive sensory panel (DSP). The same fractions were injected into a gas chromatograph-olfactometer (GCO) and the effluents evaluated qualitatively and quantitatively by four trained subjects. The GCO data was collected using a method called Osme based on a time intensity (TI) device connected to an IBM computer. The samples were analyzed by mass spectrometry (MS) to identify the odor active compounds. Correlation analysis was performed between the descriptive sensory analysis data and the intensity rates of the compounds sniffed through the GC. Chemical and sensory profiles of the samples were similar indicating that the new varieties are good representatives of "noble aroma" hops. Linalool and oxidation products of caryophyllene and humulene were important contributors to the overall aroma of the samples. Differences found seemed to be associated with the amount of oxidation products present due to different oxidative stages of the samples.

1. INTRODUCTION

Since the advent of the GC much has been learned regarding the composition of hop oil. More than 150 volatile constituents of hops have been characterized by several authors (1-4) and new compounds are reported continuously in the literature. Studies on hop oils have shown marked chemical differences among varieties, demonstrating that certain components or ratios of components are highly specific for individual varieties (5-7). The sensory properties of beer are dependent on the composition of hops and hop oil used (8-11).

Instrumental analyses are increasingly more reproducible and reliable, but they are of little importance unless their results correlate with the results of sensory judgment. A correlation of the sensory properties of hop oil with the chemical analysis may help brewers predict sensory properties of their beers as a function of hops used before conducting large scale brewing trials. No records were found in the literature describing the sensory properties of hop oils and their correlation with chemical composition.

The human nose and GC detectors vary widely in their sensitivity to different molecular species and to different compounds of the same chemical type. Most of the flavor research purporting correlation between sensory and instrumental data used the flame ionization detector (FID) response as a variable without taking into account that the FID is a detector whose response is linear with concentration; whereas, the human olfactory system is a detector whose response is usually a power function with concentration. Correlations have been made without knowing whether or not the peaks correspond to an odor active compound. Sniffing of the chromatographic effluents can help identify odor active peaks, determine their relative sensory importance, and produce a more reliable variable to be introduced into the correlation analysis.

Acree et al. (12) developed a GCO technique named CharmAnalysis™ and Grosch et al. (13) developed a similar method called AEDA. Both methods are based on the GCO analysis of serial dilutions of a sample. In CharmAnalysis, volatiles are extracted from the sample with solvents and separated by GC. The presence or absence of odor in the effluent as a function of time is recorded by the subject using a microcomputer. The data has the value of "zero" (cannot be perceived) or "one" (can be perceived) at every time during the run. A serial dilution of the sample is continued until no odor is detected at all. Combining these results in a particular way produces a graph called a charm chromatogram (14). The largest peaks in the graph correspond to the chemicals with the most intense odor. Applications of CharmAnalysis have been used to determine the odor activity of compounds in wine (15-17), grape juice (18), apples (14), crackers (19), and to determine variability in thresholds (20). Other similar methods have been developed by Scheiberle and Grosch (21-22) for food odorants and by McDaniel et al. (23) for a wine maturity study. McDaniel et al. (23) developed a technique called Osme which is similar to charm but does not determine odor thresholds. Osme is a method to evaluate the odor activity of compounds eluting from a gas chromatograph both qualitatively (descriptors) and quantitatively (intensity ratings) by human subjects.

It is commonly reported that certain German hop varieties such as Hallertauer Mittelfrüh, Spalter, or Tettnanger impart a "noble" or "traditional" hop aroma to beer which is often described as herbal/spicy. Because German varieties have low yields and high susceptibility to diseases when cultivated in the United States, hop breeders seek crosses that produce higher yields and characteristics similar to the imported varieties. Two triploids derived from a tetraploid of Hallertauer, U.S.D.A. 21455 (Mt. Hood) and U.S.D.A. 21459, developed at the Oregon State University Agricultural Experiment Station, were identified as having aroma properties similar to their parent Hallertauer Mittelfrüh (24). These two new crosses of hops were selected for study as potentially important substitutes for Hallertauer.

The objectives of this study were to 1) use the Osme method to identify odor active regions on the FID chromatograms of the oxygenated fractions of the hop oils, rate their intensities, and describe their sensory properties, 2) characterize the sensory properties of the oxygenated fractions by DSP analysis and relate these results with the GCO sniffing results, and 3) identify the odor active peaks, when possible, by GC-MS analysis.

2. MATERIALS AND METHODS

2.1 Extraction, fractionation, and general chemical analyses

The hop varieties from the 1987 crop (John I. Haas, Inc., Yakima, Wa) were analyzed approximately one year from harvest (November, 1988). The hops were pelletized, vacuum sealed in plastic bags, and held in temperature controlled storage (3-4°C) until analyzed. The American varieties were grown in Washington state and the Hallertauer hops were imported from Germany.

Hop oil was collected by steam distillation according to Likens and Nickerson (7). Alpha and beta acids were determined by the ASBC method (25), alpha acids composition by the method of Verzele (26), and hop storage index (HSI) according to Nickerson and Likens (27).

Hop oil (0.1 ml) was fractionated into oxygenated and hydrocarbon fractions according to the method of Nickerson and Likens (8). The oxygenated fraction was eluted with 10 ml of diethyl ether. Samples were concentrated with the use of a Vigreux column.

2.2 Equipment

The GC (Hewlett Packard 5890) was equipped with a 0.53 mm ID by 30 m fused silica column coated (0.50 μm) with Supelcowax 10 (Supelco, Inc., Bellefonte, PA). Injector port temperature was 200°C, detector temperature was 250°C, and split ratio was 16:1. The temperature program was 80°C for 5 min, rate A = 5°C/min, final temperature A = 155°C, rate B = 4°C/min, and final temperature B = 240°C for 60 min. Carrier gas was helium at a linear velocity of 25 cm/sec.

The equipment used to sniff the GC effluents was described by Acree et al. (28). The GC effluent was mixed with humidified air at a flow of 11 L/min. The relative humidity of the air, measured by the difference in temperature between wet and dry bulb thermometer, was 60% at the end of the sniffer and the temperature of the air was approximately 25°C. The resolution was optimized by adjusting the air flow as the sum of the linear velocity of the helium carrier gas plus makeup gas coming from the column. To record the aroma intensity of the GC effluent, panelists used a TI device consisting of a cursor with an attached scale (0=none, 7=moderate, and 15=extreme).

The TI device was connected to a computer and the data were collected through a special data-collection software program that recorded the sensory responses as a set of points that formed a peak with a maximum intensity value at the correspondent time. The times registered were coincident with the retention time of the peaks coming through the GC column.

Using the FID, a series of normal hydrocarbons were chromatographed under the same operating conditions as the stimulus samples. Retention data for the hydrocarbon runs were used to convert stimulus retention times into Kov*a*ts Indexes (KI_{20M}).

Mass spectral data were acquired on a Finnigan 4023 quadrupole mass spectrometer operated in the electron impact mode. The GC (Varian 3400) was equipped with a 0.32 mm ID by 60 m fused silica column coated (0.50 µm) with Supelcowax 10 (Supelco, Inc, Bellefonte, PA). This phase was functionally equivalent to Carbowax 20M. The operating conditions were as follows: injector port temperature = 250°C; split ratio = 50:1; temperature program = 60°C for 5 min, 5°C/min up to 155°C, 4°C/min up to 240°C. Mass spectral data were compared with reference spectra from the National Bureau of Standards and with a collection of reference spectra compiled in the Agricultural Chemistry Laboratory at Oregon State University. Off-line file searching made use of an IBM AT using combined Kov*a*ts Indexes and mass spectral file (29) for aroma compounds that was created under Borland's PARADOX database program (Borland International, Scotts Valley, CA).

2.3 Sample preparation

2.3.1 Descriptive sensory panel. Sixty µl of the oxygenated hop oil fraction from Hallertauer Mittelfrüh, U.S.D.A. 21459, and U.S.D.A. 21455 were each dissolved in 160 µl of 95% alcohol (Clear Spring, Clermont, KY). From this solution, 2.5 µl aliquots were spiked into 50 ml of spring water in 350 ml amber glasses, covered with an aluminum lid, and served at ambient temperature after standing for 30 min to equalize the headspace. The glasses were coded with three digit random numbers; the random numbers represented treatment types.

2.3.2 Osme. The oxygenated fraction was dissolved in pentane. One-half µl of n-tetradecane ($C_{14}H_{30}$) was added as an internal standard and the volume adjusted up to 1 ml. Because the proportion of oxygenated fraction was different in each variety (Table 1), the 3.5 µl volumes injected were adjusted by closing the split vent so that the same amount of each fraction was delivered through the sniffport to the subjects.

2.4 Training and testing procedure

2.4.1 Descriptive sensory panel. Ten trained panelists evaluated the aroma properties of the hop oil oxygenated fractions spiked in water; all were volunteer

TABLE 1

Chemical composition of hops

Varieties	% α-acids[1] AI	DW	% β-acids[2] AI	DW	Oil cont.[3] AI	DW	H.S.I.[4]	Cohumulone(%)[5] ratio	Oxyg. Fraction[6]	% Oxyg. Fraction
U.S.D.A. 21455	2.9	3.1	5.1	5.6	0.70	0.77	0.55	23	0.34	35.4
HALLERTAUER	4.6	5.0	3.3	3.6	0.70	0.77	0.37	33	0.12	11.7
U.S.D.A. 21459	2.0	2.2	2.9	3.2	0.30	0.33	0.55	28	0.15	31.7

1- % α-acids calculated on an "as is" (AI) and dry weight (DW) basis.
2- % β-acids calculated on an "as is" (AI) and dry weight (DW) basis.
3- Oil content (expressed in ml/100 g hops), determined on an "as is" (AI) and dry weight (DW) basis.
4- Hop storage index.
5- Expressed as % of α-acids.
6- Expressed in ml/100 g of hops.

students or faculty of Oregon State University.

Panelists were trained over a three week period to evaluate aroma intensity using a sixteen point intensity scale (0=none, 3=slight, 7=moderate, 11=large, and 15=extreme). For each sample, panelists scored aroma attributes by referencing anchored intensity standards (3=safflower oil, 7=orange drink, 11=grape juice, 15=cinnamon gum). For example, panelists would compare the intensity of an attribute to the intensity of the standard and then rate their sample relative to the standard. Trained panelists selected and rated 11 attributes: overall intensity, soapy, herbal, woody, grassy, citrus, sweet, fruity, artificial fruit, floral, and vitamin B. Panelists described vitamin B as having a meaty or brothy aroma, thiamine-like. Reference standards were provided at each session (Table 2).

For testing, three samples were presented to each panelist in random order. Panelists were seated in individual booths and instructed to evaluate the samples from left to right. Samples were evaluated at approximately 21°C.

2.4.2 Osme. Four female subjects, volunteers from OSU, participated in this section of the study. Three of them were also members of the descriptive sensory panel. For training, the panelists were familiarized with the samples and the chemicals that were found in the samples. Details on the training and methodology are cited in Sanchez (30).

For testing, each sample was evaluated by each panelist on four consecutive days. Each sniffing session took approximately 35 min. Prior to sniffing, subjects were presented with standards in order to help them describe the effluent (Table 3).

Subjects were instructed to breathe normally while sniffing the GC effluent. They moved the TI cursor according to the intensity perceived and reported a quality descriptor for that odor (Fig. 1). The odor intensity responses were registered by the computer while the odor quality descriptors were relayed verbally to the experimenter. The sensory responses collected in the computer consisted of a set of points that formed a peak with a maximum intensity value at a correspondent time. The times registered were coincident with the retention times of the peaks coming through the GC column.

Times and intensities of peaks detected at least 50% of the time for each subject were averaged. Then, times and intensities of those peaks that were detected at least for three of the four subjects were averaged again and a consensus osmegram was obtained for each variety evaluated. An example of an osmegram can be seen in Fig. 4.

Assessments by panelists were analyzed per peak across treatments by a one way anaylsis of variance (ANOVA). The F-value for testing treatment significance was calculated using the Mean Square Error as the denominator.

2.4.3 Confirmation of compounds by Osme. Several compounds thought to be

TABLE 2

Definitions of the attribute reference standards[1] used by the DSP during the evaluation of hop oil oxygenated fractions.

Attribute	Reference[1] Definition and Preparation
Overall Aroma	Total impact of all aromas.
Soapy	Aroma intensity which yielded an irritating piercing or reflex response. Reference prepared by imbibing an aroma paper[2] stick on 90% pure Methyl Laureate (Eastman Organic Chemicals, Rochester, NY).
Herbal	Primary aroma of a reference prepared by mixing 1 g each of Sassafras, Chamomile, Rosehips, Hibiscus and 2 g of Lemon Grass (Marquette Herbs, Corvallis, OR).
Woody	Primary aroma of a reference prepared by imbibing an aroma paper stick in Cedar Wood Essential Oil (Frontier Herbs, Norway, IA 52318).
Grassy	Primary aroma of a reference prepared by: 1- 50 ml solution of 0.01% of cis-3-hexenal (95%, Bedoukian Research, Inc., Danbury, CT), in spring water. 2- 60 ml of macerated straw or hay in spring water.
Citrus	Primary aroma of a reference prepared by combining two half wedges of orange, grapefruit and lemon (Sunkist Growers, Inc., Los Angeles, CA).
Sweet	Primary aroma of 10 ml of honey (Sue Bee, Grade A White, Pure Clover Honey, Sioux Honey Assn., Sioux City, IA).
Fruity	Primary aroma of a reference prepared by: 1- Three 1 cm dices of cooked, dried, apricots (Del Monte Co., San Francisco, CA). 2- One-half canned Bartlett pear (Del Monte Co., San Francisco, CA), diced in 1 cm cubes. 3- One-quarter fresh Jonathan apple diced in 1 cm cubes.
Artificial Fruit	Primary aroma of a reference prepared by: 1- 100 g of artificial fruit-flavored cereal (Fruit Loops, Kellog Col, Battle Creek, MI). 2- 15 g of Mixed Berry Jello (General Foods Co., White Plains, NY).
Floral	Primary aroma of a reference prepared by imbibing an aroma paper stick in carnation or rose essence (Uncommon Scents, Eugene, OR).
Vitamin B	Primary aroma in a reference prepared by 2 halved tablets of Stresstabs 600 (Lederle Laboratories Division, Pearl River, NY), soaked with few drops of spring water.

1- All the Reference Standards were evaluated in 350 ml amber glasses covered with an aluminum foil lid and served at room temperature.
2- Fragance Test Filters (Orlandi, Inc., Farmingdale, NY).

TABLE 3

Attribute reference standards[1] and definitions used during the sniffing of the chromatographic effluents for hop oil oxygenated fractions

Attribute	Reference Preparation
Rancid	Thirty ml of rancid oil (Saffola 100% Safflower Oil, Westley Foods, Inc., Plymouth, FL).
Cheesy	Fifty ml of a solution 0.01% of butyric acid (Aldrich, 99%, Gold Label, Milwaukee, WI).
Fresh Vegetative	Three sliced, fresh sweet peas.
Cooked Vegetative	Fifty grams of canned green beans (S&W, French Style, Fine Foods, Inc., San Ramon, CA).
Spicy	1- One cinnamon stick (Spice Islands, Specialty Brands, San Francisco, CA). 2- Three grams of nutmeg (Schilling, McCormick & Co., Inc., Baltimore, MD). 3- Three grams of anise seeds (The R.T. French Co., Rochester, NY). 4- Imbibing an aroma[2] paper stick in Eugenol (Aldrich, 99%, Milwaukee, WI).
Minty	1- Two grams of mint leaves (Nichols Garden Nursery, Albany, OR).
Fruity	1- One-half fresh Jonathan apple sliced in 1 cm cubes. 2- One-half fresh Granny Smith apple sliced in 1 cm cubes. 3- One-quarter fresh banana (Dole, Inc., Honolulu, Hawaii).
Tobacco	One Camel cigarette (R.J. Reynolds Tobacco Co., Winston, Salem, NC).
Floral	Imbibing an aroma paper stick in: 1- carnation 2- magnolia 3- rose 4- violet essences (Uncommon Scents, Eugene, OR).
Piney	Fifty ml of pine needles macerated with spring water for 1 min in a blender.
Citrus	Two half wedges of grapefruit, orange and lemon (Sunkist Growers, Inc., Los Angeles, CA).
Butter	Thirty grams of 100% butter (Darigold AA grade, Seattle, WA).
Burned Matches	One burned match. (Diamond Brands, Inc., Minneapolis, MN).
Prunes	Three 1 cm cubes of prunes (Del Monte Co., San Francisco, CA).
Cooked Fruit	Cook for 5 min: 1- Three prunes (Del Monte Co., San Francisco, CA). 2- Three dried apricots (Del Monte Co., San Francisco, CA). 3- One-half Jonathan apple diced in 1 cm cubes.
Vinyl	Plastic toy.
Musty	Five filbert halves soaked in spring water and held until mold developed on them.
Woody	Imbibing an aroma paper stick in Cedar Wood Essential Oil (Frontier Herbs, Norway, IA 52318).

1- All the Reference Standards were evaluated in 350 ml amber glasses covered with an aluminum foil lid and served at room temperature.
2- Fragrance Test Filters (Orlandi, Inc., Farmingdale, NY).

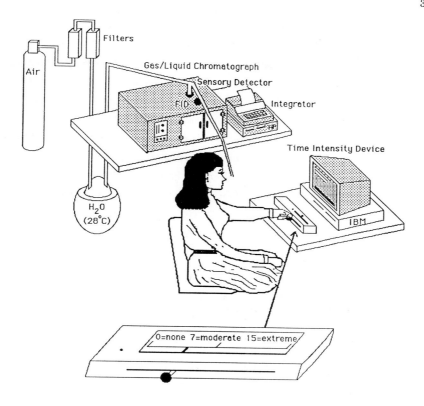

Fig. 1. Gas chromatograph set-up for GCO using the Osme method.

responsible for the odor active peaks were collected and tentatively identified by GC-MS. To confirm the sensory characteristics of these identified compounds, three of the four panelists sniffed solutions from the GC containing approximately equal concentrations of compounds in pentane as in the hop oil sample. The amounts injected were adjusted so that the peak areas for each compound in pentane were similar to the peak areas of the compounds in the hop oil sample. GC effluents from the pentane solutions were evaluated in the same way as were the hop oil samples.

2.5 Experimental design and statistical analysis

Three different analyses were applied to the data collected: analysis of variance, principle component analysis (PCA), and sensory-instrumental correlation.

2.5.1 Analysis of variance. For DSP, a completely randomized balanced block design was used with three replications.

Panelists were first evaluated for consistency of their responses by examining their individual standard deviations over replication. One panelist's data was removed because the observations resulted in high standard deviations for most of the attributes tested.

An individual ANOVA was conducted for each attribute (30): Factors tested included treatment, panelist, replication, and panelist x treatment (PxT) interaction. The treatment set consisted of the three oxygenated hop oil fractions: Hallertauer Mittelfrüh, U.S.D.A. 21459, and U.S.D.A. 21455.

2.5.2 Principal component analysis. To visualize in space the differences among samples and the correlation among attributes, DSP sample results were analyzed using PCA (31).

All statistical analyses were performed using PC.SAS (SAS Institute, Inc., Cary, N.C.).

2.5.3 Sensory-instrumental correlation. Data collected for the DSP and GC were correlated using the following analyses:

(1) Prior to correlating the sensory and instrumental data, a two sample t-test was performed for each of the attributes using data from the whole panel and data from the three common panelists. (The 'common' panelists were on the DSP and Osme panels.) This procedure was conducted to see if the opinion of the three subjects that performed the GCO differed from the opinion of the whole panel (30).

(2) A correlation matrix among each sensory attribute score (averaged over the three replications) for the three common panelists in the DSP and the odor intensity assigned for each subject to each one of the GCO peaks (averaged over those peaks that were detected at least 50% of the time) was conducted. Those peaks that were correlated with the sensory attributes with a p value ≤ 0.5 were selected as independent variables for the next step.

(3) A stepwise regression analysis was conducted for each sensory attribute determined by the three common panelists from the DSP on each of the GCO peaks that presented high correlation coefficients with the sensory attribute predicted. The procedure used a significance value of $p \leq 0.15$ to introduce, keep, or to take variables out of the model. Mallows' Cp criteria was used to establish the statistical significance of the equations (32). Cp is a measure of the bias in the regression model. When there is no bias in a model with p-1 predictor variables the expected value of Cp is p. All correlation analyses were performed using PC.SAS (SAS Institute, Inc., Cary, N.C.).

3. RESULTS AND DISCUSSION

3.1 Chemical composition of hops

It has been reported that hops with high cohumulone ratio (such as above 50%) confer harshness to beers, hence high concentrations of this compound correlate negatively with hop quality (33). All hop varieties associated with noble aroma, such as Hallertauer, have a cohumulone ratio of approximately 25% or less (34). U.S.D.A. 21455 and 21459 had cohumulone contents of 23% and 28%, respectively, which fit the characteristics of the noble aroma hop (Table 1).

The HSI is an indicator of the aging stage of hops (27). It has been reported that humulene and myrcene oxidation products increase and alpha acid content decrease as hops are aged (35). Hallertauer had the lowest HSI, which means that it was less aged than the other two varieties. That explains why it had a higher percentage of alpha acids and a lower percentage of oxygenated fraction (Table 1).

3.2 Descriptive sensory panel

The oxygenated fractions of the three varieties were quite similar in sensory quality: no one aroma was predominant. The overall intensity levels of the hop oils were rated as moderate-to-large, but the remaining attributes were a mixture of low intensity notes (Table 4). Soapy was the next highest-rated descriptor with intensity ratings of slight-to-moderate. Herbal, sweet, fruity, artificial fruit, and floral were all rated between just detectable and slight. Panelists rated the hop oils as slight in citrus aroma and as just detectable in woody and grassy notes.

3.2.1 Analysis of variance.

The treatment effect was only significant ($p \leq 0.001$) for the vitamin B attribute. Hallertauer was rated significantly higher in vitamin B character; the experimental varieties contained none of this attribute (Table 4). Although the reference standard used for vitamin B was a vitamin complex, the odor characteristic was similar to the aroma of impure thiamine, one of the components of the vitamin complex.

The PxT interaction was only significant ($p \leq 0.01$) for the vitamin B attribute. This interaction was caused by five panelists who were very sensitive to this attribute while the other four panelists did not perceive it at all.

The panelist effect was statistically significant for all the attributes except for vitamin B and fruity. This implied that summed over treatments and replications, judges differed significantly in their scores, which indicated the use of different parts of the scale.

3.2.2 Principal component analysis.

Sensory differences among the hop oils were distinguished better by PCA than by ANOVA. Four principal components (PC) accounted for 71.6% of the total variance. The contribution of each attribute to each

TABLE 4

Attribute means,[1,2] (standard deviations), and LSD[3] values from descriptive panel for hop oil oxygenated fractions

Attribute	HOP VARIETIES			LSD Values
	Hallertauer	USDA 21459	USDA 21455	
Overall Intensity	9.0 (1.63)	8.9 (1.95)	8.8 (2.66)	---
Soapy	4.2 (3.03)	4.3 (2.64)	5.1 (2.87)	---
Herbal	2.3 (2.08)	2.2 (2.08)	2.3 (2.03)	---
Woody	1.1 (1.64)	1.5 (2.14)	2.2 (2.20)	---
Grassy	1.7 (2.22)	1.4 (2.19)	1.4 (2.06)	---
Citrus	2.9 (2.57)	3.0 (2.31)	3.2 (2.17)	---
Sweet	2.4 (2.47)	2.5 (2.56)	2.2 (2.31)	---
Fruity	2.5 (2.33)	2.1 (2.46)	1.6 (1.89)	---
Artificial Fruit	2.1 (2.64)	2.6 (2.76)	2.1 (2.83)	---
Floral	1.7 (2.28)	2.8 (2.78)	2.8 (2.53)	---
Vitamin B	2.4^a (2.78)	0.0^b (0.00)	0.0^b (0.00)	1.34

^{a,b} Means with different superscripts within the same row are significantly different from one another.
[1] Sixteen point intensity scale (0 = none, 15 = extreme).
[2] Means based on average ratings by nine panelists.
[3] LSD at $p \leq 0.05$.

PC is represented by vectors with the length of each vector proportional to its relative importance in explaining the variability among the samples (Fig. 2). Those vectors that are close together are highly correlated while those in opposite directions are negatively correlated. PC1 was weighted mainly by soapy, floral, overall intensity, and artificial fruit (Fig. 2). PC2 separated the samples based on herbal, citrus, and vitamin B attributes indicating that Hallertauer had more herbal, citrus, and vitamin B character. U.S.D.A. 21459 was separated from Hallertauer by artificial fruit, sweet, and floral. PC3 separated the samples based on grassy, vitamin B, fruity, and citrus: Hallertauer was the richest in the first three attributes with U.S.D.A. 21455 being completely separated from Hallertauer by citrus (Fig. 2). PC4 separated the samples primarily on vitamin B and fruity with Hallertauer being the richest in these attributes. U.S.D.A. 21459 was widely separated from Hallertauer by woody and herbal in PC4. Overall the Hallertauer triploid varieties were very similar as shown by their proximity to each other in Fig. 2.

In Fig. 2 it is possible to see that fruity and vitamin B attributes are positively

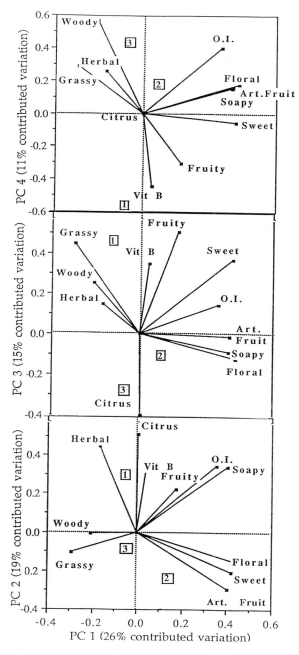

Fig. 2. PCA graphs (PC1 vs. PC2, PC3, PC4) for hop oil oxygenated fractions: 1 = Hallertauer, 2 = U.S.D.A. 21459, 3 = U.S.D.A. 21455, O.I. - Overall intensity. The contribution of each attribute to each PC is represented by vector lenght.

correlated. Herbal is negatively correlated with artificial fruit and sweet; woody and grassy are negatively correlated with floral and soapy. Soapy, overall intensity, floral, and sweet are positively correlated. Vitamin B and fruity seem to be independent of artificial fruit and floral.

3.2.3 Sensory-instrumental correlation. Stepwise discriminant analysis (36) is a procedure where variables most effective at classifying samples are selected one by one according to the contribution that each variable makes to the resolution of sample differences. The first variable chosen is the one with the highest F value.

When stepwise discrimination analysis was applied to the DSP data for the whole panel it was possible to conclude that vitamin B, soapy, and woody were the main discriminator variables among the three varieties. The mean scores for soapy and woody were highest for U.S.D.A. 21455 and 21459 and the score for vitamin B was highest for Hallertauer (Table 4).

Because of software and people constraints, it was not possible for all the members of the DSP to evaluate the GC effluents; however three subjects took part in both the DSP and GCO. The scores assigned to each attribute by these three subjects in the DSP, and the scores assigned to the odor active peaks sniffed through the GC were taken into account in the correlation.

From the correlation maxtrix, vitamin B, the main discriminator among varieties, was positively correlated ($p \leq 0.001$) with peak A in Hallertauer, and was negatively correlated ($p \leq 0.05$) with the odor intensities of peaks 9, 10, 11, and 19 in the consensus osmegrams. It was not possible to identify peak A but it was described as having a tobacco or apple character. Peaks 9, 10, 11, and 19 were identified as caryophyllene and three humulene oxidation products, respectively. All of them were described as musty/floral/spicy. When stepwise regression was applied to these variables, only peak A was included in the equation (Table 5). That is because peak A was negatively correlated ($p \leq 0.05$) with peaks 9, 10, 11 and 19. These observations confirmed the results suspected from the GC effluent sniffing results: the lower amount of caryophyllene and humulene oxidation products, as well as the presence of a unique peak with a high intensity may have contributed to the vitamin B character of the Hallertauer oxygenated fraction.

Soapy was correlated with peaks 14 and 3 in the consensus osmegrams ($p \leq 0.05$ and 0.15, respectively). Peak 14 was a unique peak in U.S.D.A. 21455 but it had a very low intensity. Peak 3 was described as floral and it was not an extremely intense peak. GCO peak intensities are shown in Table 7 and explained under the Osme section. Even though the stepwise regression equation for soapy had a significant F value ($P \leq 0.05$) and a relatively high correlation coefficient (0.60), the Cp value, 102, was very

TABLE 5

Correlation equations between the sensory attributes from DSP and the odor active peaks by GCO

Attribute	Equation (SE)[a]	$C_{(p)}$	F value Model	Cumulative R-square Model	
Overall Intensity	6.08 + 0.34 P2 + (1.56) (0.20) 0.28 P4 - 0.11 P18 (0.23) (0.13) + 0.33 PE (0.18)	2.5	4.88[1]	P4	0.508
				P18	0.633
				PE	0.703
				P2	0.829
Soapy	2.45 + 0.60 P3 + (1.06) (0.22) 0.49 P14 (0.15)	102	10.04*	P14	0.487
				P3	0.769
Herbal	-4.94 + 0.36 P1 + (1.23) (0.17) 0.42 P4 + 0.99 P5 (0.17) (0.25)	16	21.59**	P1	0.645
				P5	0.835
				P4	0.928
Woody	-5.01 + 0.89 P2 (1.95) (0.27)	1.5	10.84*	P2	0.608
Grassy	2.72 - 0.26 P12 - (0.24) (0.05) 0.18 P16 (0.03)	4.8	39.85***	P2	0.729
				P12	0.879
				P16	0.949
				-P2	0.930
Citrus	2.92 + 0.43 P5 + (0.56) (0.13) 0.12 P8 (0.04)	2.0	17.67**	P5	0.632
				P8	0.855

TABLE 5 (cont.)

Attribute	Equation	$C_{(p)}$	F value Model	Cumulative R-square Model
Fruity	-2.29 + 0.56 P4 + (1.08) (0.30) 0.35 P7 (0.19)	6.0	10.50*	P7 0.651 P4 0.778
Artif. Fruity	-0.83 + 1.14 P3 - (3.20) (0.54) 0.55 P7 (0.23)	1.4	8.72*	P7 0.554 P3 0.744
Sweet	6.20 - 9.99 P3 (1.35) (1.25)	0.9	22.5*	P3 0.641
Floral	1.55 + 0.98 PE (0.39) (0.20)	1.0	23.33**	PE 0.769
Vitamin B	0.12 + 0.69 PA (0.39) (0.12)	1.4	36.33***	PA 0.834

*,**,*** significant at ($p \leq$ 0.05, 0.01, 0.001), respectively
1 significant at ($p \leq$ 0.15)
a Standard Error (SE) for the estimated regression coefficients

high when it should be around 3 (Table 5). This indicated that the equation was not well-modeled statistically.

Woody was related ($p \leq 0.05$) to linalool (peak 2), but the descriptors assigned to linalool were floral/fruity/citrus and not woody.

The last important discriminator for the data was floral. The equation obtained was statistically valid ($p \leq 0.01$), but it may not have any sensory significance because this character was associated with peak E, which was very small and unique to U.S.D.A.

21459 (Table 5).

The equation that associated fruity with peaks 7 and 4 in the consensus osmegrams may have sensory significance ($p \leq 0.05$). Peak 7 was described as having a tobacco or dried prune character. This peak may be damascenone which has a detection threshold of 0.009 ppb in water (37) and an average group detection threshold in beer of approximately 0.3 ppm (Lederer, unpublished data). Peak 7 had high intensities in all of the samples (Table 6) and was one of the most intense in Hallertauer: This variety had a high score for PC3 that was weighted mainly by fruity (Fig. 2), so it was possible that peak 7 was a good contributor to the fruity character of the sample. Peak 4 was described as rancid and it was not rated high in intensity, nor was it identified.

The attribute grassy was associated negatively with peaks 12 and 16 ($p \leq 0.01$). Peak 12 was identified as a humulene monoepoxide III and peak 16 was tentatively identified as a humulenol isomer and was absent in Hallertauer. In addition, Hallertauer had a high score in PC3 and PC3 was also weighted in grassy (Fig. 2).

Another interesting correlation is that of citrus with peaks 5 and 8 ($p \leq 0.05$) in the consensus osmegrams. Peak 5 was described as having a citrus, minty, and spicy character. This peak was associated with citral B. Peak 8 was not identified but GC panelists agreed that it was floral. From a correlation matrix among sensory attributes by the DSP, it was determined that citrus and herbal were positively correlated ($p \leq 0.001$). It was possible that peak 5 contributed to this correlation because it was a common peak.

The objective of the correlation analysis was to improve on the usual approach to GC-sensory correlation by using the odor intensity of the active peaks and not the FID areas. Correlation equations were in agreement with the PCA results obtained by the DSP. We concluded that by using this approach meaningful equations could be obtained (Table 5).

3.2.4 <u>Requirements and limitations of sensory-instrumental correlations</u>. Correlations were extrapolated to the whole sensory panel opinion because results from a t-test showed that the attribute mean scores over treatments, replications, and panelists did not differ significantly ($p \leq 0.05$) [except for citrus, where the three panelists scored higher than the rest of the panel ($p \leq 0.001$)].

Some of the pitfalls of the correlations established in this study can be stated: 1) To assess most of the correlations, a model system containing the compounds of interest must be prepared to study the behavior of these compounds in solution. It was not known if the relative odor importance of the compounds at the dilution that the whole sample was evaluated by the DSP was the same as that established during the sniffing of the chromatographic effluent or how these compounds interact with each other, 2) statistically it would have been better to correlate both sets of data using multivariate techniques (such as canonical correlation) because they take into account all the correlations among the parameters evaluated. However, the number of observations in this study was too small to apply these methodologies, and 3) sample profiles were very similar among the three samples causing a very low variability in both sets of data. Only one attribute could be considered a good discriminator. That was one of the reasons for which a p value ≤ 0.150 was established as a limit in order to enter or reject a variable in the correlation model.

For all the reasons stated, it is important to assume that the results can be orientative but they may not reflect cause and effect.

3.3 Mass spectrometric analysis

An FID chromatogram for U.S.D.A. 21455 with the identified peaks labeled is shown in Fig. 3. The names and concentrations of these compounds are listed in Table 6 (numbers in Fig. 3 are coincident with numbers in Table 6). Those in square brackets were only tentatively identified. Considering the chemical complexity of this fraction, the identification of compounds was done mainly in the regions where odors were detected. It is important to mention that no standards were available for the majority of the sesquiterpene alcohols and they seemed to be odor active in this study. No standards were available for the confirmation of 9-methyl-decan-2-one, humulol, humulenol II, methyl-4-decenoate, methyl-4,8-decadienoate, and farnesol H; but there was very good agreement in the results of the search in the three spectral libraries and data base programs used.

It should be mentioned that no sulphur compounds were detected in these samples, but some of the odors were described as having sulphury characteristics such as the one perceived at 32:80 min (2213) in U.S.D.A. 21455 (Table 7). It is suspected that these compounds were probably at a concentration not detected by the instrument.

To improve the identification of compounds, it will be necessary to enrich the trace constituents by preparative GC and to synthesize as many compounds as possible because there are few standards available through the chemical companies.

3.4 Osme

There were striking differences between the FID chromatograms and consensus osmegrams (Fig. 4). For the FID, 41 common peaks were identified in each variety; for the consensus osmegrams, panelists identified 19 peaks for U.S.D.A. 21455, 17 peaks for U.S.D.A. 21459, and 12 peaks for Hallertauer. The low number of peaks in Hallertauer was attributed to the fact that Hallertauer had the lowest HSI; therefore it had less oxidation products than the two triploids. This was especially reflected in the region

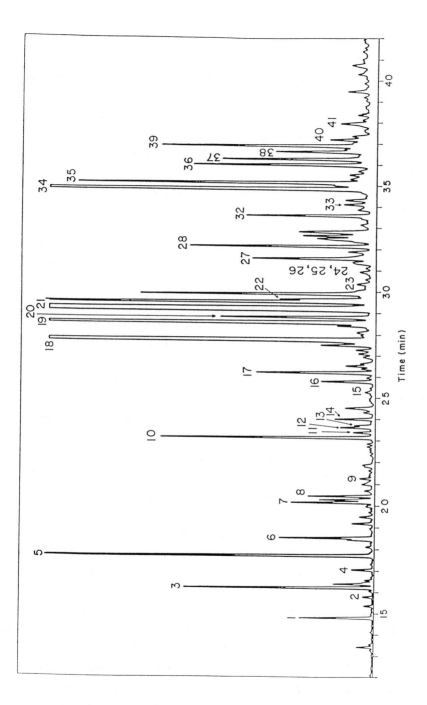

Fig. 3. FID chromatogram for U.S.D.A. 21455. Identity of each compound is listed in Table 5.

TABLE 6

Chemical Composition of the hop oil oxygenated fractions analyzed. 1 = U.S.D.A. 21455, 2 = HALLERTAUER, 3 = U.S.D.A. 21459

Compound (KI_{20M})		Concentration[1] (ppm in oil)		
		Var 1	Var 2	Var 3
1-	2-Decanone* (1518)	125.7	923.4	264.14
2-	9-Methyl Decan-2-One (1558)	44.5	61.9	8.1
3-	Linalool* (1562)	1869.9	1696.0	883.2
4-	N.I. (1588)	234.20	116.4	68.3
5-	2-Undecanone* (1611)	3738.5	5143.9	1967.3
6-	Methyl-4-Decenoate (1643)	991.2	1443.6	206.3
7-	Methyl-4,8-Decadienoate (1711)	874.2	1464.3	366.5
8-	2-Dodecanone* (1722)	692.1	797.5	494.0
9a-	Citral A (Geranial)*	156.0	80.9	60.1
9b-	Citral B (Neral)*	232.2	333.5	182.9
10-	2-Tridecanone* (1820)	2362.5	3675.1	1868.4
11-	Geranyl iso-butyrate* (1830)	194.3	59.61	62.80
12-	N.I.(similar to Geraniol) (1839)	351.0	498.3	453.0
13-	[Tridec-?-en-2-one] (1842)	178.0	114.5	136.0
14-	Geraniol* (1854)	410.6	274.8	325.8
15-	N.I. (Geraniol ester) (1888)	410.6	274.8	325.8
16-	[Sesquiterpene epoxide] (1926)	669.3	827.1	515.6
17-	Ketone (N.I.) (1942)	1582.7	730.1	1123.5
18-	Caryophyllene Oxide* (2004)	20355	2548.4	9348.9
19-	2-Pentadecanone* (2037)	8927.6	1549.7	4823.2
20-	Hum.monoepox. I* (2048)	1906.5	1325.4	1335.5
21-	Hum.monoepoxide II* (2075)	5466.3	1633.0	2818.2

TABLE 6 (cont.)

Compound (KI$_{20M}$)		Concentration[1] (ppm in oil)		
		Var 1	Var 2	Var 3
22-	Hum.monoepoxide III* (2083)	939.7	789.35	649.0
23-	[δ-Cadinol] (2103)	164.6	139.5	11.5
24-	[Epicubenol] (2112)	190.05	135.5	18.57
25-	[Hop Furanone Z] (2128)	109.8	57.1	145.8
26-	[Spathulenol] (2156)	2192.8	271.0	941.3
27-	Humulol (2161)	2192.8	2215.3	1805.4
28-	[τ-Cadinol] (2183)	2730.7	1809.3	1820.6
29-	[Sesquiterpene alcohol] (2198)	1765.5	526.5	858.3
30-	[α-Cadinol or τ-Muurolol] (2204)	1233.9	131.9	352.9
31-	[Torreyol] (2210)	1934.9	392.3	464.3
32-	[τ-Muurolol] (2244)	1595.5	1409.4	1480.8
33-	N.I. (2267)	432.0	437.7	2398.5
34-	Humulenol II (2298)	11072.3	4814.4	2157.5
35-	[Fused polyciclic alcohol] (2311)	4141.3	1941.8	1059.3
36-	[Humulenol Isomer] (2348)	2439.2	368.7	911.9
37-	Hum.diepoxide A* (2361)	1991.7	627.3	2697.6
38-	Hum.diepoxide B* (2377)	1185.7	563.7	1199.3
39-	Farnesol H (2387)	2790.4	530.7	1500.2
40-	[Sesquiterpene alcohol] (2401)	409.7	303.1	551.77
41-	N.I. (similar to Humulenol II) (2441)	1061	542.8	615.3

1- Concentration calculated using internal standard method.
(*) means that the identity was confirmed using standards.
2-Compounds in square brackets are those that were tentatively identified.
3-(N.I.) means that the compound was investigated but not identified.

392

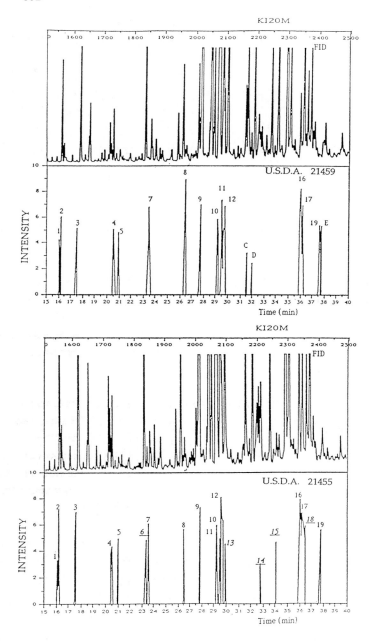

Figure 4 (continued next page)

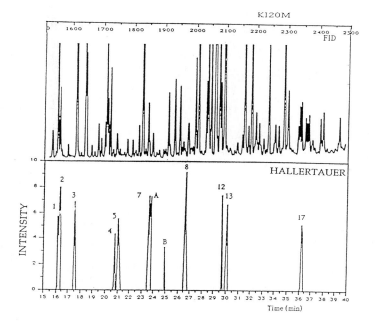

Fig. 4. Consensus osmegrams (bottom) and FID chromatograms (top) for U.S.D.A. 21459, U.S.D.A. 21455, and Hallertauer Mittelfrüh. Compounds identified in the osmegram can be found in Table 7.

where the humulene oxidation products should have occurred (between 32 and 39 min) (Fig. 4).

3.4.1 <u>Consensus peaks common to three varieties</u>. In Table 7, peaks are grouped into three categories: peaks common to all three varieties, peaks common to triploid crosses, and peaks unique to each variety. 21455 was the first variety to be evaluated; these peaks were numbered consecutively. Hallertauer and 21459 were given the same number for peaks common to 21455, but peaks unique to these varieties were labelled with letters A through E and the number 4a ("a" means uncertainty in the assignment of the peak). For Hallertauer, 4a was described using similar terms to peak 4 (Table 7), but the KI was slightly higher: peak 4a may be 4,4-dimethylfuran-2-one. Tressl (37) calls it 4-4 dimethyl-2-buten-4-olide. It is this compound which, along with its acyclic form (4-methylpent-3-enoic acid), is responsible for the cheesy-rancid odor of old hops. Nine peaks were present in all three varieties (1-8, 12, and 17) each exhibiting aroma intensities of over five on the intensity scale (Table 7). There were no significant differences ($p \leq 0.05$) among the intensities of these common peaks for the three

TABLE 7
Consensus odor active peaks detected during GC olfactometry evaluation of the three hop varieties.

Peak #	RT (min) (KI_{20M})	Most Frequent Descriptor	HALLERTAUER Odor Int.[2] (SD)[4]	% Total Area[3]	21459 Odor Int. (SD)	% Total Area	21455 Odor Int. (SD)	% Total Area	Identified Compound (KI_{20M})
			PEAKS COMMON TO ALL THREE VARIETIES						
1	16:09 (1559)	Musty-Rancid	5.7 (1.00)	3.8	4.2 (1.91)	1.6	3.3 (1.33)	2.5	
2	16:23 (1563)	Floral/Fruity/Citrus	7.9 (0.72)	13.1	6.0 (1.33)	3.1	7.1 (2.44)	4.7	Linalool (1562)
3	17:51 (1602)	Floral	6.8 (3.90)	7.6	5.1 (2.01)	3.3	6.9 (1.72)	5.0	
4	20:60 (1729)	Rancid-Cheese	4.3 (2.04)	4.0	5.0 (1.71)	5.5	4.3 (0.93)	5.2	
5	21:00 (1751)	Minty-Anise Citrus-Spicy	5.5 (0.83)	8.9	4.8 (1.31)	3.3	4.9 (1.62)	2.9	Citral B (1751)
7	23:53 (1838)	Prunes-Apple Tobacco	7.3 (2.51)	8.0	6.7 (4.12)	10.2	6.1 (0.84)	5.1	
8	26:57 (1958)	Floral	9.1 (3.33)	14.4	8.9 (3.30)	10.1	5.6 (2.41)	4.4	
12	29:67 (2083)	Musty/Floral/Spicy	7.3 (0.78)	5.1	6.8 (3.01)	10.3	8.1 (2.22)	8.3	Humulene Monoepox. III (2083)
17	36:20 (2360)	Musty/Floral/Spicy	5.1 (2.62)	8.8	6.9 (1.54)	11.8	6.9 (3.92)	5.6	
			PEAKS COMMON TO TWO VARIETIES						
13	30:00 (2095)	Vinyl-Floral	6.7 (1.53)	9.5	----	----	4.5 (1.71)	3.3	
9	27:79 (2006)	Musty/Floral/Spicy	----	----	7.0 (1.92)	7.1	7.3 (0.54)	4.9	Caryophyllene Oxide (2004)
10	29:21 (2065)	Musty/Floral/Spicy	----	----	5.8 (2.32)	7.0	5.9 (1.54)	5.2	Humulene Monoepox. I (2048)
11	29:46 (2075)	Musty/Floral/Spicy	----	----	7.2 (4.70)	8.1	4.9 (0.73)	3.1	Humulene Monoepox. II (2075)
16	36:03 (2352)	Musty/Floral/Cloves	----	----	8.2 (2.63)	7.3	7.9 (2.32)	10.2	
19	37:69 (2427)	Floral	----	----	5.3 (1.61)	5.9	5.7 (1.83)	6.0	
			PEAKS UNIQUE TO EACH VARIETY						
4a	20:75 (1734)	Rancid-Putrid Cheesy	4.3 (2.04)	4.0	----	----	----	----	
A	23:77 (1847)	Tobacco-Floral Prunes	7.2 (1.20)	13.2	----	----	----	----	
B	24:95 (1893)	Rancid Floral	3.3 (0.94)	3.5	----	----	----	----	
C	31:55 (2161)	Fresh Veg. Soapy	----	----	3.2 (2.01)	1.8	----	----	
D	31:98 (2179)	Egg Yolk	----	----	2.4 (1.30)	0.8	----	----	
E	37:74 (2433)	Musty/Floral/Spicy	----	----	5.3 (2.44)	1.7	----	----	
6	23:33 (1832)	Rancid-Violets	----	----	----	----	4.8 (1.51)	3.8	
14	32:80 (2213)	Rancid-Sulfur Putrid	----	----	----	----	3.0 (0.72)	1.2	
15	34:06 (2267)	Floral-Roses Citrus	----	----	----	----	4.6 (1.33)	1.6	
18	36:48 (2372)	Musty/Floral/Spicy	----	----	----	----	5.8 (2.44)	16.0	

[1] Compounds identified by MS and odor were confirmed by using standards.
[2] Intensities were rated using a 16 point intensity scale (0=none, 15=extreme) and averaged over subjects.
[3] Area percent calculated with the Osme data collection software.
[4] SD = Standard deviation

varieties. Peak 1, identified as 9-methyl-decan-2-one, has been reported as a hop oil component by Tressl et al. (3) and Meilgaard and Peppard (38). From our study, we suspected this compound had a very low threshold because it could be detected when the amount present was at least 100 times smaller than linalool (assuming equal FID sensitivity for each compound). No threshold data or descriptors were found in the literature for this compound, but GC panelists described it as being rancid-musty.

Peak 2, linalool, was present in high concentrations in all three samples; it has been reported to have a very low taste and olfactory threshold (39-41). For that reason it was considered a good aroma contributor to the samples. Linalool is considered one of the major compounds responsible for the floral character of beer.

Peaks 3 and 4 could be associated by GC/MS with 2-undecanone and 2-dodecanone, respectively. When a mixture of the two ketones was injected and the effluent sniffed, odor was not detected for 2-undecanone even at a concentration 1.5 times higher than that of the sample. It is reasonable to conclude that peak 3 was associated with a compound other than 2-undecanone. The compound 2-dodecanone was described as having a vinyl, fresh vegetative, and citrus character when sniffed at a very high concentration and not rancid or cheesy as detected in the sample. The reported taste threshold for 2-dodecanone is half that of the 2-undecanone (39). Because it was found in the samples in very low concentrations and the odor characteristic was different, 2-dodecanone was not the compound responsible for the odor detected for peak 4.

Peak 5 was possibly associated by GC-MS with citral B (neral). When citral was sniffed through the GC at the same concentration as in the sample, citral B was described as having a citrus character and a very low odor intensity. Because of the odor characteristic and the coincident KI_{20M} calculated for the standard, citral B is assumed to be the compound responsible for the odor detected in that region. Meilgaard (39) reported a taste threshold of 0.15 ppm for the mixture of citral isomers and described it as lemon. Peak 7 was described as having prune-apple and tobacco character; as stated earlier, damascenone may be responsible for this peak's aromas. Peak 8 had a high intensity in all the samples but it could not be identified. Peaks 12 and 17 are discussed in the humulene oxidation products section.

3.4.2 <u>Consensus peaks common to two varieties</u>. Peak 13 was common to Hallertauer and U.S.D.A. 21455; it was described as having vinyl and floral character (Table 7). It could be associated with δ-cadinol which was tentatively identified. This compound was previously reported by Tressl et al. (3), but no sensory reports were found in the literature. There was no significant difference between the intensities of this peak in the two varieties ($p \leq 0.05$). Varieties U.S.D.A. 21455 and 21459 shared five peaks (9-11, 16, and 19); all of them had intensities higher than 5 (Table 7).

Peaks 9, 10, 11, and 16 had musty/floral/spicy character and 19 was described as being floral. Peak intensities were not significantly different ($P \leq 0.05$) between either essential oil. Most of these peaks were associated with humulene and caryophyllene oxidation products that were absent or at lower concentration in Hallertauer.

3.4.3 <u>Consensus peaks unique to each variety</u>. Each variety presented a few unique odor active peaks. U.S.D.A. 21455 had four unique peaks (6, 14, 15, and 18), most of them had low odor intensity. Peak 6 was described as having rancid-violet character, peak 14 as having rancid-sulfur notes, peak 15 as having floral-rose and citrus aromas, and 18 as being musty/floral/spicy. Peak 6 was suspected to be 2-tridecanone or geranyl iso-butyrate. When these two compounds were sniffed at the same concentration as in the sample, 2-tridecanone was described as being floral/vinyl/citrus for some of the subjects. Based on the descriptors assigned to the standard and KI_{20M} proximity, 2-tridecanone was detected only by two subjects and therefore it was not a consensus peak. No odor was detected by any of the subjects for geranyl iso-butyrate, even at concentrations three times higher than in the sample. The taste threshold reported for geranyl iso-butyrate was reported to be 450 ppb in beer (16 times higher than linalool) by Peacock et al. (41). The amount of this compound in these samples was not enough to make a significant contribution to the aroma. For these reasons the odor detected was due to a compound not identified here.

Peak 14 could be associated by GC-MS with α-cadinol or torreyol; α-cadinol was reported in hop oil by Tressl et al. (3). Neither of these compounds were confirmed because there were no standards available for reference.

U.S.D.A. 21459 had three unique peaks (C, D, E), all of them with odor intensities lower than or equal to 5 (Table 7). No standards were available to confirm these compounds or to assess their odor characteristics. Peak C could possibly be associated with spathulenol or humulol. GC panelists described it as having fresh vegetable and soapy character. This compound had been described by Fukuoka and Kowaka (42) as having a hay-like odor. The taste threshold reported in beer is greater than 2 ppm (43).

Peak E of U.S.D.A. 21459 could be associated with some of the humulenol isomers and was described as having musty/floral/spicy character. Peacock et al. (9) speculated that humulenol II could be a hop flavor contributor and determined the threshold to be 500 ppb, but the compound used was a mixture of humulenol I and II so the odor and the threshold of each isomer is not known. Peacock and Deinzer (10) later reported a taste threshold of 2500 ppb for humulenol II in beer.

Hallertauer had three unique peaks: 4a, A, and B (Table 7). Peak 4a had a KI_{20M} (1734) higher than in the other varieties ($KI_{20M}=1729$) but the rancid-cheese descriptor assigned was the same. The variability could be due to a different duration of the odor in this sample, or it could be a different compound. Peak A was a unique peak with an odor intensity higher than 5; it was described as tobacco, floral, or prunes. Because of the similarities in KI_{20M}, it could be associated by GC-MS with tridec-?-en-2-one or with geraniol. No standard was available for tridec-?-en-2-one and geraniol was not considered a consensus peak because it was detected by only two subjects.

Because of the similarities in descriptors, it was possible that in Hallertauer the compound responsible for peak 7 was in higher concentration than in the other samples causing a continuous odor in this region. It was also possible that some other geraniol derivative in that region is responsible for the odor.

3.4.4 <u>Caryophyllene and humulene oxides</u>. Oxidation products of humulene, one of the major sesquiterpene hydrocarbons in hop oil, have been the focus of much attention in recent years as a possible source of the traditional noble hop aroma. That assumption was made indirectly without sensory confirmation; hops with higher concentrations of humulene oxidation products are those considered as noble hops by the beer industry. The relative contributions of these compounds to the aroma of the hop oil and finished beer is still questioned (37, 42, 43, 9, 10, 41, 44). These products are formed by oxidation of humulene during hop storage and fermentation of beer (44). It is noted that the noble hop aroma found in beer may be caused, not by these compounds directly, but by transformation products formed during fermentation.

A mixture of the three monoepoxides, composed mainly of monoepoxide II (70%), was sniffed by the panelists at concentrations similar to those found in the sample; all the subjects detected three peaks of moderate intensity and described them as musty/floral/spicy. Because the descriptors assigned to these peaks in the sample were the same as those in the standards, and the KI_{20M} were also the same, peaks 10, 11, and 12 (Table 7) were assumed to be due to humulene monoepoxide I, II, and III, respectively. Monoepoxide III probably had a much lower threshold than monoepoxide I because it was possible to detect it at concentrations less than half that of humulene monoepoxide I. Taste thresholds in beer for a mixture of monoepoxides were reported by Peacock and Deinzer (10) and Irwin (43). No data exist in the literature regarding the threshold of the humulene epoxides individually. It is important to determine if these compounds are major aroma contributors when they are in solution such as that evaluated by the DSP. Yet another aspect will be to investigate if these compounds survive the brewing process and therefore may be responsible for the noble aroma in beer. Peak 9 (Table 7) was associated with caryophyllene oxide. When the purified compound was sniffed through the GC, it was described as having a spicy/floral character similar to that of the humulene epoxides for the majority of the subjects. Because peak 9 was described with the same terms, was present in high concentration, and was similar in KI_{20M} values, caryophyllene oxide was assumed to be responsible for the odor detected in that region. No threshold information was found in the literature for caryophyllene oxide. Some authors report that this compound probably does not survive the brewing process because it has not been found in beer (9, 11).

Peak 18, as well as 17 (Table 7), may be associated with humulene diepoxides. The descriptors musty/floral/spicy assigned to the odors in this region were similar to those assigned to the humulene monoepoxides. This fact was also stated by Lam and Deinzer (45), but they could not assign a particular odor to each of the isomers because they could not isolate the diepoxides from the mixture. It has been reported that there are 12 possible isomers, depending on the location and relative configuration between the two epoxide rings (45, 44). These compounds were reported as being related to beer brewed with noble aroma varieties but no sensory information was available.

When panelists sniffed a mixture of diepoxide A and B, no odor was detected, even at concentrations 25 times higher than that found in the sample. Keeping in mind that different enantiomeric forms and isomers can have different odors (46), it is possible that the odor perceived in this region was due to one of those 12 isomers mentioned above and not due to diepoxide A or B.

3.4.5 Non-consensus peaks. Those odor active peaks that were detected at most by only two of the subjects were considered in this study as non-consensus peaks.

Non-consensus peaks arise because of individual differences among panelists. Odor thresholds for one subject vary from time to time, and the same odor sensation is described differently among people (47-49). Panelist fatigue, cultural factors, and specific anosmia are other factors contributing to individual differences (50). Individual differences exist and are the reason for using more than one panelist in a sensory evaluation. Day to day variability also exists and supports the need for replication of the experiment.

The compounds, 2-decanone, 2-tridecanone, 2-pentadecanone, and geraniol were confirmed using standards. The compound 2-decanone was detected by subjects 3 and 4 only in Hallertauer where it was present in higher concentration. The standard was described as having a floral and rancid character.

The compounds 2-tridecanone and 2-pentadecanone were described as having a vinyl, fresh vegetative, and citrus character when sniffed by the same subjects that evaluated the samples. Because of the descriptors assigned it seems that 2-tridecanone was detected by only subjects 1 and 3. For that reason 2-tridecanone was not the compound responsible for peak 6. It is believed that 2-pentadecanone was detected only by subjects 1 and 3 because they assigned the same descriptor to this peak as they did to the standard.

Geraniol was described by some of the subjects as having a floral/citrus character when it was sniffed at the same concentration as in the sample. Based on KI_{20M} proximity and odor descriptor, geraniol was detected only by subjects 1 and 4, or by subjects 1 and 2 (30).

There were some compounds such as methyl-4-decenoate (KI_{20M} = 1643) or methyl-4,8-decadienoate (KI_{20M} = 1711) for which no standards were available to confirm their odor descriptors. Both esters seemed to be in higher concentrations in Hallertauer. Esters constitute the largest single group of oxygenated hop oil components and are considered by some researchers to be the most important because of their low threshold (40, 8, 38). These compounds weren't consensus peaks because of their low concentration, or because the subjects that performed the evaluation weren't sensitive to these particular compounds.

Other compounds included a non-identified sesquiterpene epoxide (KI_{20M} = 1926), and epicubenol (KI_{20M} = 2112).

4. CONCLUSION

The two triploid Hallertau crosses are good potential noble aroma contributors to beer because their aroma profiles were very similar to that of the German Hallertauer. This conclusion was reached based upon results from the DSP and sniffing of the GC effluents.

Subtle differences found in aroma quality could be attributed to the higher oxidative stage of the triploid crosses. There were higher amounts of caryophyllene and humulene oxidation products in the crosses than in Hallertauer. Because these products were shown to be odor active, it was possible that they made an important contribution to the overall aroma profile of these samples and caused the differences found.

The methodology used in this research, once optimized, will provide good chemical and sensory descriptions of the samples, and yield better tools to correlate sensory with chemical properties.

ACKNOWLEDGMENTS

We would like to thank Morten Meilgaard, Val Peacock, and Terry Acree for their thoughtful reviews of the sensory and chemistry sections of this manuscript. Special thanks to Cheryl Houk for her 'always cheerful' technical assistance in typing, editing, and proofing of this paper, and to Don Griffin from Oregon State University, Ag. Chemistry Dept. for GC/MS analyses.

REFERENCES

1. Buttery, R.G., McFadden, W.H., Lundin, R.E. and Kealy, M.P. Volatile hop constituents: conventional and capillary gas chromatographic separation with characterization by physical methods. *J. Inst. Brew.* 70:396-401, 1964.
2. Buttery, R.G., Black, D.R., Guadagni, D.G., and Kealy, M.P. A study of the volatile oxygenated constituents in different hop varieties. *Proc. Am. Soc. Brew. Chem.* 103-111, 1965.
3. Tressl, R., Friese, L., Fendesack, F., and Koppler, H. Studies of the volatile composition of hops during storage. *J. Agr. Food Chem.* 26(6):1426-1430, 1978.
4. Tressl, R., Engel K.H., and Köppler, H. Characterization of tricyclic sesquiterpenes in hop (*Humulus lupulus*, var. Hersbrucker Spät) *J. Agric. Food Chem.* 31(4):893-894, 1983.
5. Buttery, R.G., and Ling, L.C. Identification of hop varieties by gas chromatographic analysis of their essential oils. *J. Agr. Food Chem.* 15(3):531-535, 1967.
6. Likens, S.T., and Nickerson, G.B. Identification of the varietal origin of hop extracts. *Proc. Am. Soc. Brew. Chem.* pp. 23-29, 1965.
7. Likens, S.T., and Nickerson, G.B. Identification of hop varieties by gas chromatographic analysis of their essential oils. *J. Agr. Food Chem.* 15(3):525-530, 1967.
8. Nickerson, G.B., and Likens, S.T. Gas chromatographic evidence for the occurrence of hop oil components in beer. *J. Chromatogr.* 21:1-5, 1966.
9. Peacock, V.E., Deinzer, M.L., McGill, L.A., and Wrolstad, R.E. Hop aroma in American beer. *J. Agr. Food Chem.* 28(4):774-777, 1980.
10. Peacock, V.E., and Deinzer, M.L. Chemistry of hop aroma in beer. *J. Am. Soc. Brew. Chem.* 39:136-141, 1981.
11. Peppard, T.L., Ramus, S.A., Siebert, K.J., and Witt, C.A. Correlation of sensory instrumental data in elucidating the effect of varietal differences in hop flavor in beers. *J. Am. Soc. Brew. Chem.* 47:18-22, 1989.
12. Acree, T.E., Barnard, J., and Cunningham, D.G. A procedure for the sensory analysis of gas chromatographic effluents. *Food Chemistry* 14:273, 1984.
13. Ulrich, F. and Grosch, W. Identification of the most intense volatile flavour compounds formed during autooxidation of linoleic acid. *Z. Lebensm. Unters. Forsch.* 184:277-282, 1987.
14. Acree, T.E., and McLellan, M.R. Flavor components and quality attributes. *Processed Apple Products*. Downing, Donald L., Ed. Van Nostrand Reinhold Publisher, p. 314, 1989.
15. Nelson R.R., Acree, T.E., and Butts, R.M. Isolation and identification of volatiles from Catawba wines. *J. Agric. Food Chem.* 26(5):1188, 1978.
16. Nelson, R.R., and Acree, T.E. Concord wine composition as affected by maturity and processing technique. *Am. J. Enol. Vitic.* 27(2):83, 1978.
17. Acree, T.E., and Cottreli, T.H.E. Chemical indices of wine quality. *Alcoholic Beverages*. Birch, G.G., and Lindley, M.G., Eds. Elsevier Applied Science Publishers, p. 145, 1985.
18. Braell, P.A. Chracterization of the flavor of *Vitis labrusca* using charm and SIS. Cornell: Cornell Univer.; 1986. Dissertation.
19. Yong, L.F.M., Acree, T.E., Lavin, E.H., and Butts, R.M. Aroma chemistry of crackers. In *Thermal Generation of Aromas*. Am. Chem. Soc. p. 276, 1989.
20. Marin, A.B., Acree, T.E., and Barnard, J. Variation in odor detection thresholds determined by charm analysis. *Chemical Senses* 13(3):435, 1988.
21. Schieberle, P., and Grosch, W. Bestimmung des Aromas der Krusten von Weiß- und Roggenbrot durch eine Verdunnungsanalyse der Aromaextrakte. *Z. Lebensm Unters Forsch.* 185:111, 1987.
22. Schieberle, P., and Grosch, W. Identification of potent flavor compounds formed in aqueous lemon oil/citric acid emulsion. *J. Agric. Food Chem.* 36:797, 1988.

23. McDaniel, M.R., Miranda-Lopez, R., Watson, B.T., Micheals, N.J., and Libbey, L.M. Pinot noir aroma: a sensory/gas chromatographic approach, flavor and off-flavors. *Proceedings of the 6th International Flavor Conference, Rethymnon, Crete, Greece, July 5-7.* Charalambous, G., Ed., p. 23, 1989.
24. Haunold, A., and Nickerson, G.B. Development of a hop with European aroma characteristics. *J. Am. Soc. Brew. Chem.* 45:146-150, 1987.
25. American Society of Brewing Chemists. *Methods of Analysis*, 7th. ed. HOPS-6A. The Society: St. Paul, MN., 1976.
26. Verzele, M., Van Dyck, J., and Claus, H. On the analysis of hop bitter acid. *J. Inst. Brew.* 86:9-14, 1980.
27. Nickerson, G.B., and Likens, S.T. Hop storage index. *J. Am. Soc. Brew. Chem.* 37:184-187, 1979.
28. Acree, T.E., Butts, R.M., Nelson, R.R., and Lee, C.Y. Sniffer to determine the odor of gas chromatographic effluents. *Anal. Chem.* 48:1821-1822, 1976.
29. Libbey, L.M. A paradox database for GC/MS data on components of essential oils and other volatiles. *J. Ess. Oil. Res.*, 3, May-June 1991.
30. Sanchez, N.B. Analytical and sensory evaluation of hop varieties. Corvallis: Oregon State Univ.; 1990. Thesis.
31. Johnson, R.A., and Wichern, D.W. *Applied Multivariate Statistical Analysis.* Second edition. Prentice Hall, Englewood Cliffs, New Jersey. pp. 340-377, 1988.
32. Neter, J., Wasserman, W., and Kutner, M.H. *Applied Linear Regression Models.* R.D. Irwing, Inc. Homewood, Illinois. pp. 426-428, 1983.
33. Rigby, F.L. A theory on the hop flavor of beer. *Proc. Am. Soc. Brew. Chem.* p.46-50, 1972.
34. Meilgaard, M. Hop analysis, cohumulone factor and the bitterness of beer: review and critical evaluation. *J. Inst. Brew.* 66:35-50, 1960.
35. Foster, R.T., and Nickerson, G.B. Changes in hop oil content and hoppiness potential (Sigma) during hop aging. *J. Am. Soc. Brew. Chem.* 43:127-135, 1985.
36. Afifi, A.A., and Azen, S.P. *Multivariate Statistical Analysis.* Academic Press, Inc., New York, Ch. 7, 1979.
37. Tressl, R., Friese, L., Fendesack, F., and Köppler, H. Gas chromatographic-mass spectromic investigation of hop aroma constitutents in beer. *J. Agr. Food Chem.* 26(6) 1422-1425, 1978.
38. Meilgaard, M.C., and Peppard, T.L. The flavour of beer. In *Food Flavors. Part B. The Flavor of Beverages. Developments in Food Science 3B.* Morton, I.D. and Macleod, A.J., Eds. Elsevier, New York, pp. 99-169, 1986.
39. Meilgaard, M. C. Flavor chemistry of beer: Part II: flavor and threshold of 239 aroma volatiles. *Tech. Q. Master Brew. Assoc. Am.* 12:151-168, 1975.
40. Guadagni, D.G., Buttery, R.G., and Harris, J. Odour intensities of hop oil components. *J. Sci. Fd. Agric.* 17:142-144, 1966.
41. Peacock, V.E., Deinzer M.L., Likens, S., Nickerson, G.B., and McGill, L.A. Floral hop aroma in beer. *J. Agr. Food Chem.* 29(6):1265-1269, 1981B.
42. Fukuoka, Y., and Kowaka M. Identification of compounds imparting hoppy flavor to beer. *Rep. Res. Lab. Kirin. Brewery Co.* 26:31-36, 1983.
43. Irwin, A.J. Varietal dependence of hop flavour volatiles in lager. *J. Inst. Brew.* 95:185-194, 1989.
44. Peacock, V.E., and Deinzer, M. The structures of humulene diepoxides found in hops and beer. *J. Am. Soc. Brew. Chem.* 47:4-7, 1989.
45. Lam, K.C., and Deinzer, M.L. Tentative identification of humulene diepoxides by capillary gas chromatography/chemical ionization mass spectrometry. *J. Agric. Food Chem.* 35(1):57-59, 1987.
46. Pickenhagen, W. Enantioselectivity in odor perception. In *Flavor Chemistry. Trends and Developments.* Am. Chem. Soc., Washington, DC. Ch. 12, 1989.
47. Keverne, E.B. Chemical senses: smell. In *The Senses.* Barlow, H.B., and Mollon, J.D., Eds. Cambridge University Press. p. 409, 1982.

48. Amerine, M.A., and Roessler, E.B. *Wines - Their Sensory Evaluation*. W.H. Freeman and Company, 1983.
49. Stevens, J.C., Cain, W.S., and Burke, R.J. Variability of olfactory thresholds. *Chemical Senses* 13(4):643, 1988.
50. Lawless, H.T. Exploration of fragrance categories and ambiguous odors using multidimensional scaling and cluster analysis. *Chemical Senses* 14(3):349, 1989.

SENSORY AND ANALYTICAL EVALUATION OF BEERS BREWED WITH THREE VARIETIES OF HOPS AND AN UNHOPPED BEER

Nora B. Sanchez[1], Cindy L. Lederer, Gail B. Nickerson[2], Leonard M. Libbey, Mina R. McDaniel[3]

Sensory Science Laborabory, Dept. of Food Science and Technology, Wiegand Hall, Oregon State University, Corvallis, OR 97331-6602

[1]CIATI - Bartolome Mitre y 20 de Junio (8336), Villa Regina-Rio Negro, Argentina Fax: 941-25377

[2]Agricultural Chemistry Department, Oregon State University 97331-6502

[3]Author to whom correspondence should be sent.

SUMMARY

Pilot brews made with Hallertauer Mittelfrüh, U.S.D.A. 21459, U.S.D.A. 21455 (Mt. Hood), and a beer brewed without hops were evaluated for aroma by a descriptive sensory panel (DSP). The extracts from the beers were evaluated using Osme, a GC olfactometry method: The beer extract samples were injected into the gas chromatograph-olfactometer (GCO) and the effluents evaluated qualitatively and quantitatively by four trained subjects. A time-intensity device connected to an IBM computer was used to record the odor intensities. The samples were analyzed by mass spectrometry to identify the odor active compounds. Sensory profiles of the hopped beers were similar indicating that beers brewed with U.S.D.A. 21455 and U.S.D.A. 21459 contribute "noble" hop aroma.

1. INTRODUCTION

Hops are used in beer to produce a characteristic bitter taste and distinctive hoppy aroma. Although they contribute a great deal to the overall flavor of beer, their contributions to beer aroma are still not well understood. The kettle hop aroma is quite different from the aroma of hops themselves. Hydrocarbons and oxygenated compounds contribute to the aroma of hops. Hop derived compounds remaining after evaporation, particularly the oxygenated components, are suspected to contribute to kettle hop aroma in beer (1-4). Hop aromas in beer vary depending on the hop variety used and by the method of hopping (5-14).

It is not well known which hop components contribute the most to the kettle hop aroma. A major problem is that to implicate a compound as flavor active, it is necessary to know its flavor threshold and measure how much compound is present. To do this, it is necessary to *have* some of the compound. Very few of these compounds are commercially available; they need to be synthesized which is very difficult and time consuming.

An alternative approach is to determine the odor active compounds or regions by sniffing the chromatographic effluents and then correlate these sensory results with the instrumental data (15,16).

In a previous study, Sanchez, et al. (17) found that the chemical and sensory properties of hop oils extracted from U.S.D.A. 21459, U.S.D.A. 21455, and Hallertauer Mittelfrüh hops were very similar indicating that the U.S.D.A. varieties were potentially good substitutes for Hallertauer. The next step is to compare the aroma profiles of beers brewed with these hops.

The objectives of this study were as follows:

1- To characterize, by descriptive sensory analysis, the aroma of beers brewed with U.S.D.A. 21455, U.S.D.A. 21459, Hallertauer Mittelfrüh, and a control brewed without hops.

2- To use the Osme method (17) to identify the most important odor active compounds or regions of the chromatograms corresponding to aroma extracts of these beers.

3- To identify by mass spectrometric analysis (MS) the most important odor active compounds.

2. MATERIALS AND METHODS

2.1 Preparation of pilot scale brews

In researching how different varieties of hops affect beer aroma or flavor, many authors prepared their beers by adding enough hops to produce the same BU (Bitter Units) to each one. They did not take into account that each hop has different amounts of essential oil and that within each oil the amount of oxygenated and hydrocarbon fraction is different. It is widely reported that the oxygenated fraction (3,4) is responsible for the hop aroma character in beer because these compounds have very low thresholds and they are present in considerable amounts.

Previous hop oil analyses showed that the proportion of oxygenated fraction in U.S.D.A. 21455 and 21459 was approximately three times larger than in Hallertauer (17). Based on this, beers were brewed by adding hop amounts which would provide the same amount of oxygenated fraction to each beer. The purpose of this addition was to get similar hop character intensity to compare the sensory attributes of beers brewed with U.S.D.A. 21455, U.S.D.A. 21459, and Hallertauer. Thus, beers were brewed at a commercial pilot plant (The Stroh Brewery Company, Detroit, MI) using the following amount of hops added in 40 liters of wort:

> Hallertauer..............800 g pellets
> U.S.D.A. 21455........284 g pellets
> U.S.D.A. 21459........657 g pellets

The hops were the same ones used in Sanchez, et al. (17).

Pellets were broken up before the addition to the kettle. To obtain the maximum amount of volatiles, pellets were added during the last 15 min. of the boil. A control was brewed in the same conditions as the hopped beers but no hops were added. Beers were kept at 1°C for one month until their evaluation.

2.2 Extraction of aromatic compounds

Aromatic compounds were extracted according to the methodology developed by Likens and Nickerson (2) (Fig. 1). The pentane used for extraction had been purified by stirring with concentrated H_2SO_4 for two days, washed with water, washed twice with 5% of $NaHCO_3$, washed again with water and finally redistilled and stored over Na_2SO_4.

2.3 Descriptive sensory panel (DSP)

2.3.1 Sample preparation. Two 355 ml bottles of beer were gently poured into a 2 L beaker to make a homogeneous sample. Sixty ml of each beer were poured into 355 ml amber glasses, labeled with three digit random numbers, and covered with aluminum lids and Parafilm (American National Can, Greenwich, CT).

2.3.2 Training procedure. A panel of nine subjects evaluated the beers. They were all volunteer students or faculty of Oregon State University who were highly experienced in beer evaluations.

Panelists were trained over a two week period to evaluate aroma intensity using a sixteen point intensity scale (0=none, 3=slight, 7=moderate, 11=large, and 15=extreme). For each sample, panelists scored aroma attributes by matching or extrapolating between overall intensity of intensity standards.

To describe the samples qualitatively, panelists developed their own terms. After a panel consensus, eight attributes were selected to be evaluated: Overall intensity, fruity, citrus, floral, spicy, sweet, malty, and ethanol. Reference standards were provided in each session (Table 1).

2.3.3 Experimental design and sample presentation. A completely randomized balanced block design was used with three replications. In each session all four beers were evaluated. To minimize the bias for order presentation, samples were randomized for each panelist within and across each replication. Panelists were seated in individual booths and instructed to evaluate the samples from left to right. Samples were evaluated at 21°C under red light.

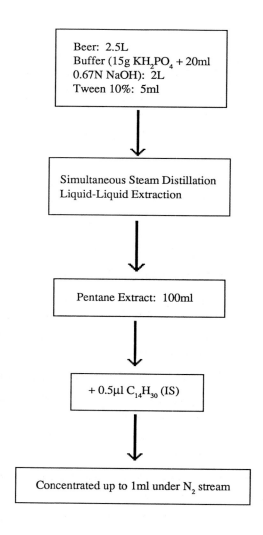

Fig. 1. Beer aroma extraction procedure.

TABLE 1.

Definitions of the attribute reference standards[1] used by the DSP during the evaluation of beers brewed with different varieties of hops and an unhopped beer.

Attribute	Reference Definition and Preparation
Overall Aroma	Total impact of all aromas.
	<u>Aroma of a reference prepared by:</u>
Fruity	Canned, one-half Bartlett pear (Del Monte Co., San Francisco, CA), diced in 1 cm cubes.
	One-quarter fresh Jonathan apple diced in 1 cm cubes.
	One-quarter fresh banana diced in 1 cm slices.
	Fresh pineapple diced in 1 cm cubes.
Citrus	Combining two half wedges of orange, grapefruit, and lemon (Sunkist Growers, Inc., Los Angeles, CA).
Floral	Imbibing an aroma paper stick in carnation or rose essence (Uncommon Scents, Eugene, OR).
	Two-three grams of dried lavender or pink roses.
Spicy	Two grams of nutmeg (Schilling, McCormick and Co., Inc., San Francisco, CA).
	Imbibing an aroma paper stick[2] in Eugenol (Aldrich, 99%, Milwaukee, WI).
	One cinnamon Stick (Spice Islands, Speciality Brands, San Francisco, CA).
Sweet	Six coffee beans (Millstone Coffee, Everett, WA).
	Ten ml of honey (Sue Bee, Grade A White, Pure Clover Honey, Sioux Honey Assn., Sioux City, IA).
	Two sliced Sathers Butterscotch Buttons (Sathers, Roundlake, Mn).
Malty	One hundred grams of Grapenuts (General Foods Corporation, White Plains, NY) wetted with spring water.
Ethanol	Ten ml 95% ethanol (Clear Spring, KY) in 50 ml of spring water

1- All the reference standards were evaluated in 350 ml amber glasses, covered with an aluminum foil lid and served at room temperature.
2- Fragance Test Filters (Orlandi, Inc., Farmingdale, NY).

Two trays were presented to the panelists, one at a time. In each tray there were two beer samples and a duplicate of each sample. These duplicates were used as warm up samples to allow panelists to practice their evaluation: During training sessions it was determined that some of the volatiles in the headspace disappeared once the lid was removed. The warm-up samples allowed panelists more time to evaluate the rapidly dissipating volatiles. Panelists took a 5 min break between trays.

2.3.4 Statistical analysis. Before analysis of the treatment data, panelists were first individually evaluated for consistency in their responses. Two panelists were removed because their observations resulted in high standard deviations in almost all of the attributes tested.

An individual analysis of variance (ANOVA) for each attribute was conducted using PC.SAS (SAS Institute, Inc., Cary, N.C.). Because each panelist replicated three times, the replications could be used to construct a three-way ANOVA (factors = panelists, replications, and treatments). Panelists and replications were treated as random sources of variation. The F tests were conducted as mentioned in Sanchez et al (17). When the interaction panelist by treatment was significant, mean scores for each panelist were graphed against treatments to determine which panelist was responsible for the interaction and to validate the significance of the treatment effect.

To visualize in space the differences among the samples and the intercorrelation among attributes, samples were analyzed using principal component analysis (PCA) (18).

2.4 Gas chromatographic analysis

The GC used was a Hewlett Packard 5890 equipped with a 0.54 mm ID by 30 m fused silica column coated (0.25 μm) with Supelcowax 10 (Supelco, Inc., Bellefonte, PA). Operating parameters for the GC were as follows: 1) Injector port temperature: 150°C, 2) Detector temperature: 250°C, 3) Split ratio: 16:1, 4) Temperature program: 45°C during 5 min., rate A = 5°C/min., final temperature A = 155°C, rate B = 4°C/min., final temperature B = 240°C during 60 min., and 5) Carrier gas: helium at a linear velocity of 25 cm/sec. The volume of sample injected was 4 μl.

Peaks were identified by MS analysis and by comparing Kovàts Indexes (KI) of some peaks with the correspondent standards Kovàts indexes. Table 6 shows standards used and their respective KI.

2.5 Mass spectrometric (MS) analysis

Mass spectral data were acquired on a Finigan 4023 quadrupole mass spectrometer operated in the electro impact mode. The operating conditions were as follows: 1) Resolution: 1000 or unit mass, 2) Ion source temperature: 145°C, 3) Electron energy:

60 eV, and 4) Transfer line temperature: 260°C. Data were acquired and stored on disks for later retrieval.

The GC used was a Varian 3400 with a 0.32 mm ID by 60 m fused silica column coated (0.25 μm) with Supelcowax 10. The operation conditions were as follows: 1) Injector port temperature: 250°C, 2) Split ratio: 50:1 and 3) Temperature program: 45°C for 5 minutes, 5°C/min up to 155°C, 4°C/min up to 240°C and maintained at 240°C for 60 min. Peak identification was only made on odor active regions of the chromatogram.

As an aid to identification of compounds, mass spectral data were compared with reference spectra form the National Bureau of Standards, and with a collection of reference spectra compiled in the Agricultural Chemistry Laboratory at Oregon State University.

2.6 Osme

The equipment and procedure used to conduct Osme were described in a previous paper (17). The GC conditions and volume of sample injected were the same as reported under the Gas chromatographic analysis section.

Four panelists, the same who evaluated the hop oils (17), evaluated the beer samples using GCO. Each sample was evaluated on each of four consecutive days. Each sniffing session took approximately 20 min. References standards were evaluated prior to each sniffing session (Table 2). Times and intensities of peaks detected at least 50% of the time for each subject were averaged. Then, times and intensities of those peaks that were detected at least for three of the four subjects were averaged again and a consensus osmegram was created for each sample evaluated. An example of a consensus osmegram can be seen in Fig. 3.

At the end of the sample evaluations, panelists evaluated a mixture of standards using GCO. Each compound in the mixture had the same concentration in pentane as in the sample. Amounts injected were adjusted so that the peak areas for each compound were similar to those for the same compounds in the samples. Effluents were described in the same way as were the beer extracts. In this way it was possible to confirm the identity and sensory properties of some of the peaks.

The mixtures sniffed contained the following compounds:
Mixture 1:
    1- Isobutanol (99%, Aldrich Chemical Co., Milwaukee, WI)
    2- Isoamyl Acetate (99%, Aldrich)
    3- Isoamyl Alcohol (99%, Aldrich)

4- Ethyl Hexanoate (99%, Aldrich)

5- Ethyl Heptanoate (99%, Aldrich)

6- Ethyl Octanoate (99%, Aldrich)

7- Ethyl Nonanoate (99%, Aldrich)

8- Linalool (97%, Aldrich).

9- Ethyl Decanoate (99%, Aldrich)

10- 2-Phenetyl acetate (99%, Aldrich)

11- 2-Phenetanol (99%, Aldrich)

12- Decanoic Acid (99%, Aldrich)

Mixture 2:

1- n-Octyl Formate

2- 2-Undecanone (98%, Fluka-Chemika Biochemika, Ronkonkoma, NY).

3- α-Humulene (99%, Fluka-Chemika)

4- 2-Dodecanone (99%, Fluka-Chemika)

5- 2-Undecanol (Eastman Organic Chemicals, Rochester,NY).

6- 2-Tridecanone (99%, Aldrich)

7- Citronellol

8- Geraniol (98%, Aldrich)

9- 2-Pentadecanone (95%, Pfaltz and Bauer, Waterbury, CT)

Mixture 3:*

1- Humulene Monoepoxide I

2- Humulene Monoepoxide II

3- Humulene Monoepoxide III

4- Humulene Diepoxide A

5- Humulene Diepoxide B

*All of the humulene components were synthesized at the Agricultural Chemistry Dept., Oregon State University.

3. RESULTS AND DISCUSSION

3.1 Descriptive sensory panel

3.1.1 <u>ANOVA</u>. No significant differences were found among the aroma of beers brewed with different varieties of hops and the unhopped control when the data was analyzed using ANOVA on each attribute. It is suspected that the unhopped beer was contaminated with hop residues probably adsorbed on the yeast, or the amount of hops added was not enough to produce an aroma difference between hopped and unhopped

indicating that the majority of fruity aroma may be a product of fermentation. Spicy, malty, and ethanol scores ranged between slight and slight-to-moderate. Across the beer samples brewed with the three hop varieties, the attribute intensity ratings were similar. The hop oil samples from the same three varieties were also similar: Vitamin B was the only attribute rated significantly different across samples (17). This suggests that the U.S.D.A. variety hops have similar aroma profiles to Hallertauer both before and after the brewing process.

There was a significant ($P \leq .01$) panelist effect for each attribute indicating that panelists used different parts of the scale. The attributes citrus and sweet had significant ($P < .05$) panelist by treatment interactions: panelists assigned the samples different trends for these two attributes. It is probable that panelists needed more training for these two attributes.

3.1.2 <u>Principle component analysis</u>. Three principle components (PC) accounted for 71.6% of the total variance (Fig. 2). The contribution of each attribute to each PC is represented by vectors with the length of each vector proportional to its relative importance in explaining the variability among the samples. PC1 was mainly weighted by overall intensity, citrus, floral and, to a lesser extent, by fruity, sweet, and ethanol. U.S.D.A. 21455 had the highest score in PC1. In Sanchez et al. (17), U.S.D.A. 21455 was rated high in PC3 indicating that this variety was high in citrus character. A comparison of the PCA's from the beer and hop oil studies indicated that U.S.D.A. 21455 was high in citrus character; therefore, the source for citrus aroma may be the hops. PC2 was weighted by spicy, sweet, and negatively by ethanol. Beer brewed with Hallertauer hops had the highest scores on PC2 indicating that it was more spicy and sweet than the other beers, while the unhopped beer was highest in ethanol of all the beers. Hallertauer hop oil was rated high in PC's containing herbal, citrus, vitamin B, and grassy aromas (17). Although the descriptors for the hop oil and beer were not identical, they were similar suggesting that the spicy, herbal, grassy, and citrus notes originated from the Hallertauer hops. PC3 was weighted mainly by malty character; the unhopped beer was the richest in this attribute. All the attributes were positively correlated except for malty which was negatively correlated with the others.

3.2 <u>Osme</u>

In Table 4 are listed the total number of odor active peaks found in the beers brewed with hops and the unhopped control. The number of peaks found in the unhopped beer was 32 percent smaller than the number found in the beers brewed with hops. The biggest odor active area corresponded to the beer brewed with U.S.D.A.

TABLE 2

Definitions of the attribute reference standards[1] used during the sniffing of the chromatographic effluents of beer extracts

Attribute	Reference Preparation
	Aroma reference prepared by:
Rancid	Thirty ml of rancid oil (Saffola 100% Safflower oil, Westley Foods, Inc., Plymouth, FL).
Cheesy, Sweaty	Fifty ml of a solution 0.01% of Butyric acid (Aldrich, 99%, Gold Label, Milwaukee, WI).
Fresh Vegetative	Three sliced fresh sweet peas.
Cooked Vegetative	Fifty grams of canned green beans (S&W, French Style, Fine Foods, Inc., San Ramon, CA).
Spicy	One cinnamon stick (Spice Islands, Specialty Brands, San Francisco, CA).
	Three grams of nutmeg (Schilling, McCormick & Co., Inc., Baltimore, MD).
	Three grams of anise seeds (The R.T. French Co., Rochester, NY).
	Imbibing an aroma[2] paper stick in Eugenol (Aldrich, 99%, Milwaukee, WI).
Corn Chips	10 g of mashed corn chips (Fritos Corn Chips, Frito Lay, Inc., Dallas, TX)
Fruity	One-half fresh Jonathan apple sliced in 1 cm cubes.
	One-half fresh Granny Smith apple sliced in 1 cm cubes.
	One-quarter fresh banana (Dole, Inc., Honolulu, Hawaii).
Tobacco	Primary aroma of one Camel cigarette (R.J. Reynolds Tobacco Co., Winston, Salem, NC).
Floral	Imbibing an aroma paper stick on: Carnation, Magnolia, Rose, and Violet essences (Uncommon Scents, Eugene, OR).
Vinyl	Ten ml of STP vinyl protectant (First Brands Corp., Danbury, CT).

TABLE 2. (cont.)

Attribute	Reference Preparation
	Aroma reference prepared by:
Citrus	Combining two half wedges of grapefruit, orange and lemon (Sunkist Growers, Inc., Los Angeles, CA).
Butter	Thirty grams of 100% butter (Darigold AA grade, Seattle, WA).
Burned Matches	One burned match (Diamond Brands, Inc., Minneapolis, MN).
Prunes	Three 1 cm cubes of prunes (Del Monte Co., San Francisco, CA).
Cooked Potatoes	Boiling one sliced potato until it is overcooked.
Musty	Soaking with spring water five halves of filberts and let stand until mold developed on them.
Skunky	Leaving one 250 ml erlenmeyer filled with beer and capped under a fluorescent light for five days.
Vitamin B	Two halved tablets of Stresstabs 600 (Lederle Laboratories Division, Pearl River, NY), soaked with few drops of spring water.
Artificial Fruit	Fifteen grams of Mixed Berry Jello (General Foods Co., White Plains, NY)
Sweet	Ten ml of honey (Sue Bee, Grade A white, Pure Clover Honey, Sioux Honey Assn., Sioux City, IA).

1- All the reference standards were placed in 350 ml amber glasses covered with an aluminum foil lid and served at room temperature.
2- Fragrance Test Filters (Orlandi, Inc., Farmingdale, NY).

beers. In Table 3 are listed attribute means and standard deviations (SD) for each variety. The overall intensity levels of the beers were rated as moderate-to-large. Fruity was the next highest-rated attribute with intensity ratings between slight-to-moderate and moderate. In the hop oil study (17), fruity was rated between just detectable and slight. Citrus, floral, and sweet in this study and the hop oil study were rated low in intensity: between just detectable and slight. Relative to the citrus, floral, and sweet descriptors that were common to both studies, fruity ratings increased substantially in the beer study

TABLE 3

Treatment means[1,2] and standard deviations (SD) for DSP evaluation of the unhopped beers and beers brewed with U.S.D.A. 21455, U.S.D.A. 21459, and Hallertauer Mittelfrüh hops.

Attribute	Hallertauer	21455	21459	Unhopped
Overall Intensity	9.5 (1.56)	9.1 (1.64)	9.4 (1.79)	9.6 (1.69)
Fruity	6.1 (2.39)	5.8 (2.33)	5.8 (2.64)	6.0 (2.80)
Citrus	1.6 (2.52)	2.7 (2.28)	1.7 (2.70)	1.3 (2.44)
Floral	2.0 (2.61)	2.8 (2.93)	2.7 (3.00)	1.9 (2.44)
Spicy	4.0 (2.46)	4.5 (3.06)	4.2 (3.13)	3.4 (2.04)
Sweet	3.1 (2.83)	2.3 (2.7)	2.8 (2.73)	2.9 (2.04)
Malty	4.6 (1.79)	4.0 (1.46)	4.1 (1.75)	5.0 (1.78)
Ethanol	5.0 (1.84)	4.2 (2.21)	4.9 (2.25)	2.5 (3.86)

[1]Sixteen point intensity scale (0 = none, 7 = moderate, 15 = extreme).
[2]Means based on average ratings by nine panelists.

21459 hops. This fact does not correlate with the overall intensity attribute determined by DSP for which the unhopped beer had the highest overall intensity. This was probably due to the higher alcoholic character in the unhopped beer.

Odors related to sulfur compounds made up the highest percentage of the total odor active area, especially for the unhopped beer (40%). These odors generally had a low intensity and they had a long duration, making the areas larger. No sulfur compounds were identified by MS and the FID detector is not very sensitive to these compounds. The association of these odors with sulfur compounds comes from the literature. The corn odor was related to dimethyl sulfide, cooked potatoes to methional, and garlic to ethyl mercaptan etc. (19). The next most important odor characteristic was fruity for the unhopped beer and floral for the hopped beers. This fact may indicate that hop compounds are responsible for the floral aroma of beers while the yeast fermentation products contribute more to the fruity character of beers.

Skunky was an attribute unique to the hopped beers produced as a consequence of light-induced oxidation. There was only one peak in each beer extract that had skunky odor. This suggests the possibility of a unique compound responsible for this defect in

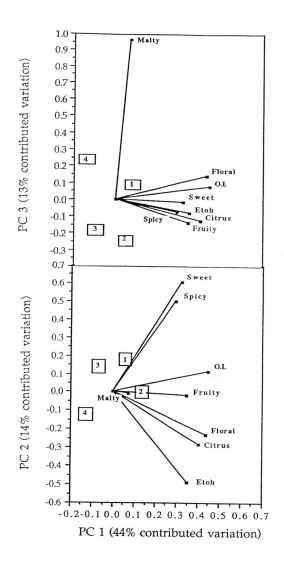

Fig. 2. PCA graphs (PC1 vs. PC2, PC3) for beers brewed with 1 = Hallertauer, 2 = U.S.D.A. 21455, 3 = U.S.D.A. 21459, and 4 = Unhopped. O.I. = Overall intensity, and Etoh = ethanol. The contribution of each attribute to each vector is represented by vector length.

TABLE 4

GCO

	USDA 21459	Hallertauer	USDA 21455	Unhopped
Number of odor active peaks	25	24	25	17
Total area[1]	21.33	15.28	18.43	10.64
% OF TOTAL PEAK AREA[2]				
Floral	26	33	28	14
Fruity	14	12	15	32
Skunky	6	5	6	0
Sweet	4	8	5	10
Musty/vinyl/ fresh vegetative	4	5	8	5
Sulfur related odors[3]	26	29	37	40
Others[4]	5	8	0	0
Floral/Fruity	9	20	10	4

[1] Calculated using DASSIE special software (Sensory Science Laboratory, Oregon State University).
[2] Calculated as area of each descriptor divided by total area.
[3] Includes corn chips, burned matches, natural gas, garlic, vitamin B, meaty, and cooked potato descriptors.
[4] Includes butter, sour, and vanilla descriptors.

beer. The concentration was not enough to alter the sensory properties of the beers as evaluated by the DSP because skunky aroma was not detected in any of the beers.

The rest of the odor characteristics only represented a low percentage of the total odor active area.

Fig. 3. shows the consensus osmegrams and FID chromatograms for the odor active peaks for the four samples. In Table 5 are listed the retention times (RT), Kováts Indices (KI), descriptors, and identified compounds of the odor active peaks detected by GC olfactometry. Compounds that have a question mark (?) are those with the KI closest to the KI of the odor, but no standard was available to confirm the odor, or the odor associated with the standard doesn't correspond with the odor detected in the samples.

Peak 6 was described as skunky. It was not possible to identify the compound associated with it. Only some sulfur ions were detected. A number of compounds have been detected in light-struck beer, the most significant being 3- methylbut-2-en-1-thiol and to a lesser extent methanethiol (20). These compounds are presumed to be major contributors to the skunky aroma. Sniffing of the chromatographic effluents may be a good approach to identify more compounds that contribute to skunky (lightstruck) aroma. For U.S.D.A. 21459, this peak was perceived as a continuous odor but had two maximum peaks (Fig. 3).

Some peaks such as 7, 18, 21, 24 and 28 were perceived as continuous odors (intensity never reached zero), but with different aroma characteristics and two maximums. For example, peak 7, in the beer brewed with U.S.D.A. 21459 hops, was described as banana and sweet solvent at the beginning turning to cardboard or vinyl at the end. In the case of peak 18, it was perceived as one peak with two maximum for U.S.D.A. 21459 beer, but for U.S.D.A. 21455 it was perceived as two different peaks (reached intensity zero).

The odor associated with peak 21 was reported previously (17) during the GCO evaluation of hop oil oxygenated fractions. In that report, this odor was described as musty-rancid and associated with the compound 9-methyl-decan-2-one. In beer it was not possible to identify the compound associated with this odor because it was present in a very low concentration, but the odor description was the same (Table 5). Because of its low threshold and ability to survive the brewing process, this compound may be important as an odor active compound, along with linalool. An interesting point is that U.S.D.A. 21459 hop oil contained the lowest amount of this compound (8.1 ppm) (17) while Hallertauer had the highest (61.9 ppm). In beers, the odor was not perceived in the beer brewed with U.S.D.A. 21459 hops, yet it was
perceived as a continuous peak in beers brewed with Hallertauer hops: This indicates that this compound is not generated during fermentation.

Peak 27 was associated with citronellol. It was described as fruity-apple. It was not found in the hop oils, but it was postulated to be an oxidation product from yeast acting on neral and geranial (Citral) (21).

On the other hand, peak 28 had a different pattern. This peak began with a rancid, cooked-vegetable odor, then changed to floral and then to prunes. It is suspected that two or three compounds were eluting at the same time in this region. One of these

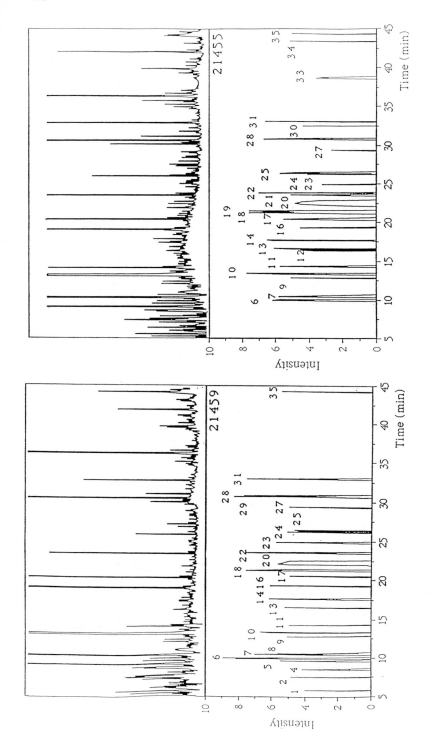

419

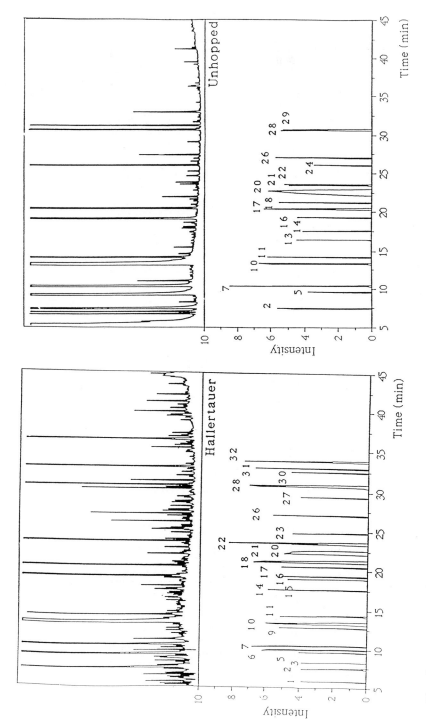

Fig. 3. Consensus osmegrams (bottom) and FID chromatograms (top) for beers brewed with U.S.D.A. 21459, U.S.D.A. 21455, Hallertauer Mittelfrüh, and unhopped beer.

TABLE 5

Consensus odor active peaks detected during GC olfactometry evaluation of the following beers: 1 - U.S.D.A. 21459, 2 - Hallertauer, 3 - U.S.D.A. 21455, and 4 - unhopped.

Peak #	RT(min)[1] (KI$_{20M}$)	Descriptor[2]	Odor Intensities[3] Varieties				Identified Compounds[4]	RT(min)[5] (KI$_{20M}$)
			1	2	3	4		
1	5:80 (991)	Butter-Sour	4.0	3.8	-	-	n-Butyl Acetate?	
2	7:51 (1050)	Fruity	4.8	3.9	-	5.6	Ethyl Butanoate?	
3	8:30 (1074)	Butter-Sour	-	3.8	-	-	-	
4	8:52 (1080)	Fruity-Fermented	4.2	-	-	-	-	
5	9:61 (111)	Musty-Vinyl	5.4	4.0	-	3.8	Isobutanol?	
6	9:94 (1123)	Skunky	8.9	6.1	6.2	-	-	
7	10:44 (1135)	Banana-Sweet Solvent	7.0	6.8	5.8	8.5	Isoamyl-Acetate	10:45 (1136)
8	10:59 (1142)	Vinyl Cardboard	5.6	-	-	-	-	
9	12:79 (1202)	Fermented Fruit	5.0	5.2	5.1	-	-	
10	13:35 (1220)	Sweet-Alcoholic	6.7	6.0	7.7	6.7	Isoamyl Alcohol	13:42 (1218)
11	14:25 (1248)	Fermented Fruit	4.9	5.1	5.7	6.2	Ethyl Hexanoate	14.26 (1246)
12	16:34 (1309)	Dusty-Musty	-	-	4.5	-	-	
13	16:52 (1315)	Fresh Vegetative-Vinyl	5.2	-	6.1	4.5	-	
14	17:56 (1350)	Corn Chips	6.1	5.9	6.5	4.1	6-Methyl-5-Hepten-2-One?	
15	18:96 (1393)	Garlic-Natural Gas	-	4.7	-	-	-	
16	19:31 (1405)	Floral-Vinyl	6.0	5.1	4.5	4.4	-	
17	20:45 (1449)	Floral-Rancid	4.9	5.1	5.5	6.4	Ethyl Octanoate	20:54 (1449)

TABLE 5 (continued)

Peak #	RT(min)[1] (KI$_{20M}$)	Descriptor[2]	Odor Intensities[3] Varieties				Identified Compounds[4]	RT(min)[5] (KI$_{20M}$)
			1	2	3	4		
18	21:22 (1478)	Cooked Potatoes	7.5	6.7	7.6	5.5	-	
19	21:44 (1486)	Dirty Socks-Sweaty	5.3	-	7.6	-	-	
20	22:40 (1519)	Vit B-Meaty	5.6	4.9	4.8	6.1	-	
21	23:48 (1557)	Musty-Vinyl	-	4.5	5.1	4.9	-	
22	23:59 (1561)	Floral/Fruity /Citrus	7.6	8.3	5.7	5.2	Linalool	23:62 (1560)
23	24:86 (1602)	Floral-Fruity	5.7	4.5	3.2	-	-	
24	26:17 (1657)	Burned Matches/Sulfury	5.0	-	4.1	3.4	-	
25	26:38 (1665)	Floral-Oxidized	4.6	-	5.7	-	-	
26	27:01 (1690)	Vit. B	-	5.6	-	5.7	-	
27	29:33 (1778)	Fruity-Apple	4.9	4.0	2.7	-	Citronellol	29:19 (1773)
28	30:69 (1831	Rancid-Cooked Vegetative	8.2	-	-	5.4	-	
29	30:82 (1836)	Floral Prunes	7.7	7.0	6.7	5.3	2-Phenylethyl-Acetate	30:70 (1831)
30	32:51 (1902)	Floral-Fruity	-	4.6	4.4	-	-	
31	33:04 (1925)	Floral-Roses	7.5	6.7	6.6	-	Phenethanol	32:98 (1924)
32	33:9 (1960)	Floral-Fruity	-	7.4	-	-	-	
33	38:74 (2158)	Artificial Fruit-Sweet	-	-	3.6	-	-	
34	43:39 (2356)	Floral-Spicy	-	-	5.1	-	-	
35	44:30 (2394)	Artificial Fruit-Candy	5.4	-	5.0	-	-	

1- Time (min) and KI20M averaged over the subjects that detected the odors. KI$_{20M}$ means Kovàts' index on Carbowax 20M column.

2- Most frequent descriptors assigned to the odors.
3- Sixteen point intensity scale (0=none, 15= extreme)
4- Those compounds with a question mark (?) were identified by MS but no standard was available to confirm this.
5- Retention time (min) and KI_{20M} of the standards.

---

compounds, most probably associated with the floral character, was 2-phenylethyl-acetate. In Hallertauer and U.S.D.A. 21455 beers, the rancid odor was perceived but the maximum of the peak was reached at the floral to prunes region. Damascenone may be responsible for the prune aroma. In Sanchez et al. (17) a hop oil compound eluting at almost the same KI (1838) as in beer (KI 1836) was described as having tobacco and prune aromas (Table 5). Tressl et al. (22) reported that damascenone elutes very close to 2-phenylethyl acetate.

The odors associated with the humulene oxidation products were not detected in any of the hopped beers, even though these compounds were identified by MS. Only one panelist, the most sensitive to these compounds, was able to detect the odors associated with these compounds describing them as spicy/musty/floral (23).

Thus some of these compounds did survive the brewing process, but they were not present in enough concentration to be important odor contributors to beer aroma. Again, no odor was perceived in the region where humulene diepoxides elute and no odor was perceived during the GCO evaluation of the standards. This fact suggests that they may not be odor active compounds.

It has to be mentioned that results obtained from Osme are highly dependent on the extraction methodology, solvents used, and amount of extract injected. Therefore, these results must not be considered absolute.

In Table 6 are listed all the compounds identified by MS analysis. By observation of concentration levels, the differences among varieties could be explained as a function of the different concentration of the compounds rather than to a specific compound. These differences in concentration were not big enough to produce sensory changes in the aroma of the beers brewed with them. Even though the chemical composition of the unhopped beer aroma extract differed from the hopped beers, the DSP found no differences in the aroma of this beer compared with the hopped ones. There are several possible explanations for this. The fusel alcohol contribution was so strong that it may have masked all hop aromas. There was a one month lapse before DSP evaluation; during that time the hop aroma may have dissipated. Hop components may have been lost to the beer cap liner (24). Panelists may have needed more training.

TABLE 6

Chemical composition of the beer aroma extract.

Compound RT(min) (KI$_{20M}$)	Concentration (ppb)[1]			
	USDA 21459	Haller-tauer	USDA 21455	Unhopped
[n-Butyl Acetate] 5.70 (985)	71	30	115	-
[Ethyl Butanoate] 7.50 (1049)	42	147	24	210
[Methyl Butanol] 8.50 (1079)	3	-	-	2
Iso-Butanol 9.7 (1098)	220	724	342	1350
Isoamyl Acetate 10.42 (1136)	390	339	1035	834
Isoamyl Alcohol 13.29 (1218)	4000	13956	12979	571
[Isobutyl Isobutyrate] 13.70 (1231)	5	1	8	-
Ethyl Hexanoate 14.22 (1247)	40	54	111	60
Ethyl Heptanoate 17.47 (1345)	21	19	46	1
[6-Methyl-5-Hepten-2-one] 17.47 (1351)	10	8	20	-
n-Octyl Formate 20.30 (1443)	8	5	18	-
Ethyl Octanoate 20.50 (1450)	78	84	239	130
[Linalool Oxide A or B] 22.08 (1508)	4	4	8	-
* Linalool 23.59 (1560)	66	101	202	1
* 2-Undecanone 5.08 (1610)	4	24	14	-

TABLE 6 (continued)

Compound RT(min) (KI_{20M})	USDA 21459	Haller-tauer	USDA 21455	Unhopped
Ethyl Decanoate 26.06 (1652)	28	25	72	45
* α-Humulene 27.05 (1690)	11	37	12	-
2-Undecanol 28.00 (1728)	6	9	20	-
Citronellol 29.20 (1773)	6	11	20	-
[Methyl Dodecanoate] 30.22 (1812)	20	40	71	-
* 2-Tridecanone 30.43 (1821)	5	13	19	-
2-Phenylethyl Acetate 30.69 (1831)	97	80	360	29
* Geraniol 31.25 (1854)	24	23	48	-
Phenylethanol 32.98 (1924)	63	128	239	7
* 2-Pentadecanone 35.68 (2032)	7	9	13	-
* Humulene Monoepox.II 36.79 (2070)	270	13	32	-
* Humulene Monoepox.III 36.92 (2082)	4	6	12	-
Decanoic Acid 43.41 (2356)	33	14	-	-
* Humulene Diepoxide A 43.89 (2377)	20	1	5	-
* Humulene Diepoxide B 44.42 (2041)	24	48	10	-

1 - Quantitation relative to internal standard.
[] - Compounds in brackets were tentatively identified.
* - Hop compounds reported previously in hop oil oxygenated fractions by the same author.

4. CONCLUSION

Based on the DSP and GCO results, beers brewed with U.S.D.A. 21459 and U.S.D.A. 21455 have similar aroma characteristics to the beer brewed with Hallertauer Mittelfrüh.

Although humulene oxidation products survived the brewing process, they were not present in enough concentration to be important contributors to hop aroma.

The results obtained are dependent on extraction methodologies and solvents used. The same compounds were found in all three varieties, but in varying concentrations for each compound. This difference in concentration was not great enough to change the sensory properties of the beers.

There were chemical differences between the hopped and unhopped beers. The consensus osmegrams also showed differences between the hopped and unhopped beers, but these differences were not detected by the DSP.

REFERENCES

1. Howard, G.A., and Stevens, A.R. Evaluation of hops. IX. Flavour of hop oil constituents. J. Inst. Brew. 65 (1959) 494.
2. Likens, S. and Nickerson, G.B. Detection of certain hop oil constituents in brewing products. Am. Soc. Brew. Chem., Proc. (1964) 5-13.
3. Buttery, D.G., Black D.R., Guadagni, D.G., and Kealy, M.P. A Study of the volatile oxygenated constituents in different hop varieties. Am. Soc. Brew. Chem., Proc. (1965) 103.
4. Guadagni, D.G., Buttery, R.G., and Harris, J. Odour intensities of hop oil components. J. Sci. Fd. Agric. 17 (1966) 142.
5. Likens, S.T. and Nickerson, G.B. Identification of the varietal origin of hop extracts. Am. Soc. Brew. Chem., Proc. (1965) p.23.
6. Peacock, V.E., Deinzer M.L., McGill, L.A., and Wrostald, R.E. Hop aroma in American beer. J. Agr. Food Chem. 28 (1980) 774-777.
7. Peacock, V.E. and Deinzer M.L. Chemistry of hop aroma in beer. J. Am. Soc. Brew. Chem. 39 (1981) 136-141.
8. Peacock, V.E., Deinzer M.L., Likens, S., Nickerson, G.B., and McGill, L.A. Floral hop aroma in beer. J. Agr. Food Chem. 29 (1981) 1265-1269.
9. Haley, J. and Peppard, T.L. Differences in utilisation of the essential oil of hops during the production of dry-hopped and late-hopped beers. J. Inst. Brew. 89 (1983) 87-91.
10. Murakami A.A., Rader S., Chicoye, E., and Goldstein H. Effect of hopping on the headspace volatile composition of beer. J. Am. Soc. Brew. Chem. 47 (1989) 35-42.
11. Irwin, A.J. Varietal dependence of hop flavour volatiles in lager. J. Inst. Brew. 95 (1989) 185-194.
12. Siebert, K.J., Ramus S. A., Peppard T.L., Guzinski J.A. and Stegink L.J. An investigation into hop fractions leading to hoppy aroma in beer. MBAA Techical Quarterly, 26 (1989) 62-69.
13. Peacock V.E., and Deinzer, M. The structures of humulene diepoxides found in hops and beer. J. Am. Soc. Brew. Chem. 47 (1989) 4.

14. Peppard, T.L., Ramus, S. A., Siebert, K.J.,and Witt,C.A. Correlation of sensory instrumental data in elucidating the effect of varietal differences in hop flavor in beers. J. Am. Soc. Brew. Chem. 47 (1989) 18.
15. Acree, T.E., Butts, R.M., Nelson, R.R., and Lee, C.Y. Sniffer to determine the odor of gas chromatographic effluents. Anal. Chem. 48 (1976) 1821.
16. Acree, T.E., Barnard, J., and Cunningham, D.G. A procedure for the sensory analysis of gas chromatographic effluents. Food Chem. 14 (1984) 273.
17. Sanchez, N., Lederer C., Nickerson, G., Libbey, L., and McDaniel, M.R. Analytical and sensory evaluation of hop varieties. Recent Developments in Food Science and Nutrition, Elsevier, Amsterdam, 1991.
18. Johnson R.A., and Wichern D.W. Applied multivariate statistical analysis. Second edition. Prentice Hall, Englewood Cliffs, New Jersey, chpt. 8, 1988.
19. Meilgaard, M. C. Flavor chemistry of beer: part II: Flavor and threshold of 239 aroma volatiles. Tech. Quart., Master Brew. Assoc. Amer. 12 (1975) 151-168.
20. Gunst, F. and Verzele, M. On the sunstruck flavour of beer. J. Inst. Brew. 84 (1978) 291-292.
21. Lam, K.C., Foster, R.T., and Deinzer, M.L. Aging of hops and their contribution to beer flavor. J. Agr. Food Chem. 34 (1986) 763-770.
22. Tressl, R., Friese, L., Fendesack, F., and Koppler, H. J. Gas chromatographic-mass spectrometric investigation of hop aroma constituents in beer. J. Agr. Food Chem. 26 (1978) 1422-1426.
23. Sanchez, N.B. Analytical and sensory evaluation of hop varieties. Corvallis, Oregon State Univ., 1990. Thesis.
24. Peacock, V.E., and Deinzer, M.L. Fate of hop oil components in beer. ASBC Journal. 46(4) (1988) 104-107.

G. Charalambous (Ed.), Food Science and Human Nutrition
© 1992 Elsevier Science Publishers B.V. All rights reserved.

NITRATE MASS-BALANCE IN THE BREWING INDUSTRY

M.MOLL[1], S.CHEVRIER[1], N. MOLL[2] and J.P. JOLY[2]

[1] Cervac-Est, 1 Allée Chaptal, 54630 Richardménil (France)

[2] Laboratoire de Chimie Organique 3, URA 486, B.P. 239, 54506 Vandoeuvre Cédex (France)

SUMMARY

The increase of nitrate in water and in cultivated plants is due to intensive agricultural practice so as to raise the agricultural yield. Nitrogen beside potassium and phosphates as fertilizers are applied in an uncontrolled manner in the fields. The consequences are the contamination of many ground water sources. The brewing water may contain high levels of nitrate, above 50 mg/l and should be reduced. Hops is an important raw-material which reaches levels of 2-18 g/kg of nitrate. Brewing liquor and hops are the main sources of nitrate in the final beer. Techniques to reduce nitrate concentration in the brewing industry are available.

Nitrate may be converted into nitrite by specific micro-organisms. Nitrite which is very reactive can interact with amino compounds as nitrosation to form N-nitroso-compounds.

Analytical procedures for the determination of nitrate and nitrite were modernized and calorimetric methods replaced by HPLC and enzymic procedures. In this study, nitrate in malt, hop, wort and beer was determined by a reversed-phase ionic HPLC procedure using a dynamically coated stationary phase. The separation of nitrate from other matrice constituents was without interferences.

1. MATERIALS

1.1 HPLC equipment

Nitrate determination in beer was performed by high-performance liquid chromatography with UV detection. The chromatographic system uncluded a Model 302 pump (Gilson), a 20 µl internal loop Rheodyne valve, a Cecil 2012 variable wavelength UV monitor (Waters) set at 212 nm and a Spectra Physics 4290 integrator.

Analytical column : 140 x 3.9 mm I.D. packed with LiChrospher

Si 300 10 μm (Merck) silanized with trichlorooctadecylsilane (1) (see methods). The precolumn (25 x 3.9 mm I.D.) was packed with 30 μm RSil C18 HL (RSL, Eke, Belgium).

1.2 Reagents

Water for the preparation of the eluents and the stock and standard solutions of KNO_3 was freshly double distilled.

Kalium nitrate (Merck) for the calibration curve of nitrate.

Tetrabutylammonium hydrogen sulfate (Aldrich) (TBAHS) used in the mobile phase for HPLC.

Hexadecyltributylphosphonium bromide (Fluka) (HTBP) used in the dynamically coating of the stationary phase.

Eluent for the dynamically coating : prepare 1 mM HTBP in $MeOH/H_2O$ (75/25)(v/v). Filter through a 0.45 μm membrane filter.

Mobile phase for HPLC : prepare 5 mM (1.7 g/l) TBAHS in water, pH 3.5 and filter through a 0.45 μm membrane filter.

Stock and standard solutions of KNO_3 : a 500 mg/l KNO_3 stock solution was prepared in bidistilled water and kept several weeks in the refrigerator. Standard solutions (2-100 mg/l) were prepared feshly by dilution of the stock solution.

Samples preparation :

Brewing liquor was directly injected into the chromatograph after filtration on membrane.

Malt, 6 raws Plaisant, was ground. 50 g were extracted with 200 ml water for 1 hour at 75°C. After cooling the mixture was filtered, the volume adjusted to 200 ml and aliquots filtered on membrane and injected into the chromatograph.

Hops Hallertau N.B., 6.2% alpha acids (2 g) were extracted in boiling water for 15 minutes (2). After filtration and adjustment to 1 liter, aliquots were injected.

Wort samples were filtered through a membrane filter and injected.

Beer samples were degassed for 10 minutes in an ultrasonic bath and filtered through a membrane filter. After a five times dilution of the filtrate, aliquots were injected.

2. METHODS

2.1 Preparation of the analytical column

The packing material used was LiChrospher Si 300 (Merck, ref. 19639, batch 703 YS).

Treatment of silica before silanization (3) : 6.00 g of the chromatographic grade silica were heated in a quartz crucible under vacuum to 100, 250, 450 and finaly 850°C during 14 hours and allowed to cool in a vacuum oven to room temperature. The dehydroxylated silica was then rehydrated by boiling in an aqueous hydrofluoric acid solution (~ 400 ppm) for 72 h, filtered, rinsed with distilled water (600 ml) and finally dried at 80°C for 72 h and then at 120°C for 24 h under vacuum.

Silanization of silica (4) : 3.6 g of rehydrated silica were added to a nitrogen purged solution of trichlorooctadecylsilane (1.0 ml) in dry 1,1,2-trichloroethane. The suspension was heated under reflux for 3 hours and allowed to cool to room temperature. The product was filtered and washed with 1,1,2-trichloroethane (50 ml), methanol (50 ml), methanol/water (70/30) (50 ml) and finally with methanol (50 ml). The silanized silica was then dried at 80°C for 14 hours under vacuum. Final weight : 3.74 g. Elemental analysis on carbon : 3.72% corresponding to an alkyl surface concentration of 2.5 to 3.5 μmoles/m^2.

Packing of the column : a 2.5 g amount of the bonded silica was suspended in a mixture of toluene/i-PrOH/36% EtOH (1/1/1)(v/v/v) by ultrasonication according to the classical slurry method (5).

2.2 HPLC procedure

Dynamically coating of the bonded silica according to (6,7). The column is first equilibrated with 100 ml MeOH/H$_2$O (75/35)(v/v) at a flow rate of 1 ml/min. The coating is conducted by elution of 200 ml of the HTPB solution at the same flow rate. The column is then rinsed with 200 ml water, conditioned with 100 ml of the mobile phase and is ready to use.

Chromatographic conditions : in all experiments the mobile phase flow rate was 1.5 ml/min. The UV detector was set at 212 nm.

3. NITRATE LEVELS IN BREWING RAW-MATERIALS

Brewing liquor

The main contribution to nitrate in beer is water. Several authors (8-15) have mentioned levels from <1 to >100 mg/l of nitrate in brewing liquors. The EEC requirements 80/778 for nitrate are : guidline 25 mg/l, maximum acceptable concentration : 50 g/l. For nitrite the maximum acceptable concentration is 0.1 mg/l. The presence of nitrite in water indicates a contamination by waste water.

The reduction of nitrate in brewing liquor can be obtained through different treatments (16-19).

- Ion-exchange (anionic type) : Nitrate is retained with sulphates and partially bicarbonates and replaced by chlorides during the regeneration with sodium chloride. The sulphate level needs to be adjusted by addition of calcium sulfate. This technique gives satisfactory results in the brewing industry.

- Biological treatments using antotrophic or heterotrophic bacterias. The last type of bacteria is the most common were ethanol or acetic acid is employed as nutritional source.

- Reverse osmosis, electrodialysis etc..

Hops (2,8-11,14,15,20-23)

Hops contain an appreciable amount of nitrate : 2 g - 18 g/kg and represent the second most important source of nitrate which is transfered to beer. The real influence of place of growth, the effect of fertilizer dosage and the hop variety on the nitrate concentration in hops is still under investigation.

The reduction of nitrate in hops can be obtained by extraction of hop products. Table 1 shows the levels of contamination of nitrate, nitrite and apparent total N-nitroso content (ATNC) in hops and hop extracts (23).

TABLE 1
Contaminants in hops and hop extracts

Product\Contamination	Sup.c.CO_2 Extract	Liq.CO_2 Extract	Ethanol Extract	Methanol Extract	Hop Pellets	Whole Hops
Nitrite	3-58	3-281	36-110	36-222	12-478	138-504
Nitrate	51-266	201-479	513-6433	3719-11402	13349-19403	7056-11608
ATNC	30-87	8-47	44-520	710-720	840-1190	809

Whole hops and hop pellets can contribute up to 20 mg/l of nitrate to beer. Ethanol extract 0.5-1.5 mg/l nitrate and CO_2 extract 0.05 mg/l nitrate. Hot water extract which is used to standardise the solvent extracts contain large amounts of nitrate up to 30 g/kg.

Malt and adjuncts (8-11,15)

Several investigations show a low contribution to nitrate in beer by these raw-materials. Table 2 summarizes the level of nitrate in malt and adjuncts.

TABLE 2

Nitrate levels in malt and adjuncts (9)

Raw-material	Nitrate (mg/kg)		Contribution to nitrate in beer (mg/l)
	Range	Average	
Malt (n = 26)	<10-45	22	2-3
Flaked barley	11-27	13	0.3
Micronized barley	25	25	0.6
Flaked wheat	20	20	0.5
Torrefied wheat	21	21	0.5
Micronized wheat	16	16	0.4
Wheat flour	14	14	0.4
Flaked corn	23-33	28	0.7
Copper syrup	7	7	neg.

Contribution from adjuncts calculated assuming 20 % of grist.
During the malting process the nitrate level in the water may affect the final nitrate concentration in malt. Other measures carried out on 12 different malts from Germany, France and Tchecoslovakia gave values between 20-138 mg/kg of nitrate (10).

Fermentation

Several authors (11-14,24) have confirmed that nitrate levels up to 200-500 mg/l in wort has no apparent effect on fermentation. The contamination of wort or yeast by nitrate reducing bacterias such as *Obesumbacterium proteus* and *Entereobacteriaceae* affects the fermentation and contribute to nitrite formation (24).

4. MASS BALANCE OF NITRATE IN A BREWERY

4.1 Analytical considerations

To know from where the contribution of nitrate in raw material is affected to wort and beer, it is necessary to dispose one accurate and simple analytical method. The most useful technique proposed in the literature is HPLC with ultraviolet absorbance, electrochemical or conductimetric detection (2,25-27). An alternate approach to the analysis of inorganic ions has been the use of reversed-phase columns and long alkyl chains ion-pairing reagents such as hexadecyltrimethylammonium bromide, tetrabutylammonium hydroxide, hexadecyltributylphosphonium bromide..., dynamically coated on the stationary phase and which would not desorb in aqueous eluents (6). The ionic interaction is achieved by the use, in the mobile phase, of a high molecular weight modifier, which in this study was 5 mM tetrabutylammonium hydrogen sulfate.

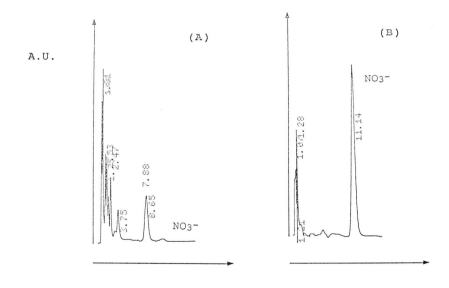

Fig. 1. Chromatograms of a malt extract (A) and a Hop extract (B). Chromatographic conditions : column 140 x 3.9 mm I.D. packed with a C_{18} stationary phase prepared in the laboratory and dynamically coated with HTPB ; mobile phase, 5 mM TBAHS, pH 3.5 at a flow-rate of 1 ml/min. ; volume injected, 20 µl ; UV detection at 212 nm.

The chromatograms represented on Fig. 1 and 2 show the well-resolved peak of nitrate at 10.63-11.21 min. in the raw-materials malt and hop and in the wort and beer. The sensitivity of the method is below 1 mg/l and the coefficient of variation was 2.5 % for the brewing liquor and 4-5% for the other samples.

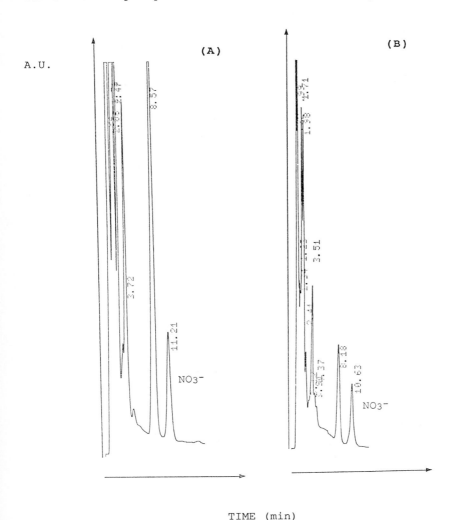

Fig. 2. Chromatograms of a wort extract (A) and a 1/5 diluted beer (B). Chromatographic conditions as in Fig.1.

4.2 Results and discussion

Nitrate determination in raw-materials of the brewery is shown below:

Brewing liquor	21 mg/l nitrate	380 hl = 798 g	65,2 %
Hops Hallertau N.B., 6,2 % alpha acids	8,2 g/kg nitrate	48 kg = 393.6 g	32.2 %
Malt 6 raws Plaisant	5 mg/kg	5800 kg = 29 g	2.4 %
Adjunct corn grits	2 mg/kg	1600 kg = 3.2 g	0.2 %
Total nitrate from raw-materials		1223.8 g	100 %

For 445 hl of wort we obtain 1223.8 g/445 hl = 27.5 mg/l of nitrate which seems an upper limit compared to the guideline of the EEC Requirements (25 mg/l of nitrate) for potable waters. The brewery may apply two modifications in the choice of raw-materials :

- treatment of brewing liquor so as to reduce the content of nitrate < 5 mg/l
- change the bitter substances by using CO_2 hop extracts. This would reduce the nitrate content by

5 mg/l nitrate x 380 hl	= 90 g	85.0 %
200 mg/kg nitrage CO_2 hop extract 45 % alpha acids, 6,6 kg	= 1.3 g	0.6 %
Malt	= 29 g	13.0 %
Adjunct	= 3.2 g	1.4 %
Total nitrate from raw-materials	223.5 g	100 %

For 445 hl we obtain 223.5 g/445 hl = 5 mg/l nitrate or a reduction of 81.7 %.

This example shows that the right choice of raw-materials and water denitrification techniques allows a valuable reduction of the nitrate content of wort and beer.

REFERENCES

1   N. Moll and J.P. Joly, Determination of ascorbic acid in bers by high-performance liqui chromatography with electrochemical detection, J. Chromatogr., 405 (1987) 347-356.

2   P. Anderegg and H. Pfenninger, Bestimmung von Nitrat in Hopfenpulver und Hopfenextrakt, Brauerei-Rundschau, 99 (1988) 133-136.
3   J. Koehler and J.J. Kirkland, Improved silica-based column packings for high-performance liquid chromatography, J. Chromatogr., 385 (1987) 125-150
4   K. Jones, Optimizationprocedure for the silanization of silicas for reversed-phase high-performance liquid chromatography. I. Elimination of non-significant variables, J. Chromatogr., 392 (1987) 1-10. II. Detaildes examination of significant variables, Ibid., 11-16.
5   J.J. Kirkland, High-permance liquid-partition chromatography with chemically bonded organic stationary phases, J. Chromatogr. Sci., 9 (1971) 206-214.
6   R.M. Cassidy and S. Elchuk, Dynamically coated columns for the separation of metal ions and anions by ion chromatography, Anal. Chem., 54 (1982) 1558-1563.
7   M. Lookabaugh, I.R. Krull and W.R. LaCourse, Determination of iodide and thiosulfate by paired-ion, reversed-phase high-performance liquid chromatography with ultraviolet absorbance, electrochemical, and conductrimetric detection, J. Chromatogr., 387 (1978) 301-231.
8   W. Postel, Nitratbestimmung und Nitratgehalt in Bier und Brauereirohstoffen, Brauwissenschaft, 29 (1976) 39-44.
9   E.D. Baxter, The importance of nitrates in brewing, Ferment, 1, 6 (1988) 31-33.
10 H. Senften and H. Pfenninger, Zum Nitratproblem, Brauerei-Rundschau, 98 (1987) 105-109.
11 F. Schur, Nitrat bei der Bierherstellung, Brauerei-Rundschau, 99 (1988) 89-95.
12 E. Schild and H. Diemer, Der Einfluss der Nitrate des Brauwassers auf den Herstellungsprozess von Würze und Bier, Brauwissenschaft, 15 (1962) 125-139.
13 K. Vogl, G. Schumann and W. Pröpsting, Über den Einfluss des Nitratgehaltes natürlicher Wässer auf den Gärverlauf von Bierwürzen, Monatsschrift für Brauerei, 20 (1967) 116-120.
14 I. Stone, C. Laschiver and L.T. Saletan, Nitrates in worts beers, and brewing, Proceeding of the American Society of Brewing Chemists, 1968, 125-131.
15 G. Cerutti and R. Pegoraro, The fate of nitrate from raw materials to beer, EBC- Symposium, Water in the brewing industry, Zoeterwoude, Monograph XIV, Verlag Hans Carl Nürnberg 1988, 114-123.
16 Degremont, Memento technique de l'eau, 9th edition, 2 volumes, Lavoisier, Paris, 1989.
17 G. Schumann, Verminderung des Nitratsgehaltes im Wasser, Brauwelt, 126 (1986) 1638-1639.
18 J. Dobias, M. Stahl and P. Fleminger, Denitrifikationsverfahren für Trinkwasser, Getränketechnik, (1985) 204-211.
19 G.Nagel, Nitratreduzierung in Trinkwasser und Brauchwasser, Brauindustrie, 70 (1986) 421-427.
20 F. Ghelch, J. Maier, G. Rossbauer, F. Zwack and D. Nast, Nitrat im Bier - ein Problem durch den Rohstoff Hopfen ?, Brauwelt, 129, (1989) 2156-2162.
21 A. Forster, Moderne Hopfung, Erläuterung am Beispiel der Nitratreduzierung, Der Weihenstephaner, 29 (1989) 16-23.
22 A. Forster, Zur Nitratdosage durch Hopfen und Hopfenprodukte, Brauwelt, 128 (1988) 188-191.

23 F.R. Sharpe, A user's view of hop products, E.B.C.-Symposium on hops, Freising Weihenstepha, Monograph XIII, Verlag Hans Carl, Nürnberg, 1987, 254-264.
24 J.P. Weiner, D.J. Ralph and L. Taylor, Nitrate and nitrite in brewery fermentation, Proceedings of the European Brewery Convention, 15th Congress, Nice, 1975, 565-579.
25 S. Donhauser, E. Geiger and K. Glas, Ionenpaarchromatographischer Nachweis von Nitrat und weiteren anorganischen Anionen,Monatsschrift für Brauwissenschaft, 42 (1989) 352-354.
26 C. Borchert, K. Jorge-Nothaft and E. Krüger Ionenchromatographische Methode zur Bestimmung des Nitratgehaltes in Brauwasser, Malz, Hopfen, Würze und Bier, Monatsschrift für Brauwissenschaft, 41 (1988) 112-115.
27 E.J. Knudson and K.J. Siebert, Application of Ion Chromatography to Beer, Wort and Brewing Water, Journal of the American Society of Brewing Chemists, 42 (1984) 65-70.

EXTRACTABILITY OF CATECHINS AND PROANTHOCYANIDINS OF GRAPE SEEDS. TECHNOLOGICAL CONSEQUENCES.

E. REVILLA[1], E. ALONSO[1], M. BOURZEIX[2] and V. KOVAC[3]

[1]Departamento de Química Agrícola, Geología y Geoquímica, Universidad Autónoma de Madrid, 28049 Madrid (Spain)

[2]Station Expérimentale de Pech Rouge-Narbonne, INRA, Bd. Géneral de Gaulle, 11100 Narbonne (France)

[3]Faculty of Technology, University of Novi Sad, 21000 Novi Sad (Yugoslavia)

SUMMARY

Grape seeds are considerably rich in catechins and proanthocyanidins, which have shown some biological properties of interest. These components are partially extracted during red and rosé winemaking and, consequently, the pomace obtained as a winery by-product contains a significant amount of these components. In this work, we have studied the extraction of these components under different conditions, using fresh seeds and those contained in the pomace obtained as a by-product of red winemaking. Results have shown that the alcoholic degree and the acidity of solutions used in extraction experiments greatly affects the extraction kinetics of these compounds. Large-scale vinifications have led to wines with a content of catechins and proanthocyanidins closely related to the quantity of grape seeds present in the must during fermentation.

1. INTRODUCTION

Catechins (flavan-3-ols) and their oligomers, known as proanthocyanidins, are natural products which have shown a number of biological properties of interest, due to their free radicals scavenger capacity (1-2) and of their positive role in atherosclerosis and other vascular diseases (3). They are also involved in chemical reactions with salivary glycoproteins which take place in the mouth, that generate the sensation known as astringency (4-6).

Mature grapes are the edible fruits which probably contain the largest amount of these substances, which are more abundant in lignified tissues. Thus, most of the catechins and proanthocyanidins of grape clusters are placed in seeds and cluster stems (7, 8). The seeds of mature grapes contain up to 28 g kg^{-1} of catechins and proanthocyanidins, depending on cultivars (8-10). These compounds are only partially extracted during red and rosé winemaking, and this fact. makes the use of pomace obtained as a winery by-product an easily available source of catechins and proanthocyanidins for several purposes, taking in mind that this by-product constitutes 10 to 20% of the weight of grapes, and that its seed content, on a wet basis, ranges from 20 to 30% (7). For this reason, the study of the factors which may affect the extraction of catechins and proanthocyanidins may be of interest for optimizing the process, avoiding the use of organic solvents, such as methanol or acetone, which are considered to be harmful to humans. We have carried out a number of experiments at laboratory scale to understand the kinetics of the extraction of catechins and proanthocyanidins of grape seeds under different conditions.

Furthermore, the content of catechins and proanthocyanidins of wines may be affected by the extent of pomace contact with must, and also with the quantity of pomace present in relation to must. For several white grape varieties it has been shown that the astringency of wines increases significatively with increased phenolic content, produced by skin contact times from one to five days (11). In the case of red wines, the content of tannins is higher as maceration time increases (12, 13), but other parameters related to the colour, like colour intensity and tint, decrease after eight days of maceration (12), and it has been proposed that this is due to the adsorption of anthocyans by skins and seeds. The ratings obtained in the sensory evaluation of experimental red wines of Carignan variety after 15 and 20 days of maceration of pomace with must were lower than those of that wine after 11 days of maceration, due to higher astringency (13). Arnold and Noble (14) have evaluated the biterness and astringency of several concentrations of grape seed phenolic extract in a model wine solution, showing that the ratings for astringency increased significatively with phenolic concentration increase, but the bitterness ratings were not significatively different to each other. Nevertheless, it should be possible to increase the content of catechins and proanthocyanidins of red wines with the addition of a supplementary quantity of grape seeds and reduction in the time of contact of pomace with must to avoid the reduction of colour intensity and tint due to the adsorption of anthocyans by pomace. Some experiments have been conducted for this purpose, and the results obtained are shown in this paper.

2. MATERIALS AND METHODS
2.1 Grapes cluster pomace

Samples (about 50 kg of pomace) were collected at Pech Rouge Experimental Cellar (INRA, France) in September 1989. Pomace of Chardonnay grapes was collected after pressing, and that of Alicante-Bouschet grapes, an intraspecific hybrid of three *Vitis vinifera* cultivars (Aramon, Teinturier and Grenache), after the thermovinification process. Once in the laboratory, seeds were separated from other pomace components (mainly skins and cluster stems), cleaned with wet filter paper and dried under CO_2 to eliminate surface water. Then seeds were placed in a plastic container and stored at a temperature below 5°C.

2.2 Extraction of catechins and proanthocyanidins of grape seeds

Extraction of Alicante-Bouschet seeds was carried out by using aqueous solutions containing 20, 40, 60 and 95% ethanol (by vol.), over periods of three, six and twelve hours at room temperature (about 20°C). For the extraction of catechins and proanthocyanidins from Chardonnay seeds aqueous solutions containing 8, 10 or 12% ethanol (by vol.) and different quantities of tartaric acid (4, 6 or 8 g dm^{-3} were used, over periods of seven, ten and 14 days at room temperature. In both cases, grape seeds (about 10 g) were placed in a glass container and a volume of the above mentioned solutions was added, so that the seed/extractant ratio was 1:4. The glass containers remained undisturbed during the experiments. Every experiment was carried out in triplicate.

After the extraction, the samples were tranferred into plastic tubes, and then centrifuged in a Jouan 2000 RS centrifuge at 4000 rpm (3000 g) for 10 minutes. The supernatants were transferred to glass flasks, and an aliquot (10 cm^3) was dealcoholized under vacuum at 30°C in a rotary evaporator (Rotavapor-R, Büchi, Switzerland). The aqueous residue was adjusted to pH 7.0 with NaOH, then diluted to 20 cm^3 with distilled water, and stored at a temperature below 5°C prior to analysis.

2.3 Wines

Seven red wines of Vranac grapes made by different procedures at Grokombinat "13. Jul", Titograd, Republic of Montenegro (Yugoslavia) in 1989 have been studied. Some characteristics of these vinifications are given in table 1. About 20,000 kg of grapes from the same vineyard were used for every experiment. The analysis were carried out in an aliquot of these wines, sampled after the spontaneous clarification took place. The determination of catechins and proanthocyanidins was carried out with an aliquot of 25 cm^3, which was conditioned by the same procedure described for seed extracts.

TABLE 1

Some characteristics of procedures used for obtaining Vranac wines.

Wine	State of grape clusters	Seeds added*	Extent of maceration (days)
V-26	entire	–	7
V-28	destemmed	–	7
V-29	destemmed	–	14
V-30	destemmed	60	7
V-31	destemmed	60	14
V-32	destemmed	120	7
V-33	destemmed	120	14

* grams of seeds added for each kg of grapes.

2.4 Conventional analysis of wines

The following parameters were determined by standard methods: colour intensity (15), tint (16), free anthocyanins (17), Folin-Ciocalteau index (18) and colouring matter qualitative estimation (19), which allows an estimation of the relative amount of red monomers, red polymers and brown polymers. The absorbance at 280 nm of wine samples diluted 1:50 was multiplied by 50 to obtain the tannic matter index.

2.5 Analysis of catechins and proanthocyanidins

The analysis of catechins and proanthocyanidins in seed extracts and wines was carried out in the ethyl acetate fraction obtained by using the wine phenolics fractionation procedure described previously (20), which involves the use of SEP-PAK C_{18} cartridges (Waters Associates, USA). The above fraction was used to analyse some catechins and proanthocyanidins by HPLC, using a Waters Associates chromatograph equipped with M6000A and M45 pumps, an U6K universal injector, a 490 programable multiwavelength visible-ultraviolet detector, a 730 data module and a 760 system controller. The HPLC separation was carried out on a 250 mm x 4.6 mm Nucleosil-5 μm C_{18} column (SFCC, France) at 32°C, using a linear gradient with a flow rate of 0.8 mL min^{-1}. Mobile phase A was 10% acetic acid and mobile phase B was deionized, distilled water. The linear gradient was started with 10% A to 82% A over 47 min., and continued with 82%

A to 100% A over 8 min. It was then run with 100% A for 10 min., and then back to initial conditions after washing for 45 min. with methanol/acetic acid/water (50:15:35). The effluent was monitored at 280 and 313 nm, with a sensitivity of 0.1 AUFS. A chromatogram of catechins and proanthocyanidins of a Vranac wine is given in figure 1. The determination of catechins and proanthocyanidins was achieved by an external standard procedure, using standards of (+)-catechin and (−)-epicatechin purchased from Fluka AG (Switzerland), and those of procyanidins B1, B2, B3, B4 and C1 kindly supplied by Dr. M. Moutounet, Institut des Produits de la Vigne, Montepellier, France. In the case of wines, the ethyl acetate fraction mentioned above was also used to determine total catechins and proanthocyanidins on the basis of their reaction with vanillin in acidic media, according to the procedure described previously (21).

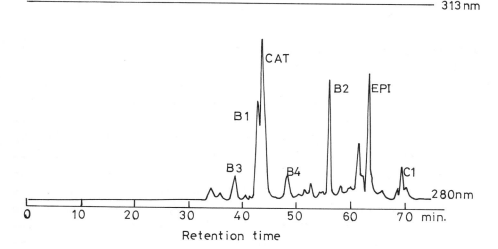

Fig. 1. HPLC chromatogram of a Vranac wine. CAT: (+)-catechin, EPI: (−)-epicatechin, B1: procyanidin B1, B2: procyanidin B2, B3: procyanidin B3, B4: procyanidin B4, C1: procyanidin C1. For separation conditions, see text.

3. RESULTS AND DISCUSSION

3.1 Extraction with ethanol

The results obtained in the extraction experiments carried out with Alicante-Bouschet seeds, using aqueous solutions containing 20, 40, 60 and 95% ethanol (by vol.) are given in table 2. As expected,

TABLE 2

Extraction of catechins and proanthocyanidins of Alicante-Bouschet seeds by using water/ethanol mixtures (mean values of three replications). Results are given in mg kg^{-1}.

ethanol (%)	time (hours)	CAT	EPI	B1	B2	B3	B4	C1
20	3	48	62	18	31	7	14	14
	6	184	250	73	96	35	48	95
	12	275	337	141	154	80	95	227
40	3	63	63	19	34	8	26	19
	6	289	374	122	206	73	152	228
	12	396	575	161	314	111	181	385
60	3	86	117	29	52	21	40	29
	6	328	493	147	279	89	189	341
	12	450	614	177	385	142	218	474
95	3	406	462	114	256	68	124	283
	6	451	618	200	453	126	235	516
	12	471	730	238	509	164	262	609

CAT: (+)-catechin; EPI: (-)-epicatechin; B1: procyanidin B1; B2: procyanidin B2; B3: procyanidin B3; B4: procyanidin B4; C1: procyanidin C1.

the extraction is more efficient when both the extraction time and the ethanol content of the extractant rise, but the extraction is not linear in any case. It is very low for the three hour experiments (except when 95% ethanol has been used), and it rises dramatically between three and six hours Although the extraction of catechins and proanthocyanidins improves between six and twelve hours, the increase in concentrations is not as high as it was between three and six hours. This can be explained by the time needed to soak the seeds with the extractant, and the effect of the extractant's saturation. As the extraction flasks remained undisturbed during the experiments, a diffusion equilibrium would be reached after a certain time, and the small increase in the extraction of catechins and proanthocyanidins between six and twelve hours in relation to that observed between three and six hours could be an index of the appearance of that diffusion equilibrium.

The results obtained in the two-way analysis of variance (table 3) have shown that there are significant differences at P=0.05 level among different times of extraction and also among different extractants. Thus, the efficiency of the extraction of catechins and proanthocyanidins of entire Alicante-Bouschet grape seeds can be considered a function of the extraction time and of the richness in ethanol in the extractant.

TABLE 3

Results of two-way analysis of variance (P=0.05) for the experiments carried out with Alicante-Bouschet seeds for periods of three, six and twelve hours using different ethanol/water mixtures.

Compound	Extraction time		Percentage ethanol	
	Sample F ratio[a]	LSD*	Sample F ratio[b]	LSD*
(+)-catechin	13.28	138	8.32	119
(-)-epicatechin	29.94	144	15.12	125
procyanidin B1	96.26	28	32.32	24
procyanidin B2	27.64	96	22.52	83
procyanidin B3	74.50	23	22.59	20
procyanidin B4	46.14	42	27.57	37
procyanidin C1	36.22	113	21.33	98

* expressed as mg Kg^{-1}
[a] Tabled F (P=0.05) for extraction time experiments: 5.14
[b] Tabled F (P=0.05) for percentage ethanol experiments: 4.76

3.2 Extraction with ethanol and tartaric acid

The results obtained in the experiments carried out with Chardonnay grape seeds show that the extraction of catechins and proanthocyanidins depends on the alcoholic degree and the content of tartaric acids of solution, and also on the extent of contact of the seeds with the extractant in some cases. Figure 2 shows the effect of alcoholic degree of solutions containing 4 g dm^{-3} of tartaric acid and of the extent of contact on the extraction of two major components of grapes seeds [(-)-epicatechin an procyanidin B2]. As can be noted, the amount of those substances extracted is higher after ten days, but in the case of procyanidin B2 there is not a significant difference at P=0.05 level between seven and ten days extraction, as has been shown by two-way analysis of variance. (table 4). Nevertheless, the increase of the content of tartaric acid in the extractant leads to a higher extraction efficiency, and there are significant differences at P=0.05 level in both cases (table 4). The other two major components [(+)-catechin and procyanidin B1] have shown a similar behaviour.

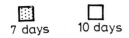
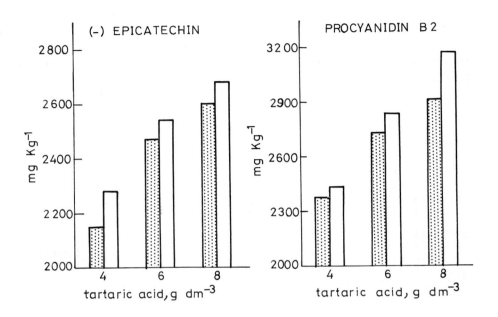

Fig. 2. **Extraction of (-)-epicatechin and procyanidin B2 from Chardonnay seeds using solutions containing 8% ethanol (by vol.) and different quantities of tartaric acid over seven and ten days.**

TABLE 4

Results of two-way analysis of variance (P=0.05) for experiments carried out with Chardonnay seeds, using solutions containing 8% ethanol (by vol.).

Compound	Extraction time		Tartaric acid	
	Sample F ratio[a]	LSD*	Sample F ratio[b]	LSD*
(-)-epicatechin	24.36	58	181.35	48
procyanidin B2	5.95	–	38.29	153

* expressed as mg kg^{-1}
[a] Tabled F (P=0.05) for extraction time experiments: 6.61
[b] Tabled F (P=0.05) for tartaric acid experiments: 5.14

A set of experiments was carried out for seven days with solutions containing 4 g dm^{-3} of tartaric acid and 8, 10 or 12% ethanol (by vol.). The four major components (procyanidin B1, procyanidin B2, (+)-catechin and (-)-epicatechin) have shown similar behaviour. The extraction efficiency rises with the alcoholic degree of solutions used in the experiment, see figure 3. The results of one-way analysis of variance have shown that there are significant differences at P=0.05 level in each case (table 5).

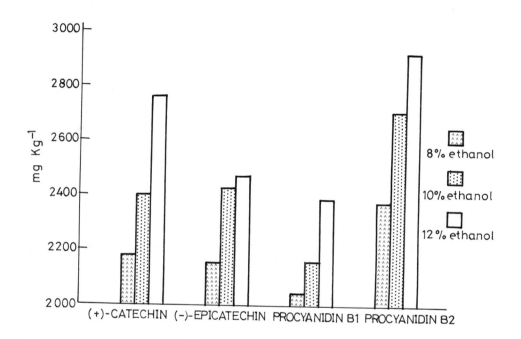

Fig. 3. Extraction of catechins and proanthocyanidins from Chardonnay seeds using solutions containing 4 g dm^{-3} of tartaric acid and different percentage of ethanol for seven days.

Supplementary experiments were carried out with different compositions of the extractant for 14 days. As a general rule, the amount of catechins and procyanidins in the extractant after that time was smaller than in the experiments carried out for seven or ten days. This fact is difficult to explain, but could be a consequence of condensation reactions which may take place in that media. Nevertheless, proving this hypothesis requires further research.

TABLE 5

Results of one-way analysis of variance (P=0.05) for experiments carried out with Chardonnay seeds using solutions containing tartaric acid (4 g dm^{-3}) and 8, 10 or 12% ethanol (by vol.) for seven days.

Compound	Sample F ratio[a]	LSD[b]
(+)-catechin	146.61	85
(−)-epicatechin	5.93	244
procyanidin B1	7.78	219
procyanidin B2	9.29	316

[a] Tabled F ratio (P=0.05): 5.14
[b] expressed as mg kg^{-1}

Anyway, the results obtained show that the concentration of organic acids in the extractant may affect the efficiency of the extraction of catechins and proanthocyanidins. So, the composition of grape musts may affect in some way the content of catechins and proanthcyanidins of wines in some way, as a consequence, the stability of colour and several related parameters.

3.3 Wines

As a general rule, the content of catechins and proanthocyanidins and other related parameters are higher in wines made with a higher quantity of pomace, when the extent of maceration is the same. If we compare the data corresponding to wines V-26, V-28, V-30 and V-32, which have been in contant with pomace for seven days, this fact may be clearly observed (Table 6).

A similar situation occurs when comparing the analytical data of wines V-29, V-31 and V-33, which have been in contact with pomace for 14 days (Table 7). These results show that the content of catechins and proanthocyanidins of wines is closely related to the quantity of pomace in contact with must during maceration, and that the presence of stems or of a suplementary quantity of seeds leads to wines richer in those compounds. However, if wines made with a similar quantity of pomace but with different extent of maceration are compared (e.g., wines V-28 and V-29, V-30 and V-31, and V-32 and V-33), the content of catechins and proanthocyanidins and other related parameters decrease with the extent of maceration, in a similar way to anthocyans (12). However, the decrease of catechins and proanthocynains may be due to reactions which lead to higher polymers, as mentioned above. Anthocyanins and acetaldehyde may be involved in these reactions (22). If we compare the experiments carried out with seven days of maceration using destemmed grape clusters, two parameters closely related to colour (colour intensity and free anthocyans) are higher in wines made with a supplement of seeds, and especially in those made doubling the quantity of seeds. In the same way, the addition of seeds leads to wines with a lower proportion of red monomers in relation to red and brown polymers, and this also shows that the addition of a supplementary quantity of seeds may be of interest in stabilitizing the colour of red wines.

TABLE 6

Some analytical data of Vranac wines made with seven days of maceration

	V-26	V-28	V-30	V-32
Colour intensity	1.463	1.428	1.795	1.540
Tint	0.62	0.63	0.59	0.61
Free anthocyans (mg dm^{-3})	360	260	320	230
Folin-Ciocalteau index	30.0	26.7	45.1	44.4
Tannic matter index	59.9	54.3	80.0	77.0
Red monomers (%)	51.3	44.4	35.5	35.5
Red polymers (%)	35.8	41.2	41.9	39.9
Brown polymers (%)	12.9	14.4	22.6	24.6
Total catechins and proanthocyanidins, colorimetric (mg dm^{-3})*	657	607	1154	2133
Total catechins and procyanidins, HPLC (mg dm^{-3})	437	322	566	794
(+)-catechin (mg dm^{-3})	120	95	135	208
(−)-epicatechin (mg dm^{-3})	66	61	86	101
Procyanidin B1 (mg dm^{-3})	105	36	116	159
Procyanidin B2 (mg dm^{-3})	66	62	106	148
Procyanidin B3 (mg dm^{-3})	29	21	33	55
Procyanidin B4 (mg dm^{-3})	26	29	48	66
Procyanidin C1 (mg dm^{-3})	25	18	42	57

* (+)-catechin equivalents.

The seven wines were submitted to a preliminary sensory evaluation by expert panelists. The best rating was obtained by wine

V-31 (made with destemmed grape clusters, doubling the quantity of seeds and with a pomace contact time of 14 days). These results suggest that the addition of a supplementary quantity of seeds may lead to more equilibrated wines, but this practice should probably be combined with a higher extent of maceration. Anyway, the influence of other enological practices, such as clarification or ageing, has not been taken into account, and these results must be validated by the sensory evaluation of finished wines.

TABLE 7

Some analytical data of Vranac wines made with 14 days of maceration

	V-29	V-31	V-33
Colour intensity	0.731	1.199	1.063
Tint	0.64	0.68	0.67
Free anthocyans (mg dm^{-3})	220	260	160
Folin-Ciocalteau index	18.3	30.8	31.0
Tannic matter index	38.0	57.5	57.5
Red monomers (%)	54.5	44.6	33.0
Red polymers (%)	34.5	39.5	42.7
Brown polymers (%)	11.0	15.9	24.3
Total catechins and proanthocyanidins, colorimetric (mg dm^{-3})*	497	1328	1672
Total catechins and procyanidins, HPLC (mg dm^{-3})	267	531	574
(+)-catechin (mg dm^{-3})	79	165	169
(−)-epicatechin (mg dm^{-3})	48	78	98
Procyanidin B1 (mg dm^{-3})	46	101	98
Procyanidin B2 (mg dm^{-3})	41	91	92
Procyanidin B3 (mg dm^{-3})	18	36	38
Procyanidin B4 (mg dm^{-3})	23	28	47
Procyanidin C1 (mg dm^{-3})	12	32	32

* (+)-catechin equivalents.

4. CONCLUSIONS

The experiments carried out with Alicante-Bouschet seeds obtained from pomace of thermovinification are a potential source of catechins and proanthocyanidins for various purposes. The use of ethanol/water mixtures appears to be of interest for the extraction of these compounds, and the efficiency of the extraction may be increased by mechanical stirring. However, the disolution of oxygen due to stirring may cause oxidative reactions which can reduce the efficiency of the process.

The presence of tartaric acid in the water/ethanol mixtures used for the extraction of catechins and proanthocyanidins from grape seeds affects its efficiency, which is increased when the concentration of tartaric acid rises. However, when the extent of maceration is longer than ten days, the extraction appears to be less efficient, and this phenomena may be due to the appearance of condensation reactions. This fact may be of importance to Enology, but their exact role requires further research.

The large-scale vinification experiments with Vranac red grapes show that the presence of an additional quantity of seeds during the fermentation with destemmed grape clusters may lead to wines with an improved sensory quality. The extent of maceration affects the final content of catechins and proanthocyanidins in wines, which is lower for wines which have been in contact with pomace for 14 days. This may be due to condensation reactions, and this may affect the stability of colour. The elucidation of this phenomena, which may be similar to that observed in the experiments of extraction with solutions containing tartaric acid mentioned above, requires further research.

ACKNOWLEDGEMENTS

The authors acknowledge financial support from Institut National de la Recherche Agronomique (France), and that of Ministerio de Educación y Ciencia (Spain) and Ministère de la Recherche et la Technologie (France) in the form of a MEC/MRT postdoctoral fellowship for one of as (E.A.).

REFERENCES

1. S. Uchida, R. Edamatsu, M. Hirazmatsu, A. Mori, G. Nonaka, I. Nishioka, M. Niwa and M. Ozaki, Med. Sci. Res., 15 (1987) 831.
2. J. Masquelier, Diétetique et Médecine, 14 (1989) 141.
3. J. Masquelier, Proc. Intern. Sympos. "L'alimentation et la consommation du vin", Verone, Italy, 1982, pp. 147-155.
4. T.N. Asquith and L.G. Butler, Phytochemistry, 25 (1986) 1591-1596.
5. J. Masquelier, Bull. OIV, 61 (1988) 554-556.
6. E. Haslam and T.H. Lilley, CRC Crit. Rev. Food Sci. Nutr., 27 (1988) 1-40.
7. V.L. Singleton and P. Esau, "Phenolic Substances in Grapes and

Wines, and Their Significance", Academic Press, New York, 1969.
8. M. Bourzeix, D. Weyland and N. Heredia, Bull. OIV, 59 (1986) 1171-1254.
9. V. Kovac, M. Bourzeix, N. Heredia and T. Ramos, Rev. Franc. Oenol., 125 (1990) 7-14.
10. E. Revilla, M. Bourzeix and E. Alonso, Chromatographia, (1991), in press.
11. V.L. Singleton, H.A. Sieberhagen, P. de Wet and C.J. van Wyk, Am. J. Enol. Vitic., 26 (1975) 62-69.
12. P. Ribéreau-Gayon, P. Sudraud, J.C. Milhé and A. Canbas, Conn. Vigne Vin, 4 (1970) 133-144.
13. M. Bourzeix, J. Mourgues and S. Aubert, Conn. Vigne Vin, 4 (1970) 447-460.
14. R.A. Arnold and A.C. Noble, Am. J. Enol. Vitic., 29 (1978) 150-152.
15. Y. Glories, Conn. Vigne Vin, 18 (1984) 253-271.
16. P. Sudraud, Ann. Technol. Agric., 7 (1958) 203-208.
17. P. Ribéreau-Gayon and E. Stonestreet, Bull. Soc. Chim. Fr., 9 (1965) 2649-2652.
18. V.L. Singleton and J.A. Rossi, Am. J. Enol. Vitic., 16 (1965) 144-158.
19. M. Bourzeix and N. Heredia, Feuillet Vert OIV nº 796 (1985).
20. E. Revilla, E. Alonso, M. Bourzeix and N. Heredia, Dev. Food Sci., 24 (1990) 53-60.
21. E. Revilla, E. Alonso, M. Bourzeix and N. Heredia, Feuillet Vert OIV nº 829 (1989).
22. P. Ribéreau-Gayon, in: P. Markakis (Ed), Anthocyanins as Food Colours, Academic Press, New York, 1982, pp. 209-244.

LOW-ALCOHOL CONTENT WINE-LIKE BEVERAGES. STORAGE STABILITY OF THOSE OBTAINED FROM DEALCOHOLIZED WINES.

M.D. SALVADOR [1](*), R. PEREZ [1], M.D. CABEZUDO[2], P. J. MARTIN-ALVAREZ[2] AND L. IZQUIERDO[1]

(1) Instituto de Agroquímica y Tecnología de Alimentos (CSIC), Jaime Roig 11, 46019 Valencia (Spain).

(2) Instituto de Fermentaciones Industriales (CSIC), Juan de la Cierva 3, 28006 Madrid (Spain).

(*) Current address: Facultad de Ciencias Químicas, Paseo de la Universidad 4, 13071 Ciudad Real (Spain)

SUMMARY

The problem of surplus wine production and falling overall wine consumption has led to the development of other possible alternatives. The trend towards the consumption of low-calory content beverages has prompted studies into the elaboration of new drinks derived from wine and/or grapes with low alcoholic content. Techniques of reducing the alcoholic content of wines are summed up.

The quality and stability of low-alcohol content beverages obtained from dealcoholized wine as affected by method of aromatization, preservation treatment and light were studied during storage for three months at 0º, room temperature and 37º. Beverages preserved by flash pasteurization (FP) or by amicrobic flitration (AF) were considered by the tasters better than those preserved by chemicals. Method of aromatization, recovered aromas (Beverage A) as opposed to original wine addition (Beverage B) affects slightly sensory quality. In general, Beverage A scores better than Beverage B. FP and AF beverages (A and B) stored in darkness at 0ºC did not show loss of quality after three months; at room temperature, they maintained their original quality intact for two months. No significant differences were observed between samples kept for one month, at room temperature, both in light and in darkness. More unfavorable conditions should be avoided.

1. STATE OF THE ART

For several decades now the wine-producing sector has been facing the serious problem of surplus production, aggravated by the worldwide trend in producing countries towards a reduction in consumption (1). Consumers' preference for fruity low-alcohol content wines has led to the manufacture of new beverages derived from wine and grape juice (2-6). This phenomenon can be partly explained by a change in life style, the dangers of alcohol when driving, and concern for health and keeping fit, together with a search for lower-calory food (7-9).

In 1970 the brewing industry launched the first alcohol-free and low-alcohol content beers, with the wine industry joining the light category later (10-12). The change in the North American market, with the appearance in California in 1983 of a new beverage called "wine cooler" (13, 14), is especially outstanding. "Wine coolers" are elaborated from a wine base, with blends of fruit juices, usually citrus fruits, and have a low alcoholic content, between 4º and 6º. These products are mild, refreshing and fruity, with a sugary aftertaste, and are generally of the sparkling type (15-17). There are other light beverages which are also obtained through dilution of wine: sangría and wine cocktails.

Another large group of low-alcohol content wine-like beverages is obtained through fermentation of the juice of grapes which have not ripened, and therefore have a low sugar content (18). It is also possible to use suitably ripened grapes and interrupt the fermentation with cold (19), or by centrifuging the yeasts (20) on reaching a moderate alcoholic grading (3%,v/v); this technique leaves an amount of remanent sugar which requires advanced technology to obtain a stable beverage. On the same lines, there have been proposals for the cryogenic concentration of grape juice to separate two fractions with different amounts of sugar and to ferment the one that is more suitable for obtaining a low alcoholic concentration (21). If it is wine that is frozen, two fractions are also obtained, one of which contains less alcohol and can be the object of later mixing with the original wine (22).

However, the most common technique employed is the elimination of the alcohol formed in fermentation, that is to say dealcoholization (23). The bibliography describes various ways of carrying out this process, but the main ones can be summed up as follows: extraction with suitable solvents, evaporating techniques, use of membranes (dialisis, inverse osmosis and pervaporation) and mixed techniques consisting of integrated operations (24-26).

The alcohol extraction mode with the greatest future is extraction with gases in supercritical condition (27-30), especially CO_2 (31-34), although this requires technology with high installation and running costs.

There is a very old precedent for use of evaporating techniques from 1908 (35) and they are without doubt the most widely used procedure nowadays to obtain light wines. As a general rule, it is prefered to work at reduced pressure so that evaporation is achieved at low temperatures. In order to do this, appropriate evaporators, vacuum distillation columns (36-45), film centrifugal evaporators (46-48) and some ones especially designed to direct the condensate's composition (49-53) are used.

The main advantages of this technique lie in the low evaporation temperature of the ethanol, which makes it possible for the wine extract not to suffer appreciable changes during the dealcoholization process, thus preserving its characteristic composition, sensorial notes, etc. Some authors, however, have noted some loss of aroma (54) as well as the risk of the appearance of a boiled taste (55) if the process is not carried out under good conditions.

Membrane technology has been successfully applied in the past few years as a substitute for conventional separation procedures. Semi-permeable membranes have been developed since 1970 which enable alcohol produced by fermentation to be separated satisfactorily (56).

Among membrane processes used in the dealcoholization of wines inverse osmosis (57-64), dialisis (55) and pervaporation (24,65,66) especially stand out. The main advantage of these processes is that work is carried out at a temperature of between 5º-10ºC and in this way heat damage to the product is avoided. However, these techniques require the use of selective membranes, with sound physico-chemical stability, and also a high flow of permeate. The use of membranes can cause problems of occlusion and slow incomplete filtration, which are countered by suitable choice of membranes or by their regeneration.

Light wine is above all a new product, which, from a sensorial point of view, possesses the characteristics of the original wine and grape juice. With the elimination of the alcohol a marked acidity and astringency may appear which must be countered by the addition of grape juice.

In some cases it is necessary to make up for loss of aroma with the addition of wine or recovered wine aromas.

In any case these beverages should be high quality (67-69), produced from appropriate technological processes, and should satisfy modern consumer taste, especially the young (70,71).

Since they are new, these beverages face a problem of identity, as well as a certain lack of credit for the term "light" because of the high number of dealcoholized products. For this reason there is a search for harmonization within the legal systems of the EC on the requirements that they should meet (72, 73).

From a technological point of view there is no one procedure that leads to the optimum beverage. Thus there is a tendency to combine the maximum number of advantages through the use of a mixture of procedures. The use of heat treatment and then membrane techniques to finish off is to be particularly recommended.

2. DEALCOHOLISATION OF COMMON SPANISH WINES BY THERMAL PROCESSING.

Since Spain is the third biggest wine producing country in the world, wine-derived drinks with low alcohol content have aroused logical interest. The best studied procedures have been the separation of fermentation alcohol by means of vacuum flash evaporation and by column distillation.

2.1 Dealcoholisation by flash evaporation

The choice of this process has been based on the good results obtained in dearomatisation of orange juice (74); orange juice is a heat-sensitive product as is wine. The method consists of evaporating part of the wine (ethanol, water and aroma) and afterwards, in a second stage, separating the aroma's components from the ethanol/water mixture. By using synthetic solutions of a similar composition to that of wine, an equation has been calculated which, when the quantity of alcohol in the batch of wine is known and the remaining alcohol which is requiered in the dealcoholised substrate, enables calculation to be made of the degree of evaporation to be applied.

$$y = 0.06\ x^2 - 4.35\ x + 103.2\ (r = 0.991) \qquad (42)$$

where: x = degree of evaporation
y = residual quantity of ethanol in the dealcoholized substrate.

Having carried out some experiments in dealcoholisation at various temperatures ranging from 35 to 90°C, the most satisfactory were obtained when working at intermediate temperatures, from 50°C to 70°C. Several writers have proposed similar temperature values (26,37,51).

The main advantages of the treatment are that it can be applied by stages, and it is an easy, quick and economical process (42).

2.2 Dealcoholisation by column rectification

Most known methods are with distillation equipment at low pressure and low temperature, protected by patents, and with little information known about them. The rectification column should have enough theoretical plates in order to achieve an efficient aroma enrichment. A heat exchanger heats the wine previously which feeds a 16 theoretical plate column (12 and 4 plates in the stripping and in the rectifying sections respectively) at two thirds height from the bottom. The vapor and the condensate travel up and down through plates to achieve the required aroma enrichment (43). Temperature equals 60°C allowed to obtain the best product from the sensorial point of view, as in similar situations (26, 32, 34, 46). A nonalcoholic fraction (aproximately, 1%, v/v) was obtained in only one stage and about a 50% of the wine volatiles remained in the condensed vapor from the top of the column (53).

The efficacy of the process depends on the degree of evaporation applied, so that with 15% evaporation the product is already dealcoholised. Installation is rather more costly and requires more careful maintennace than in the previous case. A comparative study between flash evaporation and column rectification enables the conclusion to be drawn that from these two procedures alcohol-free wines of similar characteristics were obtained, both from the chemical and sensory point of view (75).

Though light wines are products that have a short commercial life, it is of interest to find out when and in what conditions they can be kept in the stores, supermarkets, etc... without deteriorating. For this reason, various stabilisation procedures have been tried to avoid microbiological risks, and samples have been preserved cold and at rather higher temperatures, both in light and darkness, with the aim of establishing the influence on quality over time of all these circumstances.

3. MATERIALS AND METHODS

3.1 Raw material

White table wine, 11.9º (alcoholic content), from Turis (Valencia, Spain).

3.2 Equipment

Flash evaporation apparatus (Unipetkin P 20/5) modified by Salvador et al. (42) and distillation column (Unipetkin E 50) previously described (43).

3.3 Process

3.3.1 <u>Dealcoholization.</u> Wine was partially dealcoholized at 60ºC in the flash evaporator by evaporating 10.2% of its total volume. Alcoholic content of condensed vapours and of partially dealcoholized wine was 50.5º and 7.2º (alcoholic grading) respectively. In a second stage the partially dealcoholized wine was almost completely dealcoholized, 0.2 (%,v/v), in the distillation column at 60ºC by evaporating 19.7% of its volume.

3.3.2. <u>Rearomatization.</u> Two types of final beverages with about 5º (alcoholic grading) were prepared by aromatizing the dealcoholized wine through addition of a) the condensed fraction obtained in the flash evaporation, or b) original wine. In both cases the beverages were reconstituted with water up to their original volume and sweetened by addition of 21 g litre-1 of sucrose.

3.3.3. <u>Preservation treatment and bottling.</u> Three types of treatment to avoid microbial spoilage were performed: heat treatment, filtration and chemical preservation. In each case the beverages were bottled after treatment in glass bottles with crown caps. Bottles and caps had previously been sterilized.

a) Heat treatment. The beverages were heated to 92ºC for three seconds in a plate heat exchanger and immediately cooled in the final stage by exchange with water. Bottling was done in a sterile chamber with sterile air flow.

b) Filtration. The characteristics of the filtering equipment (Millipore) were: filterholder, 142 mm. diameter; filtration surface, 97 cm.2; 0.45 mesh (Durapore membrane); prefilter, AP 20. Bottling was carried out in the sterile chamber.

c) Chemical preservation. Sorbic acid (400 g litre-1) and benzoic acid (200 g litre-1) were added as potassium and sodium salts to the corresponding beverages.

3.4 Storage.

Beverages were stored at 0ºC and at room temperature. The influence of light during storage was also studied.

3.5 Chemical and microbiological analyses.

The following analyses, described elsewhere (42), were performed for all samples: alcoholic content, total acidity, volatile acidity, pH, Brix degree, hydroximethylfurfural, tartaric acid, malic acid and absorbance at 420 nm. Total cells (bacteria, yeasts and moulds) were also counted.

3.6 Sensory analysis

A 10-assessor panel evaluated the quality of the samples at the moment of bottling and after 1, 2 and 3 months of storage. In each taste-panel session the judges scored three samples according to a random block design on a scale from 1 to 5 points. The three types corresponded to the three types of preservation treatment (heat, filtration and chemicals), whereas aromatization type, temperature and storage time were the same for the three samples. All the necessary taste-panel sessions were conducted following this pattern (2 aromatization types, 2 temperatures, 4 storage times, and exposure or non-exposure to light). The scores obtained were subjected to analysis of variance study.

4. RESULTS AND DISCUSSION

4.1 Analytical characteristics of original wine and of low-alcohol content beverages

Table 1 shows the characteristics analyzed in the original wine and in the two resulting beverages flavoured by recovered aromas and by addition of the original wine respectively. The initial wine had an alcoholic content of 11.9º (%,v/v), whereas the two final beverages were adjusted to 5º (%,v/v); all other characteristics shown in Table 1 remained practically unchanged.

The composition of light wines tends to vary within very broad limits, from alcoholic grading, which can range between 4 and 7.5 or even higher, to pH, which in some cases reveals the presence of unripened grapes, e.g. values of 2.91, 2.99, 2.97 are reported by Amati (19) and Usseglio-Tomasset et al., (41), although it is more common for dealcoholized beverages' pH, and other conventional analyses, to stay close to those of a normal wine (76-78) as was the case in this study.

TABLE 1.
Analytical characteristics of the original wine and the two types of low-alcohol content beverages.

Analytical characteristics	Wine	Dealcoholized wine aromatized with recoverd aroma Beverage A	Dealcoholized wine aromatized with original wine Beverage B
Alcoholic content (%, v/v)	11.9	5.0	5.1
Total acidity^a	5.55	5.43	5.45
Volatile acidity^b	0.7	0.8	0.8
pH	3.6	3.5	3.6
oBrix	6.8	6.5	6.5
Hydroxymethyl-furfural^c	4.0	6.0	6.0
Tartaric acid^d	2.1	2.0	2.0
Malic acid^d	0.5	0.5	0.5

(a) g tartaric acid litre-1; (b) g acetic acid litre-1; (c) mg litre-1; (d) g litre-1.

Hydroxymethylfurfural content (Table 1) is slightly higher than in other cases (48), although the concentration of 4-6 mg litre-1 poses no problem.

4.2   Microbial content.

In the untreated wine 590 colonies per ml. of bacteria and 1480 of moulds and yeast were observed (Table 2). In flash pasteurized and filtered beverages no colonies were detected. Samples preserved with chemicals initially showed a minimal microbial content, which disappeared with storage. So, all preservation treatments studied rendered satisfactory results.

TABLE 2

Microbial content of original wine and beverages

Storage sample	Length of time stored	Microbial content (colonies/ml.)	
		Bacteria	Moulds and yeasts
Original wine (*)	0	590	1480
Flash pasteurized samples	1 month	nd(**)	nd
	2 months	nd	nd
	3 months	nd	nd
Filtered samples	1 month	nd	nd
	2 months	nd	nd
	3 months	nd	nd
Chemically preserved samples	1 month	18	36
	2 months	4	2
	3 months	nd	nd

(*) Before dealcoholization
(**) nd = not detected

4.3 Colour.

Absorbances at 420 nm were determined for all samples at each temperature and length of storage in dark rooms. Another set of samples had been stored at room temperature exposed to the effect of light. The absorbances of these samples were also analyzed and compared with those of samples stored in darkness at the same temperature.

Figure 1 shows that 420 nm absorption changes were not significant after 1 to 3 months storage in darkness at 0º and at room temperature. A higher storage temperature (37ºC) significantly increases absorbance value; these, however, are very unfavourable conditions for any food or beverage. Increases in absorbance are related to non-enzymatic browning.

Sunlight significantly enhanced absorbance at 420 nm of the samples stored at room temperature (Figure 2). This result was expected, given the new beverages' dependence upon common table wines.

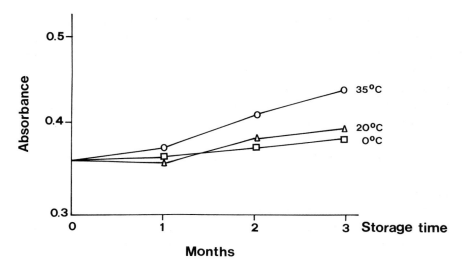

Fig. 1. Absorbances at 420 nm as affected by temperature and time

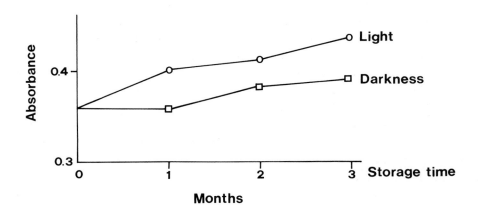

Fig. 2. Absorbances at 420 nm as affected by light. Samples stored at room temperature.

4.4   Sensorial Analysis.

4.4.1. Quality difference due to aromatization type. Analysis of variance, applied to the scores given by the tasters to the two beverages A and B (aromatized with recovered aromas or with original wine, respectively) and subject to the three preservation procedures shows significant differences in sensorial quality according to aromatization type and preservation procedure.

The upper part of Table 3 reflects the sensorial analysis of the samples just after they had been produced. In general, beverage A scores better than B, and the top score is for flash pasteurized beverage A; this is followed, in descending order, by filtered beverage A and beverage A with added chemical agents. The use of preservatives with a concentration of 160 to 770 mg litre-1 benzoic acid, or of around 200 mg litre-1 sorbic acid, each one together with SO_2 (78), is quite a widespread practice. The low scores awarded in this study by the tasters show that although the amounts used are legal, they are not to be recommended.

Very much the same can be seen with beverage B, which is similar, although somewhat inferior, in quality to A, and where the pasteurized samples score significantly higher than the others.

4.4.2. <u>Quality of beverages stored up to two months in different conditions</u> The results obtained from applying the analysis of variance again to the samples stored for 1 or 2 months in different conditions allow us to conclude (second part of Table 3) that both beverages, A and B, stabilized by any of the three procedures, maintain their original quality intact for two months, as long as they are stored in the dark; this is so whether they are stored at 0ºC or simply at room temperature.

4.4.3. <u>Sensorial control of beverages stored for 3 months</u>. All wines are very sensitive to the action of temperature and time. For this reason it is advisable to store them at temperatures below room temperature, and if they are common wines for the least time possible.

The simple act of dealcoholizing wine makes it much more vulnerable to the action of these factors (time and temperature), and so we should not have high hopes over these dealcoholized beverages' quality when they are kept for three months. In this study, however, it is our aim to obtain indicative data on their shelflife.

When we compare the data at the end of Table 3 (scores awarded by the tasters to the samples stored in darkness at room temperature and at 0ºC for 3 months) with the scores they awarded to the samples when they had just been bottled, significant changes for the worse in quality are observed.

It is obvious that although the beverages maintain their sensorial properties well for two months, if they are to be stored longer it must be at 0ºC and in darkness for quality not to fall significantly. It is observed again that the mixture of sorbic acid and benzoic acid is not suitable for this type of beverage.

TABLE 3

Mean values and standard deviation of quality scores awarded by 10-taster panel on 5-point scale.

Type of preservation	Dealcoholized wine aromatized with recovered aroma: Beverage A	Dealcoholized wine aromatized with original wine: Beverage B
Just-bottled beverages		
Flash pasteurization	3.87^a(0.81)^b	3.57 (0.77)
Amicrobic filtration	3.45 (0.91)	3.30 (0.90)
Chemical addition	3.10 (0.56)	3.00 (0.35)
Bottled samples stored up to two months in darkness		
Beverage A and beverage B, stabilized by any of the three procedures, maintain their original quality intact for 2 months when stored in darkness at 0ºC or at room temperature.		
Bottled samples stored up to three months in darkness		
Flash pasteurization 0ºC	3.50 (0.71)	3.42 (0.56)
Room temp.	2.78 (0.39)	3.00 (0.60)
Amicrobic filtration 0ºC	3.50 (0.92)	3.18 (0.64)
Room temp.	3.08 (0.70)	3.00 (0.71)
Chemical addition 0ºC	3.00 (0.62)	2.83 (0.86)
Room temp.	2.87 (0.63)	2.32 (0.68)

(a) mean value; (b) standard deviation.

In short, Fig. 3 shows that three months of refrigerated storage or two months at room temperature (in darkness) is the limit that must be adhered to in the marketing of these flash pasteurized or amicrobically filtered beverages.

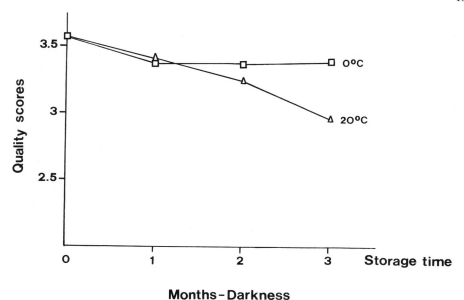

Months-Darkness

Fig. 3 Quality scores given by the tasters to pasteurized and filtered samples as affected by time and temperature.

TABLE 4

Quality score analysis of variance. Factors and interactions for which significant differences among samples were observed. Beverage A: dealcoholized wine plus its own aroma.

Source of variation	Sum of squares	Df	Mean square	Experim. F	Significance level
Exposure to light	2.72	1	3.72	8.40	* *
Time	6.31	2	3.15	7.12	* *
Time x preservation procedure	5.71	4	1.43	3.22	*
Exposure to light x preservation procedure	5.58	2	2.79	6.30	* *

At 95% confidence level, degree of freedom from error, 166. Residual variance, 0.44.

4.4.4. <u>The effect of light on sensorial characteristics</u>.
Since we were dealing with two beverages originating from wine it

was predictable that light would cause some deterioration in them. Nowadays there is no problem in getting hold of containers and packages that protect the contents from light. Some samples, however, were kept at room temperature and in light in order to discover how important it would be if these products eventually suffered the action of light during transport, in shop windows, etc.

The analysis of variance carried out on the samples stored in light and in darkness for 1, 2 or 3 months at room temperature showed significant differences in the tasters' ratings, and these must be attributed to the action of light, time and preservation procedure, both for beverage A (Table 4) and beverage B (Table 5).

TABLE 5

Quality score analysis of variance. Factors and interactions for which significant differences among samples were observed. Beverage B: dealcoholized wine plus original wine.

Source of variation	Sum of squares	Df	Mean square	Experim. F	Significance level
Time	21.41	2	10.70	26.90	* *
Preservation procedure	5.51	2	2.76	6.93	* *
Exposure to light	6.96	1	6.95	17.50	* *

At 99% confidence level, degree of freedom from error, 198. Residual variance, 0.63.

However, if we limit the experience to the samples kept for a month both in light and in darkness the differences observed between them are not very much important. Neither are there very high differences in respect of the recently-bottled beverages (Table 6).

5. CONCLUSIONS

The results presented in this paper allow us to expect that future drinks with a low alcoholic content and wine-like taste would be well accepted by potential consumers. Predictable acceptance is rather high, taking into account that wine consumer scores were about 3.6 on the scale used, which is equivalent to "like moderately". Such drinks would be obtained with relative ease, once the original wine had been dealcoholized. Aromatization could be achieved by addition of either recovered aromas or an appropriate amount of the original wine.

Table 6. Mean values and standard deviation of quality scores given by the 10 taster panel using 5 point scale. Just-bottled samples and samples stored for a month both in light and in darkness.

Type of preservation	Just-bottled samples		After one month.
	BEVERAGE A		
Flash pasteurization	3.87 (0.81)*	darkness light	3.60 (0.57) 3.05 (0.83)
Amicrobic filtration	3.45 (0.91)	darkness light	3.10 (0.66) 3.65 (0.47)
	BEVERAGE B		
Flash pasteurization	3.57 (0.77)	darkness light	3.50 (0.56) 3.30 (0.67)
Amicrobic filtration	3.30 (0.90)	darkness light	3.35 (0.67) 3.46 (0.62)

(*) standard deviation.

The resulting drinks should be protected from light to avoid changes in colour and off-flavour development. Flash pasteurization and amicrobic filtration of the drinks are a satisfactory guarantee of efficient microbiological preservation. From the sensorial point of view, both preservation procedures, followed by refrigerated storage, are preferable to chemical additions. Preservation period is three months (if pasteurized or amicrobic filtered and stored at 0ºC, in darkness), about two months at room temperature, and no longer than one month if exposure to light is not avoided. More unfavorable conditions are disapproved.

The technical characteristics of elaboration are quite similar to those followed in the industrial preparation of soft drinks.

ACKOWLEDGEMENTS

This work has been possible thanks to the financial assistance of the Spanish Comisión Interministerial de Ciencia y Tecnología (CICYT, Project ALI88-206).

REFERENCES

1. Anonimous. "World Drink Trends" NTC Publications Ltd, Oxon RG9 2BG (UK) 1990 edition.
2. E.A. Díaz Peralta, Bull. de l'OIV 53 num. 589 (1980) 224-237.
3. R. Bird, Soft Drinks Trade J. 38 (1984) 393-394.
4. B. Heilbuth, Hotelier and Caterer 19 (1986) 28-30.
5. E. Rivella, Vini d'Italia 28 (1986) 13-20.
6. E. N. Storchvoi, N.G. Sarichvili, N.N. Pavlenko, Bull. de l'OIV 685/686 (1988) 235-266.
7. H.Gounelle de Pontanel et P. Jaulmes, Med. et Nut. XIII (1977), 91-93.
8. E. Rivella, Vins moderns pour nouveaux consommateurs. Proceedings of Symposium Int. Consom. du Vin, March 15-19 (1982) 253-257.
9. M. Modot et J.-M. Mignomac, Rev. Francaise d'Oenologie, num. special, (1985) 72-73.
10. L.C. Jacobs, Food Development 15 (1981) 14-15; 18.
11. T. Stampft, Schweizerische Weinzeitung (20) (1983) 490.
12. D.L. Taylor, Food Engineering 55 (1983) 51.
13. A.S. Kiratsous, in: G. Charalambous (Ed.) Frontiers of Flavour, Elsevier Sci. Pub., The Netherlands (1988) 771-781.
14. L. Usseglio-Tommasset, M. Ubigli i R. Di Stefano, L'Enotecnico 25 (1989) 81-116.
15. L. Usseglio-Tommasset, L'Enotecnico 20 (1984) 435-438.
16. H. Petershans, German Fed. Republic Patent Application (1988) DE 37 22 535 A1.
17. R. Ferrarini i C. Riponi, Vignevini 14 (1987) 23-28.
18. H. Haushofer et W. Meier, Bull. de l'OIV 52 num.587 (1980) 40-48.
19. A. Amati, L'Enotecnico 20 (1984) 441-446.
20. C. Saez, P. Strehaiano, G. Goma et Y. Stilhart, Rev. Francaise d'Oenologie 26 (1986) 42-46.
21. T.R. Lang and D.J. Casimir, European Patent Application (1986) EP 0 177282 A2.
22. P.J. Vella, United States Patent (1985) US 4 468407
23. M. Christmann, Flüss. Obst. 53 (1986) 396-402.
24. R. Binnig, Flüss. Obst. 50, Heft 12 (1983) 666-669.
25. J.M. Barillere, J.L. Escudier, A. Samson, L. Angele et D. Thibert, Les techniques de dealcoolisation, in Institut Technique de la Vigne et du Vin, Collections Vignes et Vins, Les boissons nouvelles faiblement alcooliseés à base du vin,

(1987) 31-42.
26   A. Carnacini, N. Marignetti, A. Antonelli, N. Natali i S. Migazzi, Industrie delle Bevande XVIII (1989) 257-264.
27   A.B. Caragay, Perf. & Flavorist 6 (1981) 43-55.
28   D.R.P. Jolly, Process Biochem. Aug/Sep (1981) 22-34.
29   D.E. Blenford, The potential of Carbon Dioxide as an extraction solvent, in Progress in Food Eng. (Ed. C. Cantarelli) Foster Verlag, Kuesnacht (1983) 207-216.
30   E. Stahl and E. Willing, Pharm. Ind. 42 (1980) 1136-1139.
31   A. Muller, German Federal Republic Patent Application (1982) 3024055 A1.
32   F. Berger, B. Cerles et F. Sagi, French Patent Application (1983) FR 2 514781 A1.
33   A. Wiesenberger, R. Marr, E. Kolb, J.A. Schildmann und R. Weisrock, German Federal Republic Patent Application (1987) DE 35 42757 A1.
34   R. Zobel, E. Schutz, H.R. Wollbrecht und R. Faust, German Federal Republic Patent Application (1990) DE 38 43908 A1.
35   C. Jung, Schweizer (1908) Patent num. 44090 vom 6 März.
36   J.J. Thumm, Australian Patent (1975) 66 366
37   B.H. Deglon, Swiss Patent (1975) 564603
38   J.M. Hurley, UK Patent Application (1982) GB 2 084607
39   U. Schobinger, P. Durr, und R. Walvogel, Internationale Patentanmeldung (1982) WO 82/02723
40   A.R. Boucher, UK Patent Application (1987) US 4 643083.
41   L. Usseglio-Tommasset, M. Ubigli i R. Di Stefano, L'Enotecnico 22 (1986) 287-304.
42   M.D. Salvador, L. Izquierdo, M.I. Nadal y R. Pérez, Rev. Agroq. Tecnol. Alim. (Spain) 28 (1988) 261-273.
43   R. Pérez, M.D. Salvador, R. Melero, M.I. Nadal y F. Gasque, Rev. Agroq. Tecnol. Alim. (Spain) 29 (1989) 124-130.
44   R. Trothe, German Democratic Republic Patent (1990) DD 283153
45   S. Link, Weinwirtschaft-Technik 126 (1990) 14-15.
46   M.M. Pavlenko et V.V. Kiritsev, Method. Anal. de l'Office Int. Vigne et Vin, Doc. 1236 (1984) FV 782.
47   A.R. Boucher, United States Patent (1986) US 4 570534.
48   A.R. Boucher, (1984) GB 2 130497 A.
49   A.R. Boucher, German Federal Republic Patent Application (1985) DE 34 29777 A1.
50   G. Mehl, German Federal Republic Patent (1986) DE 3507150.
51   R. Poinsard et C. Pere-Lahaille, French Patent Application (1986) FR 84 11413.
52   A.R. Boucher, United States Patent (1988) US 4775538.
53   M.D. Salvador, L. Izquierdo, M.I. Nadal, R. Pérez, Rev. Agroq. Tecnol. Alim. (Spain) 29 (1989) 469-477.
54   U. Schobinger, Mitt. aus dem Gebiete der Lebens. und Hyg. 77 (1986) 23-38.
55   K. Wucherpfenning, K.D. Millies und M. Christmann, Weinwirschaft-Technik 122 (1986) 343; 348; 350-354.
56   E. Bermbach, K. W. Adler, und G. Burzle, German Federal Republic Patent Application (1975) 2 339206.
57   S.L. Matson, United States Patent (1988) US 4 778688.
58   Ph. Cuenat, D. Kolbe et J. Crettenaud, Rev. Suisse Vitic. Arboric. Hortic. 6 (1985) 367-371.
59   J.P. Bonnome, European Patent (1986) 0 078 226 B1.
60   J.M. Girard, Swiss Food 8 (1986) 27-30.
61   W. G. Light, United States Patent (1986) US 4 617127.

62 K. Bui, R. Dick, G. Moulin and P. Galzy, Am. J. Enol. Vitic. 37 (1986) 297-300.
63 J.M. Girard and P. Cuenat, PCT International Patent Application (1987) WO 87/03902 A1.
64 J. Dikansky et E. Terre, French Pattent Application (1989) FR 2620129 A1.
65 J.E. Escudier, Proceedings of the third Congress on Pervaporation, Ed. Bakish (1988) 387-397.
66 J.E. Escudier, Rev. des Oenologues (1991) 57-61.
67 R. Bini, Riv. Soc. Italiana Sci. Aliment. 5 (1984) 425-429.
68 U. Schobinger und P. Durr, Alimenta 22 (1983) 33-36.
69 N. Cavazzini, Riv. Soc. Italiana Sci. Aliment. 5 (1984) 429-439.
70 U. Schobinger, Zeitschrift für Obst- und Weinbau 119 (1983) 694-698.
71 Ph. Cuenat, D. Kolbe, Ch.-E. Bourgeois, Rev. Suisse Vit. Arboric. Hortic. 20 (1988) 155-159.
72 U. Schobinger, P. Durr und R. Waldvogel, Schweiz. Zeitschrift für Obst- und Weinbau 122 (1986) 98-110.
73 M. Christmann, Weinwirtschaft - Technik 125 (1989) 50; 52; 54; 58-59.
74 B. Lafuente, F. Gasque, M.I. Nadal y R. Pérez, Rev. Agroq. Tecnol. Alim. (Spain) 22 (1982) 560-574.
75 M.D. Salvador y R. Pérez, Rev. Agroq. Tecnol. Alim. (Spain) 30 (1990) 539-544.
76 Ch. Junge, Method. Anal. Office Int. Vigne et Vin, Doc. 1208/84 (1984) FV 774.
77 M.P. Sudraud, Method. Anal. Office Int. Vigne et Vin, Doc. 1210/84 (1984) FV 778.
78 P. Berta, Vignevini 16 (1989) 29-35.

SYNTHESIS OF OPTICALLY ACTIVE WHISKY LACTONE

Y. NODA, and M. KIKUCHI

Department of Industrial Chemistry, College of Engineering, Nihon University, Koriyama, Fukushima, 963 (Japan)

SUMMARY

The *cis*- and *trans*-5-butyltetrahydro-4-methylfuran-2-ones (=whisky or quercus lactones) have been identified as aroma components of aged alcoholic beverages such as whisky, brandy, and wine.

The optically active *cis*-whisky lactone have been prepared from (S)-(-)-1-(1,3-dithian-2-yl)-1-pentanol, which was obtained by the bakers yeast reduction of 1-(1,3-dithian-2-yl)-1-pentanone.

And key step lactonization employed intramolecular Wittig reaction.

INTRODUCTION

The optically active 4-substituted butanolides and but-2-enolides constitute not only versatile synthetic intermediates but are also stractural features of numerous natural products. For instance, these are found in flaver components and in insect sex pheromones.

Several methods of preparation of optically active 4-substituted butanolides and butenolides have been published.

The *cis*- and *trans*-5-butyltetrahydro-4-methylfuran-2-ones(=3-methyl octanolides)(1) have been found as aroma components of aged alcoholic beverages such as whisky, brandy, and wine[1]. These substances are extracted by whisky or other spirits from oak barrels

(1) trans whisky lactone   (1) cis whisky lactone   (2) cognac lactone

for maturing, they are known as whisky, oak, or quercus lactones[2].
Recently tetrahydro-4-methyl-5-pentylfuran-2-one(=3-methyl nonan-4-olide)(2) of the presumed *trans* configuration, has been detected in cognac and so reffered to as cognac lactone [3]. These substance as flavers are important.

We have been synthesized of insect pheromone *endo*-brevicomin [4] from (S)- α-hydroxy thioacetal(4) ,which was prepared by bakers yeast reduction of α-ketothioacetal(3).

We now report a simple and versatile synthesis of optically active *cis*-whisky lactone by using bakers yeast reduction of α-ketothioacetal(5).

RESULTS AND DISCUSSION

Our synthesis of whisky lactone 1 was straight forward, as illustrated in scheme 1.

The bakers yeast reduction of α-ketothioacetal 5 gave optically active (S)-(-)-1-(1,3-dithian-2-yl)-1-pentanol(6) in 50% yield {[α]$_D$ -30° (CHCl$_3$)}.

It was alkylated by 2-equivalent of n-BuLi and CH$_3$I to afford (7) in 75% yield.

But bakers yeast reduction of α-ketothioacetal(8) gave 7 only low yield.

7 was treated with bromoacetylbromide in the presence of pyridine in ether to give bromoacetate(9) in 70% yield {[α]$_D$ -11.1° (CHCl$_3$)}.

Treatment of 9 with neat trimethylphosphite at 110-120℃ for 3hr gave wittig reagent(10) in 80% yield {[α]$_D$ -11.1° (CHCl$_3$)}.

Hydrolysis of 10 with mercuric oxide and borontrifluoride-etherate in aqueous THF gave ketone(11) in 55% yield {[α]$_D$ -15.3° (CHCl$_3$)}.

scheme 1

Treatment of 11 with NaH in THF at 0 ℃ gave the intramolecular Wittig reaction product(12) in 80% yield. {[α]$_D$ +4.5° (MeOH)}.

Hydrogenation of 12 by sodium borohydride in the presence of nickel chloride in MeOH afforded the lactone 1 (cis:trans=85:15) Trans-1 was isolated by preparatire TLC, {[α]$_D$ -85° (MeOH), lit.[α]$_D$ -87° (MeOH)}.

The ^{1}H-NMR spectrum of the synthetic trans-whisky lactone 1 completely coincided with that of the natural one.

We are developing now synthesis of trans-whisky lactone 1 and trans-cognac lactone 2.

These synthetic route were straight forward, as illustrated in scheme 2.

scheme 2

REFERENCES
1) M. Masuda, and K. Nishimura, Chem. Lett. (1981), 1333-1336.   ref. cit. therein.
2) H. Tsukasa, Kouryou 158 (1988) 104 ref. cit. therein.
   C. Gunther, and A. Mosandl, Liebigs Ann. Chem. (1986) 2112-2122
   J. P. Marino, and R. Fernandez de la Pradilla, Tetrahedron Lett. 26 (1985) 5381-5384
   R. Bloch, and L. Gilbert, J. Org. Chem. 52 (1987) 4603-4605
   J. Salaun, and B. Karkour, Tetrahedron Lett. 29 (1988) 1537-1540
   R. M. Ortuno, R. Merce, and J. Font, Tetrahedron. 43 (1987) 4497-4506
   C. W. Jefford, A. W. Sledeski and J. Boukouvalas   Helv. Chim. Acta. 72 (1989) 1362-1370

M. Beckmann, H. Hildebrandt, and E. Winterfeldt Tetrahedron:Asym 1 (1990) 335-345

T. Ebata, K. Matsumoto, H. Yoshikoshi, K. Koseki, H. Kawakami, and H. Matsushita Heterocycles 31 (1990) 1585-1588

3) R. ter Heide, P. J. de Valois, J. Visser, P. P. Jaegers, and R. Timmer, in Analysis of Foods and Beverages, Ed. G. Charalambous, Academic Press, New York, 1978, p. 275.

4) Y. Noda, and M. Kikuchi Chem. Lett. (1989) 1755-1756

EFFECT OF COPPER, POTASSIUM, SODIUM AND CALCIUM. ON ALCOHOLIC FERMENTATION OF RAISIN EXTRACT AND SUCROSE SOLUTION

K. AKRIDA-DEMERTZI[1] AND A. A. KOUTINAS[2]
1: Department of Chemistry, University of Ioannina, P.O. Box 1186, 45110 Ioannina, Greece.
2: Department of Chemistry, University of Patras, 26110 Patras, Greece.

SUMMARY

The reduction of cell growth and fermentation rate. attributed to increase of uptake of copper, in the raisin extract alcoholic fermentation from batch to batch at the cell recycle method. at 50 ppm copper content is discussed. The effect of low concentrations of copper on biomass production as well as of copper in mixture with K, Na, Ca on cell growth and fermentation rate in the fermentation of synthetic media containing sucrose is also reported. Specifically, 5 ppm copper in the presence of K, Na, Ca at optimum concentrations 500 mg K_2O/100 g, 500 mg Na_2O/100 g. 1000 ppm Ca drastically reduces the fermentation time and increases the cell growth. Better fermentabillity observed in raisin extract compared with those obtained in synthetic media containing sucrose, may be due to the presence of Cu, K, Na, Ca at suitable concentrations. The reduction of the fermentation rate in the presence of copper was found (using ^{14}C-glucose) to be due to the reduction of glucose uptake rate.

INTRODUCTION

Raisin is used in Greece, as a raw material for potable alcohol production. According to our previous study (ref. 1) the trace element copper, a constituent of raisin, was shown to have an important inhibition effect on alcohol production. Although a number of publications have appeared discussing the effect of some trace elements in yeast cells. similar investigations concerning the trace element copper are not abundant in the literature. Specifically, the correlation between cadmium sensitivity and cadmium uptake in the strains of *S. Cerevisiae* (ref. 2), the effect of cadmium on growth and metabolism (ref. 3) as well as the different distribution of cadmium between cadmium-sensitive and cadmium-resistant strains of *S. Cerevisiae* has been discussed (ref. 4). Recently, the in vivo influence of cadmium, zinc. lead and mercury on the activities of intracellular enzymes in *S. Cerevisiae* has been studied (ref. 5). According to this work cadmium and lead cause a significant increase of the enzyme activity. while zinc and mercury do not affect the enzyme activity but intensify the effect of cadmium and lead. It is well known that the trace elements cobalt, zinc and iron promote the catalytic activity of enzymes of the yeast, whereas lead and cadmium are inhibitors (refs. 6, 7, 8, 9, 10).

Investigation of calcium and potassium, significant constituents of raisin has not been thoroughly covered in the literature. Many investigators have focused their interest in the study of the effect of calcium on alcoholic fermentation. Majorella and coworkers (ref. 11) showed that a concentration of 0.23 mol. L^{-1} calcium causes 80% reduction of cell growth. Relatively high concentrations result in an uptake by yeast cells that has a damaging effect (refs. 12, 13). According to Eilam (ref. 14) the rejection of calcium ion by *S. Cerevisiae* cells is correlated to its uptake of mono- and di-valent cations. Increased concentrations of phosphates in the fermentation media cause a reduction of the uptake of calcium (ref. 15). Calcium chloride does not affect the dehydrogenase activity but activates the enzyme decarboxylase of pyruvic acid (ref. 16). Furthermore, Norris and co-workers (ref. 13) reported that calcium protects yeast cells from the toxic effect of cadmium. Recently, the reduction of ethanol productivity and yield in *Zymomonas Mobilis* fermentation of glucose solution in the presence of calcium chloride was investigated (ref. 17). Finally, morphological changes were observed for *Z. Mobilis* (ref. 18) cells when the concentration of calcium chloride in the fermentation medium was higher than 30 mM.

Potassium and sodium are also components of raisin. Both of these elements have large significance in the life of cells. The aforementioned elements are contained in the ash of yeast (ref. 19).

On the basis of the bibliographical studies, presented above, one can conclude that a more detailed study of the effect of the trace element copper on alcohol production is necessary, since industrial ethanol production is realized by the use of the cell recycling method. The study of the effect of copper on this method is of great technological important. Likewise, the effect of metals such as calcium, potassium and sodium with or without correlation to copper is also necessary, because these elements are aboundant in raisin and other raw materials used in alcohol production.

The aims of the present investigation are to examine: (i) the effect of trace element copper on cell growth and alcohol production from raisin extract in the cell recycling method. (ii) the effect of the trace element copper on cell growth. (iii) the effect of copper in conjunction with metals such as potassium, sodium and calcium on alcohol production and cell growth.

METHODS

Preparation of raisin extract.

The extraction was carried out with hot water at 70 °C for 6h, using *Trechumena*, a Greek variety of raisin. A 5 L conical flask, loaded with the suitable amounts of pulpified raisin and distilled water, was placed in a water bath at 72 °C. The weight proportion raisin/water is related to invertsugar content in raisin extracts. The pH was adjusted to 3.2 with sulfuric acid.

Fermentation.

For batch cultivation, a fermenter of 1L capacity without stirring was used. The fermenter was loaded with 500 ml raisin extract with a density of 7 °Be. A solution of copper sulfate was added until the concentration of copper acquired the suitable value. Then 10 g pressed baker's yeast were added and the fermentation was carried out at 30 °C. After the end of the batch fermentation the culture was separated by centrifuge and when necessary, it was transferred to another fermentation batch (or batches) for further use.

Fermentations of sucrose solutions, with a density of 7 °Be were made at 30 °C, using *S. Cerevisiae* at the same concentration of cell as described above. A series of batches containing different concentrations of copper were fermented. Also fermentations were carried out in the presence of 500 mg K_2O/100 g or 500 mg Na_2O/100 g or 1000 ppm Ca. and in addition in the presence of 5 ppm copper with 500 mg K_2O/100 g and 500 mg Na_2O/100 g and 1000 ppm Ca. The pH was adjusted to 4.7 with sulfuric acid.

Ethanol Determination.

The ethanol concentration was determined using a gas chromatograph (Varian, model 3700) and porapak Q as column material with nitrogen as carrier gas (40 ml/min). The ethanol yield factor was calculated as the ratio of g ethanol/g of utilized sugar. The ethanol productivity was calculated as the g of ethanol produced per L per 24 h.

Biomass Estimation.

The biomass was determined by measuring the optical density at 700 nm. Standard curves of optical density vs wet weight (g/L) were prepared for the estimation of the biomass concentration in the sample.

Residual Sugar.

The amount of invertsugar that was not consumed during fermentation was determined using the well known Lane-Eynon analytical procedure (ref. 20). Residual sucrose was estimated by the same method after sucrose hydrolysis by hydrochloric acid solution in hot water.

Uptake of copper.

The determination of copper was carried out by atomic absorption spectrometry, using a Perkin Elmer, model 560 spectrophotometer, acetylene-air flame and copper hollow cathode lamp. The analysis was made in the ash of the yeast used.

Uptake of Glucose.

A culture of *S. Cerevisiae* prepared according to method described in the next experimental section was employed. Aerobic fermentations were carried out to determine the concentration of glucose in which the higher uptake of ^{14}C-glucose was obtained. This concentration was found to be 1000 nM. At this concentration aerobic fermentation experiments were made in the presence of ^{14}C-glucose using the following concentrations of copper: 0, 0.2, 1, 3, 5, 7, 10 and 15 ppm. In these fermentations using a suitable concentration of copper, samples were collected and the ^{14}C-glucose uptake were measured, at *S. Cerevisiae* cells obtained after filtation of samples, using the scintillation counter, Intertechnique SL 3000. The glucose uptake rate was calculated as nM glucose per min and mg dry weight *S. Cerevisiae* cells.

Growth of cultures.

Using baker's yeast a mono-cell culture was isolated and was grown on complete medium containing yeast extract agar (ref. 21). This was inoculated in a minimal liquid medium. The culture was employed in alcoholic fermentations of sucrose solutions in the presence of Cu, Ca, K, Na and their mixtures.

Determination of Potassium, Sodium and Calcium in raisin.

The treatment of samples was carried out according to our recent study (ref. 1) and the determination of K and Na was made by flame photometry, using a flame photometer Turner model 510. Calcium was determined by atomic absorption spectrometry with a Perkin Elmer instrument model 560, air-acetylene flame and hollow cathod lamp. To avoid interferences of phosphates, sulfates, aluminium and silicon, a solution of La_2O_3 treated with hydrochloric acid was used (ref. 23). This solution was added to the solution of samples in a proportion of 0.1 to 1%. For the preparation of the La_2O_3 solution, 58.64 g La_2O_3 were added to 50 ml distilled water and treated with 250 ml hydrochloric acid. This solution was diluted to 1 L.

RESULTS AND DISCUSSION.

Effect of Copper on Fermentation of Raisin Extract in Cell Recycle Method.

The fermentation of raisin extract was studied in batch system with industrial ethanol production standards. In Greece, the cell recycle method is used in raisin extract industrial scale alcoholic fermentation. The effect of copper concentration on fermentation kinetics and cell growth in the case of raisin extract medium employing the cell recycle method, is presented in figures 1 and 2 respectivelly. In figures 1 and 2 one can also observe fermentation kinetics and cell growth at the same copper content when the same yeast culture was recycled in a series of three fermentation batches (1st, 2nd, 3rd). Specifically, in Fig. 1 it is observed that the fermentation rate and fermentation time show no significant differences at copper content 5 and 50 ppm in the first fermentation batch. This difference becomes larger at 50 ppm copper content when the same yeast culture is used in the 2nd and 3rd fermentation batches. On the basis of data presented in fig. 2 one may conclude that the rate of cell growth decreases as the trace element copper content increases from 5 to 50 ppm. The decrease becomes larger in the case of 50 ppm when the same yeast culture is used in the 2nd and 3rd fermentation batches.

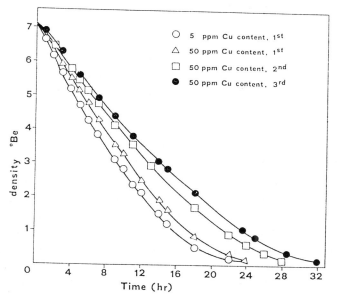

Figure 1. Kinetics of alcoholic fermentation of raisin extracts at different concentrations of copper in three fermentation batches with cell recycle.

An inspection of Table 1 and Figs. 1 and 2 shows that the increase of fermentation time, the decrease of the fermentation rate and the decrease of the rate of cell growth are related to the increase of the uptake of copper. The uptake increases as the same yeast culture is used continuously in repeated fermentation batches. Ethanol yield factor and ethanol productivity are lower when the uptake of copper increases (Table 1).

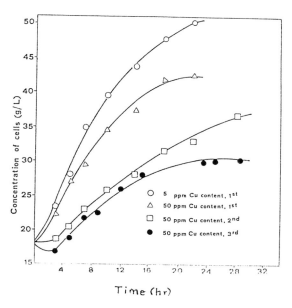

Figure 2. Concentration of cells vs time in the alcoholic fermentation of raisin extracts at different concentrations of copper in three fermentation batches with cell recycle.

Effect of copper content on cell growth and ethanol yield in fermentation of sucrose.

Fig. 3 illustrates the effect of copper content, on cell growth. One can observe that the biomass increases, in the case of sucrose synthetic media, as the concentration of copper increases from 0 to 10 ppm. For larger copper contents the biomass is reduced. A analogous behavior is also observed in ethanol production yield (Fig. 4). From the presentation of results in figs. 3 and 4 one may conclude that the biomass, as well as the ethanol yield, fall after an uptake of copper (100 ppm) by the yeast cells. Furthermore, fig. 4 shows the increase of uptake of copper with the increase of copper concentration. These results are analogous to those presented in a recent study of ours (ref. 1) concerning the effect of copper on alcoholic fermentation rate. The reduction in cell growth, ethanol yield

Table 1. Uptake of copper in the alcoholic fermentation of raisin extracts by cell recycle, as related to ethanol yield, productivity and cell growth.

batch	Concentration of copper (ppm)	Uptake of copper (ppm)	Fermentation time (h)	Ethanol productivity (g/L/24h)	Ethanol yield factor (g/g)	Cell growth (g/L)
1st	5	-	22	56.3	0.47	30.0
1st	50	203* 602	22	56.3	0.47	22.0
2nd	50	953	28	45.8	0.45	17.0
3rd	50	1276	29	44.4	0.44	16.6
4th	50	1413	32	37.5	0.43	11.0

* In the case of raisin extract fermentation baker's yeast is used.

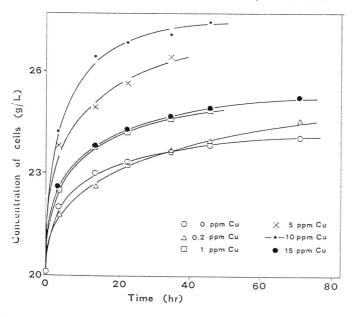

Figure 3. Concentration of cells vs time in the alcoholic fermentation of synthetic medium of sucrose carried out at various concentrations of copper.

and ethanol production rate is due to the reduction of glucose uptake rate resulting from the increase of copper concentration, as presented in fig. 5.

Effect of copper in the presence of the metals K. Na and Ca.

Since molasses and raisins are used as raw materials molasses in Greece in ethanol production, which are rich in metals such as K, Na, Ca (Tables 2 and 3), a detailed study of the alcoholic fermentation in the presence of copper and the metals K, Na and Ca in mixture or in the presence of the metals K, Na and Ca separately is also necessary.

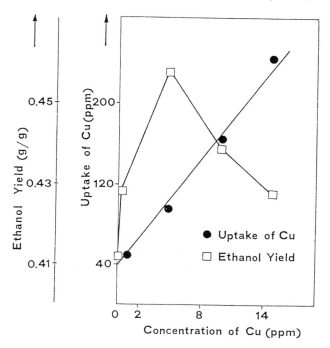

Figure 4. Uptake of copper and ethanol yield vs concentration of copper in alcoholic fermentation of synthetic medium of sucrose.

Fig. 6 indicates that a low copper concentration (5 ppm) increases the fermentation rate and reduces the fermentation time from 115 h to 37 h in the case of sucrose. The fermentation time was further decreased to 22 h when the fermentation was carried out in the presence of Cu, K, Na, Ca at concentrations shown in fig. 6. Furthemore, copper and the other metals mentioned significantly increase the cell growth, as illustrated in fig. 7. These results of the fermentation of raisin extract showed similar differences with those of sucrose solution (fig. 1 and fig. 6). The fermentation rate in the case of raisin extract, rich in copper and the metals K, Na and Ca, is higher than those of sucrose. Similar results were obtained for biomass (fig. 2 and fig. 7). Specifically, the concentration of cells is higher

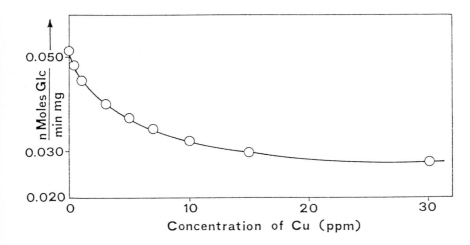

Figure 5. Glucose uptake rate by *S. Cerevisiae* vs concentration of copper in synthetic media containing glucose and ^{14}C-glucose.in raisin extract as compared to that in sucrose.

in raisin extract as compared to that in sucrose.

Fig. 8 illustrates that the metals K, Na and Ca, used separately in the fermentation of synthetic medium of sucrose, lead to a reduction of fermentation time as compared to the fermentation of synthetic medium of sucrose without these metals. Potassium has a major effect in the reduction of fermentation time. Similar results, presented in fig. 9 were obtained for cell growth. Potassium increases the cell growth more than sodium and calcium.

In Fig. 10, one observes that the fermentation time, in the fermentation of synthetic media containing sucrose, decreases as the concentration of K, Na, Ca used separately increases from 0 to 500 mg K_2O or Na_2O/100g and from 0 to 1000 ppm Ca. At higher concentrations of the aforementioned metals the fermentation time increases. The concentrations of K, Na, Ca mentioned above are optimum for the alcoholic fermentation of synthetic media containing sucrose.

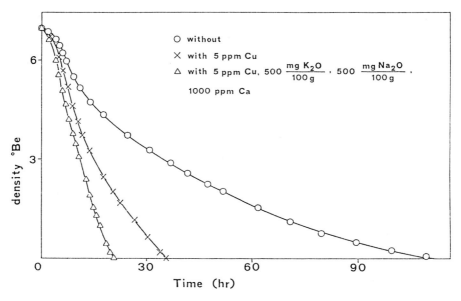

Figure 6. Effect of copper and the metals K, Na and Ca in mixture, on alcoholic fermentation of synthetic medium containing sucrose.

Table 2. Concentrations of K, Na and Ca in Greek molasses.

Sample origin	K (mg K_2O/100g)	Na (mg Na_2O/100g)	Ca (ppm)
Plati	3385.7±29.8	1560.0±18.7	5160±40.3
Xanthi	3342.0±28.4	1466.9±16.9	2284.8±35.6
Larissa	2795.7±21.5	1340.4±16.5	3608.0±35.4
Serres	1486.8±18.7	1914.1±17.2	2947.9±30.6
Orestiada	525.2±16.3	1738.7±16.3	2535.7±42.1

The results of the fermentation of raisin extract as compared to those achieved for synthetic medium of sucrose are in excellent agreement with the results reported in a recent study (ref. 22) for *Z. Mobilis*. The better results obtained for *Z. Mobilis* in the raisin extract as compared to those of synthetic media, were attributed to an unidentified factor. The results presented in this study lead to the conclusion that the

Table 3. Concentration of K, Na and Ca in various kinds of Greek raisin.

Sample kind	K (mg K_2O/100g)	Na (mg Na_2O/100g)	Ca (ppm)
Trechumena	546- 964*	19-37	1117-1634
Chondrada	746- 823	17-35	1510-1793
Piotiki dialogi	792- 842	24-43	1610-1949
Psila	757-1027	20-51	1827-3870

* Concentration ranges were obtained in all cases, from analytical results of samples collected from 5 different areas of Greece.

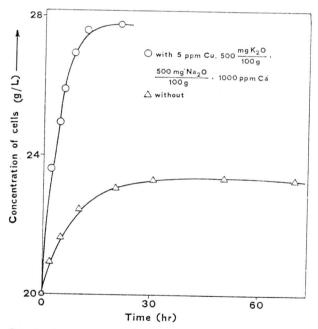

Figure 7. Effect of copper and the metals K, Na and Ca in mixture, on cell growth in alcoholic fermentation of sucrose solution

presence of Cu, K, Na and Ca in mixture and in suitable concentrations is the reason for the better vitality of cells (*Z. Mobilis* and *S. Cerevisiae*) and higher fermentation rates, in comparison to those obtained in synthetic media.

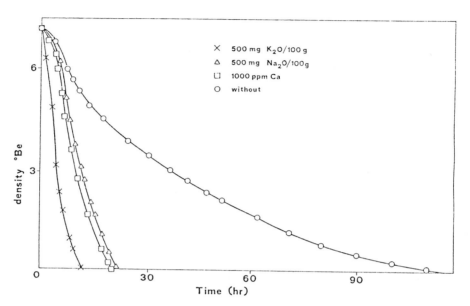

Figure 8. Kinetics of alcoholic fermentation of synthetic medium containing sucrose carried out in the presence of K or Na or Ca as compared to those obtained in their absence.

CONCLUSIONS.

Relatively high concentration of copper in raw material (raisins) of alcohol production leads to a reduction in number of fermentation batches in cell recycle method due to high uptake of copper by the yeast cells. Low concentrations of copper increases the cell growth. Also a low concentration of copper in the presence of the metals K, Na, Ca further decreases the fermentation time with an increase in cell growth. The presence of Cu, K, Na, Ca at suitable concentrations in raw materials for alcohol production is of great significance for their fermentability. The optimum concentrations of K, Na and Ca in the alcoholic fermentation are 500 mg K_2O/100 g, 500 mg Na_2O/100g and 1000 ppm Ca.

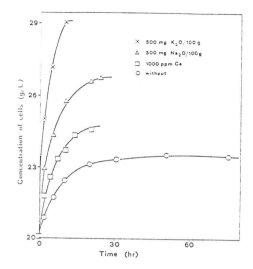

Figure 9. Cell growth vs time in the alcoholic fermentation of synthetic medium containing sucrose carried out in the presence of K or Na or Ca compared to those obtained in their absence.

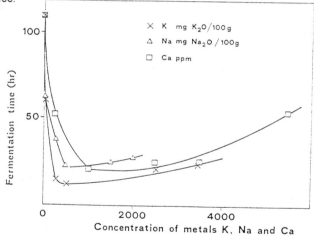

Figure 10. Fermentation time vs concentration of the metals K, Na and Ca in the alcoholic fermentation of synthetic media containing sucrose, carried out in the presence of the metals mentioned above, separately.

REFERENCES.
1. K. Akrida-Demertzi, P. G. Demerztis and A. A. Koutinas, PH and trace elements content in raisin extract industrial scale alcoholic fermentation, Biotechnol. and Bioeng. 31(7), (1988) 666-669
2. M. Joho, Y Sukenobu, E. Egashira and T. Murayama. The correlation between Cd^{2+} sensitivity and Cd^{2+} uptake in the strains of *S. Cerevisiae*. Plant and Cell Physiology, 24(3), (1983), 389-394.
3. L. Berthe-Corti, I Pietsch, M. Mangir, W. Ehrlich und E. R. Iochmann, Die Wirkung von Cadmium auf Wachstum und Stoffwechsel von *Saccharomyces* und *Rhodotorula*-Zellen. Chemosphere, 13(1), (1984), 107-119.
4. M. Joho, M. Imai and T. Murayama, Different distribution of Cd^{2+} between Cd-sensitive and Cd-resistant strains of *S. Cerevisiae*. Journal of General Microbiology. 131, (1985), 53-56.
5. H. Grafl und Schawantes, Der Einfluss von Cadmium, Zink, Blei und Quecksilber auf die Enzymaktivitat bei *S. Cerevisiae* in vivo. Zentralblatt für Mikrobiologie, 140. (1958), 3-11.
6. A.H. Cook, The chemistry and Biology of Yeasts, Academic Press, New York, (1958), 535-579.
7. I. Veliky and S. Jozei, Effect of cobalt on the multiplication of *S. Cerevisiae*. Naturwissennschaften. 51(21). (1964). 518-519.
8. R. Heldwein, H. W. Tromballa und E. Broda, Aufnahme von Cobalt, Blei und Cadmium durch Backehefe. Zeitschrift für Allgemeine Mikrobiologie, 17(4), (1977), 299-308.
9. A. I. Khrycheva, Effect of trace elements on the growth of *S Cerevisiae* biomass, Prikladnoj Biokimii Mikrobiologii. 6(3), (1970), 307-312.
10. M. L. Failla C. D. Benedict and E. D. Wainberg, Accumulation and storage of zinc by *Candida Utilis* Journal of General Microbiology, 94, (1976), 23-36.
11. B. L. Maiorella, H. W. Blanch and C. R. Wilke, Feed component inhibition in ethanolic fermentation by *S. Cerevisiae*. Biotechnology and Bioengineering, 26, (1984), 1155-1166.
12. G. M. Roomans, A.P.R. Theuvenet, T.P.R. Van Den Berg, G. W. G. H. Borst-Pauwels, Kinetics of Ca^{2+} and Sr^{2+} uptake by yeast. Effect of pH, cation and phosphate, Biochimica et Biophysica Acta, 551(1), (1979), 187-196.
13. P. R. Norris and D. P. Kelly, Accumulation of cadmium and cobalt by *S. Cerevisiae*, Journal of General Microbiology. 99(2), (1977), 3127-324.
14. Y. Eilam, The effect of potassium ionophores and potassiumon cellural calcium in the yeast *S. Cerevisiae*. Journal of General Microbiology, 128, (1982), 2611-2614.
15. J. Dyr, J. Fabianova and M. Rychtera, Regulation of ethanol and biomass formation during ethanol fermentation. The relationship between ethanol production and the growth of biomass in anaerobic process during stationary cultivation. Sbornik Vysoke skoly chemico-technologicke v Praze Potraviny, E31, (1971), 41-62.
16. T. C. Hoppner and H. W. Doelle, Purification and Kinetic characteristics of puruvate decarboxylase and ethanol dehydrogenase from *Z. Mobilis* in relation to ethanol production, European Journal of Applied Microbiology and Biotechnology, 17, (1983), 152--157.
17. P. K. Bajpai, J. B. Wallace and A. Margaritis, Effect of calcium chloride concentration on ethanol production and growth of immobilized *Z. Mobilis*, Journal of Fermentation Technology, 63(2), (1985), 199-203.
18. N. Stevnsborg and H. G. Lawford, Effect of calcium on the performance and morphology of *Z. Mobilis* ATCC 29191 in continuous ethanol fermentations, Biotechnology Letters, 8(3), (1986), 181-186.
19. A. H. Cook, The Chemistry and Biology of yeast, Academic press, New York, (1958), 535-579.
20. H. Egan, R. S. Kirk and R. Sawyer, Eds. Pearson's Chemical Analysis of Foods, 8th ed. Churchill Livingston Edinburg, (1981), 150-189.
21. H. Gutz, H. Heslot, U. Leupold and N. Loprieno. Handbook of Genetics, 1, Ed.: King R., C Plenum, New York and London. Chapter 25, (1974), 395-446.

22 A. A. Koutinas, M. Kanellaki, M. A. Typas and C. Drainas. Raisin a suitable raw material for ethanol production using *Z. Mobilis*. Biotechnology Letters, 8(7), (1986), 517-520.
23 S. L. Sang, W. C. Sheng, H. I. Shiue and H. T. Cheng. Direct determination of trace metals in cane juice, sugar and molasses by atomic absorption spectrophotometry, Taiwan Sugar, 23(1), (1976), 22-28.

G. Charalambous (Ed.), Food Science and Human Nutrition
© 1992 Elsevier Science Publishers B.V. All rights reserved.

MICROBIOLOGICAL CHANGES DURING THE RIPENING OF TURKISH WHITE PICKLED CHEESE

M. KARAKUŞ and I. ALPERDEN

TUBITAK, Department of Nutrition and Food Technology, P.O. Box 21, 41470 Gebze-Koacaeli, Turkey

1. INTRODUCTION

White pickled cheese, with an annual production of over 130,000 tonnes, stands out as the main cheese variety in Turkey Similar cheeses are extensively manufactured in the other Balkan and Middle-Eastern countries (1,2).

In Turkey as well as in some other countries, the manufacturing procedure for this type of cheese is not uniform and varies with locality and tradition. Originally Turkish white pickled cheese is manufactured from sheep's milk but nowadays cow's milk and the mixtures of both are also frequently used.

As this cheese is produced mostly by traditional methods, many problems are encountered such as non-uniform quality, flavour and texture defects. These problems are partly attributable to the fact that this kind of cheese are usually made from unpasteurized milk without the use of specific starter culture, which leads to unpredictable biochemical and microbiological changes during manufacture and ripening.

The manufacture of any kind of high quality cheese is primarily dependent on controlled fermentation of milk constituents. Degradation of lactose, fat and proteins at a certain level is necessary to obtain the desired characteristics. It is therefore essential to find out the microbial flora involved in the manufacturing and ripening processes of cheese in general, in order to prepare a specific starter culture for industrial production.

Some microbiological studies have been conducted on white pickled cheese varieties produced in different countries (1). However very scant data are available on microbiological changes which take place during the manufacturing and ripening of traditionally made Turkish white pickled cheese (3).

The present work was undertaken to follow the evolution of main groups of microorganisms and to identify lactic acid bacteria species involved in the manufacturing and ripening processes of this kind of cheese.

2. MATERIALS AND METHODS

2.1 Cheesemaking procedure

Two batches of Turkish white pickled cheese were made

according to the traditional method from raw cow's milk. Forty liters of milk obtained from a local dairy was heated to 30°C. Coagulation took place in 90 minutes after addition of rennet. The curd was cut in 1 cm cubes, left to stand for 15 minutes, transferred to a cheese-cloth lined mould. Drainage took about 4 hours. For 1 hour the curd was allowed to drain naturally, but subsequently a weight equal to the curd weight was applied. Pressed curd from the mould was then cut into rectangular pieces (8x8x7 cm), put into a brine solution of 14 % NaCl and kept overnight. Cheese blocks were then transferred into tins of about 3 kg capacity, and covered with brine. The tins were sealed and kept at ambient temperature for two days. Finally, cheese was ripened in a cold store at 5°C for 4 months.

Samples taken for microbiological and chemical analyses during manufacture were milk, curd, pressed curd and cheese on the 1st day following brining and after 15th, 30th, 60th, 90th and 120th days of ripening.

2.2 Microbiological analyses

Milk was homogenized with pepton containing physiological saline and the curd and cheese samples with 2 % sodium citrate solution (4). Dilutions of the milk, curd and cheese homogenates were plated on different selective media in order to determine the numbers of the various groups of microorganisms. The media and the incubation conditions used for different groups of microorganisms were as follows:

Total viable count on Plate Count Agar at 32°C for 48 h.
Lactic streptococci on M-17 Agar at 30°C for 48 h.
Lactobacilli on Rogosa Agar at 30°C for 72 h.
Enterococci on Slanetz-Bartley Agar at 45°C for 48 h.
Coliforms on Violet Red Bile Agar at 30°C for 24 h.
Micrococaceae on Mannitol Salt Agar at 37°C for 48 h.
Yeasts on Oxytetracycline Glucose Yeast extract Agar at 25° for 5 days.

Results are expressed as c.f.u./ml for milk and c.f.u./g for curd and cheese samples.

2.3 Identification of lactic acid bacteria

About 20 % of the colonies were picked from the M-17 agar and Rogosa agar plates using Harrison's disc procedure (5). The strains isolated were purified and identified using the criteria of Sharpe (6), Deibel and Seeley (7), Rogosa (8), and Garvie (9).

2.4 Chemical analyses

Samples of milk, curd, pressed curd and cheese were analysed for pH, total solids and salt content. Determination of total solids was carried out by heating the sample at 105°C to constant weight; pH using a combined electrode pH-meter (Metrohm 632); and salt content by the Mohr method.

3. RESULTS AND DISCUSSION

Figure 1 shows that the variations of the different groups of microorganisms followed similar patterns during manufacture and ripening process in both batches of white pickled cheese.

The total viable count which is indicative of overall changes of the microflora is found to be about 10^6 and 10^5 c.f.u./ml in raw milks used in Batch 1 and 2 respectively. In one-day-old cheeses the number reached about 10^9 c.f.u./g and then a slight decrease was observed due to the development of acidity, salt content, and other changes in the ripening cheese (Table 1).

TABLE 1
Changes in total solids, pH and NaCl content in milk (M), curd (C), pressed curd (PC) and cheeses from batches 1 and 2 during ripening over 120 days.

Samples (days)	Total solids (%)		pH		NaCl (%)	
	Batch 1	Batch 2	Batch 1	Batch 2	Batch 1	Batch 2
M	11.0	12.0	6.72	6.82	–	–
C	11.4	12.0	6.42	6.66	–	–
PC	39.5	42.6	5.56	5.44	–	–
1	40.2	40.3	5.47	5.17	3.67	3.20
15	39.6	41.4	5.12	5.16	2.97	3.88
30	39.4	37.6	5.17	5.02	3.66	4.34
60	38.5	37.2	5.23	5.26	3.65	4.11
90	41.6	38.4	5.11	5.17	3.67	4.11
120	40.1	38.4	4.80	4.86	3.65	3.74

Lactic streptococci were found to be the predominating organisms during the whole process. It is well known that these organisms play a basic role in the manufacture of most of the cheese varieties by bringing about acidification of milk and cheese through lactic fermentation. As in the case of total viable count, the number of lactic streptococci increased considerably during the manufacture, attaining a maximum in the first days of the ripening period. Then they declined slowly until the end of this period. Ergüllü (3) observed similar trends in the number of streptococci in commercially made Turkish white cheese samples. Also Lomsadze et al.(10) and Rasic (11) found that these germs predominated during manufacture and ripening of Russian and Yugoslavian white pickled cheeses respectively.

Few lactobacilli were found in the milk samples (below 10^2 c.f.u./ml in Batch 1 and about 10^3 c.f.u./ml in Batch 2). However they increased continuously during the manufacture and ripening process, appearing as the second important group of microorganisms

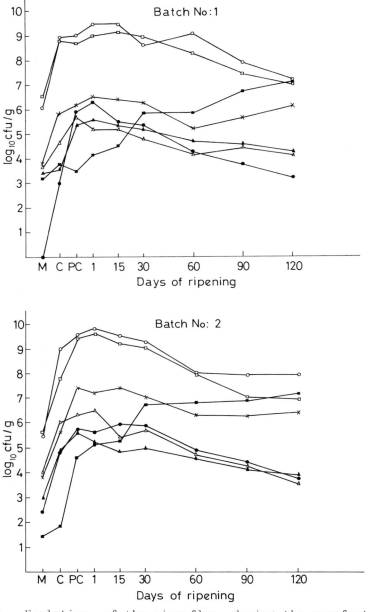

Fig. 1. Evolution of the microflora during the manufacture and ripening of Turkish white pickled cheese. Total viable count (□), lactic streptococci (○), lactobacilli (■), enterococci (X), coliforms (●), *Micrococcaceae* (Δ), yeasts (▲). (M, raw milk; C, curd; PC, pressed curd).

after 1 month of ripening. They reached levels very close to those of lactic streptococci in the 4-month-old cheese samples. The presence at high level of lactobacilli were also reported in ripened Turkish (3) and other white pickled cheeses (11,12). It seems likely that these organisms play an important role in the ripening of white pickled cheese as is the case with some other cheese varieties (13-15).

The number of enterococci was about 10^4 c.f.u./ml in the raw milk samples. Their growth was very rapid during the manufacturing stages, reaching a maximum at the beginning of ripening period. Although a slight decrease was observed during the whole period of ripening, their number persisted at a level of 10^6 c.f.u./g in the 4-month-old cheese samples. Presence of enterococci at similar levels has been detected in many varieties of cheese (14-16), as well as in white pickled cheeses (12,17). The possible contribution of enterococci to the ripening of cheese have been suggested on the basis of their numerical importance in the microflora of cheeses and their proteolytic and lipolytic activities (16,18).

Coliforms which were present in very low numbers in raw milk samples, increased rapidly during the manufacturing and the early stages of the ripening period. Thereafter their number decreased regularly to levels of 10^3-10^4 c.f.u./g in ripe cheeses. The counts of *Micrococcaceae* and yeasts followed similar development patterns; they increased notably during the manufacturing and subsequently declined during the ripening period.

In order to reveal different lactic acid bacteria species that take part throughout the manufacturing and ripening process of white pickled cheese, a total of 175 strains, isolated from the samples of raw milk, 1-day-old and 4-month-old cheeses, were identified. Isolates were obtained from colonies grown on M-17 and Rogosa agar plates. Taking into account the bacteria counts obtained on each isolation medium and the number of identified strains, the distribution of different species in the samples was estimated as percentage of total lactic acid bacteria. The data obtained for each of the two batches studied are presented in Table 2.

In agreement with the preceding results, lactic streptococci were found to constitute the major part of the lactic flora during the manufacture and ripening of cheeses in both batches. Especially in raw milk and 1-day-old cheese samples, the lactic flora was composed almost entirely of these germs. In ripened cheese samples, however, other lactic acid bacteria species belonging to the genera of *Lactobacillus* and *Leuconostoc* were also found at levels of about 5% and 3% of total lactic flora, respectively. Among the lactic streptococci the species identified were *S.lactis* and *S.lactis* subsp. *diacetilactis* in both batches. Their ratio

TABLE 2
Relative frequencies of lactic acid bacteria species present in raw milk, 1-day-old cheese and 4-month-old cheese (% of total lactic acid bacteria)

Batch no.	Bacteria species	Raw milk	Samples 1-day old cheese	4-month-old cheese
1	S.lactis	42.94	62.41	55.94
	S.lactis subsp. diacetilactis	56.92	37.59	37.29
	Leu.mesenteroides subsp. dextranicum	0.02	-	-
	Leu.paramesenteroides	0.02	-	-
	Pediococcus spp.	0.01	-	-
	Lb.casei	0.08	0.006	3.18
	Lb.plantarum	0,02	0.004	2.37
2	S.lactis	30.76	59.95	32.53
	S.lactis subsp. diacetilactis	69.24	39.97	58.68
	Leu.mesenteroides subsp. dextranicum	-	-	2.51
	Leu.mesenteroides subsp. mesenteroides	-	0.01	-
	Leu.paramesenteroides	-	0.03	0.63
	Lb.casei	-	0.03	4.39
	Lb.plantarum	-	0.005	1.26

to total lactic flora in different samples varied in similar ranges. These two species of lactic streptococci together with *S. cremoris* are the principal components of most of the starter cultures currently used in the manufacture of various fermented milk products including cheeses in which they are essentially responsible for lactic acid production. In addition, the strains of *S. lactis* subsp. *diacetylactis* contribute also to the flavour development of the products. Absence of *S.cremoris* in the samples was not surprising since its occurence in raw milk was reported to be rare or in very small numbers (19,20).

Of the other lactic acid bacteria species identified *Lactobacillus casei* and *Lactobacillus plantarum* are the only two species of this genus detected in the samples. Their part in total lactic flora was negligible in raw milk and 1-day-old cheese samples. On the other hand, in mature cheeses their relative numbers increased suggesting that they could play a role only in the last stages of the ripening. Our results are in agreement with those of Ergüllü (3) who also found that *L. casei* and *L. plantarum* constituted the major part of lactobacilli isolated from the Turkish white pickled cheese. These bacteria were also detected in large numbers during the ripening of some other cheese varieties (14,15,21,22).

Leuconostocs were present only in very small numbers in the raw milk sample of Batch 1 and in the 1-day-old cheese sample of Batch 2. However, in ripened cheese sample of Batch 2, their occurence were found to be at a noticeable level. The species identified were *Leuconostoc mesenteroides* subsp. *dextranicum* and *Leuconostoc paramesenteroides*. Presence of leuconostocs in other types of cheese is also very common (23). They can take part in the composition of some starter cultures as well where they fulfill the role of aroma producer. Also, due to their heterofermentative character, they are responsible for the formation of open texture in certain cheese varieties. Nevertheles, this is not a desirable trait in white pickled cheese.

The data reported in this study suggest that in order to formulate a specific starter for the manufacture of Turkish white pickled cheese, species belonging to lactic streptococci such as *S.lactis* and *S. lactis* subsp. *diacetilactis* should be taken into consideration. In addition to these organisms, species of lactobacilli of streptobacteria group, namely *L. casei* and *L. plantarum*, which appeared to play a certain role especially during the last stages of ripening, might be included in the composition of such a starter. Suitable strains belonging to the above mentioned species must be selected with regard to their technologically important characteristics.

REFERENCES

1   M.S.Y. Haddadin, in: R.K. Robinson (ed.), Development in Food Microbiology, Elsevier Applied Science Publishers, London, 1986, pp. 67-89.
2   M.H. Abd El-Salam, in: P.F. Fox (ed.), Cheese: Chemistry, Physics and Microbiology Vol. 2: Major Cheese Varieties, Elsevier Applied Science Publishers, London, 1987, pp. 277-309.
3   E. Ergüllü, Thesis, Aegean University, Izmir, Turkey, 1980.
4   I.D.F., Provisional International Standard 122:1984, Milchwissenschaft, 40 (1985) 533-537.
5   W.F. Harrigan and M.E. Mc Cance, Laboratory Methods in Food and Dairy Microbiology, Academic Press, London, 1976.
6   E.M. Sharpe, in: F.A. Skinner and D.W. Lovelock (eds), Identification Methods for Microbiologists, Academic Press, London, 1979, pp. 233-259.
7   R.H. Deibel and H.W. Seeley, in: R.E. Buchanan and N.E. Gibbons (eds), Bergey's Manual of Determinative Bacteriology, The Williams and Wilkins Company,Baltimore, 1974, pp.490-517.

8   M. Rogosa, in: R.E. Buchanan and N.E. Gibbons (eds), Bergey's Manual of Determinative Bacteriology, The Williams and Wilkins Company, Baltimore, 1974, pp. 576-593.
9   E.I. Garvie, Methods in Microbiol. 16 (1984) 148-178.
10   R.N. Lomsadze, G.S. Mamatelashvili, N.G. Purtseladze, L.I. Demurishvili and N.P. Mandzhavitze, Molchnaya Promyshlenost, No.12 (1976),13-15.
11   J. Rasic, Int. Dairy Cong. Section IV:2 (1962) 840-845.
12   Y. Yanai, B. Rosen, A.Pinsky and D. Sklan, J. Dairy Res., 44 (1977) 149-153.
13   B.A. Law, Progr. Ind. Microbiol., 19 (1984) 245-283.
14   T.L. Thompson and E.H. Marth, Milchwissenschaft, 41 (1986) 201-205.
15   J.A. Ordonez, R. Barneto and M. Ramos, Milchwissenschaft, 33 (1978) 609-613.
16   W.S. Clark and G.W. Reinbold, J. Dairy Sci. 49 (1966) 1214-1218.
17   M. Kıvanç, Int. J. Food Microbiol., 9 (1989) 73-77.
18   L.D.Trovatelli, A.Schiesser and S.Massa, Milchwissenschaft, 42 (1987) 717-719.
19   J.H. Galloway and R.J.M. Crawford, in: B.J.B. Wood (ed.), Microbiology of Fermented Foods, Vol. 1, Elsevier Applied Science Publishers, London, 1984, pp.111-165.
20   B.A. Law and M.E. Sharpe, in: F.A. Skinner and L.B. Quesnel (eds), Streptococci, Academic Press, London, 1978, pp. 263-278.
21   S.D. Peterson and R.T. Marshall, J. Dairy Sci., 73 (1990) 1395-1410.
22   J.A. Suarez, R. Barneto and B. Inigo, Chem. Mikrobiol. Technol. Lebensm. 8 (1983) 52-56.
23   J.J. Devoyod and F. Poullain, Le Lait, 68 (1988) 249-280.

G. Charalambous (Ed.), Food Science and Human Nutrition
© 1992 Elsevier Science Publishers B.V. All rights reserved.

PROBLEMS ASSOCIATED WITH THE PROCESSING OF CUCUMBER PICKLES: SOFTENING, BLOATER FORMATION AND ENVIRONMENTAL POLLUTION

Anne A. Guillou and John D. Floros

Purdue University, Department of Food Science,
1160 Smith Hall, West Lafayette, IN 47907-1160, USA

ABSTRACT

The traditional process of cucumber fermentation and storage was critically reviewed. Enzymatic and non-enzymatic softening, bloater formation and environmental pollution due to high salt brine disposal were identified as the most important problems. The enzymes and acids involved in softening, and the mechanism of bloater formation were examined and some solutions (firming agents, cucumber washing, brine purging, homofermentative starters and controlled fermentation) were presented. Methods to reduce environmental pollution by salt recovery, brine recycling, closed tank controlled/anaerobic fermentation and low-salt natural fermentation and storage were discussed and debated.

INTRODUCTION

Approximately 300,000 metric tons of pickling cucumbers are harvested every year in the United States and then fermented and preserved in high salt brines (USDA, 1986). The presence of NaCl in the brine creates a favorable environment for the lactic acid bacteria, suppresses the growth of spoilage microorganisms (yeasts, molds, etc.) and inhibits the softening action of pectinolytic enzymes (Bell and Etchells, 1961; Cruess, 1958). Nevertheless, the quality of fermented cucumbers is often affected by softening and bloater damage, two of the most serious problems facing the pickling industry. At the end of each storage period, the high salt brines are disposed of and the fermented cucumbers are desalted. This extensive disposal of salt creates serious environmental problems and prompted the U.S. Environmental Protection Agency to set a legal limit of 230 mg of chloride ions per liter of brine wastes (Humphries and Fleming, 1989).

Extensive research efforts have been undertaken to understand the formation of softening and bloater damage, and some methods have been developed to reduce or eliminate these defects. Similarly, research work is being performed on the environmental pollution problem, and several methods have been established to reduce the high NaCl wastes generated by the pickling industry: Salt recovery (Durkee and Lowe, 1973 and 1974); brine recycling (Geisman and Henner, 1973; Palnitkar and McFeeters, 1975); controlled fermentation (Fleming et al., 1987); anaerobic fermentation (Fleming et al., 1988); and low-salt natural fermentation and storage (Guillou, 1991; Guillou et al., 1991). The salt recovery and the brine recycling processes reduce the NaCl wastes by reusing the salt or the entire brine, respectively, in subsequent fermentations. Controlled, anaerobic and natural low-salt fermentation processes, on the other hand, reduce the NaCl wastes by using low salt brines throughout fermentation and storage. However, none of the above methods has been widely accepted commercially, mainly due to their high initial capital investment (installation cost), increased operational cost, and/or undesirable processing complexity. Pickle processing companies are looking for simpler and cost effective methods to reduce the high NaCl content of their wastes, and optimization of the overall fermentation and storage process with respect to brine salt content is necessary (Guillou, 1991).

The purpose of this work was to review the most important problems (softening, bloater formation, environmental pollution) facing the cucumber pickling industry and discuss some of the associated solutions.

TRADITIONAL FERMENTATION AND STORAGE OF CUCUMBERS

Cucumbers used in pickle manufacturing are harvested firm, green and slightly underripe. Once harvested, they are promptly transported to processing plants where they are sorted for microbial or mechanical damage and graded for size (Ayres et al., 1980). The selected cucumbers are brined in outdoor wooden or plastic vats from 2.4 to 4.3 m (8 to 14 ft) in diameter and 1.8 to 2.4 m (6 to 8 ft) in depth (Cruess, 1958). Brine (8 to 10% NaCl) is first placed at the bottom of the vats to prevent bruising of the cucumbers during their unloading. Once the tanks are filled, more brine is added to cover the cucumbers and a wooden lid is placed on top to ensure that cucumbers remain submerged. At this stage, the brine is usually pumped and circulated to mix the salt solution and dissolve any salt that remains in the solid phase.

Within one day, the salt-tolerant acid-forming bacteria naturally present in cucumbers begin to grow. Their growth induces an active on-going acid fermentation lasting three to six weeks. During this time, the initial brine concentration is maintained by adding salt to the top of each tank and regularly circulating the brine to ensure that the salt is well distributed (Binsted et al., 1962). At the end of the fermentation, the brine attains 0.5 to 1 % total acidity (expressed as lactic acid) and its pH is 3.8 or less. The color of the cucumbers changes from a bright green to an olive-green or yellowish-green and their flesh becomes translucent instead of chalky white and opaque (Cruess, 1958). At this point, the brine concentration is gradually increased to 16-18% NaCl by regular addition of salt.

The fermented cucumbers are stored in these high salt content brines for a period of time ranging from a few months to several years. Just before final packaging and distribution, the cucumbers are subjected to a desalination process. To remove the excessive amount of salt, the cucumbers are dipped into still or running water, and subsequently placed into various solutions. Distilled vinegar is used for sour pickles, spiced sweet vinegar for sweet pickles, while dill pickles are placed in dilute brines flavored with dill herbs and spices (Cruess, 1958).

MICROBIAL ASPECTS

The fermentation of brined cucumbers arises directly from the growth of various microorganisms naturally present on cucumbers. Fleming (1982) described the process of fermentation and divided it into four steps: Initiation, primary fermentation, secondary fermentation and post-fermentation.

The initiation step involves the growth of many Gram-positive and Gram-negative bacteria. Coliform bacteria usually dominate during the first few days of fermentation but disappear within a week. At this time, the lactic acid bacteria have grown to appreciable numbers and the fermentation enters its second phase, also called primary fermentation. During this phase, the lactic acid bacteria metabolize the sugars present in cucumbers into acidic compounds. The production of acids decreases the pH and increases the acidity of the brine. Thus, a low-pH-high-acidity environment is created, which inhibits any further growth of the lactic acid bacteria.

After the lactic fermentation is completed, an undesirable secondary fermentation may take place. If any fermentable carbohydrates remain in the brine, fermentative yeasts will grow even at low pH. Finally, a post-fermentation may begin when the fermentable carbohydrates are exhausted. This might be caused by the growth of oxidative yeasts on the surface of brines not exposed to sunlight. The yeasts form a thick white to grey film and utilize lactic acid as a source of energy. Their growth induces a pH increase and an acidity decrease, which may result in the growth of molds and putrefactive bacteria. Such developments cause bad odors, off-flavors, softening and overall spoilage (Etchells et al., 1975).

Species involved

Four species of lactic acid bacteria are associated with the natural fermentation of cucumbers: *Leuconostoc mesenteroides*, *Pediococcus pentosaceus* (previously called *Pediococcus cerevisiae*), *Lactobacillus brevis* and *Lactobacillus plantarum*. The main characteristics of these species are summarized in Table 1. *Leuconostoc mesenteroides* is usually the first to grow, followed by *Lactobacillus brevis*, *Pediococcus pentosaceus* and *Lactobacillus plantarum* (Fleming et al., 1985). This growth sequence is directly related to the sensitivity of each specie to acid and/or low pH. *Lactobacillus plantarum* characteristically outlasts the rest, because it is the most resistant to acids and low pH.

Metabolic pathways.

Lactic acid bacteria ferment sugars, mainly glucose and fructose in cucumbers, by using two metabolic pathways: homo- or hetero-fermentation (Fig. 1). Homofermentative bacteria, such as *Lactobacillus plantarum* and *Pediococcus pentasoceus*, metabolize carbohydrates by the glycosidic pathway and produce essentially lactic acid. Heterofermentative bacteria, like *Lactobacillus brevis* and *Leuconostoc mesenteroides*, convert glucose into lactic acid, acetic acid, ethanol and carbon dioxide, and fructose into the four previous end products as well as mannitol (Fleming et al., 1985).

Table 1: Main characteristics of lactic acid bacteria associated with the fermentation of cucumbers[a]

Properties	Microorganisms			
	L. plantarum	L. brevis	P. pentosaceus	L. mesenteroides
Morphology	Short to medium rods, single	Short rods, single or in short chains	Cocci, single in pairs or in tetrads	Cocci, in pairs
Optimum growth temperature (°C)	30-35	30	35	20-30
Growth in 8% NaCl	Yes	No	Yes	No
Glucose metabolism	Homofermenter	Heterofermenter	Homofermenter	Heterofermenter
End products	Lactic acid	Lactic acid, acetic acid, ethanol, CO_2	Lactic acid	Lactic acid, acetic acid, ethanol, CO_2
Final pH (%acidity)[b] in cucumbers	3.5 (1.04)	3.9 (1.06)	3.5 (0.90)	3.9 (1.04)

[a] Based on information given by Fleming et al. (1985) and Stamer (1979)
[b] Acidity expressed as lactic acid

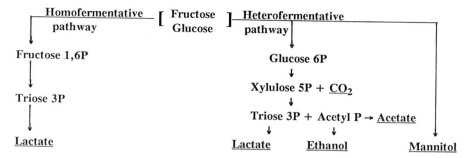

Figure 1: Major pathways for sugar fermentation by lactic acid bacteria

Salt influence.

The concentration of salt in the brine greatly influences the course of natural fermentation by controlling the microbial flora and activity. The lactic acid bacteria are only a minor component of the natural microflora found on cucumbers. Therefore, an appropriate salt concentration should not only favor the growth of lactic acid bacteria, but it should also inhibit the growth of all other microorganisms (Daeschel and Fleming, 1984). A high salt concentration in the brine (over 10% NaCl), slows down the fermentation process by reducing the activity of the lactic acid bacteria. On the other hand, a low salt concentration (below 5% NaCl) may allow microorganisms other than lactic acid bacteria to grow, thereby causing spoilage. Traditionally, concentrations of 8-10% NaCl are used, because they allow a rapid growth of the lactic acid bacteria. Such growth results in the production of acids, which decreases the pH, and inhibits the growth of any other microorganisms present on raw cucumbers.

THE SOFTENING PROBLEM

The softening of cucumbers is a recurring problem in the pickling industry. It occurs usually during the storage phase (Bell et al., 1950; Pangborn et al., 1959) and affects large and small size cucumbers (Hudson and Buescher, 1980). Various factors (pH, acidity, storage time, storage temperature) affect the texture of cucumbers and several chemical reactions are involved. In general, two different types of softening exist: enzymatic and non-enzymatic.

Enzymatic softening

Bell et al. (1950) and Lampi et al. (1958) reported that softening of cucumbers is related to the degradation of pectins by pectinolytic enzymes. Large amounts of pectins are present in the primary cell walls and the middle lamella of cucumbers. Pectins are mainly composed of linear polymers of (1→4)-α-D-galacturonopyranosyl units, esterified to some extent with methanol (BeMiller, 1986; Whistler and Daniel, 1985). Their presence contributes to the mechanical strength of the cells and facilitates the cell to cell adhesion (Van Buren, 1979).

Bell et al. (1950) and Bell (1951) were the first to report the presence of pectinolytic enzymes in mature cucumbers. Later, Etchells et al. (1958) established that a large portion of the pectinolytic enzymes present in the brine was due to fungi. They hypothetized that fungi, which grow in cucumber flowers, are introduced into the brine by the flowers that sometimes remain on the fruits. The main pectinolytic enzymes responsible for the degradation of pectins are polygalacturonase (PG) and pectinmethylesterase (PME).

Polygalacturonase (PG) is present in fungi that grow in cucumber flowers (Bell et al., 1950) and in locular tissue of mature cucumbers (McFeeters et al., 1980). This enzyme catalyzes the glycosidic hydrolysis of pectins, thereby producing monomeric D-galacturonic acid. The pectin breakdown, which results from its activity, creates an irreversible texture loss for cucumbers (Tang and McFeeters, 1983).

Pectinmethylesterase (PME) is present in the cucumber tissue (Fukushima, 1978; Haard, 1985). This enzyme cleaves the methyl ester groups from pectin polymers, thereby producing poly-D-galacturonic acid (pectic acid). Its activity depends on temperature and pH. Van Buren et al. (1962) indicated that low pH conditions increase the sensitivity of PME to high temperature. McFeeters et al. (1985) further reported that sliced cucumbers should undergo blanching at 99°C for 3 min in order to inactivate PME and inhibit its reactivation during storage.

The demethylation process induced by PME is the most important phenomenon observed in cell wall degradation during either chilling injury (Fukushima, 1978) or fermentation (Tang and McFeeters, 1983) of fresh cucumbers. McFeeters and Armstrong (1984) developed a procedure to measure the degree of pectin methylation in plant cell walls, and subsequently used it to relate pectin methylation to textural changes (McFeeters et al., 1985). They did not find any relation between pectin methylation and firmness loss in cucumbers. However, Hudson and Buescher (1986) noted that when the degree of pectin methylation is less than 13%, a linear correlation exists.

Non-enzymatic softening

Lesley and Cruess (1928) were the first to suggest that the production of acids during fermentation affects the texture of cucumbers. Bell et al. (1972) confirmed this hypothesis by studying the influence of five organic acids on the firmness of fresh-packed pickles. They found that oxalic acid had a stronger softening action than malic, citric, lactic and acetic acids. They explained these results by assuming that the reduction of calcium in cucumber tissue causes texture loss. When cucumbers are maintained in an acidified brine, calcium diffuses from the cucumber tissue into the brine, while the dissociated form of the acid present in the brine migrates toward the inside of the cucumber. Therefore, when large amounts of acid dissociate, large quantities of calcium ions diffuse outside the cucumber tissue and extensive cucumber softening occurs.

THE USE OF FIRMING AGENTS TO REDUCE SOFTENING

Once the causes of softening were identified, several methods to reduce the loss of texture in fermented pickles were established. Nowadays, the softening due to fungal pectinolytic enzymes is suppressed by washing the cucumbers before brining, and the softening due to the remaining pectinolytic enzymes (naturally present in cucumber tissue) and the acids in the brine is reduced by the use of firming agents such as calcium and alum.

Calcium

Addition of 0.2% $CaCl_2$ to the initial brine maintained the firmness of pickles and prevented softening (Fleming et al., 1987). Addition of higher concentration (0.44% $CaCl_2$) to the brine also inhibited the softening action of fungal polygalacturonase

(Buescher et al., 1979). Furthermore, Tang and McFeeters (1983) reported that the time of addition of calcium chloride to the brine is crucial. They suggested that calcium chloride is more efficient when added to the initial brine, because it can prevent but it cannot reverse the softening reactions. Guillou (1991) conducted a comprehensive optimization study on the effect of $CaCl_2$ and concluded that amounts of 0.2 to 0.3% $CaCl_2$ are necessary to prevent softening of cucumbers, particularly when low-salt brines are used for fermentation and storage.

Extensive research has been performed to understand and explain the mode of action of calcium. It has been shown that the addition of calcium to demethylated pectic substances increases the tissue firmness of snap beans (Van Buren, 1968) and inhibits the hydrolytic action of the fungal polygalacturonase in cucumbers (Bateman, 1964). Van Buren (1979) showed that calcium ions have a high affinity for the free carboxyl groups present in pectins. Interactions between calcium and carboxyl groups result in the formation of bridges between calcium and carboxyl groups. This crosslinking increases the rigidity of the polymeric network of pectins and may be responsible for the firming action of calcium (Tang and McFeeters, 1983).

However, McFeeters et al. (1985) reported that calcium prevents softening regardless of the degree of pectin methylation and Hudson and Buescher (1985) demonstrated that calcium enhances the firmness retention of cucumber tissue by reducing the solubilization and deesterification of pectin substances. These findings suggest that other kinds of interactions between calcium and polysaccharides may also be responsible for the firming action of calcium.

Alum

Alum (aluminum potassium sulfate) is a firming agent extensively used by the pickling industry. Fabian and Krum (1949) showed that its addition after desalting increases the firmness of fermented cucumbers. This result was confirmed by Buescher and Burgin (1988) in a study comparing the action of alum and calcium chloride during post-desalting treatment. They found that both compounds improved the firmness of cucumbers. However, aluminum salt seems to have the opposite effect when added to fresh pickles. Etchells et al. (1972) reported a decrease in firmness when alum was added to fresh-pack dill pickles.

THE BLOATER FORMATION PROBLEM

Bloater damage is a common defect in fermented cucumbers and it is most frequently observed in large cucumbers (Fleming et al., 1973a). Its occurrence is related to the cultivar of the cucumbers and the pre-harvest environmental conditions (Fleming et al., 1973a).

Mechanism of formation

Etchells et al. (1968) attributed bloater formation to the production of gases, mainly carbon dioxide, that are produced simultaneously by the microorganisms (as end products of metabolism) and the respiration of cucumbers. They studied the fermentation of cucumbers by pure cultures of lactic acid bacteria and proposed a mechanism of bloater development. They suggested that carbon dioxide, which is produced during fermentation, dissolves in the brine and diffuses into the cucumbers. Supersaturated levels of carbon dioxide in the brine will result in bloater damage. Furthermore, Fleming et al. (1978b) showed that bloater damage can also occur at subsaturation levels. They suggested that the critical level of carbon dioxide for bloater damage is variable, and it depends on a number of factors (brine temperature, salt concentration, initial time of CO_2 production, etc.)

Fleming and Pharr (1980) proposed a mechanism of bloater formation at subsaturation levels. They hypothesized that the movement of brine into the cucumbers clogged up the air spaces of the outer mesocarp tissue and therefore prevented the normally rapid diffusion of gases. This liquid-clogged region of tissue acts as a differentially permeable barrier to carbon dioxide and nitrogen. Carbon dioxide increases rapidly during fermentation and is diffusing from the brine into the cucumbers. Nitrogen is the most abundant gas naturally present inside the cucumbers and is diffusing outwards into the brine. Since the aqueous solubility of carbon dioxide is greater than that of nitrogen, the diffusion of carbon dioxide molecules into the cucumbers exceeds the outward diffusion of nitrogen molecules. This results in an increase in the internal pressure, which ultimately exceeds the resistance of tissue and causes bloater formation. Corey et al. (1983) confirmed the above hypothesis and reported that the diffusion rate of carbon dioxide in brined cucumber tissue is 2.4 times greater than that of nitrogen.

METHODS TO ELIMINATE BLOATER FORMATION

Several methods to reduce or completely eliminate broater formation have been suggested in the literature. The most promising ones are presented here.

Brine purging.

One method of reducing bloater damage is by purging the carbon dioxide away from the brine. Costilow et al. (1977) reported that bloater damage is greatly reduced by purging the brine with nitrogen. If the brine is regularly mixed and the purging action starts as soon as the cucumbers are covered with brine, bloater damage may be completely eliminated.

Purging with air is also an effective and less expensive method of reducing bloater formation. However, it has been shown that air purging is responsible for cucumber color loss and mold-induced softening (Fleming et al., 1975). Further research indicates that softening can be prevented by intermittent air purging, which reduces the amount of oxygen available for mold growth (Costilow et al., 1980), or by the addition of antimicrobial agents such as acetic acid (Potts and Fleming, 1982) or potassium sorbate (Costilow and Uebersax, 1982) to the brine.

Use of homofermentative starters

Etchells et al. (1968) reported that *Enterobacter*, yeasts, homo- and heterofermentative lactic acid bacteria all produce carbon dioxide. In the absence of yeasts, most carbon dioxide is produced by heterofermentative lactic acid bacteria. Thus, bloater formation can be eliminated by suppressing heterofermentation. Etchells et al. (1964) showed that microbial control in cucumber fermentation is possible, and therefore, homofermentative cultures can be used as starters in cucumber fermentations to suppress bloater damage. These starters (*Lactobacillus plantarum* or *Pediococcus pentosaceus*) are presently available on the market.

Fleming et al. (1973a and 1973b) reported that bloater damage may occur even when cucumbers are fermented by pure cultures of *L. plantarum*. Although, *L. plantarum* is an homofermentative non-gas producing bacterium, it has the ability to degrade malic acid into lactic acid and carbon dioxide (Fleming et al., 1985; McFeeters et al., 1982a). Malic acid is the major naturally occurring organic acid in cucumbers (0.2-0.3% by weight) (McFeeters et al.,1982a). McFeeters et al. (1982b) showed that during fermentation of cucumber juice by *L. plantarum*, decarboxylation of malate takes place and carbon dioxide is produced. Considerable work has been done to obtain strains of *L. plantarum* that lack the ability to degrade malate. McFeeters et al. (1984) selected two naturally occuring non-malic-acid-degrading strains, while Daeschel et al. (1984) obtained one such strain by inducing mutation of a malate decarboxylating strain of *L. plantarum*. Subsequently, McFeeters et al. (1984) used a non-malic-acid-degradative strain of *Lactobacillus plantarum* for fermentation and observed no bloater damage.

Controlled fermentation

Etchells et al. (1973) established a new procedure to ferment cucumbers that combines microbial control and brine purging. This procedure, outlined in Fig. 2, is called controlled fermentation. In comparison to the natural fermentation, this process requires several additional steps: washing of cucumbers to remove foreign material; sanitizing of cucumbers in chlorine solution and acidification of brine to suppress the growth of all natural microflora; nitrogen purging of brine to remove carbon dioxide; and finally, addition of buffer and culture to control the fermentation. The addition of buffer delays the reduction of pH, which allows the lactic bacteria to grow over a longer period of time. Therefore, the quantity of consumed and broken down sugars is increased, and the risk of a secondary yeast fermentation is drastically reduced. The cultures used for controlled fermentation are either *Lactobacillus plantarum* or *Pediococcus pentosaceus*, or a mixture of both (Fleming et al., 1985; Lingle, 1975).

Controlled fermentations have been tested successfully in industry. Wallace and Andress (1977) reported that in one commercial application, controlled fermentation of large cucumbers reduced bloater damage from 40% to 5%. Furthermore, Fleming et al. (1978a) found that this procedure also improved the firmness of small cucumbers.

THE ENVIRONMENTAL POLLUTION PROBLEM AND SOME SOLUTIONS

The natural process of fermentation and storage involves the use of high salt brines. These brines are not reused, because they contain various cucumber tissue particles, microbial cells and pectinolytic enzymes. Instead, they are disposed into ground waters at the end of each storage period. Their high salt content (16-18% NaCl) and high BOD values (10,000-15,000 ppm) contribute to water pollution (Humphries and Fleming, 1989) and adversely affect the environment. To avoid the pollution of ground waters, the U.S. Environmental Protection Agency (EPA) recently established a limit of chloride content (230mg/l) in wastewaters (Humphries and Fleming, 1989). Typical waste brines, however, contain as much as 100 times this value. Pickle processing companies must find ways to drastically reduce the amount of salt in their wastewaters. Three basic approaches have been considered to solve the problem: a) salt recovery; b) brine recycling; and c) low-salt fermentation and storage.

Salt recovery

Durkee and Lowe (1973) developed a desalination process for recovering the salt dissolved in used brines and subsequently reusing it to prepare new brines. The used brine is first brought into a submerged combustion crystallizer, which produces a slurry containing 60% NaCl and organic matter. The slurry is then introduced into an incinerator (650°C for 5 min), which purifies the salt from all organic impurities. Durkee and Lowe (1973) analyzed the composition of the recovered salt and found some chemical differences between recovered and fresh salt. The recovered salt contained carbon (from the incineration) and potassium residues in excess of the amount normally found in fresh salt.

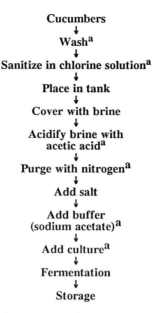

Figure 2: Flow diagram of a controlled fermentation process ([a]Steps added to the natural fermentation process)

However, fermentation proceeded normally in brines made with recovered salt and excellent quality pickles were obtained (Durkee and Lowe, 1974). No study has been done on the quality of pickles fermented in brines made with salt recrystallized and incinerated more than once.

Brine recycling

Brines used during fermentation contain various amounts of pectinolytic enzymes. These enzymes, responsible for the softening of cucumbers, must be removed or inactivated before reusing the brine for another fermentation. Geisman and Henner (1973) developed a procedure to purify the brine from all organic matter and therefore to remove the pectinolytic enzymes present. NaOH pellets were added to the used brine until a pH of 10-11 was reached and the formed precipitate was removed by filtration. The pH of the brine was then adjusted to pH=7 with concentrated HCl and the brine was reused.

In a different approach, Palnitkar and McFeeters (1975) developed a heat treatment to inactivate the pectinolytic enzymes present in brines. They used a very heat stable pectinase from *Aspergillus niger* in their tests, and reported that normal fermentation occurred with both NaOH- and heat-treated brines. Brine recycling treatments present the major advantage of being cheaper than the salt recovery process. However, there is no indication that such treatments would be successful in industrial applications. Pectinolytic enzymes more heat resistant than *Aspergillus niger* pectinase may exist and may resist the heat treatment. Furthermore, it is still unknown whether any toxic compounds accumulate throughout the recycling process.

Low-salt fermentation and storage

Fleming et al. (1987) reported that cucumbers were successfully fermented and stored in 2.6% NaCl and 0.2% $CaCl_2$ using *controlled fermentation process* (Fig. 2). However, this method requires extensive labor time and it has not been widely used in industry. Fleming et al. (1988) developed a simpler process, which they named *anaerobic fermentation*. The main steps of this process are described in Fig. 3. The authors (Fleming et al., 1988) reported normal cucumber fermentation and storage in 2.7% and 4.6% NaCl brines using the anaerobic fermentation process. They also found that butyric acid spoilage appeared when cucumbers were anaerobically fermented in 2.3% NaCl (Fleming et al., 1989). The minimum amount of NaCl required to successfully ferment and store cucumbers with the anaerobic process is still to be determined. The anaerobic process does not require as much labor or time as the controlled fermentation process. However, commercial use of the anaerobic fermentation process will imply high initial capital investment, because it involves the use of closed containers instead of the traditional open vats.

Cucumbers
↓
Wash[a]
↓
Place in closed tanks[a]
↓
Cover with brine
↓
Prepare brine (add salt
calcium acetate, culture)[a]
↓
Purge with nitrogen[a]
↓
Fermentation
↓
Storage

Figure 3: Flow diagram of an anaerobic fermentation process ([a]Steps modified or added to the natural fermentation process)

More recently, attempts have been made to reduce the amount of salt used during natural cucumber fermentation and storage by adding appropriate quantities of $CaCl_2$ and potassium sorbate in the brine (Guillou, 1991; Guillou et al., 1991). It was found that adequate concentrations of $CaCl_2$ and potassium sorbate in the brine, exhibit a synergistic effect and can minimize the amount of NaCl required to produce good quality pickles (Guillou et al., 1991). The use of several optimization methods predicted that good quality pickles can be obtained when cucumbers are naturally fermented and stored in brines containing 3% NaCl, 0.28% $CaCl_2$ and 0.28% potassium sorbate (Guillou, 1991). The validity of this prediction was experimentally confirmed. Brines made with 2% NaCl, 0.20% $CaCl_2$ and 0.30% potassium sorbate also gave good quality pickles after six months of storage. Such *low-salt matural fermentation and storage* must be tested in large industrial aplications. If the experimental results are confirmed industrially, the NaCl waste problem will be largely resolved. The desalination step could then be eliminated and the concentration of NaCl in waste waters would be drastically reduced.

A problem that may arise from the use of low-salt brines in large scale commercial applications, is freezing of brines and cucumbers during the cold winter months. Such freezing may adversly affect the quality of pickles. Research work needs to be undertaken on this issue and solutions must be found.

REFERENCES

Ayres, J.C., Mundt, J.O. and Sandine, W.E., 1980. "Microbiology of Foods", W.H. Freeman and Company, San Francisco, CA, pp 208-219.

Bateman, D.F., 1964. An induced mechanism of tissue resistance to polygalacturonase in rhizoctonia-infected hypocotyls of bean. Phytopathology, 54(4): 438-445.

Basel, R.M. and Gould, W.A., 1983. An investigation of some important storage parameters in acidified bulk storage of tomatoes. J. Food Sci., 48(3): 932-934.

Bell, T.A., 1951. Pectolytic enzyme activity in various parts of the cucumber plant and fruit. Botan. Gaz.,113: 216-221.

Bell, T.A. and Etchells, J.L., 1961. Influence of salt (NaCl) on pectinolytic softening of cucumbers. J. Food Sci., 26: 84-90.

Bell, T.A., Etchells, J.L. and Jones, I.D., 1950. Softening of commercial cucumber salt-stock in relation to polygalacturonase activity. Food Tech., 4(4): 157-163.

Bell, T.A., Turney, L.J. and Etchells, J.L., 1972. Influence of different organic acids on the firmness of fresh-pack pickles. J. Food Sci., 37(3): 446-449.

BeMiller, J.N., 1986. An introduction to pectins: structure and properties. In "Chemistry and Function of Pectins", M.L. Fishman and J.J. Jen, (Eds), Am. Chem. Soc., Washington DC.

Binsted, R., Devey, J.D. and Dakin, J.C., 1962. "Pickle and Sauce Making", 2ed, Food Trade Press LTD, London, Great Britain, Ch 9.

Buescher, R.W. and Burgin, C., 1988. Effect of calcium chloride and alum on fermentation, desalting, and firmness retention of cucumber pickles. J. Food Sci., 53(1): 296-297.

Buescher, R.W., Hudson, J.M. and Adams, J.R., 1979. Inhibition of polygalacturonase softening of cucumber pickles by calcium chloride. J. Food Sci., 44(6): 1786-1787.

Corey, K.A., Pharr, D.M. and Fleming, H.P., 1983. Role of gas diffusion in bloater formation of brined cucumbers. J.Food Sci., 48(2): 389-393.

Costilow, R.N. and Uebersax, M., 1982. Effects of various treatments on the quality of salt-stock pickles from commercial fermentations purged with air. J. Food Sci., 47(6): 1866-1874.

Costilow, R.N., Gates, K. and Lacy, M.L., 1980. Molds in brined cucumbers: cause of softening during air-purging of fermentations. Appl. Environ. Microbiol., 40(2): 417-422.

Costilow, R.N., Bedford, C.L., Mingus, D. and Black, D., 1977. Purging of natural salt-stock pickle fermentations to reduce bloater damage. J. Food Sci., 42(1): 234-240.

Cruess, W.V., 1958. Pickles. In "Commercial Fruit and Vegetable Products", 4th edition, McGraw-Hill BookCompany, Inc, New York, NY, Ch 22.

Daeschel, M.A. and Fleming, H.P., 1984. Selection of lactic acid bacteria for use in vegetable fermentations. Food Microbiol., 1(4): 303-313.

Daeschel, M.A., McFeeters, R.F., Fleming, H.P., Klaenhammer, T.R. and Sanozky, R.B., 1984. Mutation and selection of *Lactobacillus plantarum* strains that do not produce carbon dioxide from malate. Appl.Microbiol., 47(2): 419-420.

Durkee, E.L. and Lowe, E., 1973. Field tests of salt recovery system for spent pickle brine. J. Food Sci., 38(3): 507-511.

Durkee, E.L. and Lowe, E., 1974. Use of recycled salt in fermentation of cucumber salt stock. J. Food Sci., 39(5): 1032-1033.

Etchells, J.L., Bell, T.A.and Turney, L.J., 1972. Influence of alum on the firmness of fresh-pack dill pickles. J. Food Sci., 37(3): 442-445.

Etchells, J.L., Borg, A.F. and Bell, T.A., 1968. Bloater in cucumber fermentations. Appl. Microbiol., 16(7): 1029-1035.

Etchells, J.L., Fleming, H.P. and Bell, T.A., 1975. Factors influencing the growth of lactic acid bacteria during the fermentation of brined cucumbers. In "Lactic Acid Bacteria in Beverages and Food", J.G Carr, C.V. Cutting and G.C. Whiting, (Eds.), Academic Press Inc., New York, NY, pp 281-303.

Etchells, J.L., Costilow, R.N., Anderson, T.E. and Bell, T.A., 1964. Pure culture fermentation of brined cucumbers. Appl. Microbiol., 12(6): 523-535.

Etchells, J.L., Bell, T.A., Fleming, H.P., Kelling, R.E. and Thompson, R.L., 1973. Suggested procedure for the controlled fermentation of commercially brined cucumbers- the use of starter cultures and reduction of carbon dioxide accumulation. Pickle Pack., 3,4.

Etchells, J.L., Bell, T.A., Monroe, R.J., Masley, P.M. and Demain, A.L., 1958. Populations and softening enzyme activity of filamentous fungi on flowers, ovaries, and fruit of pickling cucumbers. Appl. Microbiol., 6(6): 427-440.

Fabian, F.W. and Krum, J.K., 1949. The effect of alum on microorganisms commonly found in pickles. Fruit Prod.J., 28: 358.

Fleming, H.P., 1982. Fermented vegetables. In "Economic Microbiology. Fermented Foods", A.H. Rose, (Ed.), Academic Press, New York, NY, pp 227-258.

Fleming, H.P. and Pharr, D.M., 1980. Mechanism for bloater formation in brined cucumbers. J. Food Sci., 45(6): 1595-1600.

Fleming, H.P., McFeeters, R.F. and Daeschel, M.A., 1985. The lactobacilli, pediococci and leuconostocs: vegetable products. In "Bacterial Starter Cultures for Foods", S.E. Gilligand, (Ed.), CRC Press, Inc., Boca Raton, FL, pp 97-118.

Fleming, H.P., McFeeters, R.F. and Thompson, R.L., 1987. Effects of sodium chloride concentration on firmness retention of cucumbers fermented and stored with calcium chloride. J. Food Sci., 52(3): 653-657.

Fleming, H.P., Thompson, R.L. and Monroe, R.J., 1978b. Susceptibility of pickling cucumbers to bloater damage by carbonation. J. Food Sci., 43(3): 892-896.

Fleming, H.P., Daeschel, M.A., McFeeters, R.F. and Pierson, M.D., 1989. Butyric acid spoilage of fermented cucumbers. J. Food Sci., 54(3): 636-639.

Fleming, H.P., Etchells, J.L., Thompson, R.L. and Bell, T.A., 1975. Purging of CO_2 from cucumber brines to reduce bloater damage. J. Food Sci., 40(6): 1304-1310.

Fleming, H.P., Thompson, R.L., Bell, T.A. and Hontz, L.H., 1978a. Controlled fermentation of sliced cucumbers. J. Food Sci., 43(3): 888-891.

Fleming, H.P., McFeeters, R.F., Daeschel, M.A., Humphries, E.G. and Thompson, R.L., 1988. Fermentation of cucumbers in anaerobic tanks. J. Food Sci., 53(1): 127-133.

Fleming, H.P., Thompson, R.L., Etchells, J.L., Kelling, R.E. and Bell, T.A., 1973a. Bloater formation in brined cucumbers fermented by *Lactobacillus plantarum*. J. Food Sci., 38(3): 499-503.

Fleming, H.P., Thompson, R.L., Etchells, J.L., Kelling, R.E. and Bell, T.A., 1973b. Carbon dioxide production in the fermentation of brined cucumbers. J. Food Sci., 38(3): 504-506.

Fukushima, T., 1978. Chilling-injury in cucumber fruits. VI. The mechanism of pectin de-methylation. Scientia Hortic., 9: 215-226.

Geisman, J.R. and Henner, R.E., 1973. Recycling food brine eliminates pollution. Food Engng., 45(11): 119-121.

Gould, W.A., 1983. "Tomato Production, Processing and Quality Evaluation", 2d edition, AVI Publishing Company, Inc, Wesport, Connecticut, pp 172-173.

Guillou, A.A. 1991. Minimization of the amount of NaCl used during natural cucumber fermentation and storage through multi-response optimization methods. M.S. Thesis, Purdue University, Dept. of Food Science, W. Lafayette, IN.

Guillou, A.A., Floros, J.D. and Cousin, M.A. 1991. The role of calcium chloride and potassium sorbate in reducing the amount of sodium chloride used during natural cucumber fermentation and storage. Purdue University, Agricultural Experiment Station, Paper # 13063, W. Lafayette, IN.

Haard, N.F., 1985. Characteristics of edible plant tissues. In "Food Chemistry", 2d edition, O.R. Fennema, (Ed.), Marcel Dekker, Inc., New York, NY, pp 885-886.

Hudson, J.M. and Buescher, R.W., 1980. Prevention of soft center development in large whole cucumber pickles by calcium. J. Food Sci., 45(6): 1450-1451.

Hudson, J.M. and Buescher, R.W., 1985. Pectic substances and firmness of cucumber pickles as influenced by $CaCl_2$, NaCl and brine storage. J. Food Biochem., 9(3): 211-229.

Hudson, J.M. and Buescher, R.W., 1986. Relationship between degree of pectin methylation and tissue firmness of cucumber pickles. J. Food Sci., 51(1): 138-149.

Humphries, E.G. and Fleming, H.P., 1989. Anaerobic tanks for cucumber fermentation and storage. J. Agric. Engng. Res., 44(2): 133-140.

Lampi, R.A., Esselen, W.B., Thomson, C.L. and Anderson, E.E., 1958. Changes in pectic substances of four varieties of pickling cucumbers during fermentation and softening. Food Res., 23(3): 351-363.

Lesley, B.E. and Cruess, W.V., 1928. The effect of acidity on the softening of dill pickles. Fruits Products J. & Amer. Vinegar Ind., 7(10): 12.

Lingle, M., 1975. Controlled fermentation of cucumbers: the"how's" and "why's". Food Production/Management, pp 10-13.

McFeeters, R.F. and Armstrong, S.A., 1984. Measurement of pectin methylation in plant cell walls. Anal.Biochem., 139(1): 212-217.

McFeeters, R.F., Bell, T.A. and Fleming, H.P., 1980. An endo-polygalacturonase in cucumber fruit. J. Food Biochem., 4(1): 1-16.

McFeeters, R.F., Fleming, H.P. and Daeschel, M.A., 1984. Malic acid degradation and brined cucumber bloating. J. Food Sci., 49(4): 999-1002.

McFeeters, R.F., Fleming, H.P. and Thompson, R.L., 1982a. Malic and citric acids in pickling cucumbers. J. Food Sci., 47(6): 1859-1861.

McFeeters, R.F., Fleming, H.P. and Thompson, R.L., 1982b. Malic acid as a source of carbon dioxide in cucumber juice fermentations. J. Food Sci., 47(6): 1862-1865.

McFeeters, R.F., Fleming, H.P. and Thompson, R.L., 1985. Pectinesterase activity, pectin methylation, and texture changes during storage of blanched cucumber slices. J. Food Sci., 50(1): 201-205.

Palnitkar, M.P. and McFeeters R.F., 1975. Recycling spent brines in cucumber fermentations. J. Food Sci., 40(6): 1311-1315.

Pangborn, R.M., Vaughn, R.H., York II, G.K. and Estelle, M., 1959. Effect of sugar, storage time and temperature on dill pickle quality. Food Technol., 13(9): 489-492.

Potts, E.A. and Fleming, H.P., 1982. Prevention of mold-induced softening in air-purged, brined cucumbers by acidification. J. Food Sci., 47(5): 1723-1727.

Stamer, J.R., 1979. The lactic acid bacteria: microbes of diversity. Food Tech., 33(1): 60-65.

Tang, H.L. and McFeeters, R.F., 1983. Relationships among cell wall constituents, calcium and texture during cucumber fermentation and storage. J. Food Sci., 48(1): 66-70.

USDA, 1986. "Agricultural Statistics", U.S. Dept. of Agriculture, U.S. Government Printing Office, Washington, DC.

Van Buren, J.P., 1968. Adding calcium to snap beans at different stages in processing: calcium uptake and texture of the canned product. Food Technol., 22(6): 132-135.

Van Buren, J.P., 1979. The chemistry of texture in fruits and vegetables. J. Texture Stud., 10(1): 1-23.

Van Buren, J.P., Moyer, J.C. and Robinson, W.B., 1962. Pectin methylesterase in snap beans. J. Food Sci., 27: 291-294.

Wallace, D.H. and Andres, C., 1977. Controlled fermentation of cucumbers reduces defects from 40% down to 5%. Food Processing., 38(6): 70-71.

Whistler, R.L. and Daniel, J.R., 1985. Carbohydrates. In "Food Chemistry", 2d edition, O.R. Fennema, (Ed.), Marcel Dekker, Inc., New York, NY, pp 123-125.

G. Charalambous (Ed.), Food Science and Human Nutrition
© 1992 Elsevier Science Publishers B.V. All rights reserved.

RETENTION OF ADDED ACIDS DURING THE EXTRUSION OF CORN STARCH/ISOLATED SOY PROTEIN BLENDS

J.A. MAGA and C.H. KIM

Department of Food Science and Human Nutrition, Colorado State University, Fort Collins, Colorado 80523 (United States)

SUMMARY

C_6, C_8 and C_{10} acids were added to either high or low amylose 70% corn starch/30% isolated soy protein blends and extruded with 24% moisture at 125°C. Starches with no added protein were extruded under the same conditions and served as controls. Resulting extrudates were treated with protease and amylase and the amounts of free, starch-bound and protein-bound acids were determined by gas chromatography. In starch only systems, acid retention was greatest for low amylose starch, and retention increased with chain length. The addition of isolated soy protein increased added compound retention.

INTRODUCTION

The flavoring of extruded foods has traditionally been a problem due to limited compound stability during extrusion and compound volatility immediately after exiting the die (1). Surprisingly few studies have specifically addressed this important issue (2-7).

Starch/flavor (8,9) and protein/flavor (10,11) interactions have been reported to occur in model systems. In theory, if such interactions could be encouraged during extrusion processing, added flavor compound stability and/or retention could be improved.

Therefore, the major objective of this study was to add a series of volatile acids to starch having either a high or low amylose content as well as the presence or absence of isolated soy protein, extrude under a standard set of conditions, and observe resulting acid retention in extrudates. Hopefully, the resulting information would provide a better understanding of added flavor on starch/protein interactions during extrusion processing.

MATERIALS AND METHODS

Materials

Two commercial corn starches (National Starch and Chemical Corp., Bridgewater, NJ, U.S.A.) having amylose/amylopectin ratios of 20/80 and 55/45 were used as the base materials. A commercial isolated soy protein, PP610 (Protein Technologies International, St. Louis, MO, U.S.A.) served as the protein source. Hexanoic, octanoic and decanoic acids were commercially obtained (Sigma Chemical Co., St. Louis, MO, U.S.A.). Theramyl 120 L was used for enzymatic starch digestion and Neutrase 0.5 L was employed for enzymatic protein digestion. Both were obtained from Novo Laboratories, Inc., Wilton, CT, U.S.A.

Feed Material Preparation

Starch and protein moisture contents were determined. With the starch only series, the acids were added at a level of 200 ppm each and the mixtures blended for 10 min., then the moisture content was adjusted to 24% with tap water. For the protein series, 30% dry weight isolated soy protein was dry blended for 10 min. with each of the two starches, the acids added and dry blended for 10 additional min. and then the moisture content adjusted to 24%. All mixtures were sealed in moisture proof containers and stored at 22°C for eight hours to insure equilibration.

Extrusion

A Brabender Plasticorder Model PLV 500 single screw laboratory extruder with a barrel length to diameter of 20 to 1 was used. It was equipped with a 4.80 mm diameter die opening and a 3:1 compression screw running at 120 rpm. Dough temperature just before the die exit was maintained at 125°C.

Compound Extraction

Extrudates were permitted to air dry at room temperature for 24 hours and then ground to pass through a 0.5 mm screen. Three 0.5 g ground samples of each extrudate were placed in screw cap glass culture tubes and suspended in 4 ml of deionized water. No enzyme was added to one set of tubes. This set represented "free" acids. To another set of tubes, the starch degrading enzyme Theramyl 120 L was added ("free plus starch"); and to another set of tubes, the protein degrading enzyme Neutrase 0.5 L was added ("free plus protein"). All tubes were sealed and incubated at 50°C for one hour in a vibrating water bath. The tubes were permitted to cool to room temperature and extracted with 4 ml of ether.

Gas Chromatographic analysis

A Hewlett-Packard Model 5830A gas chromatograph equipped with a Model 18850A data terminal base was used to separate and quantitate the added compounds. A two-meter glass column packed with 5% Carbowax 20 M on 80/100 mesh Gas Chrom P was used. Known quantities of the added compounds were used for identification/quantitation purposes. All quantitation data were converted to % extrudate retention.

Statistical Design and Analysis

A complete factorial design involving all variables was used. All extrusion runs were repeated and all analyses were performed in duplicate for each of the two runs. All resulting data were combined and statistically evaluated.

RESULTS AND DISCUSSION

The overall influence of starch amylose content on added acid retention is summarized in Table 1.

TABLE 1

Extrudate Percent Added Acid Retentions as Influenced by Starch Amylose Content		
Acid/Form	Amylose Content	
	Low	High
C_6		
Free	74.6	46.3
Free plus starch	47.6	45.2
C_8		
Free	80.3	52.0
Free plus starch	87.1	72.3
C_{10}		
Free	90.0	67.7
Free plus starch	103.0	86.1

First of all, it can be seen that acid retention for all acids was significantly higher in low amylose starch as compared to high amylose starch. Starch low in amylose, the straight chain fraction of starch, is proportionality higher in amylopectin, the branched chain fraction of starch. Therefore, the data in Table 1 clearly suggest that hexanoic, octanoic and decanoic acids are preferentially bound or entrapped in the amylopectin portion of starch, thereby minimizing their volatility immediately after extrusion.

Another significant observation noted from the Table 1 data is that added acid retention increased in both low and high amylose starches as chain length increased. The most probable explanation for the phenomena is that compound boiling point increases as chain length increases.

Treatment with an amylase enzyme (Theramyl 120 L) demonstrated that significantly higher amounts of octanoic and decanoic acids were preferentially part of the starch structure compared to hexanoic acid. Again, probably relative compound volatility contributed to this observation. Since hexanoic acid had the greatest volatility among the compounds evaluated, its ability to interact with starch was minimized.

The contribution of 30% isolated soy protein to both low and high amylose starch acid retention is summarized in Table 2.

The "free" data shown in Table 2 are the same as those presented in Table 1, and thus the same general conclusion apply for them in this presentation.

TABLE 2

Acid/Form	Extrudate Percent Added Acid Retentions as Influenced by Starch Amylose Content and Isolated Soy Protein Addition	
	Amylose Content	
	Low	High
C_6 Free	74.6	46.3
Free plus protein	69.2	59.1
C_8 Free	80.3	52.0
Free plus protein	100.4	65.9
C_{10} Free	90.9	67.7
Free plus protein	100.4	98.7

The inclusion of isolated soy protein at an arbitrary level of 30% did show a dramatic added acid binding effect as compared to starch along (Table 1), especially when utilized in combination with low amylose (high amylopectin) starch. For octanoic and decanoic acids, the combination of 30% isolated soy protein and low amylose starch resulted in 100% acid recoveries. Significant improvements in retention were also noted when high amylose starch and isolated soy protein were used, especially for decanoic acid.

Therefore, this study clearly demonstrated that relative to the retention of volatile acids that may have application as flavoring agents in extruded foods, the utilization of low amylose starch is preferred to high amylose starch, and that the inclusion of protein (30% isolated soy protein) significantly improves added acid compound retention in final extrudates.

REFERENCES

1. J.R. Blanchfield and C. Ovenden, Food Manufacture, 49 (1) (1974) 27-28, 51.
2. P.E. Packert and I.S. Fagerson, J. Food Sci. 45 (1980) 526-528, 533.
3. R. Delache, Gretreide Mehl. Brot., 36 (9) (1982) 246-248.
4. R.P. Lane, Cereal Foods World, 28(3) (1983) 181-183.
5. C.R. Lazarus and K.H. Renz, Cereal Foods World, 30(5) (1985) 319-320.
6. M. Mariani, A. Scotti and E. Colombo, in: J. Adda (Ed.), Progress in Flavor Research, Elsevier, Amsterdam, 1985, pp 549-562.
7. J. Chen, G.A. Reineccius and T.P. Labuza, J. Food Technol., 21 (1986) 365-383.
8. H.G. Maier, K. Moritz and U. Rummler, Starch/Starke 39 (4) (1987) 126-131.
9. E. Schmidt and H.G. Maier, Starch/Starke 39 (6) (1987) 203-207.
10. G. Jasinski and A. Kilaria, Milcwissenschaft, 40 (10) (1985) 596-599.
11. T.E. O'Neil and J.E. Kinsella, J. Food Sci., 52 (1987) 98-101.

BINDING DURING EXTRUSION OF ADDED FLAVORANTS AS INFLUENCED BY STARCH AND PROTEIN TYPES

J.A. MAGA and C.H. KIM

Department of Food Science and Human Nutrition, Colorado State University, Fort Collins, Colorado 80523 (United States)

SUMMARY

A series of C_6, C_8 and C_{10} alcohols, aldehydes and acids were added to either 100% low or high amylose corn starch or 70% low or high amylose corn starch and two 30% isolated soy proteins having different functional properties or two 30% milk protein isolates having different properties. The mixtures were adjusted to 24% moisture and extruded at 125°C. Resulting extrudates were enzymatically treated and the individual percent added compound retention determined gas chromatographically. Starch but not protein types did influence retention. Acids were bound more than alcohols with aldehydes being retained the least.

INTRODUCTION

Traditionally, extruded snack foods are flavored after extrusion, which adds to the complexity and expense of their manufacture. Pre-extrusion flavor addition has met with only limited success (1) primarily due to compound volatility as the extrudate exits the die.

Both starch (2,3) and protein (4,5) are known to bind flavorants, and thus a study was designed to investigate the roles of both starch and protein types on their ability to bind a series of flavorants having varying chain length and functional groups. Information of this type could prove useful in formulating ingredient blends with increased added volatile compound retention with extrusion processing.

MATERIALS AND METHODS

Materials

Two commercial corn starches (National Starch and Chemical Corp., Bridgewater, NJ, U.S.A.) having amylose/amylopectin ratios of 20/80 and 55/45 were used as the base materials. Two commercial isolated soy proteins, PP 610 and PP 710 (Protein Technologies International, St. Louis, MO, U.S.A.), having different functional properties and two whole milk protein isolates, TMP 1100 and TMP 1320 (New Zealand Milk Products Inc., Petaluma, CA, U.S.A.), also differing in properties served as protein sources. A series of alcohols (hexanol, octanol, decanol), aldehydes (hexanal, octanal, decanal), and acids (hexanoic, octanoic, decanoic) were commercially obtained (Sigma Chemical Co., St. Louis, MO, U.S.A.). Theramyl 120 L was used for enzymatic starch hydrolysis and Neutrase 0.5 L was employed for enzymatic protein hydrolysis. Both enzymes were obtained from Novo Laboratories, Inc., Wilton, CT, U.S.A.

Feed Material Preparation

The moisture content of all starches and proteins was determined. For the two starch only series, 200 ppm of each compound was added to each starch and the mixture was dry blended for 10 min., then the moisture content was adjusted to 24%, followed by an additional 10 min. of blending. For the protein series, 30% dry weight of each of the four proteins was dry blended with each of the two starches for 10 min., then the nine flavor compounds were added, each at 200 ppm, and the mixture dry blended for another 10 min., at which time the moisture content was adjusted to 24% with tap water and this mixture blended for an additional 10 min. All final mixtures were sealed in moisture proof containers and stored at 22°C for eight hours to insure equilibration.

Extrusion

A Brabender Plasticorder Model PLV500 single screw laboratory extruder with a barrel length to diameter of 20 to 1 was used. It was equipped with a 4.80 mm diameter die opening and a 3:1 compression screw running at 120 rpm. Dough temperature just before the die exit was maintained at 125°C. Under these conditions, a highly expanded extrudate, typical of expanded snacks, resulted.

Compound Extraction

Extrudates were permitted to air dry at room temperature for 24 hours and then ground to pass through a 0.5 mm screen. Three 0.5 g ground samples of each extrudate were placed in screw cap glass culture tubes and suspended in 4 ml of deionized water. No enzyme was added to one set of tubes. This set represented the amount of "free" (not bound) compounds present in each extrudate. To another set of tubes, the starch degrading enzyme Theramyl 120 L was added (free plus starch"). This set accounted for the amount of compounds bound by the starch portion of the extrudate. To the last set of tubes, the protein degrading enzyme Neutrase 0.5 L was added to account for the amount of compounds associated with the protein portion of the extrudates. All tubes were sealed and incubated at 50°C for one hour in a vibrating water bath. The tubes were permitted to cool to room temperature and extracted with 4 ml of ether.

Gas Chromatographic Analysis

A Hewlett-Packard Model 5830A gas chromatograph equipped with a Model 18850A data terminal base was used to separate and quantitate the added compounds. A two meter glass column packed with 5% Carbowax 20M on 80/100 mesh Gas Chrom P was used. Known quantities of the added compounds were used for identification/quantitation purposes. All quantitation data were converted to % extrudate retention.

Statistical Design and Analysis

A complete factorial design involving all variables was used. All extrusion runs were repeated and all analyses were performed in duplicate for each of the two runs. All resulting data were combined and statistically evaluated. A summary of the project design is shown in Table 1.

TABLE 1

Variables and Levels Used	
Variables	**Levels**
Starch Low amylose/amylopectin (20/80) high amylose/amylopectin (55/45)	100% or 70% 100% or 70%
Protein Isolated soy (PP 610 or PP 710) Milk protein isolate (TMP 1100 or TMP 1320)	0 or 30% 0 or 30%
Volatile compounds Hexanol, octanol, decanol Hexanal, octanal, decanal hexanoic, octanoic, decanoic acids	200 ppm each 200 ppm each 200 ppm each
All extrusion runs performed with 24% total feed moisture and the unit operating at 120 rpm and 125°C extrudate temperature.	

RESULTS AND DISCUSSION

Starch Type/Functional Group/Chain Length Interactions

The overall influence of starch amylose content on added compound retention is summarized in Table 2. Several trends are apparent from viewing these data. First of all, for each compound class, retention increased as chain length increased. This was especially true with low amylose starch and was probably associated with the fact that compound boiling point increased with chain length (Table 3). These boiling point data also correlate well with the observation that with low amylose starch, regardless of chain length, acids had the greatest retention while aldehydes had the least. Also, most compound/classes, except for C_6 and C_{10} alcohol actually bound to low amylose starch. Low amylose starch has a higher proportion of amylopectin which appears to be effective in binding most of the compounds evaluated.

A somewhat different picture appears when one looks at the influence of high amylose (low amylopectin) starch on retention in Table 2. Here compounds such as C_8 and C_{10} alcohols, C_8 acid and C_{10} aldehyde were effectively bound to starch. From this, one could conclude that they preferentially bind to amylose

TABLE 2

Extrudate Percent Added Compound Retention as Influenced by Starch Amylose Content		
Compound/Form	Amylose Content	
	Low	High
C_6 Alcohol		
Free	39.3	46.8
Free plus starch	35.8	52.8
C_6 Aldehyde		
Free	7.7	8.4
Free plus starch	9.3	10.5
C_6 Acid		
Free	74.6	46.3
Free plus starch	47.6	45.2
C_8 Alcohol		
Free	40.7	50.8
Free plus starch	51.4	65.3
C_8 Aldehyde		
Free	37.5	43.8
Free plus starch	50.1	46.3
C_8 Acid		
Free	80.3	52.0
Free plus starch	87.1	72.3
C_{10} Alcohol		
Free	57.0	32.3
Free plus starch	51.1	70.0
C_{10} Aldehyde		
Free	69.8	48.8
Free plus starch	87.5	72.0
C_{10} Acid		
Free	90.9	67.7
Free plus starch	103.0	56.1

TABLE 3

Boiling Points of Added Compounds			
Chain Length	Boiling Point (°C)		
	Alcohols	Aldehydes	Acids
C_6	158	128	205
C_8	194	171	239
C_{10}	210	208	270

since more amylose than amylopectin was present in this starch. With high amylose starch, overall, binding relative to added compound functional groups was not significantly different for alcohols and acids but was significantly lower for aldehydes, demonstrating the aldehydes were not as active as the other compound groups evaluated.

Starch Type/Functional Group/Chain Length/Protein Type Interactions

The different protein types were initially chosen because of their basic differences in structure. Soy protein has a highly dense and organized concentric structure, whereas milk protein has a more open and loose structure. One would expect that, due to structure, protein interaction with starch and added flavorants would be different with these two protein sources. In addition, each of the two proteins from the two sources had been commercially altered thereby giving them different viscosities and foaming properties. This in turn should also influence their reactivity with other components.

The influence of protein type upon the variables already discussed is summarized in Table 4; and, as can be seen, overall, the four proteins reacted in a rather similar manner. One factor not originally considered in the design of this experiment was that ingredients undergo much more stress and mechanical shear during extrusion processing compared to conventional heat processing and thus the major factor was that 30% protein was present and therefore protein type became inconsequential. Also, overall, the addition of protein appeared to minimize the influence of low versus high amylose starch that was obvious in the starch only extruded system.

As with the starch only system, C_6 aldehyde retention was quite minimal independent of starch or protein source. As shown in Table 3, this compound had the lowest boiling point of any compound evaluated, and thus volatility was probably the predominant factor contributing to its low retention. In general, with a few minor exceptions, retention for all compounds increased with increasing chain length.

Therefore, this study clearly demonstrated that compound volatility/chain length is a significant factor in both starch and starch/protein extrusion processing relative to flavorant retention. Also, in this study, protein type/modification did not significantly influence overall flavorant retention.

TABLE 4

Extrudate Percent Added Compound Retention as Influenced by Starch and Protein Types

Compound/Form	Low Amylose				High Amylose			
Protein*:	PP 710	PP 610	TMP 1100	TMP 1320	PP 710	PP 610	TMP 1100	TMP 1320
C_6 Alcohol								
Free	39.8	50.5	48.6	41.9	46.7	52.3	47.9	43.2
Free plus protein	52.1	50.2	55.6	48.4	48.0	50.1	47.0	44.6
C_6 Aldehyde								
Free	8.0	10.2	7.8	6.3	6.5	9.4	7.2	7.0
Free plus protein	9.2	10.3	7.3	6.6	7.3	9.5	8.1	10.5
C_6 Acid								
Free	36.2	74.6	21.6	33.8	37.2	46.3	13.0	26.2
Free plus protein	70.9	69.2	69.4	57.3	80.7	59.1	70.8	58.5
C_8 Alcohol								
Free	44.5	58.3	50.8	47.2	50.6	57.2	51.1	40.0
Free plus protein	63.7	60.6	64.3	55.2	58.2	59.6	55.5	64.3
C_8 Aldehyde								
Free	30.1	42.5	43.7	51.5	34.4	48.3	47.9	49.6
Free plus protein	39.5	47.7	41.9	38.7	85.7	42.5	41.4	43.0
C_8 Acid								
Free	78.0	80.3	75.8	85.3	40.4	52.0	67.5	63.2
Free plus protein	94.9	100.4	102.4	83.7	72.2	65.9	102.1	82.5
C_{10} Alcohol								
Free	56.9	72.8	59.3	53.3	45.0	38.7	48.7	29.9
Free plus protein	66.8	64.7	67.6	62.3	60.7	54.5	56.7	61.4
C_{10} Aldehyde								
Free	70.2	87.5	95.2	90.4	58.1	50.7	86.7	82.4
Free plus protein	68.0	88.4	89.5	80.7	71.0	75.6	80.8	79.3
C_{10} Acid								
Free	102.8	90.9	84.6	101.1	78.3	67.7	90.3	53.7
Free plus protein	103.0	100.4	104.4	83.0	73.8	98.7	103.1	102.4

*PP proteins are soy; TMP are milk.

REFERENCES

1. J.R. Blanchfield and L. Ovenden, Food Manufacture, 49 (1) (1974) 27-38, 51.
2. H.G. Maier, K. Mortiz and U. Rummler, Starch/Starke, 39 (4) (1987) 126-131.
3. E. Schmidt and H.G. Maier, Starch/Starke, 39 (6) (1987) 203-207.
4. G. Jasinski and A. Kilaria, Milcwissenschaft, 40 (10) (1985) 596-599.
5. T.E. O'Neil and J.E. Kinsella, J. Food Sci., 52 (1987) 98-101.

G. Charalambous (Ed.), Food Science and Human Nutrition
© 1992 Elsevier Science Publishers B.V. All rights reserved.

CAPSAICINOIDS: ANALOGUE COMPOSITION OF COMMERCIAL PRODUCTS

J.A. MAGA and H. BEL-HAJ

Department of Food Science and Human Nutrition, Colorado State University, Fort Collins, Colorado 80523 (United States)

SUMMARY

Four commercial samples of oleoresin capsicum ranging in Scoville heat units from 500,000 to 1.2 million were extracted and separated gas chromatographically into five capsaicinods (capsaicin, homocapsaicin, nordihydrocapsaicin, dihydrocapsaicin, homodihydrocapsaicin). Relative capsaicin content ranged from 1.14 to 56.92%. Next to capsaicin, homodihydrocapsaicin was the most abundant capsaicinoid (18.34-98.83%). No clear trend was apparent relating capsaicin proportion to Scoville heat units.

INTRODUCTION

Capsicum or capsaicin is the pungent sensation normally associated with various types of hot peppers, and its chemistry has been extensively reviewed (1-3). Structurally, capsaicin is known to be N-(4-hydroxy-3-methoxybenzyl)-8-methylnon-trans-6-enamide (4,5). However, at least four other compounds having similar structures have been identified in natural oleoresin extracts from hot peppers and are collectively called capsaicinoids (6). The closely related compounds are dihydrocapsaicin, nordihydrocapsaicin, homocapsaicin and homodihydrocapsaicin (Figure 1).

Various techniques, including mass fragmentography (6), mass spectrometry (7-9), gas chromatography (10-12), colorimetry (13-14), spectrophotometry (15), HPLC (16) and TLC (17,18), among others, have been used to estimate "capsaicin." Most of these procedures are rather long and involved, and therefore, the Scoville heat unit (19) subjective test has been used to evaluate pungency. Samples are diluted and the reciprocal of the dilution where pungency is detected is expressed as the Scoville heat unit. The pungency resulting from "capsaicin" is detectable at dilutions of from 1 to 15-17 million (20).

Most commercial hot pepper extracts are in the form of oleoresins, which are produced by various means (2,3). All are marketed based on their Scoville heat units, which can range from 50,000 to several million.

Therefore, the major objective of this study was to determine the relative proportions of the various capsaicinoids in a series of commercial oleoresin of capsicum samples and attempt to relate this information to their corresponding Scoville heat unit ratings.

FIGURE 1

Naturally Occurring Capsaicin Analogues

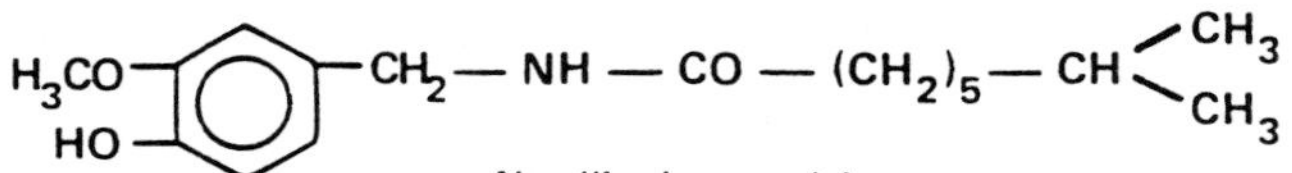

H_3CO-(benzene ring)-HO, $-CH_2-NH-CO-(CH_2)_5-CH(CH_3)_2$

Nordihydrocapsaicin

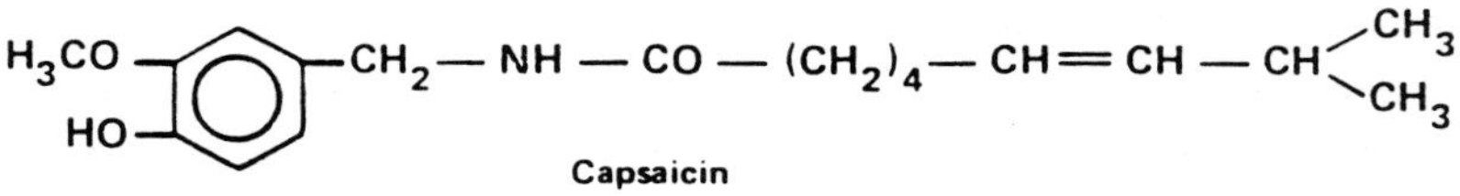

H_3CO-(benzene ring)-HO, $-CH_2-NH-CO-(CH_2)_4-CH=CH-CH(CH_3)_2$

Capsaicin

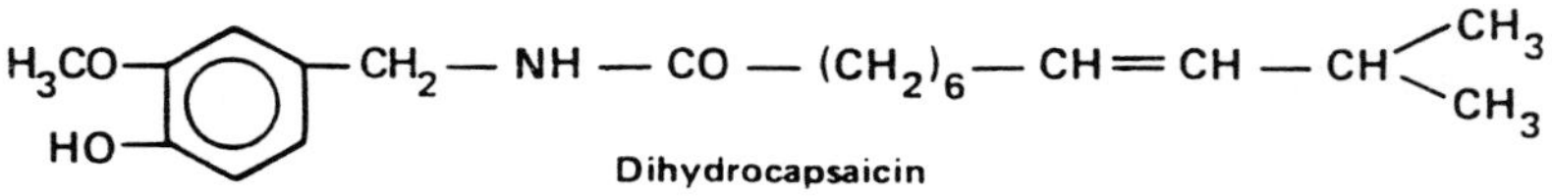

H_3CO-(benzene ring)-HO, $-CH_2-NH-CO-(CH_2)_6-CH=CH-CH(CH_3)_2$

Dihydrocapsaicin

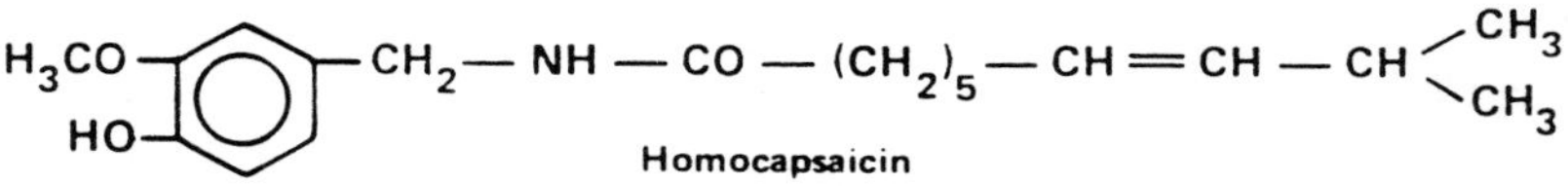

H_3CO-(benzene ring)-HO, $-CH_2-NH-CO-(CH_2)_5-CH=CH-CH(CH_3)_2$

Homocapsaicin

H_3CO-(benzene ring)-HO, $-CH_2-NH-CO-(CH_2)_9-CH(CH_3)_2$

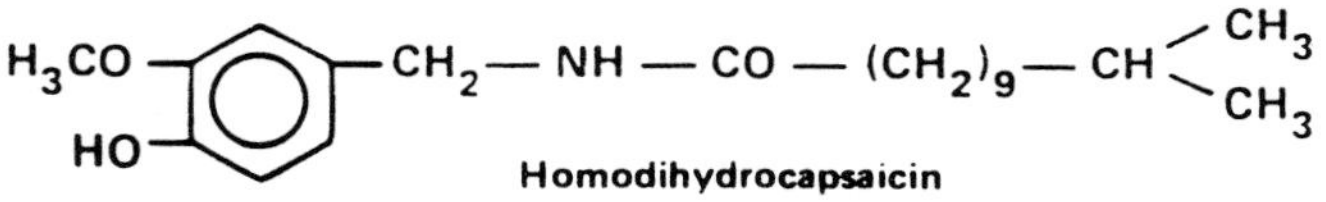

Homodihydrocapsaicin

MATERIALS AND METHODS

Oleoresin Sources

Four commercial samples, all labelled oleoresin capsicum, were obtained. Sources and Scoville heat unit ratings were as follows: Sample A. Ungerer Company, New York, NY, 500,000; Sample B. Ungerer Company, New York, NY, one million; Sample C. Fritzche Dodge and Ollcott, Inc., New York, NY, one million; and Sample D. Fritzche Dodge and Ollcott, Inc., New York, NY, 1.2 million.

Capsaicinoid Extraction and Concentration

The procedures of Kosuge et al. (21) were used to extract and concentrate the capsaicinoids present in all samples. A 25 ml oleoresin sample size was used.

Gas Chromatographic Procedure

A 0.5 µl sample of the concentrate from above was placed in a 5 ml screw cap reaction vial and 3 ml of TMS derivatizing reagent added. The mixture was capped and permitted to react at room temperature for three hours before a 3 µl sample was injected into the gas chromatograph.

A Hewlett-Packard Model 402 gas chromatograph equipped with a 2 m by 2 mm i.d. glass u-tube glass column packed with 3% SE-30 on 60/80 mesh acid washed silanized Chromosorb-W was used for separation. The column temperature was programmed from 170 to 230°C at 4°C/min. Injection temperature was 200°C while the flame ionization detector was 280°C. Helium at a flow rate of 20 ml/min. was used as the carrier. Compound identifications were based on literature values (10-12). Peak areas were calculated and reported to relative percent composition.

RESULTS AND DISCUSSION

The relative proportions of the various capsaicinoids found in the four samples are summarized in Table 1.

TABLE 1

Capsaicinoid Composition (%) of Commercial Oleoresin Capsicum Samples and their Scoville Heat Units				
Compound	Sample			
	A	B	C	D
Homocapsaicin	0.41	0.27	---	---
Nordihydrocapsaicin	13.08	22.38	0.03	13.00
Capsaicin	13.38	30.85	1.14	56.92
Dihydrocapsaicin	17.08	28.16	---	---
Homodihydrocapsaicin	66.05	18.34	98.83	30.08
Scoville Heat Units	500,000	1 million	1 million	1.2 million

Samples A and B were from one source while samples C and D were from another; and, as can be seen, they were dramatically different in capsaicinoid composition. No homocapsaicin or dihydrocapsaicin were detected in samples C and D. Perhaps the two suppliers used different hot pepper varietals, or more probably, extraction techniques used in oleoresin manufacture were different. Sample C was also rather unique in that it was almost 99% homodihydrocapsaicin. Among all samples, sample D had the highest relative proportion of capsaicin (56.92%) and also had the highest Scoville rating (1.2 million).

Samples A and D had detectable amounts of all five capsaicinoids, although the homocapsaicin levels were quite low. Interestingly, sample B, which had twice the Scoville rating of sample A, had approximately twice as much capsaicin present. However, this trend was not apparent with sample C and D, since approximately 50 times more capsaicin was present in sample D as compared to C, yet the Scoville units differed by only 200,000. Obviously, homodihydrocapsaicin makes a significant contribution to pungency.

In conclusion, dramatic differences in capsaicinoid composition were found between suppliers, probably due to differences in manufacture or perhaps sample storage/age where oxidation could become a factor. The data observed in this study would indicate that Scoville heat units can not be directly related to capsaicin level, with apparently the other capsaicinoids also contributing to pungency.

REFERENCES

1. J.A. Maga, CRC Crit. Rev. Food Sci. Nutr., 6 (1975) 177-199.
2. V.S. Govindarajan, CRC Crit. Rev. Food Sci. Nutr., 22 (1988) 109-176.
3. V.S. Govindarajan, CRC Crit. Rev. Food Sci. Nutr. 23 (1989) 207-288.
4. E.K. Nelson and L.E. Dawson, J. Am. Chem. Soc., 45 (1923) 2179-2181.
5. L. Crombie, S.H. Dandegaonker and K.B. Simpson, J. Chem. Soc., (1955) 1025-1027.
6. K.R. Lee, T. Suzuki, M. Kobashi, K. Hasegawa and K. Iwai, J. Chromatog., 123 (1976) 119-128.
7. D.J. Bennett and G.W. Kirby, J. Chem. Soc. C, (1968) 442-446.
8. S. Kosuge and M. Furuta, Agric. Biol. Chem., 34 (1970) 248-256.
9. A. Muller-Stock, R. K. Joshi and J. Buchi, J. Chromatog., 79 (1973) 229-232.
10. Y. Masada, K. Hashimoto, T. Inoue and M. Suzuki, J. Food Sci., 36 (1971) 858-860.
11. J.J. Dicecco, J. Assoc. Official Anal. Chem., 59 (1976) 1-4.
12. J. Hollo, E. Kurucz and J. Bodor, Lebensm. Wiss. Technol., 2 (1969) 19-24.
13. L.F. Tice, Am. J. Pharm., 105 (1933) 320-325.
14. H. North, Anal. Chem., 21 (1944) 934-936.
15. J.I. Suzuki, F. Tausig and R.E. Morse, Food Technol., 11 (1957) 100-107.
16. V.K. Attuquayafio and K.A. Buckle, J. Agric. Food Chem., 35 (1987) 777-779.
17. R. Rangoonwala, J. Chromatog., 41 (1969) 265-270.
18. P. Spanyar and M. Blazovich, Analyst, Lond., 94 (1969) 1084-1087.
19. W.L. Scoville, J. Am. Pharm. Assoc., 1 (1912) 453-455.
20. P.H. Todd, Food Technol., 12 (1958) 468-473.
21. S. Kosugue, Y. Inagaki and K. Uehara, J. Agric. Chem. Soc. Japan, 32 (1958) 578-585.

INFLUENCE OF CULTIVAR AND PROCESSING ON PEACH DRINK ACCEPTABILITY AND YIELD

J.A. MAGA[1] and R.A. RENQUIST[2]

[1]Department of Food Science and Human Nutrition, Colorado State University, Fort Collins, Colorado 80523 (United States)

[2]Orchard Mesa Research Center, Colorado State University, Grand Junction, Colorado 81503 (United States)

SUMMARY

Redhaven, Suncrest and Elberta peaches were processed with and without skin/pit in the presence of pectinase for five hours at 20° or 35°C. Resulting yield and overall acceptability were determined. Incubation at 35°C increased yield over 20° for all variables. The absence of skin and/or pit increased juice yield. Over all variables, Suncrest produced the most acceptable peach juice. The lower incubation temperature produced a better quality juice. The presence of skin during incubation produced a more desirable drink while the presence of peach pits detracted from juice quality. The Suncrest peach cultivar produced the best quality juice.

INTRODUCTION

Traditionally, Colorado peaches have been exclusively marketed in the fresh form and no effort has been made to utilize product deemed not appropriate for the fresh market. The amount of unmarketed peaches in Colorado amounts to approximately one million to three million pounds per year. This vast poundage currently has little or no economic value and thus represents an area worthy of investigation, since these rejects could serve as an excellent source of starting material for a variety of peach-based products that would represent an added monetary return to the grower. Other states have reported on similar projects with fruits (1).

The American public is becoming more aware of the need for good quality fruit drinks in their diet and thus the popularity of fruit-based noncarbonated drinks is increasing. The introduction of aseptic processing/packaging has also made a significant contribution to this trend.

Therefore, the major objectives of this study were to evaluate the properties of the major peach cultivars grown in the Colorado region as influenced by various processing techniques, such as the presence or absence of skin and, or pit, for the production and acceptability of a clear peach juice drink.

METHODS
Materials

Redhaven, Suncrest and Elberta peaches from the Palisade and Hotchkiss areas of Colorado which ripen early (July 27-August 13), mid-season (August 15-August 26) and late in the season (August 20-September 10), respectively, that were fully ripe but were undersized, oversized or slightly blemished for the fresh market were obtained from the sorting of freshly harvested fruit.

Processing

One of the processing variables evaluated was the presence or absence of skins and pits on resulting product quality. Therefore, 40 Kg batches of each cultivar were either manually peeled and pitted or left with the skin on and pitted and immediately ground to pass through a 2 mm sieve. The resulting pulp was immediately batch pasteurized for 30 min. at 80°C and cooled to either 35° or 20°C. The pits were saved from each cultivar and added back to one-half of the heat processed lots. Pits were not added to the remainder of each lot. A commercial pectinase enzyme (Novo Laboratories, Inc., Wilton, CT) at a level of 0.0005% (wt/wt) was added to the 35° or 20°C peach pulp and held at their respective temperatures for five hours with manual stirring every 30 min. After incubation, the mixture was filtered through Whatman No. 1 filter paper and the yield of clear juice determined, based on the original starting weight of intact peaches. After filtration, all juices were stored in glass overnight at 4°C before sensory evaluation.

A summary of the cultivar/processing variables evaluated in this study is shown in Table 1.

TABLE 1

Peach Cultivar and Processing Variables Evaluated
Cultivar: Redhaven, Suncrest, Elberta
Presence of Skin: Yes or No
Presence of Pit: Yes or No
Incubation Temperature: 20° or 35°C
Added Enzyme: Yes for all variables

Sensory Evaluation

A taste panel consisting of 20 faculty/staff members within the Department of Food Science and Human Nutrition, who ranged in age from 25-65, was used to evaluate the overall acceptability of each product. There were 12 females and 8 males on the panel. All had undergone previous instruction in sensory evaluation techniques and thus were considered to be a trained panel.

During mid-afternoon over an eight-day period, 50 ml of 4°C coded samples were presented in clear glass beakers for each of the 24 variables shown in Table 1. A maximum of six samples was randomly presented to each panel member at one session. Rinse water was presented for use between sample evaluation. The evaluations were randomly repeated so that each panel member evaluated a total of 48 samples. Data from both evaluations were averaged and the means for each variable statistically compared.

The panel was asked to rate the overall acceptability of each sample considering factors such as appearance, aroma, flavor and consistency using the 7-point hedonic scale shown in Table 2.

TABLE 2

Sensory Hedonic Scale used for Overall Acceptability
1) ____ Like extremely
2) ____ Like very much
3) ____ Like a little
4) ____ Neither like nor dislike
5) ____ Dislike a little
6) ____ Dislike very much
7) ____ Dislike extremely

RESULTS AND DISCUSSION

In any processing operation, usable product yield is an important factor to consider; and as can be seen in Table 3, the variables evaluated did significantly influence yield.

At either temperature of incubation, Suncrest had the highest juice yield ranging from 84-93% based on initial intact peach weight. In contrast, overall juice yield for Redhaven was 72-88%, while that for Elberta was the lowest, ranging from 63-75%. It should be noted that these data are for only one year and environmental factors such as moisture and temperature play an important role in determining the solids to moisture ratio in fruits.

Temperature of incubation also was found to influence juice yield, with the higher temperature (35°C) producing a better yield, probably due to a higher enzymatic activity at the higher temperature.

The presence of both skin or pit in all cases resulted in lower juice yields when compared to samples where either skin or pit were absent. Apparently, part of the enzymatic activity was being utilized to partially degrade these components resulting in the liberation of less juice from the pulp. The highest juice yield resulted when both skin and pit were removed.

TABLE 3

Influence of Cultivar and Processing Variables on Resulting Peach Juice Yield				
Cultivar	Skin	Pit	Incubation Temperature	Weight Percent Yield
Redhaven	+	+	20°C	71
	+	-	20°C	73
	-	+	20°C	73
	-	-	20°C	76
	+	+	35°C	82
	+	-	35°C	83
	-	+	35°C	86
	-	-	35°C	88
Suncrest	+	+	20°C	85
	+	-	20°C	87
	-	+	20°C	89
	-	-	20°C	91
	+	+	35°C	84
	+	-	35°C	85
	-	+	35°C	88
	-	-	35°C	93
Elberta	+	+	20°C	63
	+	-	20°C	65
	-	+	20°C	65
	-	-	20°C	71
	+	+	35°C	73
	+	-	35°C	74
	-	+	35°C	74
	-	-	35°C	75

+ : Present; - : Absent

This portion of the study clearly demonstrated that by choosing the appropriate peach cultivar (Suncrest) and removing its skin and pit, juice yields over 90% could be obtained.

The overall acceptability of resulting unsweetened peach juice served at 4°C is summarized in Table 4.

TABLE 4

Overall Acceptability of Peach Juice as Influenced by Cultivar and Processing Variables				
Cultivar	Skin	Pit	Incubation Temperature	Hedonic Score*
Redhaven	+	+	20°C	2.4
	+	−	20°C	2.0
	−	+	20°C	2.3
	−	−	20°C	2.5
	+	+	35°C	3.3
	+	−	35°C	2.7
	−	+	35°C	3.0
	−	−	35°C	3.0
Suncrest	+	+	20°C	2.4
	+	−	20°C	1.7
	−	+	20°C	2.0
	−	−	20°C	1.9
	+	+	35°C	2.8
	+	−	35°C	2.8
	−	+	35°C	3.0
	−	−	35°C	2.8
Elberta	+	+	20°C	2.7
	+	−	20°C	2.5
	−	+	20°C	2.9
	−	−	20°C	2.5
	+	+	35°C	3.5
	+	−	35°C	3.4
	−	+	35°C	3.5
	−	−	35°C	3.2

* Overall acceptability scores based on a 7-point hedonic scale with 1 being "like extremely," 4 "neither like nor dislike" and 7 being "dislike extremely."
+ : Present; − : Absent

The first obvious factor from the data shown in Table 4 is that all samples scored better than 4 (neither like nor dislike). It was also apparent that incubation at 20°C for all cultivars resulted in better products than incubation at 35°C. Several panel members commented that the 20°C products had a fresher flavor.

The presence of skin apparently contributed to product color since the panel rated these products slightly better than products that did not contain skin. However, the presence of pits was not desirable to overall acceptability and the panel characterized these products as not tasting as sweet in comparison to samples not containing pits.

Relative to cultivars, overall, both Redhaven and Suncrest were statistically the best with the Elberta cultivar being significantly lower in quality. Comments on Elberta juices included that they were not as colorful as the other two and also not as peach and sweet tasting.

In evaluating individual samples, Suncrest without pits and incubated at 20°C either with or without skin had the best overall scores. An average score of 1.7 was recorded with skin, while the without skin sample scored 1.9. Both of these scores were closest to the "like very much" descriptor of the hedonic scale.

In conclusion, this study clearly demonstrated that very acceptable peach juice can be produced from Colorado grown peaches, especially from the Suncrest cultivar.

REFERENCES

1   E.K. Heaton, T.S. Boggess, A.L. Shewfelt, K.C. Li and J.G. Woodroof, Univ. of Georgia, College of Agriculture Experiment Stations, Res. Bull. 136, 1973.

G. Charalambous (Ed.), Food Science and Human Nutrition
© 1992 Elsevier Science Publishers B.V. All rights reserved.

SUBJECTIVE AND OBJECTIVE COMPARISON OF BAKED POTATO AROMA AS INFLUENCED BY VARIETY/CLONE

J.A. MAGA[1] and D.G. HOLM[2]

[1]Department of Food Science and Human Nutrition, Colorado State University, Fort Collins, Colorado 80523 (United States)

[2]San Luis Valley Research Center, Colorado State University, Center, Colorado 81125 (United States)

SUMMARY

Five named potato varieties and eight promising experimental clones were grown at the same location and their baked aromas compared using a sensory panel as well as the levels of specific pyrazines present. Varieties/clones that scored well with the panel had the highest pyrazine concentrations (25-35 ppm), while varieties/clones that scored the lowest had significantly lower pyrazine concentrations (11-12 ppm).

INTRODUCTION

The flavor resulting from a baked potato is unique in that it is dramatically different from that of a raw potato and results solely from the dry heating process. Thus, its flavor is produced due to the thermal reactivity of the precursors present in the potato at the time of heating. The resulting flavor can be described as weak or mild yet is quite characteristic of a baked potato. However, one must assume that potato composition, as influenced by factors such as fertilization, moisture, maturity, storage, and variety, can result in different amounts of precursors and thus influence the final flavor of baked potatoes.

Various groups (1-5) have evaluated the volatiles associated with baked potatoes, with over 420 compounds being observed, of which approximately 260 have been identified. All groups have concluded that as a class, the pyrazines are major contributors to baked potato aroma. Pyrazines thought to contribute the most include 2-ethyl-3,6,-dimethylpyrazine and 2-ethyl-3,5-dimethylpyrazine (1), combinations of 2-isobutyl-3-methylpyrazine, 2,3-diethyl-5-methylpyrazine, and 3,5-diethyl-2-methylpyrazine (2), and 2-ethyl-6-vinylpyrazine along with 2-ethyl-3-methylpyrazine (3).

From a review of the literature, it was concluded that the comparison of different potato varieties relative to their baked volatile composition has not been reported, and thus became the major objective of this study. In addition, an attempt was made to correlate pyrazine concentration with the sensory evaluation of baked potato aroma.

MATERIALS AND METHODS
Potatoes

A total of five named commercial potato varieties (Russet Burbank, Russet Nugget, Russet Norkotah, Centennial Russet, Sangre) along with eight promising experimental clones (AC-81198-11, AC-80545-1, AC-78069-17, AC-77101-1, BC-0038-1, CO-80011-5, CO-81082-1, CO-79018-11) that were grown at the same location (San Luis Valley Research Center, Center, Colorado) during the 1990 summer under commercial cultivation practices were obtained after approximately one month of commercial storage.

Baking

Approximately 20 Kg of tubers from each of the 13 potato lines were individually washed under running tap water and selected so that each tuber weighed 200 ± 10 g. Each tuber was wrapped in commercial sheets (10 x 10 cm) of baking potato aluminum foil to minimize volatile loss and baked at 210°C for 70 min. Preliminary sensory trials had demonstrated that all lines were judged to be completely baked under these conditions.

Sensory Evaluation

A trained 20-member sensory panel composed of 12 women and 8 men ranging in age from 20 to 52 years was used to evaluate baked potato odor.

The individually wrapped tubers were removed from the oven, permitted to sit for 10 min. and then an intact tuber from each variety/clone was randomly presented to each panel member. They were requested to longitudinally split each tuber with a knife and immediately smell the resulting volatiles. They then recorded their impressions on the 5-point hedonic scale shown in Table 1.

TABLE 1

Hedonic Scale used for Baked Potato Volatile Evaluation	
1) ___	Like a lot
2) ___	Like a little
3) ___	Neither like nor dislike
4) ___	Dislike a little
5) ___	Dislike a lot

Pyrazine Extraction/Analysis

Baked potatoes were removed from the oven, permitted to cool at room temperature for 30 min., the foil removed, and 5 Kg were manually mashed and added to a 30 L glass distilling flask containing 12 L of freshly distilled water. The resulting slurry was steam distilled for 4 hours and 1.5 L of distillate were collected. The pH of the distillate was adjusted to 1.5 with hydrochloric acid and then extracted with freshly distilled diethyl ether (8 x 50 ml) to remove non-basic compounds. The basic fraction was liberated by adjusting the pH to 10.5 with sodium hydroxide. The basic components were extracted with diethyl ether (6 x 25 ml) and the extracts combined and concentrated on a rotary evaporator (0°C) to 1 ml. The concentrate was transferred to a 1 ml sampling vial and further reduced to 100 μl by blowing dry nitrogen gas over the liquid.

A 0.2 μl aliquot of the basic fraction was then analyzed on a Hewlett-Packard Model 5750 Gas Chromatograph equipped with a flame ionization detector. A 100 m x 0.3 mm capillary column coated with 95% Amine-200 and 5% Iqepal-880 was programmed from 90-130°C at 2°/min. The injector temperature was set at 190°C while the detector was operated at 200°C. Nitrogen, at 15 ml/min. was used as the carrier gas. Retention times and peak areas were determined with a Hewlett-Packard Model 3370B Digital Integrator. Pyrazine identification and quantitation techniques were the same as reported previously (6).

RESULTS AND DISCUSSION

The series of pyrazines shown in Table 2 was identified as being present in all 13 lines of baked potatoes. All have previously been reported in baked potatoes.

Comparison of the sensory panel scores and the total measured pyrazine concentration for all of the 13 baked potato lines are summarized in Table 3.

It is quite evident from the Table 3 data that the lines that scored in the 1-2 sensory categories had the highest level of total pyrazines. A total of four of the experimental clones and three of the named varieties fell into this category. Total pyrazine concentration for this group ranged from 25-35 ppm. Panel members commented that these products had good baked potato aromas.

As panel scores fell into the 2-3 range, total pyrazine content also fell and ranged from 17-21 ppm. Comments included that baked potatoes in this category had a weak but recognizable baked potato aroma. Three experimental clones and one commercial variety (Russet Norkotah) fell in this range.

Two lines (BC-0038-1) and Sangre (not normally used for baking) scored quite low, 4.1 and 4.4, respectively with the panel. Interestingly, both of these lines had the lowest total measured pyrazine concentrations of 11 and 12 ppm, respectively.

TABLE 2

Pyrazines Identified in Baked Potatoes
2-methylpyrazine
2,3-dimethylpyrazine
2,5-dimethylpyrazine
2,6-dimethylpyrazine
2-ethylpyrazine
2-ethyl-3-methylpyrazine
2-ethyl-5-methylpyrazine
2-ethyl-6-methylpyrazine
2,3,5-trimethylpyrazine
2,3-diethylpyrazine
2-ethyl-3,5-dimethylpyrazine
2-ethyl-3,6-dimethylpyrazine
2-ethyl-6-vinylpyrazine
2-butyl-3-methylpyrazine
2-butyl-6-methylpyrazine
2-isobutyl-3-methylpyrazine
2,3-diethyl-5-methylpyrazine
3,5-diethyl-2-methylpyrazine
2-ethyl-6-propylpyrazine
2-ethyl-3,5,6-trimethylpyrazine
2,3-dimethyl-5-butylpyrazine
2,5-dimethyl-3-butylpyrazine
2,6-dimethyl-3-butylpyrazine
2,5-dimethyl-3-isobutylpyrazine
3-isoamyl-2,5-dimethylpyrazine
2-isopropyl-3-methoxypyrazine

TABLE 3

Comparison of Sensory Scores and Total Pyrazine Concentration (ppm) of Baked Potato Volatiles		
Potato Variety/Clone	Sensory Score*	Total Pyrazines
AC-81198-11	1.1	32
CO-80011-5	1.2	35
AC-77101-1	1.4	27
CO-81082-1	1.5	25
Centennial Russet	1.1	34
Russet Nugget	1.3	30
Russet Burbank	1.3	32
AC-80545-1	2.9	15
AC-78069-17	2.2	21
CO-79018-11	2.3	20
Russet Norkotah	2.7	17
BC-0038-1	4.1	11
Sangre	4.4	12

* : 20-member trained panel using a 5-point hedonic scale with 1 being "like a lot" and 5 being "dislike a lot."

Therefore, results from this study verify the belief that pyrazines are indeed important contributors to baked potato aroma. In addition, this study clearly demonstrates that sensory panel aroma scores correlate quite nicely with total pyrazine concentration. Thus, it is proposed that potato breeders perhaps could use pyrazine concentration in promising lines of baking potatoes as a predictor of sensory potato aroma.

REFERENCES

1   R.G. Buttery, D.G. Guadagni and L.C. Ling, J. Sci. Food Agric., 24 (1973) 1125-1131.
2   S.R. Parceles and S.S. Chang, J. Agric. Food Chem., 22 (1974) 339-340.
3   E.C. Coleman and C.T. Ho, J. Agric. Food Chem., 28 (1980) 66-68.
4   C.T. Ho and E.C. Coleman, J. Food Sci., 45 (1980) 1094-1095.
5   E.C. Coleman, C.T. Ho and S.S. Chang, J. Agric. Food Chem., 29 (1981) 42-48.
6   C.E. Sizer, J.A. Maga and K. Lorenz, Lebensm. Wiss. Technol., 8 (1975) 267-269.

G. Charalambous (Ed.), Food Science and Human Nutrition
© 1992 Elsevier Science Publishers B.V. All rights reserved.

INVESTIGATION OF THE PROPERTIES INFLUENCING POPCORN POPPING QUALITY

J.A. MAGA[1] and B. BLACH[2]

[1]Department of Food Science and Human Nutrition, Colorado State University, Fort Collins, Colorado 80523 (United States)

[2]Colorado Cereals, Yuma, Colorado 80759 (United States)

SUMMARY

The roles of popcorn moisture content and storage temperature prior to popping as well as popping temperature and the amount of added oil and salt on resulting popped volume and number of unpopped kernels were evaluated. Maximum popped volume was in the 12.5-13.5% moisture range while the proportion of unpopped kernels increased with increasing moisture. Popped volume decreased while unpopped kernels increased with an increase in storage temperature. The addition of 2-4% oil maximized popped volume and minimized unpopped kernels. The addition of 2% salt gave the highest popped volume and the lowest amount of unpopped kernels. Optimum popping temperature was 180°C.

INTRODUCTION

Popcorn represents a relatively inexpensive snack food that is easily and quickly prepared. Currently, it is receiving renewed attention from health conscious consumers since it is relatively low in calories and high in dietary fiber. However, low expansion volume and the number of unpopped kernels are frequent consumer complaints (1).

Previous research has shown that moisture content of the popcorn prior to popping is the most significant factor influencing popped volume and percent unpopped kernels (2-8). In addition, popcorn maturity at harvest (2) and handling after harvest (6,8) have also been shown to influence final product quality. The time and temperature influence on popping quality have also been evaluated (3,9) along with the roles of salt, oil and storage time with microwave popcorn (4).

Although the popularity of microwave popcorn has increased, most popcorn is still popped in the conventional manner in the presence of oil and salt. Therefore, the objective of this study was to attempt to evaluate a wide variety of variables, including moisture content, storage temperature prior to popping, popping temperature, and the amount of added oil and salt on conventional popcorn popping and to measure the important consumer attributes of popped volume and the number of unpopped kernels.

MATERIALS AND METHODS

Popcorn

Commercially grown and shelled large kernel popcorn of the White Dynamite variety was obtained (Colorado Cereals, Yuma, CO) in bulk.

Moisture Analysis/Adjustments

Representative samples were ground in a Tekmar A10 analytical mill (Tekmar Company, Cincinnati, OH) and dried in an oven at 100°C for 14 hr. The moisture content of the starting material was found to be 9.5%.

It was decided to evaluate the influence of popcorn moisture content using 0.5% moisture increments from 8.0 to 18.0%. Care was taken to slowly increase or decrease moisture content from the original 9.5% to minimize stress cracks in the unpopped kernels, which has been shown to lower popped volume (6,8).

In the case of moisture contents lower than 9.5%, intact kernels were air dried in an oven at 35°C until the desired moisture contents were achieved. For moisture contents above 9.5%, the calculated amount of additional moisture was sprayed on the inside wall of a 4 L glass container half filled with kernels, sealed with a metal screw cap, and held at room temperature for two weeks to permit equilibration. The actual moisture contents were measured as described above in the moisture adjusted kernels to verify the desired 0.5% increments. A total of 21 moisture levels were evaluated.

Storage Conditions

After moisture adjustments, sealed samples were placed at one of nine temperatures (-20, 0, 20, 35, 45, 55, 65, 75, 85°C) and held there for 90 days. Storage time in the frozen state has been shown to influence the popped volume of microwave popcorn (4). These authors (4) compared one week to eight months of frozen storage. Some consumers store unpopped popcorn in the refrigerator or freezer to maintain product freshness, while others do not. Therefore, in this study, cold temperatures as well as warm to hot storage temperatures were evaluated.

Oil and Salt Additions

In a microwave popcorn study (4) varying the oil and salt levels produced variable results, but in general, increasing the salt content resulted in greater popcorn expansion while low levels (2-5%) of oil addition did not influence popped volume whereas high levels (30%) decreased volume. Therefore, in this study, 17 levels of commercial corn oil addition varying by 2% increments ranging from 0-32% were evaluated, while table salt addition ranged from 0-8% at 1% increments.

Popping Temperature

A Stir Crazy (West Bend Company, West Bend, WI) household automatic popcorn popper was used. The unit was equipped with a Teflon-lined heating base and an automatic stirring rod. A laboratory power rheostat was placed in line so that the heating element temperature could be varied. Rheostat settings were predetermined that would result in heating element temperatures ranging from 165 to 185°C in 5°C increments.

A total of 100 kernels taken directly from each storage temperature was placed in the popping unit with the appropriate oil and salt levels and permitted to pop at each temperature until no further popping was heard for 30 sec. A summary of the variables evaluated is shown in Table 1.

TABLE 1

Variables Evaluated	
Moisture Content:	8.0-18.0% at 0.5% increments (21 levels)
Storage Temperature:	-20, 0, 20, 35, 45, 55, 65, 75, 85°C (9 temps.)
Corn Oil Levels:	0-32% at 2% increments (17 levels)
Salt Levels:	0-8% at 1% increments (9 levels)
Popping Temperature:	165-185°C at 5° increments (5 temps.)

Popped Volume/Unpopped Kernels

Upon completion of the popping cycle, the product was removed from the unit and the unpopped kernels were manually separated and counted. The popped product was placed in a 500 ml graduated cylinder and the volume recorded.

Statistics

The data were analyzed using the Duncan's multiple range test ($p>0.05$).

RESULTS AND DISCUSSION

The amount of moisture present in the kernel did significantly influence both final popped volume and the percent of unpopped kernels (Table 2).

The data in Table 2 clearly show that for this variety of popcorn, optimum moisture content was in the 12.5-13.5% range. This is in general agreement with the literature (2-8). It has been postulated (3) that at low moisture contents there is insufficient superheated water within the kernel for complete expansion; whereas at high moistures, expansion is decreased due to the fact that the excess moisture weakens the pericarp thus causing an early release of pressure.

When one looks at the percent unpopped kernel data presented in Table 2, it can be seen that it does not follow the same trend as for volume. Overall, the proportion of unpopped kernels actually increased as moisture content increased. A similar trend was noted for microwave popcorn (4). Therefore, the fewest unpopped kernels were present in popcorn that had 8.0 to 13.5% moisture (2-4% unpopped), whereas 13-15% unpopped kernels were present in the high moisture (17.0-18.0%) samples. Perhaps as moisture content increases, the pericarp is softened to such an extent that the moisture is lost before it can be converted to superheated steam and thus no expansion can occur.

TABLE 2

Influence of Kernel Moisture Content on Popcorn Popped Quality		
% Moisture	Popped Volume (ml)*	% Unpopped Kernels*
8.0	300 e	2 a
8.5	320 e	2 a
9.0	350 d	3 a
9.5	380 d	2 a
10.0	405 c	3 a
10.5	405 c	3 a
11.0	410 b	4 a
11.5	420 b	4 a
12.0	420 b	4 a
12.5	465 a	4 a
13.0	470 a	4 a
13.5	465 a	3 a
14.0	440 b	5 b
14.5	420 b	5 b
15.0	420 b	7 b
15.5	420 b	7 b
16.0	400 c	9 c
16.5	390 c	10 c
17.0	370 d	14 d
17.5	370 d	13 d
18.0	350 d	15 d
* : Values in a column with the same letter are not significantly different (p>0.05).		

The influence of storage temperature prior to popping is summarized in Table 3.

TABLE 3

Popped Popcorn Quality Versus Storage Temperature		
Storage Temperature (°C)	Popped Volume (ml)*	% Unpopped Kernels*
-20	475 a	0 a
0	470 a	1 a
20	440 b	3 b
35	430 b	3 b
45	425 b	4 b
55	400 c	10 c
65	380 c	14 c
75	350 d	32 d
85	290 e	47 e
* : Values in a column with the same letter are not significantly different (p>0.05).		

It can be seen from Table 3 that popped volume decreased and the proportion of unpopped kernels increased as storage temperature increased. These data would indicate that frozen storage results in a superior product than room temperature or higher storage. A possible explanation would be that in frozen storage most of the moisture is initially immobilized and thus not free to interact and weaken the pericarp; whereas at higher storage temperature, pericarp weakening results in the premature release of moisture thus decreasing expansion volume and increasing the probability of having no popping at all.

From Table 4, it can be seen that the amount of oil used in preparation also influenced product quality.

Maximum quality was observed with the addition of 2-4% corn oil. When no added oil was present or when high levels of oil (24-32%) were used, popped volume dropped significantly and the proportion of unpopped kernels increased. In all probability, low amounts of oil coat the kernel surface and provide a medium for more efficient heat transfer thus resulting in better product quality. However, at high oil additions, the kernels were actually covered with oil which apparently interfered with moisture release and thus lowered product quality.

TABLE 4

\multicolumn{3}{c}{Popped Popcorn Quality Versus Added Oil Level}
% Added Oil	Popped Volume (ml)*	% Unpopped Kernels*
0	340 d	32 d
2	475 a	2 a
4	470 a	2 a
6	455 b	5 b
8	450 b	6 b
10	450 b	5 b
12	410 c	10 c
14	400 c	10 c
16	400 c	12 c
18	390 c	12 c
20	370 c	13 c
22	370 c	13 c
24	350 d	19 d
26	350 d	22 d
28	340 d	24 d
30	310 e	35 e
32	300 e	38 e

* : Values in a column with the same letter are not significantly different ($p>0.05$).

The amount of added salt also influenced product quality (Table 5). As can be seen, increasing the salt level up to 2% resulted in a significant improvement in volume and reduction in the number of unpopped kernels. However, as salt content was further increased (3-8%), product quality deteriorated. Apparently salt can influence heat transfer which in turn influences popping efficiency.

One would assume that popping temperature would impact popping quality, and as can be seen in Table 6, this was the case.

Maximum volume and the minimum number of unpopped kernels occurred at a popping temperature of 180°C while very poor quality product occurred when the popping temperature was low (165°C). At lower temperatures, apparently not enough superheated steam is produced to cause maximum expansion; whereas at higher temperatures, the steam escapes too soon to result in maximum expansion.

TABLE 5

Influence of Salt Addition on Popcorn Popped Quality		
% Added Salt	Popped Volume (ml)*	% Unpopped Kernels*
0	400 d	7 b
1	420 c	5 b
2	460 a	2 a
3	440 b	6 b
4	440 b	6 b
5	440 b	7 b
6	430 b	8 b
7	420 c	9 c
8	400 d	10 c
* : Values in a column with the same letter are not significantly different ($p>0.05$).		

TABLE 6

Influence of Popping Temperature on Popped Popcorn Quality		
Popping Temperature (°C)	Popped Volume (ml)*	% Unpopped Kernels*
165	240 d	58 d
170	400 c	14 c
175	450 b	12 c
180	470 a	3 a
185	440 b	9 b
* : Values in a column with the same letter are not significantly different ($p>0.05$).		

In conclusion, this study clearly demonstrates that what on the surface may appear to be minor differences in formulation or heating can result in significant difference in popped popcorn quality.

REFERENCES

1   R.F. Schiffmann, Microwave World, 7 (2) (1986) 5-8, 15.
2   C.C. Haugh, R.M. Lien, R.E. Hanes and R.B. Ashman, Trans. Am. Soc. Ag. Eng., 19 (1) (1976) 168-171, 176.

3   R.C. Hoseney, K. Zeleznak and A. Abdelrahman, J. Cereal Sci., 1 (1983) 43-52.
4   Y.E. Lin and R.C. Anantheswaran, J. Food Sci., 53 (1988) 1746-1749.
5   C.A. Flood and G.M. White, Trans. Am. Soc. Ag. Eng., 27 (2) (1984) 561-565, 571.
6   G.M. White, I.J. Ross and C.G. Poneleit, Trans. Am. Soc. Ag. Eng., 23 (5) (1980) 1272-1276.
7   G.M. White, I.J. Ross and C.G. Poneleit, Trans. Am. Soc. Ag. Eng., 24 (2) (1981) 466-468, 475.
8   R.M. Lien and C.C. Haugh, Trans. Am. Soc. Ag. Eng., 18 (5) (1975) 855-858.
9   T.H. Roshdy, K. Hayakawa and H. Daun, J. Food Sci., 49 (1984) 1412-1414, 1418.

G. Charalambous (Ed.), Food Science and Human Nutrition
© 1992 Elsevier Science Publishers B.V. All rights reserved.

SPAGHETTI PRODUCTS CONTAINING DRIED DISTILLERS GRAINS

K. VAN EVEREN, J.A. MAGA and K. LORENZ

Department of Food Science and Human Nutrition, Colorado State University, Fort Collins, Colorado 80523 (United States)

SUMMARY

Sorghum, rye, red wheat, and white wheat dried distillers grains (DDG) were incorporated into a spaghetti formulation at 0, 5, 10, 15, 20, and 30% levels of substitution for durum semolina. Compositional, functional, and sensory evaluations were conducted on the spaghetti products. Spaghetti containing DDG had significantly higher levels of protein and crude fiber than the 100% durum semolina control as indicated by compositional analysis. Cooking quality of the supplemented spaghetti samples was acceptable, but lower than that of the control. This study demonstrated that spaghetti can be produced containing DDG with improved nutritional value and reasonable consumer appeal.

INTRODUCTION

Dried distillers grain (DDG) is the major byproduct after fermentation of cereal grains in the production of alcohol. It is a byproduct from a process in which starch in grain is the energy source and is depleted in the fermentation process due to enzymatic activity. Because of this, other components such as protein, fat, fiber, and ash are concentrated, thus making DDG a viable source of nutrients for humans. Traditionally, DDG has been used mainly as animal feed and has found little application for human consumption.

The incorporation of dried distillers grain into various food products such as cookies (1), breads (2-4), muffins (5), and extruded foods (6) has been evaluated. Dried brewers spent grain, which is the byproduct from beer production, has also been incorporated into numerous foods such as cookies (7-9), muffins (9), and breads (10, 11). Thus it would appear that the evaluation of DDG in cereal based foods has been extensively covered. Only corn distillers grain has been used in spaghetti, however (12).

It was the objective of this study to determine if various other types of DDG can be successfully incorporated into spaghetti, resulting in a product of higher nutritional value and good consumer acceptability.

MATERIALS AND METHODS
Sample Identification

Four types of dried distillers grain were used in this study: hard red wheat, hard white wheat, rye, and sorghum. The samples were obtained from the Fibertein Corporation, Wheatridge, CO. The distillers grains had a range of particle sizes. Some particles were too large to fit through the spaghetti die. Therefore, only grain that was 600 microns or smaller in size was used. The separation was done by passing the distillers grain through a 600 micron sieve. The durum semolina which was used as the control and was replaced by the distillers grain at the 5, 10, 15, 20, and 30% levels was from the North Dakota Mill and Elevator, Grand Forks, ND.

Spaghetti Processing

Durum semolina spaghetti samples were made from the standard formulation shown in Table 1, utilizing a Pasta Matic Model 700 pasta machine. In addition to the durum semolina control, 5, 10, 15, 20, and 30% of the durum semolina flour was substituted with hard red wheat, hard white wheat, rye or sorghum distillers dried grain.

TABLE 1

Ingredient	Control	DDG Levels of Substitution				
		5%	10%	15%	20%	30%
Durum Semolina Flour (g)	454	431.3	408.6	385.9	363.2	317.8
DDG[a] (g)	--	22.7	45.4	68.1	90.8	136.2
Water (Distilled) (ml)	67.2	var[b]	var[b]	var[b]	var[b]	var[b]

[a]Type of DDG

[b] Amount of Water (ml) Used

	5%	10%	15%	20%	30%
Sorghum	137.0	144.3	160.0	159.0	179.0
Rye	163.6	183.7	195.8	197.0	228.9
White wheat	151.1	181.0	179.1	195.4	233.6
Red wheat	156.6	173.5	179.1	193.7	228.8

Flour/DDG blends were dry blended in the pasta machine for three min. before the required amount of distilled water was slowly added. The DDG influenced water absorption. As the level of DDG addition increased, more water was required to produce a machineable dough. The control was used as a reference. After completion of water addition, all doughs were mixed for seven min. before being extruded through a 1.59 mm spaghetti die to produce spaghetti.

After extrusion, the samples were permitted to air dry at room temperature (22°C) for 24 hours before packaging in plastic bags and stored at room temperature.

Proximate Composition

The proximate composition of the distillers grains, the durum semolina control spaghetti, and the spaghetti supplemented with DDG were determined. Samples were prepared for analysis by grinding to a uniform particle size using a Udy Laboratory Mill (Udy Labs, Fort Collins, CO) with a 1 mm sieve.

The following compositional analyses were performed on the distillers grains and the dried spaghetti products using AACC methods (13): moisture by AACC method 44-19; crude fat by method 30-20 with petroleum ether as the extracting solvent; protein by the Kjeldahl method (method 46-12, NX 5.7); crude fiber by method 32-15; ash by method 08-01. Phytic acid was determined according to the procedure of Wheeler and Ferrel (14). Two replications were done on each sample and all data are expressed on a 14% moisture basis. Color measurements were made using the Hunter Color Difference Meter.

Physicochemical Properties

The cooking quality of the spaghetti samples was determined by methods used by the Northern Crops Institute at North Dakota State University (15).

Ten g of spaghetti were added to a beaker containing 30 ml of boiling distilled water. The samples were cooked 12 min. under continuous boiling conditions. The 300 ml volume was maintained at all times. At the end of 12 min., the sample was removed and drained immediately through a Buchner funnel. The beaker and spaghetti were rinsed with distilled water (20 ml) to capture any remaining particles.

Cooked weight was determined by weighing the rinsed spaghetti after a 2.5 min. draining period. Cooking loss was determined by evaporating the cooking water overnight in an air oven at 110°C. After complete evaporation of the cooking water, the beakers were placed in a desiccator to cool. The beakers were then weighed and the difference between the empty weight and the beaker with the residue is the weight of the residue.

The firmness of the cooked spaghetti was measured with a Tensile Testing Machine (type T50021T20K--J. J. Lloyd Instruments Ltd., England) according to manual directions. A special plexiglass tooth was designed according to the methods of Walsh (16) to imitate the action of a tooth. Cooked spaghetti was tested using a 100 newton load cell adjusted times .04. The crosshead speed was 100 mm/min. with a paper/crosshead ratio of 1:1. Twenty tests were done per sample two hours after cooking. Each test used a three-inch length of spaghetti in which the plexiglass tooth cut through the sample.

Sensory Evaluation

Sensory evaluation was done on cooked spaghetti using a 13-member trained taste panel, consisting of males and females in the 21-27 year age group, from a sensory evaluation class at Colorado State University. Evaluations were performed on spaghetti supplemented with the 4 types of distillers dried grains at the 15 and 30% levels of substitution. The ranking test method, which involves a series of samples to be judged and their quality selected, was employed involving a questionnaire and a 7-point hedonic scale. The samples were given to the taste panelists one at a time in a double blind manner; neither the investigator nor the taste panel members knew which product they were testing.

Statistical Analysis

Statistical analysis was performed on all the data: fat, protein, moisture, crude fiber, ash, phytic acid, cooked weight increase, cooking loss, firmness, and sensory evaluation using the SPSS-X program on the Cyber 205 computer at Colorado State University.

RESULTS

Proximate Composition

Proximate composition of sorghum, rye, white wheat, and red wheat DDG are given in Table 2. Crude fat of the distillers grains were significantly different ($p<0.05$) from that of the 100% durum semolina control. The DDG were also significantly different ($p<0.05$) from each other with the sorghum DDG having the highest amount of fat at 9.2% and the rye having the least at 4.8%.

The protein contents of the distillers grains were more than twice that of the durum semolina (11.6%). The white wheat DDG had the highest amount of protein at 28.3%. All the protein levels were significantly different ($p<0.05$) from each other except for the sorghum and rye distillers grains.

The crude fiber value of the distillers grains were very high compared to the durum semolina. All the samples were significantly different ($p<0.05$) from each other except for the red and white wheat distillers grains.

All the distillers grain samples had a high ash content, with sorghum DDG having the highest at 4.3%. The durum semolina had the least amount at 1.4%. All the grains were significantly different ($p<0.05$) from each other.

Phytic acid was measured because of the concern over its ability to form insoluble compounds with calcium and iron (17). There was no detectable amount of phytic acid in the durum semolina. The white wheat DDG was significantly higher in phytic acid ($p<0.05$) than all the other samples. The sorghum and red wheat DDG were not significantly different ($p<0.05$) from each other as were the rye and red wheat distillers grains.

TABLE 2

Proximate Composition of Durum Semolina and Dried Distillers Grains[a]

	Durum Semolina	Type of Distillers Grain			
		Sorghum	Rye	White Wheat	Red Wheat
Moisture	5.8±1.8[a]	6.3±5.7[a]	6.7±2.3[a]	5.2±1.6[a]	6.8±2.1[a]
Crude Fat	0.78±0.06[a]	9.2±0.19[b]	4.8±0.10[c]	6.3±0.06[d]	7.0±0.09[e]
Protein	11.6±0.03[a]	22.8±0.07[b]	23.5±0.04[b]	28.3±0.05[c]	19.4±0.69[d]
Crude Fiber	0.81±0.01[a]	14.7±0.16[b]	39.2±1.8[c]	27.8±0.62[d]	26.6±0.13[d]
Ash	1.4±0.13[a]	4.3±0.11[b]	2.3±0.03[c]	2.8±0.15[d]	2.0±0.16[e]
Phytic Acid	0.0±0.0[a]	0.36±0.01[c]	0.26±0.08[b]	0.54±0.02[d]	0.32±0.01[bc]

[a]Means in a row followed by same letter are not significantly different from one another ($p<0.05$).

Proximate compositions of spaghetti products containing various amounts of DDG are shown in Table 3. The amounts of crude fat, protein, crude fiber, and ash increased as the amount of each of the DDG samples in the blend increased. This was expected based on proximate compositions of raw materials.

Hunter Color Values

As the percentage of DDG in the blends increased, the color of the spaghetti, made with each of the four distillers grains, darkened. Hunter Lab color data of all the samples can be seen in Fig. 1.

At the 5 and 10% levels of replacement, spaghetti made with red wheat, rye, and sorghum DDG were quite dark compared to the control. The spaghetti made with white wheat DDG was much lighter in color compared to spaghetti made with the three other types of distillers grains. Spaghetti made with white wheat DDG at the 5 and 10% levels looked most similar to the control, which was made from durum semolina.

Cooked Weight

Cooked weight increase is a measure of water absorption characteristics of the spaghetti sample. The cooked weight increase should be 3.0-3.5 times the dry weight (15). The product should hold its shape and be free from slime. It should not stick together during or after cooking. At the 5% level of substitution, the sorghum DDG substituted spaghetti was the only sample with a 3.0-3.5 times dry weight increase, which was not significantly ($p<0.05$) different from the control. At the higher levels of DDG substitution, all the samples were below the suggested dry weight increase. In general, as the percent DDG increased, the cooked weight increase decreased. All the samples held their shape during and after cooking except the sorghum and red wheat samples, which fell apart slightly. All the samples were a little slimy to the touch except for the white wheat DDG substituted spaghetti.

Cooking Loss

Cooking loss is the percent solids lost to the cooking water. It should not be more than 9% (15). The sorghum DDG spaghetti samples were all under 9% losses except with substitution at the 20 and 30% level at which the water was cloudy and tended to boil over. The sorghum DDG spaghetti samples had significantly ($p<0.05$) higher cooking losses than the control. The rye DDG substituted spaghetti samples were all under 9% except at the 30% level where the water was slightly cloudy. The rye DDG spaghetti samples had significantly ($p<0.05$) higher cooking losses when compared to the control. The white wheat DDG spaghetti samples were under the 9% cooking loss value but were significantly ($p<0.05$) higher than the control. None of the water was cloudy or boiled over. The red wheat DDG spaghetti samples were under the 9% level except at the 30% level of substitution. At this level, the water was cloudy and tended to boil

TABLE 3

Proximate Compositions of Spaghetti Products with Varying Amounts of DDG

DDG		Replacement Level				
		5%	10%	15%	20%	30%
Crude Fat (%)	Sorghum	1.2±0.09[a]	1.4±0.13[a]	1.7±0.04[b]	2.2±0.09[c]	3.7±0.11[d]
	Rye	0.63±0.07[a]	1.1±0.13[b]	1.2±0.09[bc]	1.4±0.14[c]	1.8±0.25[d]
	White Wheat	0.76±0.06[a]	0.96±0.13[ab]	1.2±0.15[b]	1.5±0.04[c]	2.0±0.07[d]
	Red Wheat	0.87±0.28[a]	1.2±0.07[b]	1.3±0.06[bc]	1.6±0.04[c]	2.0±0.23[d]
Protein (%)	Sorghum	12.3±0.05[a]	12.9±0.06[b]	12.9±0.11[b]	13.7±0.14[c]	14.6±0.03[d]
	Rye	12.1±0.04[a]	12.4±0.05[a]	13.1±0.04[b]	13.6±0.05[c]	14.3±0.22[d]
	White Wheat	12.6±0.03[a]	13.3±0.08[b]	14.1±0.06[c]	14.3±0.04[c]	17.6±0.14[d]
	Red Wheat	11.9±0.02[a]	12.3±0.12[b]	12.6±0.34[b]	13.1±0.07[c]	13.9±0.01[d]
Crude Fiber (%)	Sorghum	1.1±0.03[a]	1.5±0.12[b]	2.2±0.10[c]	2.6±0.42[d]	3.0±0.03[e]
	Rye	1.3±0.10[a]	2.3±0.02[b]	3.3±0.04[c]	5.0±0.01[d]	7.3±0.02[e]
	White Wheat	1.2±0.05[a]	2.2±0.03[b]	3.2±0.01[c]	4.9±0.09[d]	6.8±0.08[e]
	Red Wheat	1.8±0.02[a]	3.5±0.04[b]	5.3±0.16[c]	7.0±0.03[d]	11.4±0.05[e]
Ash (%)	Sorghum	2.4±0.07[a]	3.7±0.16[b]	3.8±0.54[b]	4.2±0.32[b]	4.3±0.06[b]
	Rye	2.2±0.45[a]	2.2±1.8[a]	1.2±0.05[ab]	1.6±0.13[b]	1.2±0.22[b]
	White Wheat	1.4±0.09[a]	1.4±0.11[a]	1.6±0.10[a]	3.5±0.18[b]	5.7±0.47[c]
	Red Wheat	1.0±0.11[a]	1.2±0.06[a]	1.2±0.38[a]	1.2±0.25[a]	1.4±0.06[a]
Phytic Acid (%)	Sorghum	0.01±0.02[a]	0.02±0.03[a]	0.01±0.01[a]	0.01±0.01[a]	0.02±0.04[a]
	Rye	0.01±0.01[a]	0.02±0.34[a]	0.02±0.17[a]	0.02±0.23[a]	0.04±0.02[a]
	White Wheat	0.03±0.01[b]	0.02±0.04[a]	0.04±0.10[b]	0.01±0.25[a]	0.05±0.01[b]
	Red Wheat	0.01±0.02[a]	0.01±0.01[a]	0.01±0.11[a]	0.02±0.01[a]	0.07±0.02[b]

[a]Means in a row followed by same letter are not significantly different from one another ($p<0.05$).

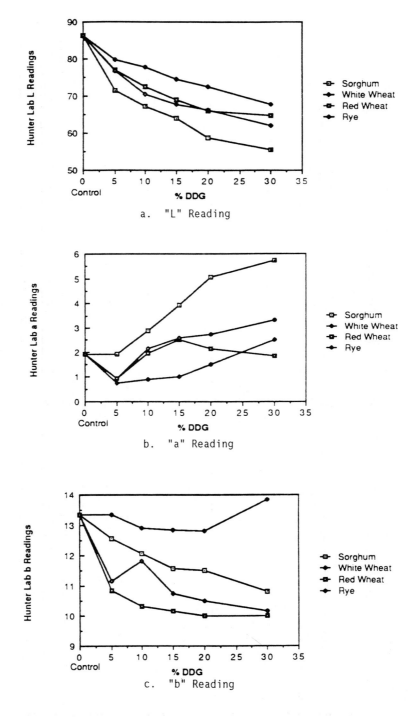

Fig. 1. Hunter Lab Readings of the DDG.

TABLE 4

Increase in Weight During Cooking (Times Dry Weight)[a]

DDG	Replacement Level				
	5%	10%	15%	20%	30%
Sorghum	3.0±0.02[c]	2.9±0.05[c]	2.8±0.06[b]	2.9±0.04[b]	2.8±0.06[b]
Rye	2.8±0.09[ab]	2.6±0.04[a]	2.7±0.04[b]	2.6±0.02[a]	2.6±0.03[a]
White Wheat	2.9±0.05[bc]	2.9±0.04[bc]	2.8±0.09[b]	2.7±0.07[a]	2.5±0.02[a]
Red Wheat	2.8±0.03[a]	2.8±0.08[b]	2.6±0.12[a]	2.7±0.05[a]	2.6±0.06[a]

Control = 3.1±0.07
[a]Means in a column followed by same letter are not significantly different from one another (p<0.05).

TABLE 5

Cooking Losses of Spaghetti Samples[a]

DDG	Replacement Level				
	5%	10%	15%	20%	30%
Sorghum	7.3±0.47[c]	7.5±0.11[b]	8.1±0.06[b]	11.0±0.09[d]	13.8±0.16[d]
Rye	6.3±0.06[a]	6.3±0.07[a]	6.4±0.06[a]	8.3±0.04[b]	9.3±0.08[b]
White Wheat	6.9±0.03[b]	7.7±0.04[b]	8.7±0.02[c]	8.7±0.07[c]	8.7±0.09[a]
Red Wheat	6.3±0.04[a]	6.1±0.10[a]	6.6±0.13[a]	7.2±0.06[a]	10.6±0.35[c]

Control = 4.9±0.17
[a]Means in a column followed by same letter are not significantly different from one another (p<0.05).

over. All the red wheat DDG spaghetti samples had values significantly (p<0.04) higher than the control.

Firmness

Firmness of the cooked spaghetti samples was measured to determine differences between the control and spaghetti substituted with the five different levels of DDG. Firmness values for all the spaghetti samples did not show any major trends, and, therefore, no conclusions could be drawn. However, as the level of DDG increased, the spaghetti samples became softer to the touch.

Sensory Evaluation

Sensory evaluation was performed on spaghetti samples substituted at the 15 and 30% levels with the four types of distillers grains. The two levels of substitution were chosen in order to reduce the number of samples presented at one time.

Question one asked the taste panel how smooth (1 in score) or gritty (7 in score) the spaghetti samples are. The control had a significantly (p<0.05) better score at both the 15 and 30% levels of substitution (Fig. 2). The spaghetti samples containing white wheat DDG had the best scores at both the 15 and 30% levels, while the red wheat DDG spaghetti samples had the worst ratings.

Question two asked the taste panel whether the cooked spaghetti samples had a desirable flavor with 1 being the most desirable and 7 being the least desirable. The control had a significantly (p<0.05) better score in comparison with both the 15 and 30% levels (Fig. 3). At the 15% level, the white wheat DDG spaghetti had the most desirable score and the red wheat DDG spaghetti had the least desirable score. At the 30% level, the rye and white wheat DDG spaghetti had the most desirable score and the red wheat DDG spaghetti had the least desirable score.

Question three had the taste panel rate the cooked spaghetti products on overall acceptability with 1 being the most acceptable and 7 being the least acceptable. Compared to the control, the 15 and 30% levels of substitution had a significantly (p<0.05) lower acceptability rating (Fig. 4). At both the 15% and 30% level, the white wheat DDG spaghetti sample had the best acceptability rating and the red wheat DDG spaghetti had the worst.

Question four asked the taste panel if they would recommend the cooked spaghetti products with 1 highly recommending and 7 disclaiming the product. The control had significantly (p<0.05) better recommendations than the products containing distillers grains (Fig. 5). At the 15% level, the white wheat DDG spaghetti had the best score while the red wheat DDG spaghetti had a significantly (p<0.05) poorer score, which was the same at the 30% level.

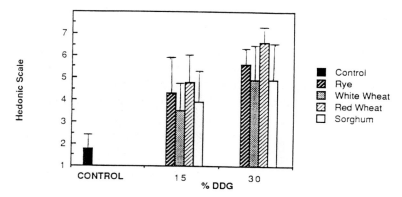

Fig. 2. Question one: How smooth is the texture of the cooked spaghetti.

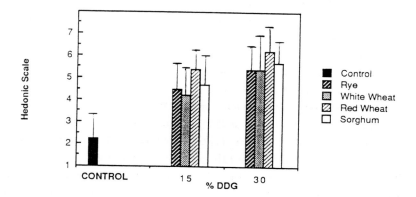

Fig. 3. Question two: How desirable in flavor is the spaghetti.

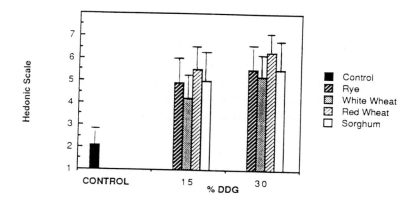

Fig. 4. Question three: How acceptable overall are the spaghetti.

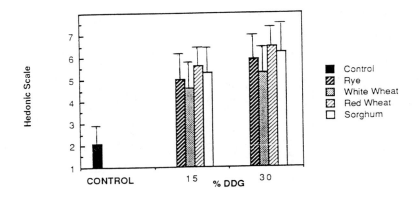

Fig. 5. Question four: Can the spaghetti be recommended?

Overall, the taste panel liked the white wheat DDG spaghetti products the most and the red wheat DDG spaghetti the least (by taking an average of all the questions).

CONCLUSIONS

Sorghum, rye, white wheat, and red wheat distillers dried grains (DDG) with varying compositions were added at the 5, 10, 15, 20, and 30% levels to a spaghetti formulation. The control consisted of 100% durum semolina. The distillers grains had higher fat, protein, crude fiber, ash, and phytic acid than the control. As the percentage of DDG increased in the spaghetti, the percentage of these components increased. Cooking qualities of the spaghetti containing DDG decreased as the percentage of DDG increased. Sensory evaluation of the spaghetti samples containing DDG was performed with the products containing 15 or 30% levels of DDG. Scores were poor overall for the DDG containing spaghetti samples.

The spaghetti samples containing DDG had a higher nutritional value than the control, and more so as the percentage of DDG in the sample increased. However, at the higher levels of DDG, the spaghetti products were unacceptable to the consumer indicating the possibility of having a spaghetti product with a low level of DDG yet still having a higher nutritional value.

REFERENCES

1 B.A. Rasco, S.E. Downey and F.M. Dong, Cereal Chem., 64 (1987) 139-143.
2 M.M. Morad, C.A. Doherty and L.W. Rooney, Cereal Chem., 61 (1984) 409-414.
3 C.C. Tsen, J.L. Weber and W. Eyestone, Cereal Chem., 60 (1983) 295-297.
4 C.E. Walker, Farm, Ranch, and Home Quarterly, Fall 1980, 3-5.

5   N.R. Reddy, M.D. Pierson and F.W. Cooler, J. Food Quality 9, (4), 1986, 243-249.
6   D.J. Wampler and W.A. Gould, J. Food Sci., 49 (1984) 1321-1322.
7   L.T. Kissel and N. Prentice, Cereal Chem., 54 (1979) 261-266.
8   N. Prentice, L.T. Kissell, R.C. Lindsay and W.T. Yamazaki, Cereal Chem., 55 (1978) 712-721.
9   N. Prentice, Bakers Digest, 52 (1978) 22-23.
10 J.W. Finley and M.M. Hanamoto, Cereal Chem., 59 (1980) 89-91.
11 P.C. Dreese and R.C. Hoseney, Cereal Chem., 59 (1982) 89-91.
12 Y.V. Wu, V.L. Youngs, K. Warner and G.N. Bookwalter, Cereal Chem., 64 (1987) 434-436.
13 AACC, Approved Methods of the AACC, American Association of Cereal Chemists, The Association, St. Paul, MN, 1982.
14 E.L. Wheeler and R.E. Ferrel, Cereal Chem. 48 (1971) 312-320.
15 B.J. Donnelly, A Manual on Objective Tests for Spaghetti Products, N. Dakota State University, Fargo, ND, 1986.
16 D.E. Walsh, Cereal Sci. Today, 16 (1971) 202-205.
17 E.N. Whitney and E.M.N. Hamilton, Understanding Nutrition, West Publishing Co., St. Paul, MN, 1981, p. 429.

COMPARISON OF PREFERENCES FOR SALTY AND UMAMI FLAVOURS BETWEEN TWO ETHNIC GROUPS OF DIFFERENT DIETARY HABITS

M. LOUISE LAW and J.R. PIGGOTT

Department of Bioscience and Biotechnology, University of Strathclyde, 131 Albion Street, Glasgow G1 1SD (Scotland)

SUMMARY

Flavour potentiators such as MSG, IMP and GMP not only potentiate the flavours of foods at subthreshold levels and favourably alter preferences for foods, but also have their own distinctive palatable taste, umami, at higher than threshold levels. A sensory study was carried out to investigate whether any differences exist in preference for salty and umami flavours between two ethnic groups of different dietary habits. Preference for the flavour of natural and pure flavour potentiators was also investigated. Malaysian assessors significantly preferred the umami flavour of the flavour potentiators in comparison with the Scottish assessors who significantly preferred the salty flavour. The Malays showed significant preference for the flavour of pure flavour potentiators to natural ones whereas the Scots showed no significant difference in preference for them.

1. INTRODUCTION

A flavour potentiator is a compound which, when used in small quantities, produces no sensory response of its own, but modifies through intensification or some form of masking the sensory properties of the food system to which it has been incorporated (1). Flavour potentiators can favourably alter the preference for foods by enhancing desirable flavours and/or suppressing undesirable off-flavours (2,3). Flavour potentiators such as monosodium glutamate (MSG), inosine 5'monophosphate (IMP) and guanosine 5'monophosphate (GMP) not only potentiate the flavour of food at subthreshold levels but also have their own distinctive, delicious, savoury, palatable tastes at suprathreshold levels (4). These tastes extend the taste realm beyond the four basic tastes (5) and are referred to as umami by the Japanese, who have used natural sources of flavour potentiators in their cooking since ancient times (4). Umami is an integral part of cuisines worldwide, from the dashi and tan broths of Japan and China to the bouillon of Europe and fish sauces of South East Asia (6).

Flavour potentiators can be obtained from a wide range of natural sources, including yeast extract. It is the natural presence of nucleotides, a significant amount of glutamate and other amino acids which give yeast extracts their flavour potentiating properties (7).

Nutritional studies (8) showed that rats on a moderate or high protein diet preferred umami flavours, with consumption of the umami solution having a reducing effect on NaCl intake. No such preference for the umami solution was shown in rats fed a low protein diet. There has been speculation that a similar effect might be observed in man.

The aim of the work described here was to investigate whether any differences exist in preference for umami or salty flavours between two ethnic groups of different dietary habits, and to compare liking of the two groups for natural and pure flavour potentiators.

2. EXPERIMENTAL

2.1 Materials

Hedonic functions of taste substances cannot be predicted from the degree of liking in a model system or simple aqueous solution, but must be evaluated in foods or flavoured solutions compatible with added tastes (9). The umami and salty taste substances were therefore incorporated into a soup food system containing vegetables. Yeast extracts with varying NaCl and flavour potentiator levels were used to compare hedonic scores for soups containing high and low concentrations of NaCl and flavour potentiators, and pure flavour potentiators were used to compare these with the natural materials contained in the yeast extract.

Bouillon base (P.1970, instant), Paselli maltodextrin (MD20), vegetable (2M-44444), chicken (Y342.04.370) and beef (Y42.08.128) flavours, yeast extracts YEP LOC (38% NaCl, 5% MSG), YEP 990C (10% NaCl, 3% IMP, 3% GMP, 5% MSG) and YEP 770C (38% NaCl, 2% IMP, 5% MSG), MSG, IMP and GMP were supplied by Quest International Flavour Centre (Bromborough Port, Wirral, Merseyside, L62 4SC, England). Bouillon base (37.5 g), maltodextrin (7.5 g) and vegetable, chicken or beef flavour (7.5 g) were mixed with 2.5 litres of water and 0.533 kg each of carrots, onions and potatoes. Flavour potentiators were added, each soup mixture was simmered for 30 minutes and then blended for approximately 2 minutes using a Kenwood Quisine Food Processor with large cutting blades at speed setting 2, as follows:

Soup 1 - Yeast extract YEP LOC (5 g) providing a low flavour potentiator concentration (0.059 g kg^{-1} MSG) and a high NaCl concentration (0.45 g kg^{-1}).

Soup 2 - Yeast extract YEP 990C (5 g) providing a high flavour potentiator concentration (0.059 g kg^{-1} MSG, 0.036 g kg^{-1} IMP and 0.036 g kg^{-1} GMP) and a low NaCl concentration (0.12 g kg^{-1}).

Soup 3 - Yeast extract YEP 770C (5 g) providing a high flavour potentiator concentration (0.059 g kg^{-1} MSG, 0.024 g kg^{-1} IMP) and a high NaCl concentration (0.45 g kg^{-1}).

Soup 4 - No additions to the basic ingredients.

Soup 5 - Flavour potentiators (0.25 g MSG, 0.15 g IMP, 0.15 g GMP) providing a high flavour potentiator concentration (0.059 g kg^{-1} MSG, 0.036 g kg^{-1} IMP and 0.036 g kg^{-1} GMP), and 0.5 g NaCl providing a low concentration (0.12 g kg^{-1}).

2.2 Assessors

Scottish and Malaysian ethnic groups were chosen for this study, because they have substantially different dietary habits and a sufficient number of each group where readily available and willing to take part. Scottish people on the whole have a generally higher protein diet than Malaysians, who tend to eat a high carbohydrate diet, having rice with all main meals including breakfast. Additionally many Malaysian residents of the UK follow a vegetarian diet, further limiting protein consumption. Twenty-nine Scottish students took part in the experiment, 17 female and 12 male, and twenty-five Malaysians, 7 female and 18 male. The ages of both groups ranged from 20 - 24 years.

2.3 Sensory Analysis

Individual assessors were given 30 ml of each coded soup formulation at 60 - 66 °C in white foamed polystyrene cups (Insulpak Ltd., Tower Close, Huntingdon, England) and were asked to taste each sample and indicate their degree of liking using a nine-point hedonic scale (10), ranging from 'Dislike extremely' (1) to 'Like extremely' (9). Individual tasting booths were used and data recorded using the PSA-System (Oliemans Punter & Partners, Utrecht, The Netherlands). The Malaysian students were only asked to taste soup samples made using vegetable flavour, whereas the Scottish students tasted all the soups. Data were analysed by one way analysis of variance using MINITAB.

3. RESULTS AND DISCUSSION

Analyses of variance of the hedonic scores are shown in Tables 1 and 2. Comparison of the results for soups 1 and 2 showed that the Malaysians preferred the umami flavour of the flavour potentiators to the salty flavour, when added to vegetable soup. In contrast, the Scottish assessors showed no significant preference, while the high salt-high flavour potentiator and low salt-low flavour potentiator soups were moderately liked and disliked, respectively, by both groups. The Malaysian assessors preferred the flavour of the pure flavour potentiators to the natural ones, whereas the Scottish assessors showed no significant difference in preference.

TABLE 1

Mean hedonic scores for Malaysian and Scottish assessors for vegetable flavour soup formulations.

Sample	Formulation	Malays[1]	Scots[2]	F_{52}^1
1	High NaCl Low FP	3.96	5.52^b	9.95++
2	Low NaCl High FP	6.76^a	5.21^b	11.28++
3	High NaCl High FP	6.44^a	6.69	0.49
4	Low NaCl Low FP	4.68	4.45	0.16
5	Low NaCl High Pure FP	7.48	5.31^b	22.75+++
df		4,120	4,140	
F		17.81+++	6.34+++	

^{a,b}means of samples which did not receive significantly different hedonic scores.
+, ++, +++ indicates significance at the 5%, 1% and 0.1% levels, respectively.
FP flavour potentiator.
^{1}LSD = 0.64.
^{2}LSD = 0.58.

The Scottish assessors showed no significant preference for salty and umami flavours in the vegetable and chicken flavoured soups, whereas they showed a significant preference for the salty flavour in the beef flavoured soup. For the vegetable and beef flavoured soups there was no difference in preference for the natural or pure flavour potentiators. Conversely there was a marked increase in preference for the chicken flavoured soup containing the pure flavour potentiators. This suggested that the chicken flavour was best enhanced by the pure flavour potentiators.

TABLE 2

Mean hedonic scores for Scottish assessors for chicken and beef flavour soup formulations.

Sample	Formulation	Chicken[1]	Beef[2]
1	High NaCl Low FP	3.24^a	6.24^{bc}
2	Low NaCl High FP	3.03^a	5.59^d
3	High NaCl High FP	5.10	6.69^b
4	Low NaCl Low FP	3.14^a	4.38
5	Low NaCl High Pure FP	5.89	5.72^{cd}
F_{140}^4		13.53+++	6.81+++

a,b,c,d means of samples which did not receive significantly different hedonic scores.
+, ++, +++ indicates significance at the 5%, 1% and 0.1% levels, respectively.
FP flavour potentiator.
[1] LSD = 0.62.
[2] LSD = 0.60.

The results of this study do not accord with previous reports (8) that rats on a moderate or high protein diet preferred umami flavours, whereas this study has shown that Scottish assessors, having a generally higher protein diet than Malaysians, have preferred salty flavours. This probably rather reflects a learned preference for the generally high salt content of the Scottish diet.

4. CONCLUSIONS

A group of Malaysian students significantly preferred soups containing high levels of flavour potentiators and low levels of salt, in contrast to a group of Scottish assessors who preferred a soup formulated with high levels of flavour potentiators and high levels of salt. The Malaysian assessors preferred pure flavour potentiators to natural ones in yeast extracts, whereas the Scottish assessors showed no significant preference.

REFERENCES

1. A. Kuninaka, in: M.S. Peterson and A.H. Johnston (Eds), Encyclopedia of Food Science, Avi Publishing, Westport, Connecticut, 1978, pp. 279-284.
2. K.N. Hall, in: M.S. Peterson and A.H. Johnston (Eds), Encyclopedia of Food Science, Avi Publishing, Westport, Connecticut, 1978, pp. 559-561.
3. S. Yamaguchi, in: J.C. Boudreau (Ed.), Food Taste Chemistry, American Chemical Society, Washington, D.C., 1979, pp. 33-51.
4. A. Kuninaka, in: R. Teranishi, R.A. Flath and H. Sugisawa (Eds), Flavour Research Recent Advances, Marcel Dekker, New York, 1981, pp. 305-353.
5. R.H. Cagan, K. Tori and M.R. Kare, in: L.J. Filer, S. Garrantini, M.R. Kare, W.A. Reynolds and R.J. Wurtzman (Eds), Glutamic Acid: Advances in Biochemistry and Physiology, Raven Press, New York, 1979, pp. 1-9.
6. Y. Kawamura, Food Technology International Europe, (1990) 151-155.
7. G. Schmidt, Food Flavourings Ingredients Packaging and Processing, 9(5) (1987) 25-30.
8. S. Kimura, Y. Yokomukai and M. Komai, in: Y. Kawamura and M. Kare (Eds), Umami: A Basic Taste: Physiology, Biochemistry, Nutrition, Food Science, Marcel Dekker, New York, 1987, pp. 611-634.
9. S. Yamaguchi, in: Y. Kawamura and M. Kare (Eds), Umami: A Basic Taste: Physiology, Biochemistry, Nutrition, Food Science, Marcel Dekker, New York, 1987, pp. 41-73.
10. E. Larmond, Laboratory Methods for Sensory Evaluation of Food, Publication 1637, Research Branch Canada Department of Agriculture, Ottawa, 1977.

G. Charalambous (Ed.), Food Science and Human Nutrition
© 1992 Elsevier Science Publishers B.V. All rights reserved.

ENZYMATIC HYDRATION OF (4R)-(+)-LIMONENE TO (4R)-(+)-α-TERPINEOL

K.R. CADWALLADER[1] and R.J. BRADDOCK[2]

[1]Department of Food Science, Louisiana State University, Baton Rouge, LA 70803 USA

[2]University of Florida, IFAS, Citrus Research and Education Center, Lake Alfred, FL 33850 USA

SUMMARY

The enzyme-catalyzed hydration of the citrus by-product, limonene, to the important flavor and aroma chemical, α-terpineol, was investigated. Particulate-associated α-terpineol dehydratase was recovered from Pseudomonas gladioli, solubilized, and partially purified using detergent extraction and gel filtration.

Activity of α-terpineol dehydratase was low in non-aqueous solvents. α-Terpineol dehydratase was characterized in buffers containing 0.1% (w/v) Triton X-100. In 10 mM MES, 10 mM BIS-TRIS PROPANE buffer, the pH optimum was 5.5 and the stability optimum was pH 8.0. The temperature optimum at pH 7.0 was 25°C in 10 mM HEPES buffer. Using temperature-activity data for 10-25°C, E_a and Q_{10} of α-terpineol dehydratase were determined to be 21.6 ± 2.9 kJ·mol^{-1} and 1.37 ± 0.07, respectively. Activity was inhibited by Triton X-100. The effects were an increase in apparent K_m and decrease in apparent V_{max}. Average apparent K_m of α-terpineol dehydratase was 2.18 ± 0.19 mM in 10 mM HEPES buffer, pH 7.0 containing 0.1% (w/v) Triton X-100.

α-Terpineol dehydratase stereospecifically catalyzed the hydration of (4R)-(+)-limonene to (4R)-(+)-α-terpineol or (4S)-(-)-limonene to (4S)-(-)-α-terpineol. The enzyme was also stereoselective, since the rate of hydration of (4R)-(+)-limonene was approximately ten times faster than the rate of hydration of (4S)-(-)-limonene.

INTRODUCTION

In recent years, there has been increasing consumer preference for food products containing "natural" flavors over those containing artificial (synthetic) flavors. This preference has led to an increased demand for natural flavor and aroma chemicals (1, 2). Biotechnological processes (processes involving the use of microorganisms, plant cell cultures, or enzymes) offer many possibilities for the production of natural flavor and aroma chemicals.

In addition to their use for production of flavor and aroma chemicals, biotechnological processes provide simple systems for studying the biosynthetic pathways involved in the formation of many important flavors and aromas. These processes have several advantages over alternate physical or chemical processes, the most important advantage being their ability to catalyze specific reactions which may not be possible with less selective processing methods. Another advantage is that biotechnological processes generally can be accomplished under mild conditions (i.e., ambient temperature, atmospheric pressure, and pH values near 7). This automatically results in lower energy consumption and decreased substrate and product damage.

The suitability of a process for the production of flavor and aroma chemicals depends on the market demand (total usage), commercial value (price) of the product and the technological state of the process. The use of a biotechnological process for the production of α-terpineol from limonene has economic potential. α-Terpineol is an important flavor and aroma chemical. Its annual consumption for flavor purposes has been estimated at over 13,000 kg, which places it among the top 30 most commonly used flavors (2).

Citrus essential oils are unusual because they contain pure (4R)-(+)-limonene at concentrations approaching 95% for orange and grapefruit oils (3). In addition to its high chemical and enantiomeric purity, limonene derived from citrus is in abundant supply, with 8.7 million kilograms being recovered during the 1988-89 Florida processing season (4). Limonene from citrus is also relatively inexpensive, the price being approximately 25% lower than the price of α-terpineol (5).

Presently, α-terpineol is commercially available only in racemic form, which is primarily recovered as a by-product from the pulp and paper industry. The properties of flavor and aroma compounds often depend on their enantiomeric purity. For example, (4R)-(-)-carvone has properties characteristic of spearmint oil; whereas, the properties of (4S)-(+)-carvone resemble caraway oil. Biotechnological processes are usually stereospecific; therefore it may be possible to produce pure (4R)-(+)-α-terpineol from (4R)-(+)-limonene by using this type of process.

Kraidman et al. (6) have shown that <u>Cladosporium</u> spp. (T_{12}) converts (4R)-(+)-limonene into pure (4R)-(+)-α-terpineol. Similarly, <u>Penicillium digitatum</u> (DSM 62840) was shown to produce (4R)-(+)-α-terpineol from either (4R)-(+)-limonene or racemic limonene (7). This could be explained by the exclusive hydration of (4R)-(+)-limonene. Cadwallader et al. (8) demonstrated that

Pseudomonas gladioli produces pure (4R)-(+)-α-terpineol from (4R)-(+)-limonene; however, the yield of α-terpineol was low due to the utilization of limonene by the bacterium for metabolic purposes. An enzyme, α-terpineol dehydratase (α-TD), has been isolated from P. gladioli, which catalyzes the hydration of limonene to α-terpineol (9). These researchers found that the enzyme was particulate-associated and could be extracted with 2.0% (w/v) Triton X-100 and 0.5 M sodium trichloroacetate. α-TD solubility was maintained during gel filtration by inclusion of 1.0% (w/v) Triton X-100. Suitability of an enzyme for the production of flavor and aroma chemicals depends on its physical and kinetic properties. It is necessary to isolate and characterize enzymes to relate these properties to important parameters affecting reactions.

Stability should be high under the process conditions which may include extremes of pH and temperature, as well as the presence of solvents or other protein denaturants. Enzymes should also be highly specific for the reaction of interest so that side products are minimized. When it is desirable to produce pure enantiomers from enantiomerically pure substrates, then the stereospecificity of the enzyme is important. Stereoselectivity is important when inexpensive racemic compounds are used as substrates instead of more expensive pure enantiomers.

The above discussion particularly relates to the importance of this study, which has the major objective of characterizing some of the physical and kinetic properties of α-TD.

ENZYME PROPERTIES

Determination of the kinetic properties of α-terpineol dehydratase was complicated because limonene was insoluble in the enzyme medium. The potential of using water-miscible organic solvents to dissolve limonene in the enzyme reaction medium was examined. Formamide, dimethylformamide, ethanol, 2-propanol, and acetonitrile inactivated α-TD at the concentrations required to solubilize limonene (25-50%). Since water is a co-substrate of α-TD, it was originally thought that the observed decrease in activity was due to decreased water activity and subsequent shift in reaction equilibrium; however, α-TD did not catalyze the reverse reaction when glycerol was used to lower the water activity.

The effects of various nonpolar solvents on α-TD activity were similar to the effects observed with water-miscible solvents. Enzyme activity was assayed in 1:1 mixtures consisting of nonpolar solvent plus aqueous enzyme solution. No activity was detected in any of the solvents tested: n-hexane, diethyl ether, dichloromethane, chloroform, and limonene. In fact, enzyme reactions could be stopped by addition of equal volumes of nonpolar solvents to aqueous enzyme assay solutions. Because of the adverse affects of solvents on α-TD, kinetic properties were determined in aqueous medium containing 0.1% (w/v) Triton X-100. Detergent was included in the medium to maintain the solubility of the enzyme; however, the solubility of limonene at this detergent concentration was very low.

Since α-TD assay was based on a one point determination, the linearity of the reaction was verified as a function of incubation time and enzyme concentration. Appearance of α-terpineol as a function of time for three concentrations of enzyme is shown in Fig. 1. Rate of α-terpineol formation was constant for all three concentrations of enzyme up to 2.5 min. Unless otherwise stated, α-TD assays were done using 2 min incubations. Initial velocity as a function of α-TD concentration is shown in Fig. 2. α-TD was present in "catalytic" amounts at all protein concentrations examined.

pH and Temperature Dependency of α-TD

The pH profile of α-TD was determined in 10 mM MES, 10 mM BIS-TRIS PROPANE buffer containing 0.1% (w/v) Triton X-100 (Fig. 3). The apparent pH optimum of α-TD dehydratase occurred at pH 5.5, while the apparent stability optimum occurred at pH 8.0. The low activity observed below pH 5.0 was probably due to enzyme inactivation rather than the formation of an improper ionic form of the enzyme, since the enzyme was very unstable below this pH. At the pH of highest enzyme stability, the activity was about one-third as high as that observed at the apparent pH optimum. It is apparent that a slightly acidic environment increased α-TD activity, at the same time lowering its stability. From these results, it was decided that all other kinetic experiments would be performed at pH 7.0, since at this pH both the activity and stability of α-TD were reasonably high.

Effect of temperature on the activity of α-TD in 10 mM HEPES buffer, pH 7.0 containing 0.1% (w/v) Triton X-100 is shown in Fig. 4. The apparent temperature "optimum" occurred at 30°C. The true optimum is the maximum temperature at which the enzyme exhibits a constant activity over a time of at least as long as the assay time (9, 10). This was determined by pre-incubating the enzyme at

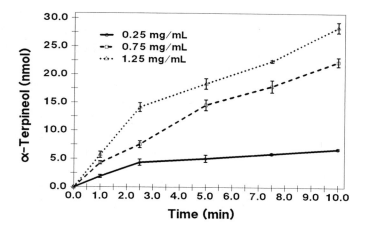

Fig. 1. Formation of α-terpineol versus time for three concentrations of α-TD. (Error bars represent standard deviations, n = 4.)

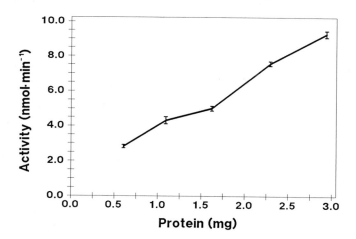

Fig. 2. Initial velocity as a function of α-TD concentration. (Error bars represent standard deviations, n = 4.)

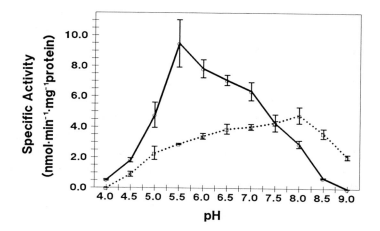

Fig. 3. Effect of pH on α-TD activity (30 min assay) and stability in 10 mM MES, 10 mM BIS-TRIS PROPANE buffer containing 0.1% (w/v) Triton X-100; activity at 25°C versus pH (—o—) and activity at pH 7.0 after 25°C pre-incubation of enzyme at indicated pH values for 30 min (♦♦♦□♦♦♦). (Error bars represent standard deviations, n = 4.)

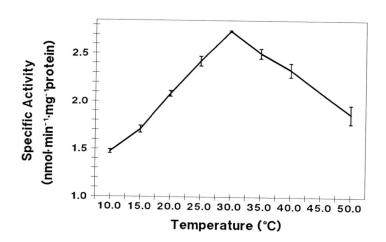

Fig. 4. Effect of temperature on α-TD activity. Activity was assayed (2 min) at indicated temperatures after 2 min preincubation. (Error bars represent standard deviations, n = 4.)

various temperatures for 2 min and then assaying for activity for 2 min at 20°C. The enzyme appeared to be completely stable to 25°C, but began to denature at 30°C. Therefore, the true temperature "optimum" of the α-TD under these conditions was 25°C instead of 30°C.

The average Arhennius activation energy (E_a) from duplicate determinations was 21.6 ± 2.9 kJ·mol^{-1}. The E_a of α-TD falls within the range of E_a values (8-50 kJ·mol^{-1}) reported for other enzymes (11, 12). The average Q_{10} for the temperature range 10-25°C was 1.37 ± 0.07. The Q_{10} of α-TD was smaller than Q_{10} values for most chemical and enzymatic reactions, which generally fall in range from 2-3 (11). The low Q_{10} indicates that activity of α-TD was not as sensitive to temperature changes as some other enzymes.

Effect of Triton X-100 on Kinetic Constants of α-TD

Effect of varying the Triton X-100 concentration on Henri-Michaelis-Menten plots is shown in Fig. 5. All plots appear to follow Henri-Michaelis-Menten kinetics (i.e., their curvature is constant); however, the activity was inhibited by the presence of 0.1 and 0.5% (w/v) Triton X-100. Kinetic parameters, K_m and V_{max}, were determined using Lineweaver-Burk double reciprocal plots (Fig. 6). The K_m and V_{max} determined under the conditions of this study are apparent values, since the enzyme and limonene were not actually soluble in the medium but instead were suspended in detergent micelles. As a consequence of including Triton X-100 in the medium, the apparent V_{max} decreased and the apparent K_m increased. The effect of Triton X-100 was uncharacteristic of classical enzyme inhibition (e.g., competitive, noncompetitive, uncompetitive, or irreversible inhibition), since none of these result in a simultaneous decrease in V_{max} and increase in K_m. The degree of inhibition was not proportional to the concentration of detergent in the medium. The value of K_m in the absence of detergent was approximately half the value of K_m in 0.1 or 0.5% detergent. The V_{max} in the absence of detergent was twice as large as the V_{max} in 0.1 or 0.5% detergent. Apparent K_m or V_{max} values determined in 0.1 and 0.5% detergent were not significantly different ($\alpha = 0.05$).

Similar results were observed concerning the effect of Triton X-100 concentration on the catalytic activity of α-TD (13), where α-TD activity in detergent concentrations above 0.1% (w/v) was shown to be insensitive to differences in detergent concentration up to 5.0% (w/v). Detergent concentrations between 0.1 and 5.0%

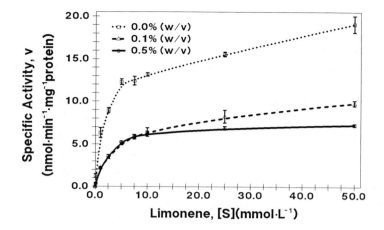

Fig. 5. Effect of Triton X-100 concentration on Henri-Michaelis-Menten (v versus [S]) curves for α-TD. (Error bars represent standard deviations, n = 4.)

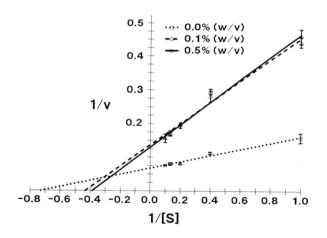

Fig. 6. Lineweaver-Burk double reciprocal (1/v versus 1/[S]) plots of data in Fig. 5 for limonene concentrations from 1 mM to 10 mM.

(w/v) decreased α-TD activity by 30%.

Replication of apparent K_m in the absence of Triton X-100 was difficult because enzyme solutions varied considerably in their composition. Ultrafiltration and Spectra/Gel D chromatography were used to reduce the Triton X-100 concentration in enzyme solution, but it was not possible to completely remove the detergent (9). Although these solutions contained less than 0.01% (w/v) Triton X-100, slight differences in detergent concentration had a dramatic effect on the results. The most common problem encountered was that the velocity became constant at limonene concentrations higher than 2.5-10 mM, indicating substrate saturation. Average of three replicates of apparent K_m in the presence of 0.1% (w/v) Triton X-100 was 2.18 ± 0.19 mM. Comparison of apparent V_{max} values obtained for different enzyme solutions was not possible because the exact amount of α-TD in each solution was unknown.

Stereospecificity and Selectivity of α-TD

Ideally, the stereoselectivity of α-TD should be determined by comparing the V_{max}/K_m ratios for both limonene enantiomers. This approach was not practical because pure (4S)-(-)-limonene is not commercially available. Commercial (4S)-(-)-limonene contained over 10% of the R enantiomer. The stereoselectivity of α-terpineol dehydratase was alternatively determined by incubating the enzyme with racemic limonene and measuring the conversion rate of each limonene enantiomer.

These studies determined that α-terpineol dehydratase catalyzed the hydration of (4R)-(+)-limonene at a faster rate than (4S)-(-)-limonene. In initial studies, enzyme solutions (10 mM HEPES buffer, pH 7.0 containing 0.1% (w/v) Triton X-100) were incubated with 0.2 mM racemic limonene at 25°C for various times and the relative concentration of each limonene enantiomer was determined by chiral GC (Fig. 7). α-TD stereospecifically converted (4R)-(+)-limonene to (4R)-(+)-α-terpineol and (4S)-(-)-limonene to (4S)-(-)-α-terpineol. These results were expected since Cadwallader et al. (8) reported that P. gladioli produces pure (4R)-(+)-α-terpineol from (4R)-(+)-limonene.

Plots of relative amounts of each limonene and α-terpineol enantiomer as a function of time (Fig. 8) were used to estimate the relative percent concentration of each α-terpineol enantiomer at the indicated times (Table 1). It is apparent from the increase in the relative percent concentration of (4R)-(+)-α-terpineol that the rate of hydration of (4R)-(+)-limonene decreased as a result of its

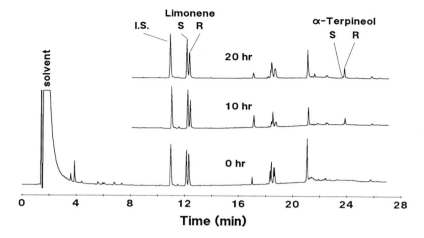

Fig. 7. GC profile of change in concentration of limonene and α-terpineol enantiomers during the course of the hydration of 0.2 mM racemic limonene by α-TD. GC conditions were as follows: 30 m x 0.254 mm i.d. Cyclodex B fused silica column (J&W Scientific, Inc., Folsom, CA); 1 μL injection with 1:100 split; helium carrier gas at 1.26 mL·min^{-1}; 200°C injector 250°C FID detector; column temperature programmed from 70°C to 200°C at 5°C·min^{-1} with a 10 min initial hold and 5 min final hold; internal standard (I.S.) was (1S)-(-)-cis-pinane at 10 ppm.

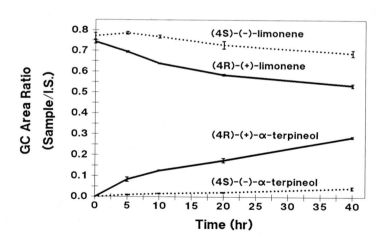

Fig. 8. Change in concentration of limonene and α-terpineol enantiomers during the course of the hydration of 0.2 mM racemic limonene by α-TD. (Error bars represent standard deviations, n = 4.)

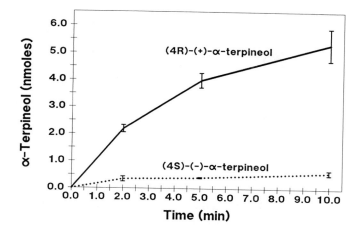

Fig. 9. Formation of α-terpineol enantiomers during the course of the hydration of 50 mM racemic limonene by α-TD. (Error bars represent standard deviations, n = 4.)

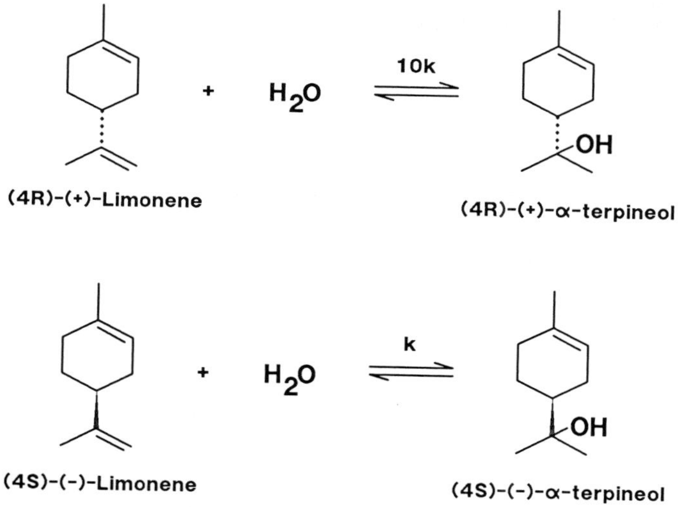

Fig. 10. Stereo-specificity and -selectivity of α-TD. Note that k represents the rate constant for the hydration of (4S)-(-)-limonene.

decreasing concentration. In order to more accurately estimate the stereoselectivity of α-terpineol dehydratase, initial kinetic rates at low limonene concentration (Fig. 8) were measured. Other enzyme assays were done using 50 mM limonene with 5 ppm n-decanol as internal standard. GC conditions were the same as in Fig. 8 except for the following: 1 µL injection with 1:10 split; helium carrier gas at 0.92 mL·min^{-1}; column temperature isothermal at 115°C. Appearance of α-terpineol enantiomers as a function of time at a constant concentration of racemic limonene (50 mM) is shown in Fig. 9. The relative percent concentration of (4S)-(-)-α-terpineol at 5 and 10 min was 9.2 and 10.2, respectively. At 2 min, the relative percent concentration was 13.7. From the curvature of both plots, it appeared that the concentration of the S-enantiomer at 2 min was overestimated. Replications of the experiment using different enzyme solutions gave an average relative percent concentration of 10.3 for (4S)-(-)-α-terpineol at 2 min. It was concluded from these results that α-terpineol dehydratase stereoselectively catalyzed the hydration of (4R)-(+)-limonene approximately ten times faster than (4S)-(-)-limonene (Fig. 10).

TABLE 1

Relative percent concentration of α-terpineol enantiomers as a function of time for the hydration of 0.2 mM racemic limonene by α-terpineol dehydratase at 25°C.

Time (hr)	Relative percent concentration[a]	
	(4S)-(-)-α-terpineol	(4R)-(+)-α-terpineol
0	0.0	0.0
5	10.8	89.2
10	11.3	88.7
20	11.4	88.6
40	13.3	86.7

[a] Relative percent conc. = $\dfrac{\text{Conc. of pure α-terpineol enantiomers}}{\text{Total conc. of α-terpineol}}$

CONCLUSIONS

α-TD activity is low in non-aqueous solvents. A slightly acidic environment increased α-TD activity, and at the same time, decreased its stability. The activity decrease at low pH was probably due to denaturation instead of improper enzyme ionization. α-TD was heat labile. α-TD activity was insensitive to temperature change as indicated by the low E_a (21.6 ± 2.9 kJ·mol^{-1}) and Q_{10} (1.37 ± 0.07) values.

Triton X-100 inhibited α-TD, causing an increase in the apparent K_m and decrease in apparent V_{max}. The average apparent K_m of α-TD in 0.1% (w/v) Triton X-100 was 2.18 ± 0.19 mM. The numerical value of K_m is important for design of an enzymatic conversion process, since an enzyme is most efficient at substrate concentrations near K_m.

α-TD stereospecifically catalyzed the hydration of (4R)-(+)-limonene to (4R)-(+)-α-terpineol and the hydration of (4S)-(-)-limonene to (4S)-(-)-α-terpineol. The enzyme was stereoselective, with the rate of (4R)-(+)-limonene hydration being approximately ten times faster than the rate of (4S)-(-)-limonene hydration.

Use of a natural process for the production of (4R)-(+)-α-terpineol from (4R)-(+)-limonene has economic potential because the annual consumption of α-terpineol is high; while at the same time, it has greater commercial value than limonene. Commercial value of pure (4R)-(+)-α-terpineol is unknown because it is not available. An additional use of α-TD could be for the resolution of commercial racemic limonene (dipentene) into pure (4S)-(-)-limonene; while at the same time producing 90% pure (4R)-(+)-α-terpineol.

Florida Agricultural Expt. Station Journal Series No. R-01620.

REFERENCES

1. J. Buchel, Perfumer & Flavorist, 14 (1989) 22-26.
2. F.W. Welsh, W.D. Murray, and R.E. Williams, Crit. Rev. Biotechnol., 9 (1989) 105-169.
3. P.E. Shaw, J. Agric. Food Chem., 27(2) (1979) 246-257.
4. Anon., in: Statistical Summary 1988-89 Season, Florida Citrus Processors Association, Winter Haven, FL, 1989, p. 1D.
5. Anon., in: H. Van, C.A. Deyrup, and M. McCoy (Eds), Chemical Marketing Reporter, Vol. 238 (12), Schnell Publishing Co., Ltd., New York, 1990, pp. 38, 40, 44.
6. G. Kraidman, B.B. Mukherjee, and I.D. Hill, Bacteriol. Proc., 69 (1969) 63.

7   W.R. Abraham, H.M.R. Hoffmann, K. Kieslich, G. Reng and B. Stumpf, in: CIBA Foundation Symposium III. Enzymes in Organic Synthesis, Pitman, London, 1985, pp. 146-157.
8   K.R. Cadwallader, R.J. Braddock, M.E. Parish, and D.P. Higgins, J. Food Sci., 54 (1989) 1241-1245.
9   K.R. Cadwallader, R.J. Braddock, and M.E. Parish, J. Food Sci., 1991 (Submitted).
10 I.H. Segel, Biochemical Calculations, 2nd ed., John Wiley & Sons, Inc., New York, 1976.
11 J.R. Whitaker, Principles of Enzymology for the Food Sciences, Marcel Dekker, Inc., New York, 1972.
12 A. White, P. Handler, and E.L. Smith, Principles of Biochemistry, 3rd ed., McGraw-Hill, Inc., New York, 1964.
13 K.R. Cadwallader, Ph.D. dissertation, University of Florida, Gainesville, FL., 1990, 157 pp.

INTERESTERIFICATION OF PALM OIL MID FRACTION BY IMMOBILIZED LIPASE IN N-HEXANE; EFFECT OF LECHITIN ADDITION

L. MOJOVIC and S.SHILER-MARINKOVIC

Biochemistry Engineering Department, Faculty of Technology and Metallurgy, P.O. Box 494, 11001 Belgrade (Yugoslavia)

SUMMARY

Regiospecific interesterification of triacylglycerols of palm oil mid fraction with stearic acid by lipase from Rhizopus arrhizus immobilized on inorganic support was studied, for the purpose of cocoa butter-like fat production. Addition of 5% of crude soybean lechitin on the mass of immobilized enzyme caused valuable increase of stearic acid content in interesterified triacylglycerols. It is considered that lechitin acts as a surface active agent and forms reverse micellar system arround immobilized and hydrated enzyme in n-hexane.

1. INTRODUCTION

It is known that properties of fats and oils, nutritional, physical and chemical, depend upon the structure and distribution of the fatty acyl groups in the triacylglycerols (1). Therefore, the production of fats with desired physical and chemical properties by replacing the fatty acyl groups of triacylglycerols with other fatty acyl groups is of great importance and interest from an industrial viewpoint. Using technique of enzymatic interesterification to alter a distribution of fatty acyl groups among the tryacylglycerols has valuable advantages compared with conventional chemical methods. These are possibilities of using mild reaction conditions and production of useful triacylglycerols which are unobtainable by chemical interesterification. It is allowed by the specifity of enzymes, e.g. lipases. In the enzymatic interesterified fats, acyl groups retain their nature cis-position.

Producing fats with highly desirable physico-chemical properties, the so called cocoa butter substitutes, has become very popular area of biotechnological research. Tanaka et al. (2-3) have studied production of cocoa butter-like fat from olive oil and stearic acid or palmitic acid by enzymatic interesterification in an organic solvent system using immobilized 1,3 regiospecific lipase from Rhizopus delmar. Palm oil mid fraction is very convenient substrate for cocoa butter-like fats production because it is inexpensive and has appropriate triacylglycerols composition (4).

It is known that lipase act on the surface of oil droplets in the aqueous system (5). Previously used, water type emulsions (6) are not convenient for fats interesterification or enzymatic acyl exchange of triacylglycerols. These reactions are based on the manipulation of the chemical equilibrium of a thermodynamically reversible reaction (7) and require low water content (8-10). By using organic solvents for lipase catalyzed reactions, it is relatively easy to achieve an optimal low water content necessary for shifting the reaction. However, choice of appropriate solvent which would solubilize the substrate and would not affect the enzyme is of great importance (11,12). Many attempts to protect the enzyme from solvent nonpolar environment and to enhence its stability by appropriate immobilization method have been done (1,3,13-16). It has been shown that the dispersion degree of lipase into organic solvent in which substrate was solubilized affects the rate of acyl exchange (2).

This paper describes regiospecific interesterification of triacylglycerols of palm oil mid fraction with stearic acid in n-hexane by lipase from Rhizopus arrhizus immobilized on inorganic support. Addition of crude soybean lechitin as a dispersion agent was also studied.

2. MATERIALS

Refined Malaysian palm oil (importer "Vital" Vrbas, Yugoslavia) was used in this experiments. Palm oil mid fraction was obtained by double stage fractionation of palm oil according to procedure described by Tanaka et al. (17). Purified sn-1,3 regiospecific lipase from Rhizopus arrhizus (400,000 units/mg) was purchased from Sigma (St.Louis MO). The enzyme was stored as a suspension in ammonium sulphate at 4^0C. Celite (545, Serva, Germany) was used as a carrier for immobilization of the lipase. Stearic acid (90% purity) was purchased from Sigma. Sigma olive oil emulsion was used for determination of lipolytic activity of the lipase. Crude soybean lechitin was a gift from "Soko Štark" (Belgrade, Yugoslavia) confectionery factory. Silica gel for column chromatography (70-230 mesh) was purchased from Kemika (Zagreb, Yugoslavia) and used for separation of triacylglycerols from the reaction mixture. All other chemical used were reagent grade.

3. METHODS

3.1 Immobilization of lipase

Lipase was immobilized on celite by adsorbtion. Appropriate amount of inorganic support was mixed throughly with lipase solution in 0,3 M TES buffer (pH=6,5). Mixture of immobilized enzyme was dried in vacuum oven at 40^0C overnight. Before use, the immobilized enzyme was hydrated by addition of a known amount of destilled water.

3.2 Enzymatic interesterification reaction

The interesterification reaction of palm oil mid fraction and stearic acid by immobilized lipase was carried out in Erlenmeyer flasks (100 ml volume) with shaking (130 strokes per minute) within 20 hours. One gram of the substrate (palm oil mid fraction) and various amounts of stearic acid (0,4-1,2 g) were dissolved in water saturated n-hexane (4 ml). Concentration of the substrate (palm oil mid fraction) in n-hexane was about 27 % (w/w). 0,1 g of the celite immobilized lipase of various actvities was added in the substrate reaction mixture. Degree of substrate conversion was followed during the time course of the reaction. The influence of the addition of various amounts of dispersion agent (lechitin) was also studied.

3.3 Analytical methods

Lipolytic activity of immobilized lipase was determined by olive oil emulsion. Amount of free fatty acids released from the olive oil emulsion was determined by titration with 0,05 M NaOH (18). Activities were expressed in IU (International Units) where 1 IU is defined as a amount of enzyme required to produce 1 μmol free fatty acid per minute.

Progress of the lipase catalysed interesterification reaction e.g. substrate conversion was followed by determination of stearic acid content incorporated in triacylglycerols of palm oil mid fraction. Triacylglycerols were isolated from the reaction mixture by silica gel column chromatography according to method described by Quinlin and Weiser (19). Separated triacylglycerols were hydrolysed and free fatty acids are formed and esterified with boron trifluoride (20). Acyl composition was determined by Gas Chromatograph (Varian 1400-FID) equipped with hydrogen ionization detector. A stainless steel column (L=2m, ID=2mm) was packed with 4% Carbowax 20 M on Chromosorb W AW (80-100 mesh). The temperatures of the injection and column were 200^0 C and 180^0 C. Flow rates of nitrogen, hydrogen and air were 25 ml/min, 25 ml/min and 250 ml/min, respectively.

4. RESULTS AND DISCUSSION

4.1 Optimization of the reaction conditions

To optimize enzymatic interesterification reaction conditions an optimal water content of celite immobilized lipase and an optimal mass ratio of palm oil mid fraction and stearic acid was studied. Activity of immobilized enzyme to achieve the highest degree of substrate conversion was also studied.

4.1.1 Effect of water content. It was studied by hydratation of vacuum dried immobilized enzyme with various amounts of destilled water and following the substrate conversion. As shown in Fig. 1. the highest percent of stearic acid in interesterified triacylglycerols was attained with addition of 0,1 ml H_2O/g of immobilized enzyme. Macrae (1) has found similar optimal degree of enzyme hydratation (about 10 %) studying the interesterification of palm oil mid fraction with lipase from Aspergillus niger. Tanaka et al. (2) have proposed immobilized enzyme activation by addition of glycerol instead of water or buffer, and in such way, they achieved higher yield of interesterified triacylglycerols. Matsuo et al. (21) insist on preparing active interesterification catalysts containing a very low amount of water (about 2%) by slow controlled drying of mixtures of diatomaceus earth and lipase solution. Chi et al. (22) consider that effective water content also depends on the type of inorganic carrier. Hoq et al. (24) have found an optimal water content in the reaction system for synthesis triacylglycerols in membrane reactor about 4%. Generally considered, a certain water content is necessary for enzyme activation and shifting the biocatalytic reaction, and is specific for various applicable systems. So it should be experimentally determined for each system.

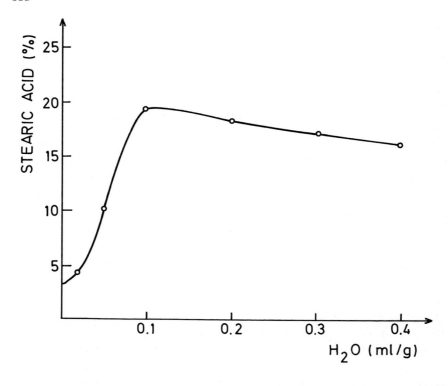

Fig. 1. Effect of water addition (ml H_2O/g of immobilized enzyme) on the interesterification reaction. Reaction conditions: t=40°C, τ=20h, V=130 strokes/min, 1g palm oil mid fraction, 0,7g stearic acid, 0,1g celite immobilized enzyme A=22 IU, 4ml water saturated n-hexane.

4.1.2 <u>Effect of mass ratio of palm oil mid fraction and stearic acid</u>. Ammount of 1g of palm oil mid fraction was interesterified with various amounts of stearic acid. As shown in Fig. 2., not quantitatively important increase in the degree of stearic acid incorporation was noticed above 0,7:1 mass ratio of stearic acid and palm oil mid fraction. Therefore, this mass ratio was used in further investigations.

4.1.3 <u>Effect of immobilized enzyme activity</u>. Interesterification reaction was studied with various added immobilized enzyme activities. The highest achieved stearic acid content in triacylglycerols was about 35% with addition of 120 IU immobilized enzyme per gram palm oil mid fraction, as shown in Fig.3. The relationship is not linearely proportional, and increase of the added immobilized enzyme activity above 120 IU does not cause higher substrate conversion.

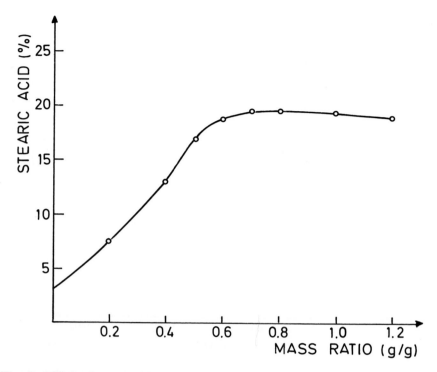

Fig. 2. Effect of mass ratio of stearic acid and palm oil mid fraction (g/g) on the interesterification reaction. Reaction conditions: $t=40^0C$, $\tau=20$ h, $v=130$ strokes/min, 1g palm oil mid fraction and various amounts of stearic acid, 0,1g celite immobilized lipase A=22 IU, 4ml water saturated n-hexane.

Time course of the interesterification reaction with the highest achieved stearic acid content (120 IU of enzyme added per 1g of palm oil mid fraction) is shown in Fig.4.

The highest substrate conversion was attained during first six hours of the reaction. Equilibrium state is established after 12-14 hours of the reaction. Decrease in the triacylglycerol content from 94% (at the beginning of the reaction) to 76% at the end of the reaction time is due to the hydrolytic reaction that occured, however. It was estimated that yield of interesterified triacylglycerols was 80,8%.

Yokozeki et al. (3) have achieved a maximum of about 40% of incorporated stearic acid in olive oil triacylglycerols. From the practical viewpoint for cocoa butter-like fats, amount of 33-36% of stearic acid (amount present in cocoa butter triacylglycerols) is sufficient. Tanaka et al. (2) have used 8000 IU of free lipase from Rhizopus delmar for interesterification of 10g olive oil triacylglycerols. Much greater consumption of the lipase in this system may be explained with the fact that lipase was not previously immobilized on inorganic support, but disperser (celite, sand, silica gel) was added separately. It is possible that all lipase in that system was not adsorbed at an interface, and due to that was not active.

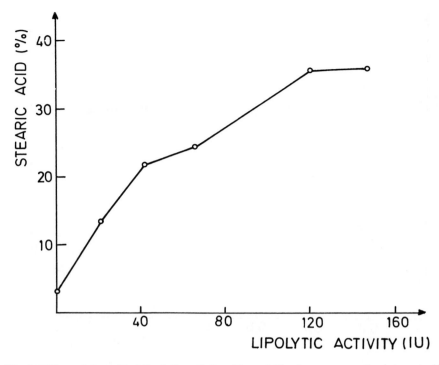

Fig. 3. Effect of the added lipolytic activity of immobilized enzyme on the interesterification reaction. Reaction conditions: t=40⁰C, τ=20h, v=130 strokes/min, 1g palm oil mid fraction, 0,7g stearic acid, 4ml water saturated n-hexane, 0,1g celite immobilized enzyme of various activities.

4.2 Effect of the lechitin addition

As it is known that the dispersion degree is of great importance for lipase biocatalytic activity, addition of crude soybean lechitin was studied. Time course of the interesterification reaction with and without lechitin addition was investigated. As it is shown in Fig.5., addition of 5% of the crude lechitin on the mass of immobilized enzyme caused valuable increase of stearic acid content in interesterified triacylglycerols from 21% (without addition) to 35%. This effect is considered of great importance, it enables achievement of interesterification conversion with substantially lower amount of enzyme involved. It is considered that lechitin acts as a surface active agent and forms reverse micellar system arround celite immobilized and hydrated enzyme in n-hexane. In such way, it protects immobilized enzyme from the nonpolar solvent environment and probably increases surface area between enzyme and substrate.

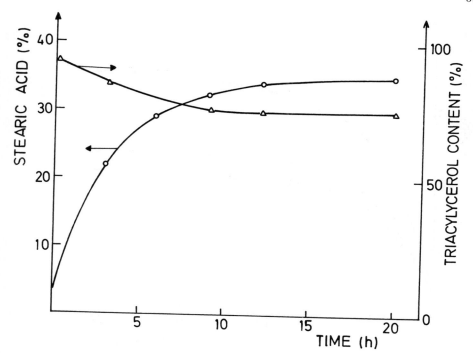

Fig.4. Time course of the interesterification reaction. Reaction conditions: t=40 °C, τ=20h, v=130 strokes/min, 1g palm oil mid fraction, 0,7g stearic acid, 0,1g celite immobilized lipase A=120 IU, 4ml water saturated n-hexane

Reverse micellar system has been developed for lipase biocatalytic reactions (15,16). The most common system is reverse micellar system with bis (2-ethylhexyl) sodium sulfosuccinate (AOT) in isooctane. However, such synthetic chemical have a limited use in food industries, while phospholipids are considerd usueful as surfactants for food systems.

Our further studies on the use of phospholipids reverse micellar system of enzyme immobilized on inorganic support for cocoa butter-like fat production are in progress. Data on this subject will be published in the near future.

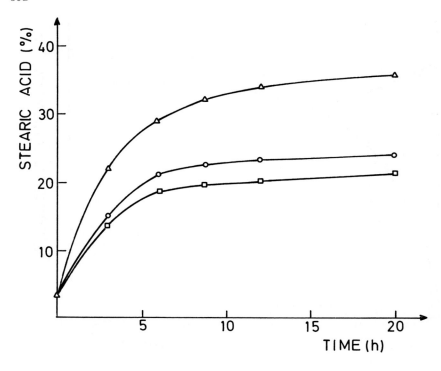

Fig.5. Effect of lechitin addition on the interesterification reaction (-□- without lechitin, -o- with 2% of the lechitin, -△- with 5% of the lechitin). Reaction conditions: $t=40^0C, \tau=20h$, $v=130$ strokes/min, 1g palm oil mid fraction, 0,7g stearic acid, 0,1g celite immobilized lipase A=48 IU, 4ml water saturated n-hexane.

5. CONCLUSIONS

The main conclusions that can be derived from the experimental results obtained are:

1. The highest substrate conversion, measured by the content of the stearic acid incorporated in triacylglycerols of the palm oil mid fraction was achieved with mass ratio of palm oil mid fraction and stearic acid 1:0,7; hydratation of celite immobilized lipase by addition of 0,1ml H_2O/g of the immobilized enzyme, and with addition of 120 IU of immobilized lipase per gram of palm oil mid fraction. The stearic acid content achieved was about 35%, what is sufficient for the purpose of cocoa butter-like fat production. The yield of interesterified triacylglycerols was 80,8%.

2. Addition of the crude lechitin in the reaction mixture enhenced degree of interesterification. This effect is considered of great importance, because it enables

achievement of the same interesterification conversion with substantially lower amount of enzyme involved. It is considered that lechitin protects immobilized enzyme from the nonpolar environment forming the reverse micellar system arround celite immobilized and hydrated enzyme in n-hexane.

REFERENCES

1. A.R.Macrae in: Biocatalysts in Organic Synthesis, Eds.J.Tramper, H.C.Van der Plas and P.Linko, Elsevier, Amsterdam, 1985, pp.195-208.
2. T.Tanaka, E.Ono, M.Ishihara, S.Yamanaka and K.Takinami, Agric. Biol. Chem. 45 (1981) 2387-2389.
3. K.Yokozeki, S.Yamanaka, K.Takinami, Y.Hirose, A.Tanaka, K.Sonomoto and S.Fukui, European J. Appl. Microbiol. Biotechnol. 14 (1982) 1-5.
4. A.R.Macrae, JAOCS, 60 (1983) 291-294.
5. G.Benzonana and P.Desnuelle, Biochim. Biophys. Acta, 105 (1965) 121-136.
6. R.W.Stevenson, F.E.Luddy and H.L.Rothbart, JAOCS, 56 (1979) 676-680.
7. K.Martinek, A.N.Semenov and I.V.Berezin, Biochim. Biophys. Acta, 658 (1981) 355.
8. S.Kyotani,H.Fukuda,Y.Nojima and T.Yamane, J.Ferment. Technol. 66 (1988) 567-575.
9. H.L.Goderis, G.Ampe, M.P.Feyten, B.L.Fouwe, W.M.Guffens, S.M.Van Cauwenbergh and P.P.Toback, Biotechnol. Bioeng, 30 (1987) 258-266.
10. T.Yamane, Y.Kojima, T.Ichiryu, M.Nagata and S.Shimitzu, Biotechnol. Bioeng. 34 (1989) 838-843.
11. A.Zaks and A.M.Klibanov, Science, 224 (1984) 1249.
12. C.Laane, S.Boeren, K.Vos and C.Veeger, Biotechnol. Bioeng. 30 (1987) 81-87.
13. S.T.Kang and J.S., Biotechnol. Bioeng. 33 (1989) 1469-1476.
14. M.B.Stark and K.Holmberg, Biotechnol. Bioeng. 34 (1989) 942-950.
15. D.Han and J.S.Rhee, Biotechnol. Bioeng. 28 (1986) 1250-1255.
16. S.Morita, H.Narita, T.Matoba and M.Kito, JAOCS, 61 (1984) 1571-1574.
17. Y.Tanaka, Y.Irianatsu, A.Noguchi, T.Kobayashi, European Patent 0 237 307 (1981).
18. N.W.Tietz and E.A.Fiereck, Clin. Chim. Acta, 13 (1966) 352.
19. P.Quinlin and H.J.Weiser, JAOCS, 35 (1958) 325.
20. L.D.Metcalfe, A.A.Schmitz and J.R.Pelka, Anal. Chem. 38 (1966) 514.
21. T.Matsuo, N.Sawamura, Y.Hashimoto and W.Hashida, US PAtent 4 420 560 (1983).
22. Y.M.Chi, K.Nakamura and T.Yang, Agric. Biol. Chem 52 (1988) 1541-1550.
23. M.M.Hoq, T.Yamane and S.Shimizu, JAOCS 61 (1984) 776-781.

G. Charalambous (Ed.), Food Science and Human Nutrition
© 1992 Elsevier Science Publishers B.V. All rights reserved.

POTENTIAL APPLICATIONS FOR SUPERCRITICAL CARBON DIOXIDE SEPARATIONS IN SOYBEAN PROCESSING

Ž.L. NIKOLOV[1,2], P. MAHESHWARI[1], J.E. HARDWICK[2], P.A. MURPHY[1,2], and L.A. JOHNSON[1,2]

[1]Department of Food Science and Human Nutrition, Iowa State University, Ames, Iowa 50011 (USA)

[2]Center for Crops Utilization Research, Iowa State University, Ames, Iowa 50011 (USA)

SUMMARY

Two potential applications of supercritical carbon dioxide (SC-CO_2) were studied: deacidification of vegetable oil and removal of off-flavor compounds from soybean flour. To evaluate the feasibility of deacidifying vegetable oils by using SC-CO_2, the solubilities of myristic, stearic, oleic, and linoleic acid were measured at three different pressures and temperatures, and compared with the literature data on solubility of vegetable oil. The effect of intermolecular interaction in the liquid phase on fatty acid solubility was investigated by measuring solubilities of synthetic mixtures of olive oil and oleic acid.

The efficiency of SC-CO_2 in desorbing the off-flavors from defatted soybean flour at 27.6 MPa and 40°C was investigated. The extraction of soy flour with water saturated SC-CO_2 reduced the usual grassy-beany flavor of hexane-defatted flour. Butanal, pentanal, and hexanal were identified as the off-flavor compounds extracted by the moist SC-CO_2. The extraction with supercritical CO_2 did not affect the solubility of soy proteins determined from the nitrogen solubility index.

1. INTRODUCTION

Various economic, environmental and social factors have motivated government agencies and industry to search for cheaper and safer extraction and separation technologies. The cost of energy was initially the incentive to develop more flexible and energy efficient processes based on supercritical fluid technology. The more recent interest in supercritical fluid separations stems from the increased scrutiny of traditional solvents, increased government regulations regarding solvent residues and fugitive hydrocarbons in the environment, increased performance demands on the product, and increased consumer's concern for possible harmful residues in foods (1,2).

Over the last ten years supercritical carbon dioxide (SC-CO_2) has emerged as an ideal solvent for a variety of extraction and separation applications. It is an inert, nontoxic, nonflammable, and inexpensive compound which is accepted as a harmless ingredient of foods and beverages (1). This solvent is particularly suitable for extraction and separation of compounds which decompose before reaching their normal boiling points. One of the significant advantages of the SC-CO_2 processing is that the solvent can be easily, quickly, and completely separated from accompanying solute, thus significantly reducing contamination of the product with a residual solvent. Several actual and potential commercial applications of SC-CO_2 separations include extraction of fragrances and flavors from liquids, decaffeination of tea and coffee, deodorization of oils, extraction of oil seeds, fractionation of highly unsaturated methyl esters derived from fish oil triglycerides, and separation of organic materials from water (3).

Supercritical CO_2 has been used in extraction of a variety of oil-bearing materials ranging from oilseeds (4-9) to algae (10). The extracted oil from the oilseeds was of comparable tocopherol and free fatty acid content as the hexane-extracted oil. A significant reduction of phosopholipids and glycolipids was achieved in SC-CO_2-extracted oils indicating that the degumming step can be omitted during the oil refining (6,7,11,12). However, the oxidative stability of SC-CO_2-extracted oil was also reduced because of lower levels of phosopholipids (4,13). The fractionation power of supercritical CO_2 has also been demonstrated in several cases such as the separation of alkyl esters derived from fish oil (2, 14-17) and the removal of mono- and diglycerides from triglycerides (18). Although the supercritical fluids exhibit some attractive separation properties, they should not be considered as "magic solvents," and the commercial viability of a particular SC fluid application has to be evaluated on a case-by-case basis (2).

The aim of our study was to assess the feasibility and merits of supercritical CO_2 in 1) deacidification of (crude) vegetable oils and 2) the removal of off-flavors from soybean flour.

1.1 <u>Solubilities and fractionation of fatty acids and triglycerides</u>
Many studies which reported solubilities of fatty acids and triglycerides in supercritical CO_2 were performed with a major interest in modeling of their behavior in the supercritical phase rather than in evaluating their potential to be fractionated. Therefore, previous work pertinent to our investigation will be briefly reviewed here.

Chrastil (19) measured solubilities of five triglycerides and two fatty acids in SC-CO_2 in the pressure range of 8 to 25 MPa and temperature between 40 and 80°C. The experimental data suggests that under certain processing conditions, fatty acids have much higher solubilities than their corresponding triglycerides. Supercritical CO_2 with ethanol as an entrainer has been employed to deacidify palm oil (20). The amount of free fatty acids in the oil was reduced from 3 to 0.1 wt% by using a multistage counter-current extractor operated at 13.7 MPa and 80°C. Bamberger et al. (21) measured the solubilities of three triglycerides (trilaurin, trimyristin, and tripalmitin) and their corresponding fatty acids at 313 K and at pressures between 8 and 30 MPa. The solubilities of fatty acids or their triglyceride homologous series decreased with increasing molecular weight. The solubilities of fatty acids were higher than their corresponding triglycerides at the same reduced density but, the solubilities of palmitic acid and trilaurin were similar. This group also studied the solubilities of triglyceride mixtures in CO_2 and found that the intermolecular interactions in the liquid phase affected the solubility of individual triglycerides in the supercritical phase. Recently, it was demonstrated that a complex mixture of triglycerides such as butterfat can be fractionated into two, four, or even eight fractions depending on the processing temperature and pressure (22-24). An extensive study of application of the SC-CO_2 in deacidification of olive oil was published by Brunetti et al.(25). These authors measured solubilities of four fatty acids and two triglycerides at 20 and 30 MPa in the temperature range between 35 and 60°C. The data suggested that, at 60°C and 20 MPa, SC-CO_2 had a higher selectivity for fatty acids than triglycerides. A deacidification of olive oil samples was performed at various fatty acid content and it was concluded that the process was feasible especially for oils with relatively high free fatty acids. White (26), and Kramer and Thodos (27) also measured the solubilities of selected fatty acids at pressures ranging from 14 to 50 MPa and temperatures ranging from 35 to 65°C. White (26) investigated the solubilities of even-numbered saturated fatty acids, C_{10} through C_{18}, whereas Kramer and Thodos (27) compared solubilities of stearic acid and 1-Octadecanol.

The published experimental data on fatty acid solubilities varies significantly due to the difference in experimental conditions and the purity of the compounds used. Therefore, to evaluate the feasibility of deacidifying vegetable oils by using SC-CO_2, we measured the solubilities of myristic, stearic, oleic, and linoleic acid and compared them to the average solubility of vegetable oils obtained from del Valle and Aguilera (28).

1.2 Off-flavor removal

The current annual world production of soy protein ingredients (flours, concentrates and isolates) for food is estimated at about 1 billion pounds with 75% produced alone in the United States. More than 95% of the soybean meal produced annually in the U.S. (apr. 45 billion pounds) is used to supply protein in animal feeds and it constitutes the largest portion of the monetary value of soybeans. In spite of its high-protein quality and low cost compared to animal protein, the soy meal has not been accepted in human foods due to off-flavors associated with it. Most of the edible protein is used to replace more expensive animal protein in meats and to a lesser extent in dairy-type products. The use of soy protein in dairy products has considerable potential for replacing increasingly expensive imported sodium caseinate. But, to achieve its acceptance in human foods, the flavor problem must be resolved.

There were a number of attempts to find a good and practical method for removing off-flavors. Two processing methods have shown a potential: steam treatment and solvent extraction. Steam treatment is used commercially (29) but it reduces the solubility of the proteins and, thus, limits the functional properties of concentrates and isolates made from them. Extraction with alcohols, such as ethanol and isopropanol, is being used to prepare bland soy concentrates (30-32). The most efficient removal of off-flavor compounds was achieved by extraction of defatted flakes with hexane-ethanol mixtures.

However, none of the treatments completely eliminate off-flavors and all denature protein. An additional problem with the solvent extraction approach is the need to eliminate all residual solvent which increases the processing cost and may cause further denaturation of soy proteins.

Most of the research addressing the effect of supercritical SC-CO_2 extraction on the flavor of soybean and corn proteins has been performed at the U.S. Department of Agriculture's National Center for Agricultural Utilization Research in Peoria, IL. Christianson et al. (6) studied the use of SC-CO_2 in place of hexane for corn oil extraction and production of a food-grade germ flour. Full-fat, dry-milled corn germ samples containing 3.5 and 8% moisture were extracted at 50°C and pressures of 34.5 and 66.2 MPa. It was found that the moisture levels did not affect the oil yield, but the flavor scores of the corn germ samples with 8% moisture were significantly better than those with 3.5% moisture. It should be noted that this group (6) used dry SC-CO_2 and by the end of extraction the final moisture level of the germ was very low (2.0-3.5%). Christianson et al. (6) also determined the nitrogen solubility index (NSI), which is a measure of protein solubility, and concluded that significant denaturation of proteins in the SC-CO_2-extracted samples had occurred. Eldridge et al. (33) varied the processing conditions (temperature, pressure and moisture) for SC-CO_2 extraction of full-fat soybean flakes to produce defatted protein products with improved flavor characteristics and high protein solubilities. A constant moisture of the sample during the extraction was maintained by adding a water-saturated glass-wool plug at the inlet of the extractor. They observed that the presence of moisture in the flakes caused denaturation of lipoxygenase that led to improved flavor. However, at higher moisture content (11.4%) and temperatures above 80°C protein solubility index (NSI) was reduced. According to these authors, high protein solubility and good flavor scores can be obtained at pressures greater than 83 MPa, temperatures about 80°C, and moisture levels between 10.5 and 11.5%. The usual grassy/beany and bitter flavors of hexane-defatted soybean flours were minimally detectable when extracting under these conditions.

The most recent work from the same group dealt with the effect of SC-CO_2 extraction on the flavor of corn distillers' grains. Wu et al. (34) improved the flavor profile of corn distillers' dried grains by treating it with SC-CO_2. They reported that SC-CO_2 extraction with water as an entrainer was more effective in reducing the fermented flavor from the corn distillers' grains than the extraction with 95% ethanol alone or with SC-CO_2-ethanol mixture. As before, the extractions were performed at rather high pressures (64-83 MPa) and temperatures (82-103°C).

The goal of our study was to examine the efficiency of SC-CO_2 in desorbing the off-flavors from defatted soybean flour at lower temperature and pressure. We also attempted to identify and quantify the removed off-flavor compounds as a result of the CO_2 extraction.

2. MATERIALS AND METHODS
2.1 Equipment

The supercritical fluid extraction system used in this work was custom assembled. A schematic diagram of the flow-through apparatus is shown in Figure 1. Carbon dioxide with 99.9% purity was delivered to a single-stage gas booster Model AGD-62 (Haskel Inc., Burbank, CA). The carbon dioxide was compressed in a stainless-steel surge

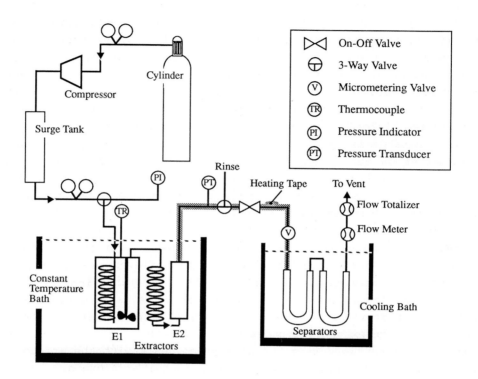

Fig. 1. Schematic process diagram for supercritical fluid extraction.

tank, which was maintained at a pressure around 48 MPa. The operating pressure of supercritical carbon dioxide was controlled by an Alphagaz Model 2612 regulator (Cooks Inc., Algona, IA). The carbon dioxide was heated to the process temperature by flowing through a stainless-steel coil before contacting the samples in the extractors (E1 or E2). The temperature in the water bath was controlled to ±0.3°C by a Fisher immersion circulator and it was recorded with a mercury thermometer to ±0.1°C.

The extraction vessel (E1) used was a 300 mL Magnedrive II assembly (Autoclave Engineering, Erie, PA). This vessel was used in the extraction experiments with oleic acid-olive oil mixtures and served as water saturator in the experiments with soybean flour. Solubility measurements of fatty acids were carried out in a 20-cm long and 1-cm internal diameter (i.d.) stainless-steel column (E2) (Alltech, Deerfield, IL). The soy flour extraction was performed in a similar column of the same length and 2.2 cm in internal diameter.

The SC-CO_2 was expanded across a micrometering valve Model 10VRMM-2812 (Autoclave Eng., Erie, PA). An on/off valve Model 10V-2075 (Autoclave Eng., Erie, PA) was installed upstream from the micrometering valve for complete gas shut-off. The precipitated solute was collected in glass-tube separators which were immersed in a zero or subzero temperature ethylene glycol bath. All stainless-steel lines and valves were heated with heating tapes at 20 to 30°C above the process temperature to avoid precipitation of the extracted material in the lines and the valves. The amount of CO_2 consumed during the process was measured by Omega mass flow controller Model FMA767-I and DP-350 totalizer (Omega Eng., Stamford, CT) calibrated for carbon dioxide use.

2.2 Materials

Fatty acids used for solubility measurements were purchased from Sigma (St. Louis, MO) and were of the following purity: myristic acid (99-100%); stearic acid (99%); oleic acid (99%); and linoleic acid (99%). The olive oil samples used for deacidification experiments were from a 100% pure cold-pressed olive oil (Bertolli, Lucca, Italy). Soybeans flour was prepared by grinding soybeans, variety Vinton 81, in a high-speed mill, Magic Mill III Plus, (Salt Lake City, UT). The flour was cold defatted with hexane. After evaporation of residual hexane from the flour at room temperature, moisture was determined to be 5%. Butanal and pentanal (98+% pure) were purchased from Polyscience Corp. (Niles, IL), and hexanal (99% pure) was obtained from Aldrich (Milwaukee, WI). Carbon dioxide (Matheson Gas Products, 99.9% pure) was used as received. All other chemicals used in this work were reagent grade.

2.3 Extraction procedures

2.3.1 Fatty Acid Solubility.
Between 5 and 10 g of solid fatty acids (myristic or stearic acid) were packed in the extractor (E2) in three alternating layers of glass wool and solid sample to minimize the channelling of SC-CO_2. In the case of liquid samples (oleic and linoleic acid), approximately 5 g of sample was soaked in the glass wool and packed in the column following the same procedure as for the solid samples. The system was then pressurized and allowed to equilibrate for at least one hour before opening the micrometering valve to start the flow of SC-CO_2.

The SC-CO_2 flow rate was kept below 0.4 g/min at all pressures and temperatures. This flow rate was determined to be low enough to insure that equilibrium was attained between the sample and the SC-CO_2 flowing through the system. The extraction was performed with various amounts of CO_2, depending on the solubility of the acid, and ranged between 4.5 and 70 g of CO_2. The solubility measurements for most of the acids were done in triplicate. Whenever the operating pressure or temperature was changed, the first run of the extraction was discarded.

The amount of extract collected in the glass-tube separators was weighed to ± 0.1 mg. The residual fatty acid that precipitated in the valves and the lines was solubilized and rinsed with 15 to 20 mL of hexane. Hexane was evaporated in a water bath at 50°C and the weight of the residue was determined. Solubilities of the various acids were expressed as weight percentage based on the total mass of carbon dioxide used in the extraction. The total mass of CO_2 consumed was calculated from the standard (101.3 kPa, 273 K) volume of CO_2 measured by the flow totalizer.

Solubilities of oleic acid-olive oil mixtures were measured using a 50 g sample in the extractor vessel (E1). The mixture in the reactor was continuously agitated at 500 rpm during the extraction experiment. All other procedures were as described above.

2.3.2 *Off-flavor Removal*. Defatted soybean flour (25-30 g) was packed in three alternating beds in the extractor (see 2.1). Downstream from the extractor-E2 (Fig. 1), a 10 cm long and 0.7 cm i.d. stainless-steel column was connected containing 0.75 g Tenax-GC, 20/35 mesh polymer packing (Alltech, Deerfield, IL). The U-tube separators were also filled with the Tenax (10 g) to ensure adsorption of the volatiles and eliminate their loss to the environment with exiting CO_2. Dry and water-saturated SC-CO_2 were used at a pressure of 27.6 MPa and a temperature of 40°C to remove off-flavor compounds. The water-saturated CO_2 was prepared by bubbling the SC-CO_2 through the extraction vessel (E1) that contained about 150 mL deionized water at 40°C. The flow rate of CO_2 was maintained below 0.4 g/min. Because the concentration of off-flavor compounds in the flour was very small, the extraction experiments were performed using a total of 900 g CO_2 in order to accumulate a sufficient amount of extract for further analysis. On the completion of the experiment, the lines were rinsed with double-distilled diethyl ether to remove the residual volatiles in the lines. A control run using gaseous CO_2 was performed at 4.1 MPa and

40°C. All operating conditions during the control run were the same as in the extraction experiment.

After the extraction of the soy flour with SC-CO_2, the layers of flour were removed from the column, separated and stored at 5°C for analysis. The extracted volatiles that were trapped on the Tenax-GC in the extractor and the U-tube were eluted with approximately 50 mL of double distilled ether. The ether was evaporated using a Vigreux (Pyrex) distillation column. The residue left in the round bottle flask was immediately frozen at -18°C to avoid the loss of volatiles.

2.4 Analytical methods

2.4.1 Gas Chromatography.

The headspace gas chromatographic (GC) analysis was performed on the control as well as SC-CO_2-treated soy flour. The volatiles extracted from the flour were analyzed using Varian 3400 gas chromatograph (Sunnyvale, CA).

A 30 m capillary DB-WAX column (J & W Scientific, Folsom, CA) was used for GC analysis. The column temperature was maintained at 40°C for 8 minutes of analysis time. The injector temperature was set at 210°C, and temperature of the flame ionization detector (FID) was 250°C. Hydrogen at a rate of 4 mL/min was used as a carrier gas, and 30 mL/min for the FID. Nitrogen was used as a make-up gas at 26 mL/min and the air flow rate was set at 300 mL/min.

For headspace analysis, 1 g of flour was weighed in a 50 mL glass vial. The SC-CO_2-treated flour was analyzed separately for the volatiles present in the top, middle, and the bottom layers of flour. A water slurry containing 1 g flour and 3 mL of water was also prepared for headspace analysis. After the sample preparation, the glass vials were kept in an oven at 37°C for at least one hour to equilibrate.

Five mL of headspace gas of the dry and water-slurried soy flour was injected into the GC. The injection time was two minutes, the splitter was turned off and the analyte was cryofocussed using liquid nitrogen (Wilson et al., 1990). The headspace analysis was performed in triplicate in each case. Butanal, pentanal and hexanal were used as external standards. The volatile compounds were identified from their retention times and quantified by their peak areas.

The extract collected from the Tenax column and the U-tubes were analyzed directly using capillary GC. About 0.5 µL cryofocussed sample of extract was injected in the GC under the conditions described above. This GC analysis was performed in triplicate.

2.4.2 Total Protein and NSI Determination.

The total protein determination and nitrogen solubility index (NSI) of defatted soy flour were expressed on a dry-weight basis. The moisture content was determined by drying the defatted soy flour in vacuum oven at 80°C for 5 hr, AOAC 925.09 (36). Control as well as SC CO_2-treated soy flour were analyzed in duplicate for total N content by Kjeldahl AOCS Method Ac 4-41 (37), using a N-conversion factor of 5.71. The official AACC Method 46-23 (38) was modified to estimate NSI from a sample size of 2.5 g. The layers of SC-CO_2-treated soy flour were mixed for NSI determination. The analysis was performed in triplicate for control as well as SC-CO_2-treated soy flour.

The level of significance for the difference between untreated and the SC-CO_2-treated samples was determined by the Students' t-test (39).

2.4.3 <u>Sensory Evaluation</u>. A triangle test (40) was performed to determine the difference between the control and the SC-CO_2-treated soy flour. Fifteen panelists familiar with soybean flavor were chosen. The panelists received three coded samples in 20-mL glass vials containing 2 g of dry soybean flour. The panelists were told that two (control) samples were the same and one was treated differently. They were asked to identify the odd sample based on its odor, and to comment on the type of difference between the samples. The level of significance for correct response was determined using the statistical chart of Larmond (40).

3. RESULTS AND DISCUSSION

3.1 <u>Solubility of Fatty Acids in SC CO_2</u>

The effects of pressure and temperature on the solubilities of the four fatty acids are plotted in Fig. 2. The solubility isotherms for individual fatty acids showed an increase of solubility with increase of pressure at all temperatures. Myristic acid had the highest solubility at the pressures and temperatures studied, followed by linoleic, oleic and stearic acid. The solubility isotherms of stearic acid at 40 and 50°C are reported in Figs. 2a and 2b because reliable solubility measurements at 60°C were difficult to obtain due to precipitation of stearic acid in the lines and the micrometering valve. The solubility of stearic acid was much lower than the other three fatty acids probably due to the difference in physical state. At the process temperatures below 50°C, stearic acid was probably in a solid state whereas the other three fatty acids, including myristic acid, were liquid. Bamberger et al. (21) recently determined experimentally that myristic acid (mp 54 °C) is a liquid at 15 MPa and 40°C in the presence of SC-CO_2. Our solubility data of

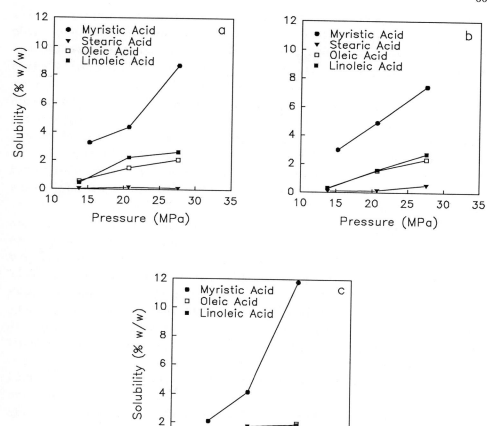

Fig. 2. Solubility isotherms of fatty acids in SC-CO_2 as a function of pressure: (a) 40°C; (b) 50°C; and (c) 60°C.

stearic acid is 2-5 times lower than those reported by Chrastil (19), White (26), and Kramer and Thodos (27), and an order of magnitude lower than those of Brunetti et al. (25) under the same experimental conditions. A review of the literature data for various fatty acids reveals that stearic acid had the largest reported discrepancies in solubility (41). The solubility of myristic acid was in the range of reported values in the literature (21,25,26). Oleic acid solubilities shown in Fig. 2 agree with the values of Nilsson et al. (18) and with the solubilities measured by Chrastil (19) at pressures below 20 MPa. Both Chrastil (19) and Brunetti (25) found oleic acid solubilities at 25 and 30 MPa, respectively, and 60°C that were almost four times higher than our values. This discrepancy could be, in part, explained by the lower purity of their starting material (18). Linoleic acid had a very similar solubility to oleic acid as would be expected on the basis of similar molecular weight and structural characteristics. Slightly higher solubility of linoleic acid than oleic acid may be attributed to the approximately 30% higher vapor pressure of linoleic acid than that of oleic acid (42). Myristic acid (C14:0) has a higher solubility in $SC-CO_2$ than any of C_{18} fatty acid because of its significantly higher vapor pressure compared to the other three fatty acids (42,43).

At lower pressures, below 15 MPa, the solubilities of the liquid fatty acids (myristic, oleic and linoleic) were found to decrease with increasing the temperature. Such behavior is termed retrograde behavior (44) and it has been explained in terms of temperature effect on the vapor pressure of the solute and on the density of $SC-CO_2$ (45). Vapor pressures of the fatty acids increase exponentially with temperature whereas the density of $SC-CO_2$ decreases almost linearly under operating conditions used in this work (42,43,46). Therefore, at lower pressure where the fluid is highly compressible, the density of $SC-CO_2$ decreases significantly with small increases in temperature. At higher pressures, temperature affects the density slightly and the solubility increases with temperature as does the vapor pressure (47). Retrograde behavior was not observed for stearic acid which with the increase of temperature from 40 to 50°C exhibited an increase in solubility. A temperature of 50°C is probably close to the depressed melting point of stearic acid which offsets the negative temperature effect on CO_2 density. Similar observations were made about another solid fatty acid, palmitic acid, which solubility also increased with a temperature increase between 35 and 50°C (25). Brunetti et al. (25) suggested that compounds which are solids under experimental conditions tend to show an increase of solubility with an increasing temperature.

To eliminate the effect of pressure on the density, solubility isotherms in Fig. 3 were plotted versus density instead of against the pressure. The difference of solubilities between C-18-fatty acids in Fig. 3 at a particular density is mainly due to vapor pressure effect and, therefore, by increasing the temperature at constant density the solubility should be expected to increase. The solubility of each fatty acid increased proportionally to the density of the supercritical fluid (44). The small decrease of solubility observed for stearic acid at SC-CO_2 density of 0.9×10^{-3} (kg/m^3) (Fig. 3a) was probably due to an experimental error in determining the extracted amount. The standard deviation (n=3) of the average solubility of stearic acid at this particular density was unusually high, almost 45%. An order of magnitude higher vapor pressure of myristic acid than vapor pressures of other three acids (42,43) is reflected in its higher solubility as shown in Figs. 2 and 3. The greater effect of temperature on the solubility of stearic acid (solid) than on the solubilities of the other (liquid) acids, as discussed above, is more apparent from solubility isotherms given in Figs. 3a and 3b.

In Fig. 3 solubility isotherms of vegetable oils were also plotted for comparison with fatty acid isotherms. The solubility values of the oil for operating conditions in this work were calculated from a model developed by del Valle and Aguilera (28). Their model-equation was based on experimental solubilities of three vegetable oils, including soybean oil, and estimates triglyceride solubilities as functions of temperature and SC-CO_2 density. By comparing the solubility isotherms of liquid fatty acids and vegetable oil shown in Fig. 3, it can be concluded that deacidification of oils would be possible. Higher temperatures and lower densities (lower pressure) would favor selectivity of CO_2 for fatty acids. The proper extraction conditions should be chosen to achieve good yield of fatty acids and satisfactory selectivity. Based on the relative solubilities of vegetable oil and liquid fatty acids, it appeared that pressure between 15 and 20 MPa and temperatures at or above 50°C would result in higher selectivity for fatty acids than the oil. For example, at 50°C and 15 MPa the solubility of pure myristic acid relative to that of vegetable oil was 30 times larger. For both oleic acid and linoleic acid, solubilities are about 7 times larger. At a higher pressure (20

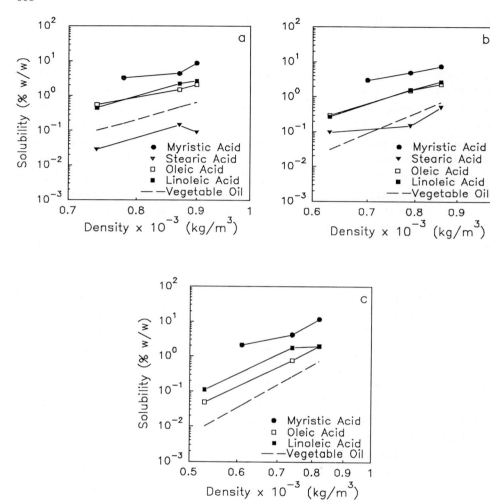

Fig. 3. Solubility isotherms of vegetable oil and fatty acids in SC-CO_2 as a function of density: (a) 40°C; (b) 50°C; and (c) 60°C.

MPa), the relative solubilities were somewhat lower--13, 4.5, and 4.5 for myristic, linoleic, and oleic acid, respectively. But, at 20 MPa and 50°C the extraction yields (g FA/g CO_2) of these three fatty acids were almost 50% higher than that at 15 MPa.

Therefore, operating conditions need to be optimized depending on the main objective of the extraction, i.e., fractionation vs oil deacidification. If fractionation of fatty acids is the goal, then lower pressure and higher temperatures would be favored. For deacidification of vegetable oils, higher pressures, as suggested above, would probably be preferred because of better yields. Stearic acid was not analyzed here because interaction with vegetable oil (triglycerides) would probably change its physical state that would probably result in a different solubility than estimated in this study.

3.2 Solubility of oleic acid-olive oil mixture

Because the solubility of pure components does not take into account the possible effect of intermolecular interaction in the liquid phase, we investigated the effect of olive oil on oleic acid solubility. Two synthetic mixtures, one containing 10 wt% and the other 50 wt% of oleic acid in pure olive oil, were used as model systems. The effects of temperature, pressure, and feed composition on the selectivity of SC-CO_2 for oleic acid is summarized in Table 1. The solubility of the mixture measured at constant pressure decreased when the temperature was raised from 40 to 60°C. The solubility of 50%-mixture displayed retrograde behavior at all pressures investigated in this work.

As previously discussed, the temperature effect on the solubility of the mixture was greater at lower pressures. At constant temperature (40 or 60°C), the change of pressure by 7 MPa affected the amount of the total extract by a factor of 2 and in two cases almost by a factor of 3. The oleic acid concentration in the feed affected the composition of the extract. The highest selectivity of CO_2 for oleic acid was obtained for the 10% mixture at 20.7 MPa. In general, the SC-CO_2 selectivity for oleic acid was higher at 20.7 than at 27.6 MPa.

Our experimental observations using oleic acid-olive oil mixtures agree well with those reported by Brunetti et al. (25) who also found that the mixture solubility decreased with decreasing the fatty acid concentration in the feed mixture. On the other hand, they have found that the distribution coefficient, which is a measure of the SC-CO_2 selectivity, increased significantly with the decrease of free fatty acid content in the feed (25). This behavior was explained by the lower association of oleic acid in the mixture due to the "dilution" effect of the "solvent" oil. Although we did not measure the fatty acid concentration in the residue, we came to the same conclusion based on mass balance considerations. The amount of oleic acid extracted from the 50 wt% mixture, as calculated from the data in Table 1, was almost the same as that obtained for pure oleic acid. This indicates that the dilution effect of the olive oil triglycerides did not play a role at such a high concentration. The results obtained with these oleic acid-olive oil mixtures confirmed our previous conclusion based on the comparison of the solubilities of pure components (Fig. 3), that myristic, oleic, and linoleic acid can be extracted from vegetable oil at operating pressures between 15 and 20 MPa and an operating temperature around 50°C.

TABLE 1
Extraction of oleic acid from oleic acid-olive oil mixtures.

PRESSURE (MPa)	TEMP (°C)	OLEIC ACID IN MIXTURE (wt %)	MIXTURE SOLUBILITY (wt %)	OLEIC ACID IN EXTRACT (wt %)
20.7	60	10.0	0.27	83
27.6	60	10.0	0.87	56
13.8	40	50.0	0.62	87
13.8	60	50.0	0.30	84
20.7	40	50.0	1.2	87
20.7	60	50.0	0.91	90
27.6	40	50.0	2.3	78
27.6	60	50.0	2.1	83

Therefore, studies with pure compounds provide useful information about the effects of pressure and temperature (extraction conditions) on their solubility although the effect of intermolecular interaction in the liquid phase between the components of the system, including SC-CO_2, should also be taken into account before a conclusion is made about feasibility of deacidification process.

3.3 <u>Off-flavor removal</u>

Our preliminary work in which we compared the extraction of defatted soybean flour with dry and moist SC-CO_2 indicated that more efficient removal of off-flavors was achieved by using water saturated $SC-CO_2$. This observation is in agreement with the results of Christianson et al. (6) and Eldridge et al. (33) who also found that the flavor improvement of $SC-CO_2$-extracted protein was directly related to the moisture content of the corn and soy protein samples. Therefore, we further studied and measured the effect of the water-saturated $SC-CO_2$ on the desorption of soybean off-flavor compounds.

The results of total volatiles present in the soy flour before and after the $SC-CO_2$ are shown in Fig.4.

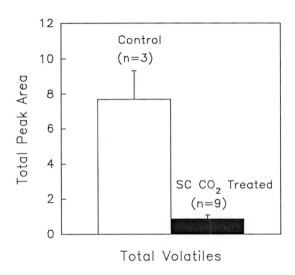

Fig. 4. Headspace analysis of the control and $SC-CO_2$ treated defatted soybean flour for the total volatiles.

Headspace analysis revealed about an eleven-fold reduction in volatiles for the samples treated with the supercritical CO_2. When soy flour was flushed with gaseous CO_2 (see 2.3.2), no change in volatile content was measured. Butanal, pentanal, and hexanal were identified as the off-flavor compounds removed during extraction (Fig. 5). The amounts of all three compounds were significantly reduced after $SC-CO_2$ extraction. $SC-CO_2$ was more effective in desorbing butanal and pentanal than hexanal from the protein. This effect could probably be explained by the expected higher solubility of butanal and pentanal compared to hexanal in the $SC-CO_2$. Butanal and pentanal concentrations were reduced 55 and 75 times, respectively, whereas hexanal concentration was reduced only three-fold. The effect of moisture on the extraction efficiency is probably related to the higher polarity of the moist CO_2 due to entrained water as well as to enhanced mass transfer due to "swelling" of the flour (48). The moist SC-CO_2 may favor a shift in the predicted Schiff's base equilibrium, thus, allowing more free aldehyde to be removed. The difficulty in removing hexanal compared to its lower MW counterparts suggests that these SC-CO_2 conditions are not yet maximized to break the stronger hydrophobic binding of hexanal to the soy proteins. Since we only have a minimal understanding of soy flavor and protein interaction, it is difficult to draw a clear picture of what SC-CO_2 is doing at the molecular level (51).

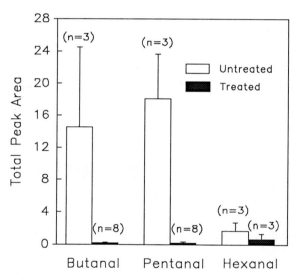

Fig. 5. Off-flavor compounds identified in the untreated and SC-CO_2 treated soybean flour. Bars represent standard deviation.

The results of GC analysis were confirmed by the triangle sensory testing. Thirteen out of fifteen panelists found that treated soy flour with moist SC-CO_2 was different ($\alpha=0.001$) than the untreated flour. The panelists commented on the lower, less strong or lack of beany flavor of the treated flour. However, some of the panelists detected fishy odor in the SC-CO_2-extracted soy flour.

The NSI values of untreated and SC-CO_2-treated soy flour samples are given in Table 2. The NSI value of the dry SC-CO_2-treated soy flour was found to be significantly ($\alpha=0.05$) lower than the untreated flour. But, there was no significant ($\alpha=0.05$) difference between the

TABLE 2

Effect of dry and moist SC-CO$_2$ extraction on nitrogen solubility index.

Analysis	Untreated Flour	Treated Flour
Total protein (%)	43.7^a ± 1.7	43.9^b ± 5.3
NSI (%), moist SC-CO$_2$	67.0^c ± 6.4	63.1^d ± 7.6
NSI (%), dry SC-CO$_2$	67.0^c ± 6.4	50.4^e ± 0.3

^{a}n=4; ^{b}n=7; ^{c}n=4; ^{d}n=7; ^{e}n=2;

NSI values of the treated and untreated flour with moist SC-CO$_2$. The total protein values of the untreated and the SC-CO$_2$-treated soy flour were also not significantly different. These results agree with the previous report by Christianson et al. (6) that the NSI value of corn germ flour extracted with dry SC-CO$_2$ was significantly lower than that of the hexane extracted material. The initial moisture of 8% in the corn germ helped the extraction of off-flavors, but the concomitant removal of water dried the sample and apparently affected protein solubility. This conclusion is supported by the subsequent work of this group where moist SC-CO$_2$ was used throughout the extraction of soybean flakes (33). Eldridge et al.(33) found that higher moisture content of soy flakes caused denaturation of lipoxygenase and a decrease in NSI. We also believe that the change in protein solubility was caused primarily by the higher temperatures of extraction (above 80°C) used in that study (49). Our work indicates that extraction of defatted flour at lower temperatures and pressures is effective in off-flavor removal without denaturing protein.

Although the SC-CO$_2$-extraction technology was found to be effective in removing the off-flavor compounds from soy proteins, its commercialization will depend on the processing concept. If soy oil is extracted with supercritical CO$_2$ instead of hexane, the processing conditions at the end of the extraction can be adjusted for optimum off-flavor removal in the same reactor without increasing significantly the cost of the meal. On the other hand, upgrading the soy meal ($0.20/kg) or food-grade flours (0.30 - 0.70/kg) in a separate process would not be very attractive since the added cost due to SC-CO$_2$ processing would be between $0.40 and $0.60/kg of feed (50). Therefore, unless soybean extraction is performed with supercritical solvents, only the higher value products such as protein isolates ($2.0-2.50/kg) would probably be able to bear the increased cost of the off-flavor removal.

ACKNOWLEDGEMENTS

The authors thank Cathy Hauck for helping with NSI, GC, sensory, and statistical analysis, and Nancy Morain with the preparation of this manuscript.

This work was supported by grants from Iowa Soybean Promotion Board, Center for Crops Utilization Research, and the Iowa Agriculture and Home Economics Experiment Station.

This is Journal Paper No. J-14564 of the Iowa Agriculture and Home Economics Experiment Station, Projects 2935 and 2164.

REFERENCES

1. F. Temelli, R. Braddock, C.S. Chen, and S. Nagy, in: B.A. Charpentier and M.R. Sevenants (Eds), Supercritical Fluid Extraction and Chromatography, ACS Symposium Series 366, ACS, Washington, DC, 1988, pp.109-126.
2. V.J. Krukonis, in: B.A. Charpentier and M.R. Sevenants (Eds), Supercritical Fluid Extraction and Chromatography, ACS Symposium Series 366, ACS, Washington, DC, 1988, pp. 26-43.
3. M. Zou, S.B. Lim, S.S.H. Rizvi, and J.A. Zollweg, in: K.P. Johnston and J.M.L. Penniger (Eds), Supercritical Fluid Science and Technology. ACS Symposium Series 406, ACS, Washington, DC, 1989, pp. 98-110.
4. J.P. Friedrich, G.R. List, and A.J. Heakin, J. Am. Oil Chem. Soc., 59 (1982) 288.
5. E. Stahl, E. Schütz, and H.K. Mangold, J. Agric. Food. Chem., 28 (1980) 1153.
6. D.D. Christianson, J.P. Friedrich, G.R. List, K. Warner, E.B. Bagley, A.C. Stringfellow, and G.E. Inglett, J. Food Sci., 49 (1984) 229.
7. M. Taniguchi, T. Tsuji, M. Shibata, and T. Kobayashi, Agric. Biol Chem., 49 (1985) 2367.
8. G.R. List, J.P. Friedrich and J. Pominski, J. Am. Oil Chem. Soc., 61 (1984) 847.
9. M. Fattori, N. R. Bulley, and A. Meisen, J. Am. Oil Chem. Soc., 65 (1988) 968.
10. J.T. Polak, M. Balaban, A. Peplow, and A.J. Philips, in: K.P. Johnston and J.M.L. Penniger (Eds), Supercritical Fluid Science and Technology. ACS Symposium Series 406, ACS, Washington D.C., 1989, pp. 449-467.
11. E. Stahl, K.W. Quirin, and H.K. Mangold, Fette Seife Anstrichm., 83 (1981) 472.
12. G.R. List and J.P. Friedrich, J. Am. Oil Chem. Soc., 66 (1989) 98.
13. G.R. List, and J.P. Friedrich, J. Am. Oil Chem. Soc., 62 (1985) 82.
14. W. Eisenbach, Ber. Bunsenges. Phys. Chem., 88 (1984) 882.
15. W.B. Nilsson, E.J. Gauglitz, Jr., and J.K. Hudson., J. Am. Chem. Oil Soc., 63 (1986) 470.
16. W.B. Nilsson, E.J. Gauglitz, Jr., J.K. Hudson., V.F. Stout,and

J. Spinelli, J. Am. Chem. Oil Soc., 65 (1988) 109.
17. S.S.H. Rizvi, R.R. Chao, and Y.J. Liaw, in: B.A. Charpentier and M.R. Sevenants (Eds), Supercritical Fluid Extraction and Chromatography, ACS Symposium Series 366, ACS, Washington, DC, 1988, pp. 89-108.
18. W.B. Nilsson, E.J. Gauglitz, Jr., and J.K. Hudson., J. Am. Chem. Oil Soc., 68 (1991) 87.
19. J. Chrastil, J. Phys. Chem., 86 (1982) 3016.
20. G. Brunner and S. Peter, Chem. Ing. Tech., 53 (1981) 529.
21. T. Bamberger, J.C. Erickson, C.L. Cooney, and S.K. Kumar, J. Chem. Eng. Data, 33 (1988) 327.
22. G. Biernoth and W. Merk, U.S. Patent 4,504,503, (1985).
23. A. Shishikura, K. Fujimoto, T. Kaneda, K. Arai, and S. Saito, Agric. Biol. Chem., 50 (1986) 1209.
24. J. Arul, A. Boudreau, J. Makhlouf, R. Tardif, and M.R. Sahasrabudhe, J. Foos Sci., 52 (1987) 1231.
25. L. Brunetti, A. Daghetta, E. Fedeli, I. Kikic, and L. Zanderighi, J. Am. Oil Chem. Soc., 66 (1989) 209.
26. T.M. White, M.S. Thesis, University of Wisconsin-Madison, Madison, WI, 1990.
27. A. Kramer and G. Thodos, J. Chem. Eng. Data, 34 (1989) 184.
28. J.M. del Valle and J.M. Aguilera, Ind. Eng. Chem. Res., 27 (1988) 1553.
29. A.K. Smith and S.J. Circle, in: A.K. Smith (Ed), Soybeans: Chemistry and Technology, Vol. 1, AVI, Westport, CT, 1978, pp. 339-344.
30. A.C. Eldridge, J.E. Kalbrenner, H.A. Moser, D. Honig, J.J. Rackis, and W.J. Wolf, Cereal Chem. 48 (1971) 640.
31. J.J. Rackis, J.E. McGee, and D. Honig, J. Am. Oil Chem. Soc., 57 (1975) 249.
32. E.C. Baker, G.C. Mustakas, and K.A. Warner, J. Agric. Food Chem., 27 (1979) 971.
33. A.C. Eldridge, J.P. Friedrich, K. Warner, and W.F. Kwolek, J. Food Sci., 51 (1986) 584.
34. Y.V. Wu, J.P. Friedrich, and K. Warner, Cereal Chem., 67 (1990) 585.
35. L.A. Wilson, I.D. Turner, C.A. Pesek, and H.J. Duncan, J. Agric. Food Chem., submitted for publication.
36. Association of Official Analytical Chemists, K. Helrich (Ed.) 15th edition, Vol 2., AOAC, Inc. Arlington, VA, 1990, p. 777.
37. Official and Tentative Methods of the American Oil Chemists' Society, W.E. Link (Ed.), 3rd ed., AOCS, Champaign, IL, 1971.
38. Approved Methods of the American Association of Cereal Chemists, W.C. Schaefer (Ed), AACC, Inc., St. Paul, MN, 1969.
39. R.G.D. Steel and J.H. Torrie, Principles and Properties of Statistics, McGraw-Hill, New York, 1980.
40. E. Larmond, Laboratory methods for sensory evaluation of food, Canadian Government Publishing Center, Ottawa, Canada, 1977.
41. P. Maheshwari, M.S. Thesis, Iowa State University, Ames, IA, 1991.
42. T.E. Daubert and R.P. Danner, Physical and Thermodynamic Properties of Pure Chemicals, Hemisphere, New York, 1989.
43. W.S. Singleton, in: K.S. Markley, (Ed.), Fatty Acids: Their Chemistry, Properties, Production, and Uses, Interscience, New York, 1960, pp.499-511.
44. R.T. Marentis, in: B.A. Charpentier and M.R. Sevenants, (Eds.), Supercritical Fluid Extraction and Chromatography. ACS Symposium Series 366, ACS, Washington DC, 1988, pp. 127-144.
45. S. Peter and G. Brunner, Angew. Chem. Int. Ed. Engl. 17 (1978) 746.
46. S. Angus, B. Armstrong, and K.M. de Reuck, International

Thermodynamic Tables of the Fluid State of Carbon Dioxde, Pergamon, Oxford, U.K., 1976.
47. Wong, J.M. and K.P. Johnston, Biotechnol Progress 2(1):29 (1986).
48. S. Peter, Ber. Bunsenges. Phys. Chem., 88 (1984) 875.
49. J.K.P. Weder, J. Am. Oil Chem. Soc., 61 (1984) 673.
50. J.M. Moses and T.J. Cody, Jr., American Oil Chemist's Society Meeting, May 1984, Dallas, TX.
51. S.F. O'Keefe, A.P. Resurreccion, L.A. Wilson and P.A. Murphy, J. Agric. Food Chem., 39 (1991) in press.

G. Charalambous (Ed.), Food Science and Human Nutrition
© 1992 Elsevier Science Publishers B.V. All rights reserved.

EFFECTS OF GLUCOSE OXIDASE-CATALASE ON THE FLAVOR STABILITY OF MODEL SALAD DRESSINGS

D.B. Min and B.S. Mistry

Department of Food Science and Technology, The Ohio State University, 2121 Fyffe Road, Columbus, OH 43210.

ABSTRACT

The effects of glucose oxidase-catalase on the flavor stabilities of model salad dressings were determined by measuring peroxide values. Further, the effects of pH, temperature and glucose on the activity of glucose oxidase-catalase in model salad dressings were studied by measuring the reduction of dissolved oxygen. As the pH increased from 3, 4, 5, to 6, the amount of dissolved oxygen of the dressing decreased significantly ($\alpha = 0.05$). As the temperature increased from 10, 20 to 30°C, the amount of dissolved oxygen decreased significantly ($\alpha = 0.05$). As the temperature increased from 30, 40 to 50°C, the amount of dissolved oxygen decreased. As the concentration of glucose increased from 0 to 0.5%, the amount of dissolved oxygen decreased significantly ($\alpha = 0.05$). There was no significant difference ($\alpha = 0.05$) in dissolved oxygen reduction among the samples containing 0.5, 1.5, or 2.0% glucose.

As glucose oxidase-catalase increased from 0 to 0.1, 0.2 and 0.3 units/g, the peroxide values decreased significantly ($\alpha = 0.05$). As glucose oxidase-catalase increased from 0.3 to 0.7 units/g, peroxide values increased significantly ($\alpha = 0.05$). In salad dressings containing no glucose, the glucose oxidase-catalase acted as prooxidant; as the enzyme increased from 0 to 0.2 and 0.3 units/g, peroxide values increased ($\alpha = 0.05$).

INTRODUCTION

Salad dressings and mayonnaises are prepared with vegetable oils and soybean oil is the major oil for dressings in the United States. Soybean oil contains a large amount of linoleic and linolenic acids which readily react with the dissolved oxygen in the dressing to produce undesirable volatile compounds (1, 2). List and Erickson (3) and Min and Wen (4) reported that the flavor quality of oils can be improved by eliminating dissolved oxygen in oils. Vacuum packaging and nitrogen blanketing have been partially effective in reducing the oxygen content in foods and improving the oxidative stability of food (5,6). Antioxidants such as BHA, BHT and propyl gallate are also added to the foods containing fats to improve the oxidative stability. Since the reaction of 2 molecules of glucose and 1 molecule of oxygen in the presence of glucose-oxidase-catalase produces 2 molecules of gluconic acid (7), it is possible to eliminate the dissolved oxygen in foods using the enzymes in the presence of glucose before the oxygen reacts with oils to produce undesirable volatile compounds. Information on the application of a biochemical method to effectively reduce the dissolved oxygen in salad dressings is not available.

This paper reports the feasibility of application of the enzyme system, glucose oxidase-catalase, on the improvement of flavor stability of model salad dressings.

MATERIALS AND METHODS

Materials

The materials used for model salad dressings were refined, bleached and deodorized soybean oil from Capital City Products (Columbus, OH), β-D-glucose from Sigma Chemical Co. (St. Louis, MO), xanthan gum from Kelco (San Diego, CA), acetic acid-sodium acetate buffer and citric acid-sodium hydroxide buffer which were prepared according to the method of Gottschalk (8), and glucose oxidase-catalase (23,000 units/g) from Sigma Chemical Co. (St. Louis, MO).

Preparation of the model salad dressing

The model salad dressing consisted of 30% soybean oil (w/v), 1% glucose, 0.35% xanthan gum (w/v) and acetic acid-sodium acetate buffer made to volume. Xanthan gum and soybean oil were initially mixed with a Nuova II stirrer for 30 minutes at room temperature. Simultaneously, glucose was dissolved in acetic acid-sodium acetate buffer at pH 5.0. The solution of glucose in the buffer was slowly added to the suspension of xanthan gum in soybean oil. The mixture was brought to the desired volume with the acetic acid-sodium acetate buffer and vigorously stirred with a Nuova II stirrer for 45 minutes. The macroemulsion was then homogenized at 2,600 psi with a laboratory scale, mechanical, multi-stage valve homogenizer (Foss America, Inc., NY) to obtain the model salad dressing.

A. Effects of pH, temperature and glucose on the activity of glucose oxidase-catalase in model salad dressings

Determination of the depletions of dissolved oxygen

The activity of glucose oxidase-catalase can be determined by measuring the rate of depletion of oxygen (7). The depletion of dissolved oxygen in the salad dressing was measured with a YSI Model 53 Biological Oxygen Analyzer equipped with a Model 5301 Standard Bath Assembly and a YSI 5331 Oxygen Probe which is a specially designed Clark type polarographic electrode (Yellow Springs, OH). The Oxygen Probe was connected to the Model 53 Oxygen Analyzer which provided a polarizing voltage, meter readout, and recorder signal. The Oxygen Analyzer was connected to a Fisher 5000 Recorder. The Oxygen Probe was inserted into the dressing sample bottle and the depletion of dissolved oxygen was determined in duplicate.

Effect of pH on the activity of glucose oxidase-catalase

Salad dressings at pH 2 and 3 were prepared in duplicate using citric acid-sodium hydroxide buffers; and at pH 4, 5 and 6 were prepared in duplicate using acetic acid-sodium acetate buffers. Stock solutions of glucose oxidase-catalase were prepared in pH 2, 3, 4, 5 and 6 buffers. To study the effects of pH on the activity of the enzyme in the model salad dressing during storage, 0.025 units of glucose oxidase-catalase/g of salad dressings were added to 8 g of salad dressing, and the sample was transferred into a 10 ml serum bottle. The bottle was immediately sealed air-tightly with rubber septa and aluminum cap. The control samples containing no glucose oxidase-catalase were also prepared. The effects of pH on the activity of glucose oxidase-catalase were determined by measuring the depletion of dissolved oxygen in the samples every 7 minutes for 42 minutes at 35°C by the Oxygen Analyzer.

Effect of temperature on the activity of glucose oxidase-catalase

Eight grams of the salad dressing at pH 5 containing 0.025 units of glucose oxidase-catalase/g of dressing were transferred into 10 ml serum bottles and the bottles were air-tightly sealed with rubber septa and aluminum caps. Control samples containing no glucose oxidase-catalase were also prepared. All samples were prepared in duplicate. The sample bottles were stored at 10, 20, 30, 40 and 50°C and the effects of temperatures on the enzyme activity were determined by measuring the depletion of dissolved oxygen in the sample bottles every 7 minutes for 42 minutes using the Oxygen Analyzer Probe.

Quantitative effects of glucose on the activity of glucose oxidase-catalase

To determine the quantitative effects of glucose on the activity of glucose oxidase-catalase, model salad dressings containing 0, 0.5, 1.0, 1.5 and 2.0% of glucose were prepared. The activity of the enzyme was determined by measuring the depletion of dissolved oxygen in the salad dressings in duplicate. The dissolved oxygen was measured immediately after the addition of 3 units of glucose oxidase-catalase/g to the salad dressings and every 24 hours for 5 days at 35°C. Graphs of 2.303 log $(C_0)/(C)$ as a function of time (t) for salad dressings containing 0.5, 1.0, 1.5 and 2.0% glucose were plotted, where C_0 = initial concentration of oxygen (uM) and C = concentration of oxygen (uM) at time t (sec). The reaction order was evaluated from the graphs and the apparent rate constants ($k\ sec^{-1}$) were determined from the slopes of the graphs.

B. Effects of glucose oxidase-catalase on the flavor stabilities of model salad dressings

To study the quantitative effects of glucose oxidase-catalase on the flavor stability of salad dressings, model salad dressings containing 0, 0.1, 0.2, 0.3, 0.5 and 0.7 units of glucose oxidase-catalase/g of salad dressings were prepared. The samples (30 g) were weighed into 35 ml serum bottles which were then sealed air-tightly with Teflon-lined rubber septa and aluminum caps. All samples were prepared in duplicate and then stored at 45°C in an incubator under dark for 5 days.

Measurement of flavor stabilities of model salad dressings

To determine the peroxide values of the model salad dressing, the dressings in the serum bottles were frozen for 2 days at -20°C after the storage. The samples were then allowed to thaw in the refrigerator for 24 hrs to break up the salad dressing into separate layers of oil and water. This broken emulsion was then centrifuged using a Sorvall Superspeed RC2-B automatic, refrigerated centrifuge (Ivan Sorvall, Inc., Newton, CT) at 15,000 rpm for 40 min. at -2°C. After centrifugation, 5 ml of the oil which was separated from the salad dressing was pipetted into a 125 ml flask and the peroxide value was determined by the AOCS (9) method. The peroxide values in 5 replicate salad dressings were measured to determine the coefficient of variance for the analytical reproducibility of peroxide determination of salad dressings.

Effects of glucose oxidase-catalase on the emulsion stabilities of model salad dressings

To study the effects of glucose oxidase-catalase on the emulsion stabilities of model salad dressings, salad dressings containing 0, 0.1, 0.2, 0.3, 0.5 and 0.7 units of glucose oxidase-catalase/g were prepared. The emulsion stabilities were determined by freeze-thawing the salad dressings, centrifuging to separate the oil from the emulsion, and measuring the oil recovered.

Effects of glucose oxidase-catalase on the salad dressings containing no glucose

To study the effects of glucose oxidase-catalase on the flavor stabilities of model salad dressings containing no glucose, salad dressings containing 0, 0.1, 0.2 and 0.3 units of glucose oxidase-catalase/g were prepared. The flavor stabilities of the samples were determined in duplicate by measuring peroxide values every 2 days for 10 days.

Statistical Analysis

The depleted oxygen and peroxide values reported in this manuscript are the means of duplicate samples. If the means were significantly different from each other, Tukey's range test was used to determine which samples were different at $\alpha = 0.05$ (10).

RESULTS AND DISCUSSION

A. Effects of pH, temperature and glucose on the activity of glucose oxidase-catalase in model salad dressings

Determination of the dissolved oxygen in the model salad dressing

The dissolved oxygen content in the model salad dressings was 20 ppm. The coefficient of variance for the measurement of dissolved oxygen in 5 replicate salad dressings was 3.0%. The coefficient of variance indicate that the measurement of dissolved oxygen with the YSI Oxygen Analyzer was a good analytical method for the determination of glucose oxidase-catalase activity in salad dressings.

Effect of pH on the glucose oxidase-catalase activity

The effects of pH 2, 3, 4, 5 and 6 on the depletion of dissolved oxygen in model salad dressings containing 0.025 units of glucose oxidase-catalase/g are shown in Figure 1. As the pH increased from 3, to 4, 5, 6, the depletion of dissolved oxygen in salad dressings increased. That is, the activity of glucose oxidase-catalase increased as the pH increased. Tukey's test in Table 1 shows that as the pH of the salad dressings increased from 3, to 4, 5, 6, the depleted dissolved oxygen increased significantly ($\alpha = 0.05$). However, at pH 2 and 3, the depletion of dissolved oxygen in the products was very low, which suggests that enzyme may have been inactivated at pH 2 and 3.

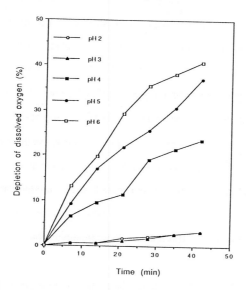

Figure 1. Effects of pH on the depletion of dissolved oxygen in dressings containing 0.025 units of glucose oxidase-catalase/g during storage for 42 minutes at 35°C.

Table 1. Tukey's range test for the effects of pH on the depletion of dissolved oxygen in salad dressings containing 0.025 units of glucose oxidase-catalase/g during storage for 42 minutes at 35°C.

pH	Mean Depleted Oxygen[a] (%)	Tukey's Grouping[b] ($\alpha = 0.05$)
2	1.65	A
3	1.60	A
4	15.23	B
5	22.89	C
6	29.56	D

a: Means of depleted oxygen of samples after 0, 7, 14, 21, 35, and 42 minutes of storage as shown in Figure 1.

b: Means with the same letter are not significantly different at $\alpha = 0.05$.

The amounts of dissolved oxygen in the dressings containing no enzyme at pH 2, 3, 4, 5, and 6 were the same during the storage period of 42 minutes (data not shown). Therefore, the differences in the depleted dissolved oxygen in the salad dressings containing the enzyme at pH 4, 5, and 6 (Figure 1) were due to the presence of glucose oxidase-catalase.

Effect of temperature on the activity of glucose oxidase-catalase

The effects of 10, 20, 30, 40 and 50°C on the activity of 0.025 units of glucose oxidase-catalase/g in the model salad dressings are shown in Figure 2. As the storage temperature increased from 10, to 20, 30°C, the depletion of dissolved oxygen increased. As the temperature increased from 30, to 40, 50°C, the depletion of dissolved oxygen decreased. The decrease in the rate of depletion of dissolved oxygen at 40 and 50°C may be due to the increase in the amount of denatured enzyme (7). The optimum temperature for the activity of glucose oxidase-catalase was 30°C.

Tukey's test show that the mean of depleted dissolved oxygen in the sample stored at 30°C was the highest and was significantly different from the means of depleted dissolved oxygen in samples stored at 10, 20, 40, and 50°C at $\alpha = 0.05$ (Table 2). The model dressings containing no enzyme stored at 10, 20, 30, 40, and 50°C during the short time storage for 42 minutes had practically the same amount of dissolved oxygen. Therefore, the differences in the depleted dissolved oxygen of the salad dressings containing the enzymes at 10, 20, 30, 40, and 50°C (Figure 2) were due to the glucose oxidase-catalase.

Quantitative effects of glucose on the activity of glucose oxidase-catalase

The plot of 2.303 log (C_o: initial concentration of dissolved oxygen) / (C: concentration of dissolved oxygen at time t) versus time (sec) for the salad dressing containing 0.5% glucose and 6 units of glucose oxidase-catalase/g is shown in Figure 3. The plots for the salad dressings containing 1.0, 1.5 and 2.0% glucose were very similar to Figure 3. The linear regression

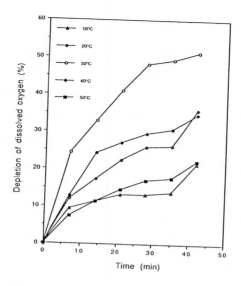

Figure 2. Effects of temperature on the depletion of dissolved oxygen in dressings containing 0.025 units of glucose oxidase-catalase/g during storage for 42 minutes at 35°C.

Table 2. *Tukey's range test for the effects of temperature on the depletion of dissolved oxygen in salad dressings containing 0.025 units of glucose oxidase-catalase/g during storage for 42 minutes.*

Temperature (°C)	Mean Depleted Oxygen[a] (%)	Tukey's Grouping[b] ($\alpha = 0.05$)
10	13.37	A
20	22.99	B
30	40.23	C
40	27.72	B
50	15.95	A

a: Means of depleted oxygen of samples after 0, 7, 14, 21, 28, 35, and 42 minutes of storage as shown in Figure 2.

b: Means with the same letter are not significantly different at $\alpha = 0.05$.

equations and the correlation coefficients for the depletion of dissolved oxygen in salad dressings containing 0.5, 1.0, 1.5 and 2.0% glucose were y = -0.082 + 0.026 x (r^2 = 0.99), y = -0.045 + 0.024x (r^2 = 0.99), y = -0.070 + 0.025x (r^2 = 0.99) and y = -0.064 + 0.020x (r^2 = 0.99), respectively; where y = the concentration of dissolved oxygen (uM) and x = time t (sec). The high correlation coefficients of the linear regression lines indicate that the depletion of dissolved oxygen in the salad dressings containing 0.5, 1.0, 1.5 or 2.0% glucose was a first order reaction.

The slopes of the regression lines (k sec^{-1}) for salad dressings containing 0.5, 1.0, 1.5 and 2.0% glucose were 0.026, 0.024, 0.025 and 0.020 sec^{-1}, respectively. The similar slopes of the regression lines indicate that the apparent rate constant (k sec^{-1}) for the depletion of dissolved oxygen in samples containing 0.5, 1.0, 1.5, or 2.0% glucose did not change.

The reaction catalyzed by glucose oxidase-catalase is a second order reaction (7). However, for commercial purposes such as desugaring of eggs to prevent Millard reaction, hydrogen peroxide is added to supply excess oxygen so that the removal of glucose by glucose oxidase-catalase is an apparent first order reaction or pseudo first order reaction (11, 12).

The effects of 0, 0.5, 1.0, 1.5 and 2.0% glucose on the depletion of dissolved oxygen in salad dressings containing 3 units of glucose oxidase-catalase/g during 5 days storage at 35°C are shown in Figure 4. The depleted dissolved oxygen in the control samples containing 0% glucose after 1 day and 5 days of storage was 4% and 22%, respectively. However, the depleted dissolved oxygen in the samples containing 0.5, 1.0, 1.5 and 2.0% glucose after 1 day and 5 days of storage was approximately 87% and 92%, respectively. After 30 days of storage, 97% of dissolved oxygen was depleted in the products containing 0.5, 1.0, 1.5 or 2.0% glucose, whereas only 25% of the dissolved oxygen was depleted in the sample containing no glucose (data not shown).

Tukey's range test shows that the depletion of dissolved oxygen in salad dressings containing no glucose was lowest and significantly different from the salad dressings containing 0.5, 1.0, 1.5 or 2.0% glucose at α = 0.05 (Table 3). The dissolved oxygen depletion among the samples containing 0.5 to 2.0% glucose was not significantly different at $\alpha = 0.05$.

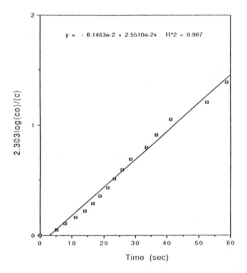

Figure 3. Determination of apparent rate constant (k sec-1) for the depletion of dissolved oxygen in the presence of 6 units of glucose oxidase-catalase/g of salad dressing containing 0.5% glucose.

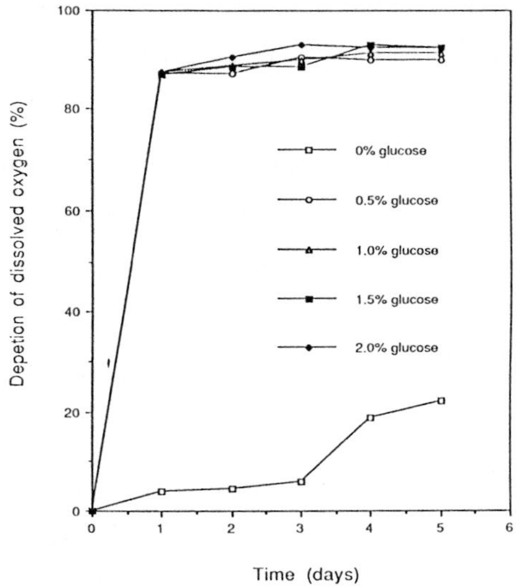

Figure 4. Effects of 0, 0.5, 1.0, 1.5 and 2.0% glucose on the depletion of dissolved oxygen in salad dressings containing 3 units of glucose oxidase-catalase/g during storage for 5 days at 35°C.

Table 3. Tukey's range test for the effects of 0, 0.5, 1.0, 1.5 and 2.0% glucose on the depletion of dissolved oxygen in salad dressings containing 3 units of glucose oxidase-catalase/g during storage for 5 days at 35°C.

Glucose (%)	Mean Depleted Oxygen[a] (%)	Tukey's Grouping[b] ($\alpha = 0.05$)
0	11.02	A
0.5	89.00	B
1.0	89.78	B
1.5	89.86	B
2.0	91.10	B

a: Means of depleted oxygen of samples after 0, 1, 2, 3, 4, and 5 days of storage as shown in Figure 4.

b: Means with the same letter are not significantly different at $\alpha = 0.05$.

The results show that glucose oxidase-catalase effectively reduced dissolved oxygen in salad dressings. Glucose oxidase-catalase showed maximum activity at pH 6 and at 30°C in the salad dressings. Glucose at 0.5% levels was sufficient to remove 92% of dissolved oxygen in the salad dressing in 5 days of storage.

B. Effects of glucose oxidase-catalase on the flavor stabilities of model salad dressings

Measurements of flavor stabilities of model salad dressings

The coefficient of variance for the measurements of peroxide values in 5 replicate salad dressings was 2.0%. The coefficient of variance indicates that the peroxide value analysis of the dressing was good in reproducibility.

Effects of glucose oxidase-catalase on the flavor stabilities of model salad dressings

The peroxide values of the salad dressings containing 0, 0.1, 0.2, 0.3, 0.5 and 0.7 units of glucose oxidase-catalase/g are shown in Table 4. As the level of enzyme in the salad dressing increased from 0 to 0.1 units, the peroxide value decreased by 14%. Tukey's test shows that there was a significant difference in peroxide values between the control dressing containing no enzyme and the salad dressing containing 0.1, 0.2, or 0.3 units of enzyme at $\alpha = 0.05$ (Table 4). When the concentration of the enzyme increased from 0.3 to 0.5 and 0.7 units, the peroxide values of the salad dressings increased significantly ($\alpha = 0.05$). The enzyme acted as prooxidant above 0.5 units/g.

Effects of glucose oxidase-catalase on the emulsion stabilities of model salad dressings

When the salad dressings containing 0, 0.1, 0.2, 0.3, 0.5 or 0.7 units of glucose oxidase-catalase were freeze-thawed to recover the oil for peroxide value determination, the oil recoveries in the products containing 0.2, and 0.3 units of the enzyme/g were approximately 55% after 5 days of storage. However, the oil recoveries in products containing 0.5 and 0.7 units of enzyme/g

Table 4. Tukey's range test for the effects of 0, 0.1, 0.2, 0.3, 0.5 and 0.7 units of glucose oxidase-catalase/g on the peroxide values in salad dressings during storage for 5 days at 45°C.

Enzyme unit/g	Peroxide Values						
	Day 0	Day 1	Day 2	Day 3	Day 4	Day 5	Mean*
0	0.8	1.85	3.01	3.25	3.52	3.70	3.07^a
0.1	0.8	1.59	2.60	2.80	3.03	3.19	2.64^b
0.2	0.8	1.35	2.90	2.99	3.01	3.61	2.64^b
0.3	0.8	1.30	2.40	2.62	2.81	3.39	2.51^b
0.3	0.8	1.30	2.40	2.62	2.81	3.39	2.5^a
0.5	0.8	2.76	10.27	12.24	13.58	16.91	11.25^b
0.7	0.8	5.61	17.38	24.38	27.00	30.91	21.06^c

*Means of peroxide values are the average of peroxide values after 0, 1, 2, 3, 4 and 5 days of storage. Means with the different letters in the group containing 0, 0.1, 0.2, and 0.3 units/g and in the group containing 0.3, 0.5 and 0.7 units/g are significantly different at $\alpha = 0.05$.

were only 11 and 5%, respectively, after 5 days of storage. Therefore, the emulsion stability of the product increased as the concentration of the enzyme in the salad dressing increased. The decreases in oil recoveries in products containing 0.5 and 0.7 units of the enzyme/g indicate that glucose oxidase-catalase was acting as an emulsifying agent in the salad dressing. Mistry and Min (13, 14) and Yoon and Min (15) reported that emulsifiers such as monoglycerides, diglycerides and phopholipids acted as prooxidants in oils.

Effects of glucose oxidase-catalase on the salad dressings containing no glucose

To verify the prooxidant property of glucose oxidase-catalase in model salad dressing containing no glucose, 0.1, 0.2 and 0.3 units of glucose oxidase-catalase/g were added to the dressing. In the dressing containing no glucose, glucose oxidase-catalase would not exhibit enzymatic activity to reduce the dissolved oxygen, it would only act as an emulsifier. As the concentration of glucose oxidase-catalase in salad dressings containing no glucose increased from 0 to 0.1, 0.2, and 0.3 units, the peroxide values increased. The peroxide values of salad

Table 5. Tukey's range test for the effects of 0, 0.1, 0.2 and 0.3 units of glucose oxidase-catalase/g on the peroxide values in salad dressings containing 0% glucose during storage for 10 days at 45°C.

Enzyme (units/g)	Means of Peroxide Values*	Tukey's Grouping** ($\alpha = 0.05$)
0	9.75	A
0.1	10.52	A
0.2	12.55	B
0.3	13.70	C

* Means of peroxide values are the average of peroxide values after 0, 2, 4, 6, 8, and 10 days of storage.
** Means with the same letter are not significantly different at $\alpha = 0.05$.

dressings containing 0.2 and 0.3 units of glucose oxidase-catalase were significantly higher than the control at $\alpha = 0.05$ (Table 5). The results indicate that 0.2 and 0.3 units of the enzyme/g acted as prooxidants in model salad dressings containing no glucose.

The prooxidant activity of glucose oxidase-catalase in salad dressings containing no glucose may be due to its emulsifying properties. Mistry and Min (13, 14) and Yoon and Min (15) reported that emulsifying agents such as mono- and di-glycerides, fatty acids and phospholipids acted as prooxidants at certain concentrations in soybean oil. The prooxidant activity of glucose oxidase-catalase may be partly due to the presence of the catalase which is hemoprotein. This hemoprotein would then become an efficient heme catalyst for the oxidation of fatty acids of soybean oil in the salad dressings; thereby decreasing the oxidative stabilities of these salad dressings. Tappel (16) and Eriksson et al (17) showed that the hemoproteins such as catalase and peroxidase, increased linoleic acid oxidation. Tappel (16) postulated that hematin compounds initiate a chain reaction by causing breakdown of linoleate peroxides into 2 free radicals. Eriksson et al (17) suggested that there was an increased unfolding of the hemoprotein causing a greater exposure of the heme groups to linoleic acid.

REFERENCES

(1) S. Fore, M. Legendre and G. Fisher. J. Am. Oil Chem. Soc., 55 (1978), 482.

(2) D. Min and D. Ticknor. J. Am. Oil Chem. Soc. 59 (1982), 226.

(3) G. List and D. Erickson. Handbook of Soy Oil Processing and Utilization. D. Erickson (Ed.)., Am. Oil Chem. Soc., Champaign, IL, 1980.

(4) D. Min and J. Wen. J. Food Sci. 48 (1983), 1429.

(5) L. Aho and O. Wahlroos. J. Am. Oil Chem. Soc., 44 (1967), 65.

(6) D. Min, S. Lee, J. Lindamood, K. Chang and G. Reineccius. J. Food Sci. 54 (1990), 1222.

(7) J. Whitaker. Principles of Enzymology for the Food Sciences. Marcel Dekker, Inc., NY, 1972.

(8) D. Gottschalk. Buffers for pH and Metal Ion Control. D. Perrin and B. Dempsey (Ed)., Halstead Press, NY, 1961.

(9) AOCS. Official and Tentative methods. 3rd Ed. Am. Oil Chem. Soc., Champaign, IL, 1980.

(10) SAS. SAS User's Guide, SAS Institute, Inc., Cary, N.C, 1985.

(11) R. Baldwin, H. Campbell, R. Thiessen and G. Lorant. Food Tech., 7 (1953), 275.

(12) C. Zapsalis and R. Black. Food Chemistry and Nutritional Biochemistry. John Wiley & Sons, 1986.

(13) B. Mistry and D. Min. J. Food Sci. 52 (1987), 786.

(14) B. Mistry and D. Min. J. Food Sci. 53 (1988), 1896.

(15) S. Yoon and D. Min. Korean J. Food Sci. and Tech., 19 (1987), 23.

(16) A. Tappel. Arch. Biochem. Biophys., 44 (1953), 378.

(17) G. Eriksson, P. Olsson and S. Svensson. Lipids, 5 (1970), 365.

G. Charalambous (Ed.), Food Science and Human Nutrition
© 1992 Elsevier Science Publishers B.V. All rights reserved.

FATTY ACID COMPOSITION OF THE TOTAL, NEUTRAL AND PHOSPHOLIPIDS OF THE BRAZILIAN FRESHWATER FISH *COLOSSOMA MACROPOMUM*

Everardo Lima Maia and Delia B. Rodriguez-Amaya

Departamento de Ciência de Alimentos, Faculdade de Engenharia de Alimentos, Universidade Estadual de Campinas, C.P. 6121, 13081 Campinas, SP., Brasil.

SUMMARY

Pond-raised *Colossoma macropomum* fillets were analyzed in terms of the lipid content and fatty acid composition. The total lipids (6.0±0.9%) consist of 90.7% of neutral lipids and 8.7% phospholipids. Of 41 fatty acids identified by GC-MS in the total lipid fraction, the principal components are: 18:1ω9 (40.1±1.2%), 16:0 (28.8±1.2%), 18:0 (9.8±0.4%), 18:2ω6 (8.9±0.3%) and 16:1ω7 (6.3±0.1%). The saturated monoenoic, dienoic and polyunsaturated fatty acids account for 40.2, 47.5, 8.9 and 2.5%, respectively. The ratio of ω3 to ω6 PUFA is very low (0.1), with only 0.1 and 0.8%, respectively, of 20:5ω3 and 22:6ω3. A modification of the diet appears necessary. The neutral lipid fraction reflected the total fatty acid composition. The phospholipids contain higher levels of PUFA, the major fatty acids being 16:0 (18.6±0.3%), 18:1ω9 (17.9±2.9%), 18:0 (10.7±1.1%), 22:6ω3 (10.6±1.7%), 18:2ω6 (9.9±0.6%). Aside from 22:6ω6, 20:4ω6, 22:5ω6, and 20:3ω6, all below 1% in the total and neutral lipids, reach 9.1, 3.9 and 3.4, respectively.

1. INTRODUCTION

Although South America has the richest ichtofaunal diversity among the continents and various native fish species have excellent potential for aquaculture, developments to date have been slow and aquaculture production has rarely progressed beyond the pilot stage (1). In recent years, however, renewed attention and significantly greater interest has been directed towards culturing indigenous fish species. Studies on the lipid chemistry of these species should contribute substantially to improvement in aquaculture, leading to the production of fishes of high quality and optimum lipid composition for human nutrition and health.

Since the polyunsaturated fatty acids (PUFA) of the ω3 family have been associated with the prevention of cardiovascular disease, extensive investigation has been conducted to determine the fatty acid composition of fish and fish oils. The total lipid content and fatty acid composition of fish have been shown to vary with different species or within a species as a function of diet, temperature or seasonal influence, development stage, sex, etc.

In Brazil, the beneficial effects of ω3 PUFA have also been divulged, but information on the fatty acids of Brazilian fishes is lacking. Only two reports were encountered in the literature, in both of which packed columns were used. Castelo et al. (2) and Maia et al. (3) determined the fatty acid composition of the total lipids of *Colossoma macropomum* from the Amazon and *Prochilodus scrofa* from São Paulo state, respectively.

Although fish consumption in the other areas of Brazil has been based principally on marine species, the Amazonian region relies on freshwater fishes from the rivers. Well appreciated for its meat-like flavor, *Colossoma macropomum* Cuvier 1818 is captured in large quantities and is considered of major economic importance. It is popularly known as "tambaqui" in Brazil, "cachama" in Venezuela, "gamitama" in Peru and "cachama negra" in Colombia (1). It has great potential for aquaculture because of its adaptability to different diets, excellent growth rates, tolerance to low oxygen conditions, facility of capture. Their reproduction in tanks has been studied. Production of this fish in other parts of Brazil is therefore viable. The present paper deals with the lipid class contents of *C. macropomum* and the corresponding fatty acid composition.

2. MATERIALS AND METHODS

2.1. Samples

The fish were reared in a pond, measuring 8 m in width, 20 m in lenght and 1.5 m in depth, at the Centro de Pesquisa e Treinamento em Aquicultura (CEPTA), Pirassununga, São Paulo. After reaching the adult stage, the fish were fed with a maintenance diet consisting of 10% fish flour, 33% soybean meal, 17% wheat meal, 38% corn, 1% each of vitamin and mineral premix, 50 g choline chloride, 50 g vitamin C and 0.8 g Gentian Violet. Three sample lots were collected in March, April and May 1990. The water temperature (^{o}C) during this period was: March, 25.8±0.9 (n=8); April, 23.0±2.9 (n=10); May, 17.5±1.8 (n=11).

Each sample lot consisted of 6 fish. The fish were captured in the morning and first placed in pails containing water at ambient temperature before being iced to diminish activity. The iced fish were immediately transported to the Food Analysis Laboratory in Campinas where they were eviscerated, skinned, filleted and homogenenized in a food grinder. Analyses were initiated on the same day. All analyses for each lot were completed within a week, the sample being kept at $-20^{o}C$.

2.2. Moisture and Lipid Determination

Moisture content was determined by the method of Umemoto (4) and the total lipids by the method of Bligh and Dyer (5).

The lipids extracted according to Bligh and Dyer were fractionated in a silica gel column, 30 cm × 2 cm i.d. glass column wet packed with 25 g silica gel (70-230 mesh) in chloroform up to a height of about 11 cm, a 1 cm layer of sodium sulfate being added to the top. The adsorbent was previously washed with methanol and then with chloroform to remove interfering impurities. After addition of each solvent, the mixture was agitated with a magnetic stirrer for an hour. The washed adsorbent was then allowed to dry in a vacuum dessicator.

An accurately weighed aliquot of the lipid extract was applied on the column; the neutral lipids were eluted with 200 mL of 20% acetone in chloroform and the phospholipids by 200 mL of methanol. This elution pattern was established by preliminary tests. The fractions collected from the column were monitored by TLC on silica, using iodine as general spray reagent, molybdenum blue for phospholipids and anthrone-sulfuric acid and phenol-sulfuric acid for glycolipids. The developing solvents were petroleum ether:ethyl ether:acetic acid (100:30:1) for neutral lipids and chloroform:methanol:H_2O (65:25:4) for the phospholipids (6). The neutral and phospholipid contents were determined gravimetrically and expressed as percentages of the total lipids.

2.3. Fatty Acid Determination

The total lipid, neutral lipid and phospholipid fractions were saponified and methylated according to the procedure of Metcalfe et al. (7) except that the methylating reagent BF_3-methanol was substituted with NH_4Cl-H_2SO_4-MeOH as suggested by Hartman and Lago (8). The modified method was shown to be equivalent to that of Metcalfe et al. (9).

Gas chromatography was conducted on a Varian model 3300 gas chromatograph with a flame ionization detector and fused silica capillary columns (50 m × 0.2 mm i.d.) (WCOT, SGE, USA) of Carbowax 20M and SE-54. The operating conditions for the Carbowax 20M column were: detector temperature, $280^{o}C$; injection port temperature, 250°C; split injection at 100:1 ratio; column temperature, 200°C for 42 min, programmed at 2°C/min up to 210°C with a final hold time of 25 min; carrier gas, hydrogen at 0.8 mL/min; make-up gas, nitrogen at 30 mL/min. For the SE-54 column, the conditions were: detector temperature, 280°C; injection port temperature, 250°C; Grob type splitless injection, with hexane as solvent and splitless period of 0.75 min; column temperature, 50°C for 6 min, programmed at 40°C/min up to 170°C, then at 2°C/min up to 230°C; carrier gas, hydrogen at 0.8 mL/min; make-up gas, nitrogen at 30 mL/min. Retention times and peak area percentages were computed automatically by a computing integrator Varian 4290. Quantitation was accomplished with the Carbowax 20M column and the results were submitted to multiple comparison by the Tukey's test at 5% level.

Conclusive identification of the fatty acids was achieved by a combination of several parameters: (1) comparison of retention times and spiking with standard methyl esters; (2) separation factors (10); (3) equivalent chain lenght values (ECL) (11-14); (4) semilogarithmic plots of retention times or ECL values versus number of carbons; (5) order of elution on the SE-54 and Carbowax 20M columns; (6) mass spectra obtained with a gas chromatograph-mass spectrometer Shimadzu QP 2000A (electron impact, ionization voltage at 70eV). Thirty-eight individual fatty acid standards (Sigma and Polyscience, USA) were utilized, along with PUFA-1 and PUFA-2 of Supelco (USA) and cod liver oil from Sigma (USA) as secondary standards.

3. RESULTS AND DISCUSSION

The *Colossoma macropomum* fillets (three sample lots, equivalent to 18 fish ranging in weight from 600 to 1115g) presented an average of 74.2% (73.1 - 75.5%) moisture and 6.0% (4.9 - 6.8%) total lipids (Table 1).Of the latter, 90.7% (88.7 - 92.0%) were neutral lipids and 8.7% (7.5 - 10.1%) were phospholipids. An attempt was made to separate and quantity glycolipids but they were not detected.

The complexity of the composition required the concerted use of several parameters to confirm the identity of the fatty acids. In most papers in the literature, the identification is based solely on comparison of the retention times with those of standards, sometimes complemented by semi-log graphs. Since this

TABLE 1

Moisture and lipid contents of *Colossoma macropomum* fillets.

Catch date	Weight/fish (g)	Moisture[a] (%)	lipid (%)		
			Total	Neutral lipids[b]	Phospholipids[b]
4/1990	905±130	73.1±1.6	6.3±0.1	91.3±0.6	8.3±0.4
5/1990	894±102	74.0±0.3	6.8±0.0	92.0±0.3	7.5±0.1
6/1990	861±176	75.5±0.2	4.9±0.2	88.7±0.6	10.1±0.6
general means ± SD	887±132	74.2±1.3	6.0±0.9	90.7±1.6	8.7±1.2

[a]Means and standard deviations of triplicate analyses for moisture and duplicate analyses for lipids. Each sample lot consisted of 6 fish.
[b]Percentage of the total lipid content.
SD = standard deviation.

is the first detailed characterization of the lipids of a Brazilian fish, rigorous identification of the fatty acids was undertaken, various chromatographic criteria being used along with the mass spectra (15-19). Also, a large number of fatty acid standards and secondary standards were utilized.

Of the 41 fatty acids found in the total lipid fraction of *C. macropomum*, the principal were 18:1ω9 (40.1±1.2%), 16:0 (28.8±1.2%), 18:0 (9.8±0.4%), 18:2ω6 (8.9±0.3%) and 16:1ω7 (6.3±0.1%) (Table 2). In general, the fatty acid profile fits into the typical pattern for freshwater fish where 18:1ω9 is usually the major constituent (20). Saturated fatty acids, which can range from 9% to 36% of the total lipid fatty acids of temperate freshwater fish (21, 22), tend to be slightly higher and can reach 45% in tropical fishes (21, 23). The saturated fatty acid content of *C. macropomum* came up to 40.2%. The monoenes, dienes and PUFA accounted for 47.5, 8.9 and 2.5%, respectively. The ratio of ω3 to ω6 PUFA, however, was only 0.1, lower than the 0.5-3.8 range found for freshwater fishes. The range for marine fishes is 4.7 to 14.4 (20).

The pond-raised *C. macropomum* analyzed in this study presented 0.1 and 0.8%, respectively, of 20:5ω3 and 22:6ω3, the two PUFA considered to be of major importance in terms of human health. The fatty acid composition of the diet was also determined and found to be: 12:0 (tr); 13:0 (tr), 14:0 (1.4 ±0.1%), 14:1ω5 (tr), i-15:0 (tr), 15:0 (0.3±0.0%), 15:1ω9 (tr), i-16: (tr), 16:0

TABLE 2

Fatty acid composition (%) of the total lipids of *Colossoma macropomum* fillets.

Fatty acid	April[a]	May[a]	June[a]	General means ± SD
12:0	tr	tr	tr	tr
14:0	1.5a	1.4a	1.1b	1.3 ± 0.2
14:1ω5	0.1a	tra	0.1a	0.1 ± 0.1
15:0	0.1a	0.1a	0.1a	0.1 ± 0.0
15:1ω9	tr	tr	tr	tr
i-16:0	tr	nd	tr	tr
16:0DMA	0.3a	0.2b	0.3a	0.3 ± 0.1
15:2ω5	0.1	nd	nd	tr
16:0	29.1a	29.8a	27.4a	28.8 ± 1.2
16:1ω7	6.3a	6.4a	6.3a	6.3 ± 0.1
i-17:0	tr	tr	tr	tr
ai-17:0	0.1a	tra	0.1a	0.1 ± 0.1
16:2ω5	tr	nd	nd	nd
17:0	0.2a	0.2a	0.1a	0.2 ± 0.1
17:1ω9	0.1a	0.2a	0.1a	0.1 ± 0.1
16:3ω3	tr	tr	tr	tr
18:0DMA	tr	tr	0.1	tr
18:1DMA	0.1a	tra	0.1a	0.1 ± 0.1
18:0	10.3a	9.8a	9.4a	9.8 ± 0.4
18:1ω9	38.8b	41.2a	40.2ab	40.1 ± 1.2
18:1ω5	0.1	tr	tr	tr
18:1ω3	tr	nd	tr	tr
18:2ω6	8.7a	9.2a	8.7a	8.9 ± 0.3
18:3ω6	0.1a	tra	0.1a	0.1 ± 0.1
19:0	tr	tr	tr	tr
18:3ω3	0.6a	0.5b	0.5b	0.5 ± 0.1
18:4ω3	0.1a	tra	0.1a	0.1 ± 0.1
20:0	0.1a	tra	0.1a	0.1 ± 0.1
20:1ω9	1.1a	1.0a	1.0a	1.0 ± 0.1
20:2ω9	0.1a	tra	0.1a	0.1 ± 0.1
20:2ω6 + 20:3ω9	0.5a	0.5a	0.5a	0.5 ± 0.0
20:2ω3	tr	nd	tr	tr
20:3ω6	0.5a	0.5a	0.5a	0.5 ± 0.0
20:4ω6	0.6a	0.6a	0.8a	0.7 ± 0.1
20:3ω3	tr	nd	tr	tr
20:4ω3	tr	nd	tr	tr
20:5ω3	0.2a	trb	0.1b	0.1 ± 0.1
22:0	nd	tr	tr	tr
22:4ω6	0.1	tr	tr	tr
22:3ω3	0.3	nd	nd	0.1 ± 0.2
22:5ω6	0.3a	trb	0.3a	0.2 ± 0.2
22:5ω3	0.1	tr	tr	tr
22:6ω3	0.9a	0.6b	0.9a	0.8 ± 0.2

[a]Means of duplicate analyses. Each sample lot consisted of 6 fish. Values in the same horizontal line not showing the same postscript are significantly different (P≤0.05).
tr = trace; nd = not detected; SD = standard deviation; DMA = dimethyl acetal; i = iso; ai = anteiso.

(19.0±0.8%), 16:1ω7 (1.6±0.0%), 16:2ω4 (0.1±0.0%), 17:0 (0.3±0.0%), 17:1ω9 (0.1±0.0%), 16:3ω3 (tr), 17:2ω5 (tr), 18:0 (2.9±0.1%), 18:1ω9 (25.0±0.2%), 18:2ω6 (44.8±0.1%), 18:3ω6 (0.1±0.0%), 18:3ω3 (2.6±0.0%), 18:4ω3 (tr), 20:0 (0.3±0.1%), 20:1ω9 (0.4±0.0%), 20:2ω6 + 20:3ω9 (tr), 20:4ω6 (tr), 20:5ω3 (0.1±0.1%), 22:0 (0.3±0.1%), 22:6ω3 (0.4±0.2%), 24:1ω9 (tr). Thus, although rich in fatty acids of the ω6 series, the feed was poor in ω3 fatty acids. A modification of the diet appears to be necessary to correct this deficiency.

Using a column packed with 17% PEGS in chromosorb W, Castelo et al. (2) identified 22 fatty acids in a sample of C. macropomum from the Amazon, of which the major constituents were: 18:1ω9 (43.8%), 16:0 (19.0%), 18:0 (15.0%), 18:2ω6 (12.6%) and 16:1ω7 (4.4%). Thus, in terms of the principal fatty acids, the data are coherent with the present results.

Since the neutral lipids comprised 90.7% of the total lipids, this fraction as expected reflected the total lipid composition, the major fatty acids being 18:1ω9 (40.9±0.8%), 16:0 (28.5±0.6%), 18:0 (10.2±0.7%), 18:2ω6 (8.6±0.1%), and 16:1ω7 (6.6±0.4%) (Table 3).

The composition of the phospholipids was markedly different, with a pronounced increase in the proportion of the PUFA (Table 4). There was a substantial lowering of 18:1ω9 (17.9±2.9%), making 16:0 (18.6±0.3%) the major fatty acid although it also decreased in relation to the total and neutral lipids. The 18:0 level (10.7±1.1%) was maintained while 18:2ω6 (9.9±0.6%) increased slightly. The fatty acids 22:6ω3, 20:4ω6, 22:5ω6 and 20:3ω6, all below 1% in the total and neutral lipids, reached 10.6, 9.1, 3.9 and 3.4%, respectively. The total monoenoic fatty acid content was only 21.5 while the PUFA level came up to 29.2%, equalling the saturated fatty acid percentage (29.7%). The higher proportion of PUFA in the phospholipid fraction has been reported in marine species (24-26) and in freshwater fishes (27-30).

Some statistically significant differences were seen between the three sample lots in the fatty acid composition of the total, neutral and phospholipids. However, the standard deviations were quite small.

TABLE 3

Fatty acid composition (%) of the neutral lipids of *Colossoma macropomum* fillets.

Fatty acid	April[a]	May[a]	June[a]	General means ± SD
12:0	tr	tr	tr	tr
13:0	tr	tr	tr	tr
i-14:0	tr	tr	tr	tr
14:0	1.4a	1.2a	1.2a	1.3 ± 0.1
14:1ω5	0.1a	0.1a	0.1a	0.1 ± 0.0
i-15:0	tr	tr	tr	tr
ai-15:0	tr	tr	tr	tr
15:0	0.1a	0.1a	0.1a	0.1 ± 0.0
16:0	27.9a	28.5a	29.2	28.5 ± 0.6
16:1ω7	6.2b	6.6ab	7.1a	6.6 ± 0.4
i-17:0	tr	tr	tr	tr
ai-17:0	0.1a	0.1a	tra	0.1 ± 0.1
16:2ω5	tr	nd	tr	tr
17:0	0.2a	0.2a	0.1b	0.2 ± 0.1
17:1ω9	0.1a	0.1a	0.1a	0.1 ± 0.0
16:3ω3	tr	tr	tr	tr
18:0	11.0a	9.9b	9.8b	10.2 ± 0.7
18:1ω9	40.4a	41.8a	40.5a	40.9 ± 0.8
18:1ω5	0.1	tr	tr	tr
18:1ω4	tr	tr	tr	tr
18:1ω3	tr	tr	tr	tr
18:2ω6	8.6a	8.7a	8.6a	8.6 ± 0.1
18:3ω6	0.1a	0.1a	0.1a	0.1 ± 0.0
19:0	tr	tr	tr	tr
19:1ω9	tr	tr	tr	tr
18:3ω3	0.6a	0.4b	0.5ab	0.5 ± 0.1
18:4ω3	0.1a	0.1a	0.1a	0.1 ± 0.0
20:0	0.1a	0.1a	0.1a	0.1 ± 0.0
20:1ω9	1.4a	1.1a	1.1a	1.2 ± 0.2
20:1ω7	tr	tr	tr	tr
20:2ω9	0.1a	0.1a	0.1a	0.1 ± 0.0
20:2ω6				
20:3ω9	0.5a	0.4a	0.4a	0.4 ± 0.1
20:3ω6	0.4a	0.3a	0.3a	0.3 ± 0.1
20:4ω6	0.2a	0.2a	0.2a	0.2 ± 0.0
20:3ω3	tr	tr	tr	tr
20:4ω3	tr	tr	tr	tr
20:5ω3	tr	tr	tr	tr
22:1ω11	0.1	tr	tr	tr
22:4ω6	tr	tr	tr	tr
22:5ω6	0.1	tr	tr	tr
22:5ω3	tr	tr	tr	tr
22:6ω3	0.3a	0.1b	0.1b	0.2 ± 0.1

[a]Means of duplicate analyses. Each sample lot consisted of 6 fish. Values in the same horizontal line not showing the same postscript are significantly different (P≤0.05).
tr = trace; nd = not detected; SD = standard deviation; DMA = dimethyl acetal; i = iso; ai = anteiso.

TABLE 4

Fatty acid composition (%) of the phospholipids of *Colossoma macropomum* fillets.

Fatty acid	April[a]	May[a]	June[a]	General means ± SD
14:0DMA	nd	tr	tr	tr
14:0	0.4a	0.3b	0.2c	0.3 ± 0.1
15:0	tr	tr	tr	tr
15:1ω7	0.7b	1.1a	0.9ab	0.9 ± 0.2
16:0DMA	5.6ab	5.3b	6.1a	5.7 ± 0.4
16:0	18.9a	18.6a	18.3a	18.6 ± 0.3
16:1ω7	2.2a	2.0ab	1.6b	1.9 ± 0.3
i-17:0	nd	tr	tr	tr
ai-17:0	tr	tr	tr	tr
17:0	0.3a	0.1b	trc	0.1 ± 0.1
17:1ω9	trc	0.3a	0.2b	0.2 ± 0.1
16:3ω3	tra	0.1a	0.1a	0.1 ± 0.1
18:0DMA	1.2a	1.2a	1.3a	1.2 ± 0.1
18:1DMA	1.0a	1.0a	1.0a	1.0 ± 0.0
18:0	12.0a	10.3b	9.8a	10.7 ± 1.1
18:1ω9	20.0a	19.0a	14.6b	17.9 ± 2.9
18:2ω6	9.9b	10.6a	9.3c	9.9 ± 0.6
18:3ω6	nd	tr	tr	tr
18:3ω3	tr	0.2	tr	0.1 ± 0.1
20:1ω9	1.0a	0.8b	0.6c	0.8 ± 0.2
20:1ω7	nd	tr	tr	tr
20:2ω9	nd	tr	tr	tr
20:2ω6 + 20:3ω9	1.9a	1.9a	1.9a	1.9 ± 0.0
20:2ω3	tr	tr	tr	tr
20:3ω6	3.2a	3.6a	3.5a	3.4 ± 0.2
20:4ω6	8.1b	9.1a	10.0a	9.1 ± 0.9
20:3ω3	nd	tr	nd	nd
20:4ω3	nd	tr	tr	tr
20:5ω3	1.5a	1.2a	1.3a	1.3 ± 0.1
22:4ω6	0.8a	1.0a	1.0a	0.9 ± 0.1
22:5ω6	2.9c	3.8b	4.9a	3.9 ± 1.0
22:5ω3	trb	0.9a	0.9a	0.6 ± 0.5
22:6ω3	9.5b	9.7b	12.5a	10.6 ± 1.7

[a]Means of duplicate analyses. Each sample lot consisted of 6 fish. Values in the same horizontal line not showing the same postscript are significantly different (P≤0.05).
tr = trace; nd = not detected; SD = standard deviation; DMA = dimethyl acetal; i = iso; ai = anteiso.

ACNOWLEDGMENT

The authors wish to thank the Fundação de Amparo à Pesquisa do Estado de São Paulo (FAPESP) for the financial support, the Centro de Pesquisa e Treinamento em Aquicultura (CEPTA) for furnishing the fish samples, the Instrumentos Científicos CG Ltda for putting at our disposition the GC-MS unit and Luiz K. Hotta for the statistical analysis.

REFERENCE
1. U. Saint-Paul, Infofish Int., March/April (1991) 49-53.
2. F.P. Castelo, D. Rodriguez-Amaya and F.C. Strong III, Acta Amazonica, 10 (1980) 557-576.
3. E.L. Maia, D.B. Rodriguez-Amaya and J. Amaya-Farfán, J. Food Chem., 12 (1983) 275-286.
4. S. Umemoto, in: M. Okada, S. Hirao, E. Noguchi, T. Sozuki, and M. Yokosuki (Eds.), Utilization of Marine Products, Overseas Technical Cooperation Agency, Tokyo, 1972.
5. E.G. Bligh and W.J. Dyer, Can. J. Biochem. Physiol., 37 (1959) 911-917.
6. J.J. Johnston, H.A. Ghanbari, W.B. Wheeler and J.R. Kirk, J. Food Sci., 48 (1983) 33-35.
7. L.D. Metcalfe, A.A. Schmitz and J.R. Pelka, Anal. Chem., 38 (1966) 514-515.
8. L. Hartman and R.C. Lago, Lab. Prac., 22 (1973) 475-476, 494.
9. E.L. Maia and D.B. Rodriguez-Amaya, VI Encontro Nacional de Analistas de Alimentos, Curitiba, Brasil, October 7-11, 1990, Abstract 17.
10. M. Kates, Techniques of Lipidology, North Holland Publishing Co., Amsterdam, 1972.
11. T.K. Miwa, K.L. Nikolajczak, F.R. Earle and I.A. Wolff, Anal. Chem., 32 (1960) 1739-1742.
12. H.L. Hansen and K.J. Andresen, J. Chromatogr., 34 (1968) 246-248.
13. C.D. Bannon, J.D. Craske and L.M. Norman, J. Chromatogr., 447 (1988) 43-52.
14. W.W. Christie, J. Chromatogr., 447 (1988) 305-314.
15. R. Ryhage and E. Stenhagen, in: F.W. McLafferty (Ed.), Mass Spectrometry of Organic Ions, Academic Press, New York, 1963, pp. 399-452.
16. B. Hallgren, R. Ryhage and E. Stenhagen, Acta Chem. Scand., 13 (1959) 845-847.
17. L.R. Alexander and J.B. Justice Jr., J. Chromatogr., 342 (1985) 1-12.
18. A.J. Fellenberg, D.W. Johnson, A. Poulos and P. Sharp, Biomed. Environ. Mass Spectrom., 14 (1987) 127-129.
19. Z.M.H. Marzoaki, A.M. Taha and K.S. Gromaa, J. Chromatogr., 425 (1988) 11-24.
20. R.G. Henderson and D.R. Tocher, Prog. Lipid Res., 26 (1987) 281-347.
21. R.G. Ackman, Comp. Biochem. Physiol., 22 (1967) 907-922.
22. F.D. Gunstone, R.C. Wijesundera and C.M. Scrimgeour, J. Sci. Food Agric., 29 (1978) 539-550.
23. P.G.V. Nair and K.J. Gopakumar, J. Food Sci., 43 (1978) 1162-1164.
24. R.F. Addison, R.G. Ackman and J. Hingly, J. Fish. Res. Bd. Can., 25 (1968) 2083-2090.
25. R.G. Ackman, in: J.J. Connel (Ed.), Advances in Fish Science and Technology, Fishing News (Books) Ltd., London, 1980, pp. 86-103.
26. S. Sasaki, T. Ota and T. Takagi. Nippon Suisan Gokkaishi, 55 (1989) 1655-1660.
27. J. Mai and J.E. Kinsella, J.Food Sci., 44 (1979a) 1101-1105.
28. J. Mai and J.E. Kinsella, J. Food Biochem., 3 (1979b) 229-239.
29. T. Ohshima, H.D. Widjaja, S. Wada and C. Koizumi, Bull. Jap. Soc. Sci. Fish., 48 (1982) 1795-1801.
30. S. Satoh, T. Takeuchi and T. Watanabe, Bull. Japan Soc. Sci. Fish., 50 (1984) 79-84.

CAROTENOID COMPOSITION OF THE TROPICAL FRUITS *EUGENIA UNIFLORA* AND *MALPIGHIA GLABRA*

MARIA LUCIA CAVALCANTE[1] and DELIA B. RODRIGUEZ-AMAYA[2]

[1]Departamento de Nutrição, Universidade Federal de Pernambuco. 50739 Recife, PE., Brasil.

[2]Departamento de Ciência de Alimentos, Faculdade de Engenharia de Alimentos, Universidade Estadual de Campinas, C.P. 6121, 13081 Campinas, SP., Brasil.

SUMMARY

Lycopene (73.0 µg/g) is the principal carotenoid of *Eugenia uniflora* from Pernambuco, Brasil; substantial amounts of γ-carotene (52.7 µg/g) and β-cryptoxanthin (47.0 µg/g) are also present. Other carotenoids encountered are phytofluene, ζ-carotene and rubixanthin. With a mean total carotenoid content of 225.9 µg/g and vitamin A value of 991 RE/100 g, this fruit proves to be carotenoid- and provitamin A-rich. In *Malpighia glabra*, only three carotenoids (α-carotene, β-carotene and β-cryptoxanthin) are found at levels higher than 0.04 µg/g, with β-carotene as the major carotenoid. The β-carotene content of the samples from the Northeastern states of Pernambuco and Ceará is 5-6 times greater than that of the samples from the colder state of São Paulo (4.0 µg/g). *M. glabra* from Pernambuco is much lower in total carotenoid content (30.5 µg/g) than *E. uniflora*, but the vitamin A value (454 RE/100g) is not proportionately much lower.

1. INTRODUCTION

Sustained interest on carotenoids is evident in the literature. In developed countries, this is mostly due to the various physiological functions attributed to these compounds, especially inhibition of cancer, which are not restricted to vitamin A-active carotenoids. In developing countries, the emphasis remains to be the continued existence of vitamin A deficiency, thus underlining the necessity of determining accurately the provitamin A content of foods.

Unlike temperate fruits, which are mostly colored by anthocyanins, numerous tropical fruits are carotenogenic. Various tropical fruits have already been investigated, but many are still awaiting analysis to establish the carotenoid composition. This type of work is especially important since these fruits thrive in regions where the vitamin A problem occurs.

In Brazil, vitamin A deficiency is severe in certain areas of the Northeast where potential sources of provitamin A can be tapped. Two popular fruits of this region, *Eugenia uniflora* and *Malpighia glabra*, were therefore analyzed in the present study.

The production of these fruits and their utilization in the form of juice, frozen pulps and other processed products have increased markedly in recent years. They are also attracting attention in foreign markets. *Malpighia glabra*, known as West Indian Cherry or "acerola" in Portuguese, has drawn considerable interest because of its very high vitamin C content. The carotenoid composition of both fruits has not been determined.

2. MATERIALS AND METHODS

Eugenia uniflora, "pitanga" in Portuguese, was taken from three sites, all in the state of Pernambuco: (a) a food processing plant located in the municipality of Bonito where it serves as raw material for juice and frozen pulp; (b) street markets in the city of Recife, the fruits coming from the town of Pandalho; and (c) home gardens in Recife and the town of Itamaracá. The fruits were ripe, brilliant wine red in color, with an average diameter of 1 cm and average weight of 6 g.

Starting with 2,000 tons at the processing plant, 6 sample lots of 3 kg each were collected as the fruits passed by in the selection and washing conveyors. These lots were combined, two at a time, to make 3 lots of 6 kg each. A 2 kg portion from each lot was deseeded and homogenized in a blendor. Two 5 g samples were taken from each homogenized lot for analyses. Five kg sample lots were collected from the other sources, from each of which two 5 g samples were taken for analyses after deseeding and homogenization.

Sample lots of 0.5 to 1.5 kg were collected from home gardens, street markets and supermarkets in three states. The fruits were ripe, having on the average 1.5 cm in diameter and 4 g in weight. Those coming from the Northeastern states (Pernambuco and Ceará) were bright red while those from the Southeast (São Paulo) were dark red. Samples of 20 g from deseeded and homogenized lots were taken for quantitative analyses.

The carotenoid composition was determined according to procedures described in detail previously (1). Briefly, this involved exhaustive extraction with cold acetone, transfer to petroleum ether, saponification with an equal volume of 10% methanolic KOH overnight at room temperature, concentration and chromatographic separation on a MgO:Hyflosupercel column (1:2) developed with increasing concentration of ethyl ether (1-9%) and acetone (1-30%) in petroleum ether. The last fraction was eluted with pure acetone or 10% water in acetone. Fractions were rechromatographed on another MgO:Hyflosupercel column (1:1) for the less polar carotenoids and neutral alumina (activity II - III) for the more polar pigments to check the purity. Provitamins were rechromatographed on a Ca(OH)$_2$ column to verify the existence of cis-isomers. The separated carotenoids were quantified spectrophotometrically. Confirmation of the identity of the carotenoids was based on the UV-visible absorption spectra, chromatographic behaviour on column and TLC, specific group chemical reactions (e.g. acetylation with acetic anhydride, methylation with acidified methanol, iodine catalyzed isomerization, reduction with sodium borohydride, epoxide tests). Necessary precautions to prevent isomerization and oxidation of carotenoids during analysis were taken (e.g. protection from light and high temperature, analysis time as short as possible).

The vitamin A values were calculated using the NAS-NRC (2) ratio of 6 μg β-carotene to 1 RE (retinol equivalent), taking into consideration accepted bioactivities (100% for β-carotene and 50% for β-cryptoxanthin and γ-carotene).

Vitamin C was determined using a 2,4-dinitrophenylhydrazine method (3). All other determinations were undertaken using standard procedures of the AOAC (4).

3. RESULTS AND DISCUSSION

3.1. Carotenoid Composition of *Eugenia uniflora*

Seven carotenoids were identified in *Eugenia uniflora* (Table 1). Identification of phytofluene, β-carotene, ζ-carotene and lycopene was based on their typical absorption spectra (5) complemented by their chromatographic behaviour. The absence of substituents was demonstrated by TLC on silica gel plates developed with 3% methanol in benzene, where the carotenes ran with the solvent front and the xanthophylls retained according to the type, number and location of the substituents. β-cryptoxanthin was confirmed by the following parameters: (a) chromophore identical to β-carotene as shown by the absorption spectrum; (b) Rf value on the silica plate indicative of a monohydroxy β-carotene derivative; (c) positive response to acetylation and negative to methylation, reflecting the nonallylic position of the hydroxyl group. The following properties identified rubixanthin: (a) absorption spectrum resembling that of γ-carotene; (b) chromatographic behaviour compatible with a monohydroxy derivative of γ-carotene; and (c) positive reaction to acetylation and negative to methylation. An unidentified carotenoid was also detected. It showed a broad spectrum similar to those of ketocarotenoids with the maximum at 430 nm in petroleum ether. However, it responded negatively to reduction with sodium borohydride.

TABLE 1

Carotenoid composition (μg/g) and vitamin A value (RE/100 g) of *Eugenia uniflora* from Pernambuco, Brazil.

Carotenoid/ Vitamin Value	Industrial lot[a]	From home gardens[a]	From street markets[a]	General mean ± SD
Phytofluene	11.6±0.5	16.4±0.7	11.4±0.5	13.1±2.4
β-Carotene	8.1±0.6	12.5±0.8	8.2±0.6	9.5±2.1
ζ-Carotene	3.6±0.5	6.6±0.4	4.8±0.6	4.7±1.6
Unidentified[b]	2.8±0.5	3.7±0.7	3.6±0.3	3.4±0.4
β-Cryptoxanthin	44.8±2.0	49.2±0.7	47.0±1.0	47.0±2.2
γ-Carotene	50.4±0.8	58.2±0.7	49.4±1.2	52.7±4.0
Lycopene	71.8±1.1	73.7±1.5	73.5±0.4	73.0±1.4
Rubixanthin	21.5±1.0	25.3±1.6	22.4±1.9	23.1±2.2
Total Carotenoid	214.6±3.8	243.0±2.0	220.2±2.0	225.9±12.8
Vitamin A value	928±29	1,104±16	939±20	991±83

[a] Results are means and standard deviations of 6 analyses.
[b] Calculated on the basis of the β-carotene absorption coefficient.

Lycopene was the principal carotenoid pigment, but substantial amounts of γ-carotene and β-cryptoxanthin were also found. The high total carotenoid content and vitamin A value, derived from β-carotene, γ-carotene and β-cryptoxanthin, place this fruit among the rich sources of provitamins A and carotenoids in general.

There was good agreement of the results of the samples collected from different localities in the state of Pernambuco. Understandably, the sample lots freshly collected from home gardens and at optimum ripeness presented higher levels of all carotenoids.

3.2. Carotenoid Composition of *Malpighia glabra*

Only three carotenoids were detected in the West Indian cherry at levels higher than 0.04 µg/g (Table 2). β-Carotene and β-cryptoxanthin were identified as described for *Eugenia uniflora*. α-Carotene was confirmed by its typical absorption spectrum and chromatographic behaviour.

TABLE 2

Carotenoid composition (µg/g) and vitamin A value (RE/100 g) of *Malpighia glabra* from three Brazilian states.

Carotenoid/Vitamin Value	Pernambuco	Ceará	São Paulo
α-Carotene	0.1±0.1	trace	trace
β-Carotene	25.8±4.4	21.5±0.9	4.0±0.6
β-Cryptoxanthin	3.6±0.7	2.1±0.4	0.5±0.2
Total Carotenoid	30.5±4.4	23.5±0.8	4.5±0.7
Vitamin A value	454±86	375±15	72±8

[a] Results are means and standard deviations of 18 analyses of fruits from Pernambuco and 4 analyses each for fruits from Ceará and São Paulo. Pernambuco is a major commercial producer of this fruit; it is not commercially produced in Ceará and São Paulo.

The principal carotenoid was β-carotene, which together with the small amount of β-cryptoxanthin, gave a vitamin A value of 454 RE/100 g for the fruits from Pernambuco.

The samples from Ceará, which is a neighbouring state of Pernambuco, exhibited a composition very similar to that obtained for those coming from Pernambuco. Notably, the carotenoid content of the cherries from the colder state of São Paulo was much lower, the β-carotene concentration being 5-6 times less than those of the Northeastern fruits. This result confirms previous observations, in relation to guava (6) and papaya (7), that the fruits produced in the hot and sunny Northeastern region have higher contents of β-carotene and other carotenoids.

Ironically, it is in the Northeastern state that serious cases of vitamin A deficiency have been reported. This indicates that a part of the population do not have access to vitamin A sources. It is also true, however, that in certain poor areas of this region, there is generalized undernutrition and parasitic infestation, conditions which hinder the absorption and utilization of provitamins.

Considerable concern has been expressed in the literature in recent years about the importance of separating the cis-isomers of α- and β-carotene, considering that they are less potent than the corresponding trans forms. β-Carotene of both *E. uniflora* and *M. glabra* and β-cryptoxanthin and γ-carotene of the former were rechromatographed on a Ca(OH)₂ column to verify the existence of cis-isomers but they were not found.

The carotenoid compositions and vitamin A values of some tropical fruits from different states in Brazil (6-10) are presented in Table 3 for comparison. Also included are the data on

TABLE 3

Comparison of some tropical fruits in terms of the carotenoid composition and vitamin A value.

Fruit, cultivar source	N[a]	Principal carotenoid (µg/g)	Total Carotenoid Content (µg/g)	Vitamin A Value (RE/100g)
Tree tomato				
São Paulo	3	β-Cryptoxanthin (13.9)	24.3	248
Malaysia	1	β-Cryptoxanthin (12.4)	18.3	203
Guava				
IAC-4, São Paulo, variety undefined,	4	Lycopene (53.4)	62.1	62
Pernambuco	3	Lycopene (53.4)	70.0	198
Mango				
Bourbon, São Paulo	5	β-Carotene (8.1)	14.3	138
Haden, São Paulo	5	β-Carotene (6.6)	13.9	115
Extreme, São Paulo	5	β-Carotene (25.5)	30.5	431
Golden, São Paulo	5	β-Carotene (18.0)	24.0	307
Tommy Atkins, Mato Grosso	5	β-Carotene (13.1)	19.2	224
Black-gold mango, Malaysia	1	β-Carotene (6.2)	6.2	103
Papaya				
Common, São Paulo	5	β-Cryptoxanthin (8.1)	13.0	112
Solo, Bahia	5	Lycopene (21.0)	34.2	124
Formosa, Bahia	5	Lycopene (19.1)	33.0	99
Formosa, São Paulo	5	Lycopene (26.5)	47.8	193
Tailândia, Bahia	5	Lycopene (40.0)	60.3	137
Papaya, Malaysia	1	Lycopene (20.0)	41.2	171
Papaya exotica, Malaysia	1	Lycopene (23.3)	37.6	120
Spondias lutea,				
Pernambuco	4	β-cryptoxanthin (16.5)	25.9	187
Watermelon, Malaysia	1	Lycopene (53.0)	61.7	99

Data taken from references 6-11 for comparison. Except for the Malaysian samples, all the other data refer to samples from Brazil.
N - number of sample lots analyzed. All results refer to edible portion.

the three fruits (mango, papaya and tree tomato), out of 12 fruits analyzed in Malaysia, which showed the highest vitamin A activity and the fruit (watermelon) which exhibited the highest total carotenoid content (11). *E. uniflora* markedly surpassed the most carotenoid-rich fruits (guava and watermelon) and the one with the highest vitamin A activity (mango cultivar Extreme) in the list. It is worth remembering, however, that the mango samples came from São Paulo; the same cultivar grown in the Northeast could yield fruits with higher carotenoid/provitamin A content.

For a more complete characterization pf the samples analyzed, determinations which are commonly carried out with fruits were also accomplished. The results are presented in Tables 4 and 5.

TABLE 4

Some properties of the *E. uniflora* samples analyzed.

	Industrial lot[a]	From home gardens[a]	From street markets[a]	General mean ± SD
pH	3.1±0.1	3.2±0.0	3.9±0.1	3.4±0.3
°Brix (20°C)	10.2±0.1	12.5±0.2	9.7±0.3	10.8±1.1
Reducing sugar (%)	5.1±0.2	6.2±0.2	5.1±0.2	5.5±0.5
Total sugar (%)	6.1±0.1	6.3±0.2	6.1±0.4	6.2±0.1
Vitamin C (mg/100g)	15.4±0.1	17.2±0.7	16.4±0.3	16.3±0.7

[a]Results are means and standard deviations of 6 analyses.

TABLE 5

Some properties of the *M. glabra* samples analyzed.

	Pernambuco	Ceará	São Paulo
pH	3.4±0.2	3.9±0.1	3.3±0.1
°Brix (20°C)	5.9±0.4	5.3±0.4	5.8±0.5
Reducing sugar (%)	2.7±0.1	2.2±0.1	2.4±0.4
Total sugar (%)	3.2±0.2	3.1±0.1	3.3±0.2
Vitamin C (mg/100g)	2,808±96	1,949±32	1,640±26

[a]Results are means and standard deviations of 18 analyses of fruits from Pernambuco and 6 analyses each for fruits from Ceará and São Paulo.

ACKNOWLEDGMENT

The authors acknowledge with gratitude the financial support given by the Financiadora de Estudos e Projetos (FINEP).

REFERENCES

1. D.B. Rodriguez, L.C. Raymundo, T.C. Lee, K.L. Simpson and C.O. Chichester, Ann. Bot., 40 (1976) 615-624.
2. NAS-NRC, Recommended Dietary Allowances, 9th edn., National Academy of Science, Washington, D.C., 1989, pp. 78-92.
3. R. Strohecker and H.M. Hening, Analisis de Vitamines. Metodos Precisos, Editorial Paz, Madrid, 1967, pp. 296-311.
4. AOAC, Official Methods of Analysis, 14th edn., Association of Official Analytical Chemists, Arlington, VA, 1990.
5. B.H. Davies, in: T.W. Goodwin (Ed.), Chemistry and Biochemistry of Plant Pigments, Academic Press, London, 1976, pp. 38-65.
6. M. Padula and D.B. Rodriguez-Amaya, Food Chem., 20 (1986) 11-19.
7. M. Kimura, D.B. Rodriguez-Amaya and S. Yokoyama, Lebensm. Wiss. Technol, (in press).
8. D.B. Rodriguez-Amaya, P.A. Bobbio and F.O. Bobbio, Food Chem., 12 (1983) 61-65.
9. H.T. Godoy and D.B. Rodriguez-Amaya, Lebensm. Wiss. Technol, 22 (1989) 100-103.
10. D.B. Rodriguez-Amaya and M. Kimura, Cienc. Tecnol. Aliment., 8 (1989) 148-162.
11. E.S. Tee and C-L. Linn, Food Chem., 41 (1991) 309-339.

FOOD EMULSIONS IN EXTRUDED GLASSY MATERIALS

FOUAD Z. SALEEB
JOHN L. CAVALLO
SUSAN VIDAL
GENERAL FOODS USA, 250 NORTH STREET, WHITE PLAINS, NY 10625

SUMMARY

This paper provides a method for fixing volatile oils/flavor ingredients in the form of droplets in homogeneous high density glassy substrates produced via a continuous melt extrusion process. The substrates required for this process consist of a dry blend of a major component (high molecular weight) and a minor component (low molecular weight) food grade ingredients that were fed to an automated extruder at a preset temperature and screw profile. A highly viscous but homogeneous melt is produced in about 1 minute that entraps the flavor ingredient in the form of fine droplets. On emerging from the die the melted mass is transferred into a glassy substrate of very desirable encapsulating properties. The physical chemical factors responsible for the stability of these glassy systems will be discussed in this article.

Introduction

The delivery of flavors has long been a problem facing many consumer products provided by the food, agricultural, pharmaceutical and cosmetic industries. Flavor is a small part by weight of these products but is the most essential attribute for product acceptability and consumer appeal. Most flavors are made up of mixtures of fairly labile compounds that are sensitive to heat, light, oxygen and moisture. In particular, in the food industry, the delivery of flavors in dry products is even more complicated by the hydrophilic nature of common food ingredients such as sugars and acids (hygroscopic) as well as the sorption/redistribution of flavors between different fat and non- fat phases during storage. The general term of encapsulation is used here to describe steps taken to protect volatile flavors from losses, oxidation, degradative reactions as well as convenient means of storing, shipping and delivering many reactive food ingredients and/or essential oils.

Spray drying is the most widely used technique to produce dried foods (e.g. milk, cheese, fruit juices, modified starches etc.) as well as flavors for many consumer products. Various carriers and blends of carriers are used to entrap flavors in the form of droplets as well as in the interstitial spacings between the carrier molecules. During the last two decades many chemically modified starches were suggested and produced by various manufacturers to replace polymeric natural, but generally expensive ingredients such as gum arabic and gelatin (1, 2). The modified starches offer other advantages such as good emulsifying capacity, good film forming properties, stability and more important less sensitivity to moisture. However, most of these special starches are not considered natural ingredients.

Spray dried products, in spite of their extensive use in many products, have some major drawbacks, namely:

a) <u>Particle size</u>: usually all spray drying produce primary particles ranging from few microns to less than hundred micron in diameter. They are fairly fine powders that have to be dealt with in processing (flow characteristics, caking, etc.)

b) <u>Surface area</u>: as a consequence of particle size, spray dried products have a fairly large external surface area that would enhance the rate of oxidation and/or flavor losses under a given storage condition.

c) <u>Absolute/structural density</u>: during the relatively fast evaporative drying of fine aqueous droplets in a hot tower, the carrier materials form a solid thin shell almost instantanously. Besides the presence of surface oil and evaporative flavor losses, the capsule walls are structurally imperfect showing cracks, and various microscopic defects that facilitates further flavor losses, oxidation and moisture transfer.

Encapsulation via extrusion is a process that was developed more than 30 years ago to overcome some of the shortfalls of spray drying (14). Several patents and related publications are available describing the recent optimization of essential oils encapsulation in sugar melts (3-6).

Fundamentally, the encapsulation of water insoluble essential oils via extrusion is based on hard candy technology (7-9). An aqueous solution of carbohydrates, mainly, sucrose, corn syrup solids and/or maltodextrins is cooked until its water content is reduced to or below about 6% (boiling point of 120°C). At this point, the heating is stopped, an emulsifier and the flavor oil are added and the hot melt is vigorously stirred to give a uniform dispersion of the oil droplets. The reactor, a sealable steam-jacketed vessel fitted with an extrusion die, is then pressurized and the hot melt is extruded into cold isopropyl alcohol. The cold alcohol bath cools the extruded filaments as well as wash the surface oil. All the above extrusion techniques are batch processes applicable only for water insoluble oils in which the oils are exposed to excessive heat (>100°C) for extended periods during the homogenization and the extrusion period of each batch.

Our recent work resolved most of the shortfalls of the previous extrusion work (10). The present process is a continuous one that does not require a cooking step and can be used for water soluble as well as water insoluble flavors in which the flavor oil is only exposed to heat (<120°C) in a pressure tight environment for less than 1 minute. The basic physical and chemical characteristics of this new extrusion encapsulation technology is given in details elsewhere (11). Briefly, the ingredients required to form the glass is a dry-blend of low molecular weight minor ingredient(s) (20-30%) and a high molecular weight major ingredient(s). These dry powders with or without flavors are feed automatically to a multi-zone extruder provided by a specified die. The temperature through the extruder is regulated so that the low molecular weight fraction (e.g. maltose, citric acid, malic acid, sorbitol, etc.) melts first. As these components melt, the major component will dissolve into the minor component, forming a viscous homogeneous fluid which enrobes the flavor droplets (added with powder but preferably metered into the middle of the extruder). The die openings provide the shape and dimension of the required product. Upon emerging from the die the melt solidifies quickly in air to form a hard homogeneous, high density glass, with a final moisture content of approximately 3-6%. Very soft as well as very hard glasses can be produced by selecting the type and composition of the dry ingredients, as well as the level of flavorant (water soluble or insoluble). It should be mentioned that water and other water soluble flavor components and carriers usually act as plasticizers, reducing the glass transition temperature (Tg) of these extruded food glasses.

The present paper gives the composition and processing parameters required to provide very stable flavor oils produced by this inexpensive continuous extrusion process. The glass transition temperature of various glasses as well as the role of water as a plasticizer will be discussed. The role of emulsifiers on oil droplet size will be given as it relates to product application.

Experimental

Extruders: Two types of extruders were used.

a) Brabender Extruder (manufactured by Brabender Corp., South Hackensack, N.J.)

is a single screw within a 0.75 inch diameter barrel. It has 3 independently controlled zones in addition to the die-head. The extruder has a screw ratio of 2:1 and can use either a single hole (up to 1/4" diameter) or a multiple hole die (down to 1/16" diameter each). The dry blend is fed to the extruder at the rate of 2-3 lb./hr.

b) Werner Pfleiderer twin screw extruder model WP-C37 (manufacture by Werner Pfleiderer Corp., Ramsey, NJ) is a fully automated extruder. Four zones were used at controlled temperatures plus the die compartment. The latter is equipped with a multi hole horizontal plate with hole diameters down to 0.018". The carrier dry mix is fed at the rate of ~12-20 lb./hr. The flavors were injected into the second barrel/section downstream via a high pressure macro-piston pump to deliver the flavor at a prefixed rate. The temperature settings, screw profile, die temperature, screw speed and pressure inside the extruder are set and/or determined by the nature of the carrier as well as the die hole size.

Thermal Analysis Techniques

The glass transition temperature (Tg) for the samples prepared were determined by a Dupont 912 DSC (Differential Scanning Calorimeter). The sample to be studied (~20 mg) is hermatically sealed in an aluminum pan and cooled to 0°C with liquid nitrogen. The sample is then heated to approximately 150°C at a rate of 5°C/minute. All samples were run in duplicate to verify the reproducibility of the technique.

TMA (Thermomechanical Analysis) was determined by a Dupont 943 system. A sample of the material to be studied is placed in a quartz glass cell. A quartz wide end probe (0.28 cm^2) is placed on top of the sample supporting a 100 g load. The sample is then cooled to -20°C with liquid nitrogen. The heating chamber is then screwed into place setting a controlled temperature environment. The sample is then heated to 120°C at a rate of 5°C/minute.

Scanning Electron Micrographs (SEM)

The extruded samples investigated were fractured to produce clean cross-sectional surfaces. These particles were then mounted on SEM stubs with a colloidal Ag adhesive and sputter-coated. Approximately 500A of Au-Pd was applied using a Denton vacuum, "Desk II" cold sputter unit. The fractured surfaces exposing the evacuated oil cell were then imaged using a Cam Scan, Series 4 SEM with a LaB$_6$ crystal electron source at 10 kV. Artifacts due to exposure of the sample to ambient humidity and/or drying were avoided by performing all operations as quickly as possible.

Encapsulating Materials

Maltodextrins, corn syrup solids, food acids, mono and disacchrides as well as the flavors used in this work were commercially available products.

The oil droplet size in the finished products was determined after dissolving the glassy carrier in water using a Brinkmann Model 2010 particle size analyzer.

Results and Discussion

Figure 1 shows a typical DSC thermogram and its derivative for an extruded sample of a corn syrup solids carrier containing on a dry bases 6% glucose, 25% maltose and 69% maltotriose and higher polymeric maltodextrins.

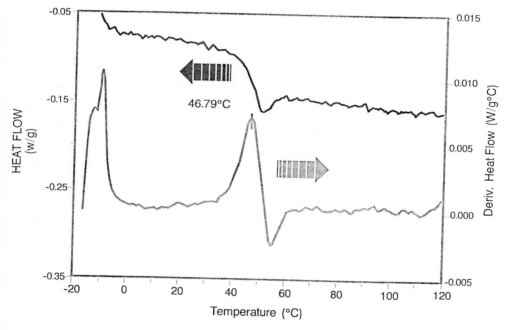

Fig. 1   DSC thermogram showing heat flow versus temperature for an extruded glassy material containing corn syrup solids and maltodextrins.

The thermogram shows the heat flow as a function of temperature. Transitions will occur, in general, as either first or second order depending on the transformation that occur at a particular temperature. As shown in Figure 1, only a second order glass transition occurs at 46.7°C. At this temperature the sample is transformed from an amorphous solid (glass state) into an amorphous liquid (rubber).

It is worth mentioning that moisture plays an important role in determining the value of the glass transition temperature in these food glasses. It has been demonstrated that for low moisture glassy systems, (2-7% total moisture) a 1% increase in the moisture level reduces the Tg by about 5-10°C. Water as well as water soluble flavorants act as plasticizer for these mostly carbohydrate glassy substrates. For the sample shown in Figure 1, the moisture level was found to be 3.5%.

Figure 2 shows the TMA softening profile for the same carbohydrate extruded sample shown in Figure 1. Starting at about 50°C a significant dimensional change in the material is evident indicating the onset of softening. Within a

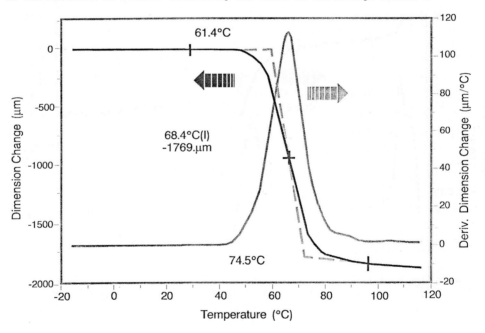

Fig. 2   TMA softening profile of the same material as in Fig. 1.

temperature range of about 20°C, the hard glass is soft enough to achieve approximately a 90% penetration by this probe (100 g/0.28cm^2). The significant dependence of melt viscosity of these systems on temperature is very important in the manufacturing of these glasses by extrusion. They are fairly fluid in the extruder but harden quickly on exposure to atmospheric temperature. Cold alcohol baths are not required to harden these glasses as needed by other processes (7-9). The almost complete penetration of the TMA probe through the sample indicates an almost homogeneous glass structure compared with many polymeric food glasses.

It is interesting to note that the onset of the softening temperature determined by TMA always occurs at a higher temperature (on the average 10-15°C) than the Tg determined by DSC. Since hard glassy materials will have very little molecular mobility below Tg, significant dimensional changes are noticeable only at temperatures several degrees above the Tg of the material. At Tg the viscosity of the rubbery state may be as high as 10^{15} poise and decreases exponentially as the temperature increases.

Tg and Composition

As mentioned in the introduction section, this dry powder extrusion technique is capable of producing food glasses of varying degrees of hardness to withstand different storage conditions for various product applications.

Table I shows the Tg values for varying glassy blends of Lodex 10 (a maltodextrin produced by Amaizo Co.) and citric acid monohydrate. The results demonstrate that when citric acid monohydrate (a low molecular weight, low Tg ingredient) is added to Lodex 10 (a high molecular weight, high Tg ingredient) it produces on extrusion homogeneous glasses possessing glass transition temperatures intermediate between those of the starting materials. For this

TABLE 1

Tg values for various blends of Lodex 10 and citric acid.

COMPOSITION %		Tg (°C)
Citric Acid Monohydrate	Lodex 10	
100	0	10
50	50	30
20	80	52
0	100	110

particular system, the greatest overall depression in Tg of Lodex occurs when approximately 20% of the high molecular weight Lodex is replaced with citric acid monohydrate (Tg is reduced from 110°C to ca. 51°C). Further addition of citric acid monohydrate results in a continuous depression of the Tg, approaching the 10°C, the Tg of the citric acid monohydrate glassy phase.

The results discussed above demonstrate the importance of both glass composition and moisture content in determining the physical and processing conditions of these unique substrates. For efficient encapsulation of a volatile oil within a glassy material the melt should be soft enough at the lowest temperature possible in the extruder. But for this system to be stable, the glass must have a Tg above the storage conditions. This is an important consideration when these glassy systems are to be used in mixtures with other food ingredients (i.e., sugars, acids, etc.). Softening of these glasses can lead to caking and agglomeration of the product on storage. To assure that the system remain stable while delivering a high fix of oil, glasses which perform best will be those where the Tg is as high as possible above storage temperature.

From a screening point of view, stable food glassy systems have been prepared in a small single barrel extruder using as little as one pound of material. In a typical example, 125 g of maltose-monohydrate and 375 g of Lodex 10 were blended together and 17.6 g of ethylbutyrate (a flavor enhancer) is added. The admixture was fed through the extruder so that a uniform rope is obtained which is allowed to cool to room temperature. The product (Tg $\sim$ 80°C) is a very homogeneous glassy material with the ethyl butyrate flavor entrapped within it. On a weight basis the sample entrapped more than 95% of the added flavor in a very stable form (for several months).

Many samples have also been prepared containing blends of food acids and corn syrup solids. A typical example is a 5% citric acid, 24% maltose, and 71% polysaccharides. This sample, prepared in the large WP extruder where orange oil was metered at the rate of 8% by weight is able to entrap orange oil at a 94% efficiency. Scanning electron microscopy (SEM) showed that the entrapped essential oils appear like an emulsion of varying droplet sizes (1-50µ), uniformly distributed in a homogeneous glassy matrix. The degree of subdivision of the flavor oil is determined by the nature of the oil, degree of shear and temperature in the extruder and level of fix.

The efficiency to fix and stabilize large quantities of liquid oil within a glass and deliver the oil in the form of a dry material is the major advantage of this technology for use in various products.

In certain cases, a controlled droplet size and size distribution in glass matrix is needed to achieve a given end point in a product. A typical example is to obtain opacity in a beverage. Addition of an emulsifier to the essential oil produces a fine emulsion when the oil phase is mixed with the melted substrate during extrusion. Choosing the optimal HLB (Hydrophilic-Lipophilic Balance) of the emulsifier for the particular oil assures a fine oil dispersion within the glass. In a typical example, orange oil containing 10% by weight emulsifier (7% hexaglycerol distearate and 3% sulfoacetate of fatty glycerides) was extruded at the level of 7% in a glass of similar composition as provided in Figs. 1 & 2 above. Glasses formed from this composition are very stable with an average droplet diameter on the order of 4.6μ. A Brinkmann particle size analyzer was used to determine the oil droplet size after dissolving the extruded glass in water as shown in Figure 3. No change in average diameter or size distribution was noticeable for up to 24 hours from dissolution. However, on stand for 3 days, the average droplet size was reduced down to 1.5μ (See Fig. 4).

A scanning electron micrograph (SEM) of the above sample is shown in Fig. 5. In this picture, an extruded rod ~ 0.5mm diameter using WP-C37 was fractured and observed by the electron microscope. A fairly homogeneous glassy substrate forming a continuous phase is seen enrobing oil droplets of relatively narrow

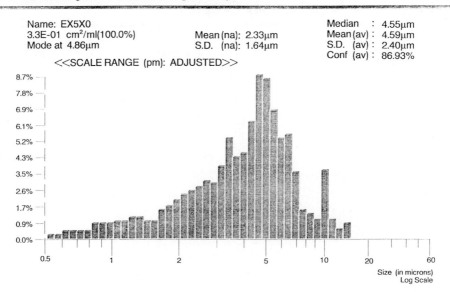

Fig. 3   Particle size analysis of oil droplets in water.

size distribution. No fractures or grain boundaried can be seen even at this high magnification (2000X).

Helium density measurements showed that this sample has a density of 1.45g/cc., a fairly high density for a carbohydrate glass containing 7% orange oil of a density of less than 1 g/cc (0.84g/cc at 20°C). The high density of the continuous phase explains the exceptional stability of these systems when stored at temperatures below their Tg. Very little flavor losses and oxygen uptakes were observed experimentally. In contrast to extruded systems, spray drying has been used extensively to encapsulate orange oil . Starch dextrins were found to have a lower encapsulating efficiency than systems utilizing gum arabic. When one compares the encapsulating efficiencies between systems prepared using gum arabic, corn dextrin or tapioca dextrin at a 20% orange oil level, the efficiencies were 83.5, 64.0, and 75% respectively. Furthermore, less surface oil was found on the samples prepared using gum arabic. The favorable attributes of the spray dried gum arabic system relate to its enhanced emulsifying properties. Improvements in the efficiency and stability of spray dried citrus oil were reported by Trubiano and Lacourse, (12), when chemically modified starches were

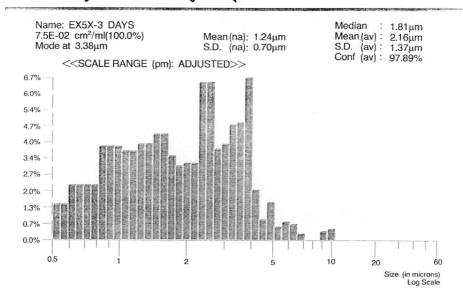

Fig. 4   Particle size analysis of oil droplets in water after 3 days.

used instead of regular dextrins. Finer emulsions were produced (2u droplets) that are more stable with respect to both droplet coalescence and oil oxidation due to the lower citrus oil content on the surface of the spray dried powders. However, as shown by Westing, et.al. (13) spray dried citrus oils have shelf lives much shorter than extruded flavors, even when the oil droplet mean diameter of the extruded flavor is larger than these for spray dried systems. Using extrusion for flavor encapsulation reduces and/or eliminates oxidation, loss of oil and extend shelf life.

In summary, this work illustrates the production of fairly stable encapsulated flavors in food glassy substrates that can be obtained by a continuous extrusion process utilizing powder blends of various food ingredients. As this technique eliminates the need for the candy cooking as well as the emulsification steps essential for current encapsulation techniques (3, 9, 10) it lends itself to the entrapment of various water soluble, water insoluble, liquid and solid flavorants. The unlimited options available to use various carrier ingredients and their blends provide glasses of varying degrees of hardness exhibiting very low to fairly high glass transition temperatures.

Acknowledgment

The authors would like to thank Kraft General Foods for permission to publish this work and the technical assistance provided by Mrs. M. Rosolen for the Thermal Analysis work and Mr. W. Popp for his SEM photographs.

662

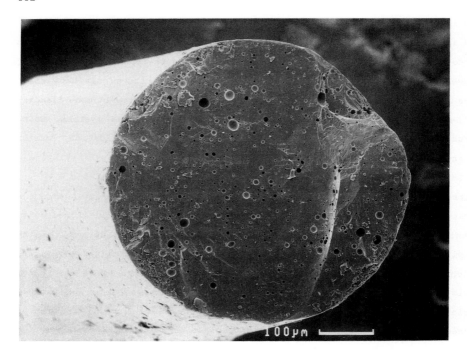

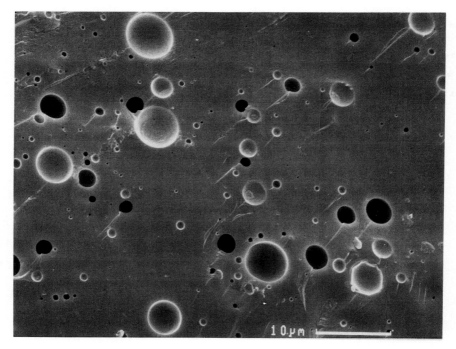

Fig. 5   SEM of extruded rod 0.5mm diameter. a) 140X, b) 2000X.

REFERENCES

1. C. G. Caldwell and O. B. Wurzburg, Polysaccaride Derivatives of Substituted Dicarboxylic Acids (1953) U.S. Patent 2,661,349.
2. P. C. Trubiano, in: O.B. Wurzburg (Ed), Modified Starches, Properties and Uses, CRC Press, Inc., Boca Raton, 1986, Chapter 9.
3. J. L. Dziezak, Food Technol., 42 (1988) 136.
4. D. H. Miller and J. R. Mutka, Preparation of Solid Essential Oil Flavor Composition, (1986) U.S. Patent 4,610,890.
5. J. M. Barnes and J. A. Steinke, Encapsulation Matrix Composition and Encapsulate Containing Same, (1987) U.S. Patent 4,689,235.
6. J. R. Mutka and D. B. Nelson, Food Technol., 42 (1988) 154.
7. E. E. Beck, Essential Oil Composition and Method of Preparing the Same, (1972) U.S. Patent 3,704,137.
8. H. E. Swisher, Solid Flavoring Composition and Method of Preparing the Same, (1957) U.S. Patent 2,809, 895.
9. H. E. Swisher Solid Essential Oil Flavoring Composition and Process for Preparing the Same, (1962) U.S. Patent 3,041,180.
10. F. Z. Saleeb and J. G. Pickup, Fixation of Volatiles in Extruded Glass Substrates, (1989) U.S. Patent 4,820,534
11. F. Z. Saleeb, et.al. (to be published).
12. P. C. Trubiano and N. L. Lacourse, in: S.J. Risch and G. A. Reineccius (Eds), Flavor Encapsulation, ACS Symposium Series #370, Washington D.C. 1986, Chapter 6.
13. L. L. Westing, G.A. Reineccius and F. Caporaso, ibid., Chapter 12.
14. B. Makower, Food Technol., 10 (1956).

G. Charalambous (Ed.), Food Science and Human Nutrition
© 1992 Elsevier Science Publishers B.V. All rights reserved.

AN OVERVIEW OF ASEPTIC PROCESSING OF PARTICULATE FOODS

Nikolaos G. Stoforos

National Food Processors Association, 6363 Clark Avenue, Dublin, CA 94568 (USA)

ABSTRACT

Recently developed procedures in designing aseptic processes for foods containing discrete particles are presented. The use of liquid crystals as temperature sensors for particle surface temperature measurements is discussed. Liquid-particle heat transfer coefficients during tubular flow heating in a holding tube simulating system are presented. An experimental methodology for particle residence time distribution measurements is outlined. A mathematical model for microbial destruction and quality factors retention calculations is presented. The effects of various product and processing parameters on process optimization, based on maximum thiamine retention, are briefly discussed.

INTRODUCTION

One way of extending the shelf life of perishable foods is thermal processing, the process in which the food is exposed to elevated temperatures for sufficient period of time to inactivate the agents of spoilage. Contrary to other means of food preservation (*e.g.*, drying, freezing, chemical additives, etc.) which control the microbial population in the food by limiting microbial growth, the lethal time-temperature conditions encountered during thermal processing are capable of destroying the microorganisms. However, while microbial destruction is being achieved during heating, quality degradation also occurs and should be of particular concern to the process designer (1), (2). In general, food quality is better preserved in thermal processes with high heat transfer rates from the heating medium to the food and the accompanied increased optimum processing temperature (3). This is due to the different reaction rate constants that characterize microbial and quality factor (*e.g.*, color, flavor, nutrient, etc.) destruction (4). Consequently, for traditional, in-container, processing, food quality becomes a function of container size and geometry. On the contrary, aseptic processing (a process in which the food and the container are sterilized separately followed by packaging in a sterile environment) results in product quality independent of the size of the container. Uniform and improved product quality, continuous operation, energy and packaging cost reduction, and the choice of a variety of packaging materials are among the factors which make aseptic processing commercially attractive despite high capital investment costs (5)-(8).

The food sterilization unit of an aseptic system consists of a heating section (*e.g.*, scraped-surface heat exchanger with steam as the heating medium) designed to rapidly increase the temperature of the food, a holding section (*e.g.*, a holding tube) where the food is held, by virtue of its transit time, for a prespecified time necessary to achieve commercial sterility, and a cooling section (*e.g.*, scraped-surface heat exchangers with water as the coolant) used to rapidly bring the food to the filling temperature. In principle, any pumpable food can be processed in aseptic systems. Nevertheless, the engineering analysis of such systems for liquid/particulate foods becomes far more complicated, compared to homogeneous foods, due to the appearance of the liquid-particle film heat transfer coefficient. The mechanism of heat transfer in aseptic processing of particulate foods is similar to the one that occurs during traditional processing of canned liquid/particulate foods under agitation: The fluid surrounding the particles is heated by convection from an outside heat source; convection also takes place at the fluid-particle interface, while heat is accumulated into the particles by conduction. Therefore, much can be learned about aseptic processing by studying in-container processes (9). However, there is an attribute unique to aseptic processing, namely the residence time distribution of the various food elements in the various components of the process system. Except for the ideal case of plug flow, different fluid elements or particles travel through the various sections of the aseptic system with different velocities. This results in a distribution of the residence times. Knowledge of the residence time for the fastest moving element, within each section, with a high degree of accuracy is essential in order to design a safe process with high quality product. Liquid to particle film heat transfer coefficient and particle residence time distribution are two key factors in establishing aseptic processes for particulate foods (10). Presumably, parameters that affect the above two factors (*e.g.*, particle size, fluid viscosity, etc.) can be set as critical control points. Knowledge of the liquid-particle heat transfer coefficient and the particle residence time distribution is also essential in mathematical modeling of heat sterilization in aseptic systems. Information drawn from mathematical models and validated by inoculated experimental pack is considered an acceptable and rather necessary part of the filing procedure to the regulatory agencies (11)-(13).

A number of researchers have concentrated their efforts in studying the liquid-particle film heat transfer coefficient, (14)-(26), determining the particle residence time distribution (27)-(41), or developing mathematical models for aseptic processing (20), (22), (23), (33),

(42)-(58). The objective of this paper is to present an overview of our work in studying aseptic processes for foods containing discrete particles, including results of our approach in studying liquid-particle heat transfer coefficients, particle residence time distribution, and mathematical modeling of aseptic processing. Space limits the discussion of the work of other researchers.

LIQUID-PARTICLE FILM HEAT TRANSFER COEFFICIENT

The determination of the film heat transfer coefficient at the liquid-particle interface during aseptic processing poses a unique challenge to the investigators. The problem is to directly or indirectly monitor the temperature of moving particles without interfering with particle motion. The magnitude of the liquid-particle film heat transfer coefficient, h_p, depends on the relative fluid to particle velocity. In the general heat transfer literature, classical correlations for h_p have been developed for fluids past stationary particles (59), (60). Following this approach, a number of researchers determined h_p by measuring the particle temperature on stationary particles (16), (19)-(24). However, data obtained with stationary particles cannot be used in aseptic system unless the relative liquid to particle velocity can be quantified. In addition, conservative h_p estimates through the above analyses (for zero fluid velocity), resulting in a microbiologically safe but overprocessed product, might negate the quality advantages of aseptic processing. A method to monitor particle temperatures for tubular flow heating with thermocouples has been suggested, (17) and (18), by pulling the thermocouple wire, attached to the monitored particle, towards the direction of flow in a way such as to simulate the motion of the unmonitored particles.

In addition, indirect methods for h_p determinations have been proposed. The basic idea behind these methods is that the percent retention of a heat-labile substance, after thermal processing, depends on the temperature experienced by that substance. This temperature, for the system under consideration, is a function of h_p. Hence, by measuring the viable spore concentration, after simulated food particles with immobilized microbial spores were processed through an aseptic system, the h_p value was determined (14), (15). Presumably, any heat-labile substance other than microbial spores, e.g., chemical substances, (61) and (62), or enzymes, (63), can be used. The above methods do not restrict particle motion. Nevertheless, the implementation of this concept involves lengthy experimentation (starting from determining kinetic parameters on heat destruction of the labile substances). In addition, variations, experimental or inherited, are amplified through the process of h_p

determination (recall that mass average survival concentrations are correlated through h_p). Therefore, the applicability of these methods is restricted to situations when direct temperature measurements are impracticable (14).

A method of measuring surface temperature data on moving particles without interfering with the particle motion has been developed for axially rotating liquid/particulate canned foods, (64) and (65), and extended to aseptic processing of particulate foods (25), (26). This method will be outlined in the remaining portion of this section.

The approach consisted of using liquid crystals to monitor particle surface temperatures. Liquid crystals are cholesteric compounds that exhibit the flow properties of a liquid and the optical properties of a crystal. At its phase transition temperature, the liquid crystal scatters available white light into spectral components. Phase transitions occur between −20 and 255 °C depending on the particular liquid crystal. During heating of a black surface coated with liquid crystal, the surface color changes from black to red, yellow, green, blue, violet, and finally returns to black (outside the phase transition temperature range the liquid crystal layer is transparent). This color sequence is reversed upon cooling. Therefore, the color of a liquid crystal coated surface becomes a function of the surface temperature.

Simulated food particles (acrylic spheres) coated with liquid crystals, initially held at approximately 4 °C, were processed in a transparent acrylic tube using water or 25% NaCl solution with or without 0.1% CMC (carboxymethyl cellulose), at room temperature, as the carrier fluid. The colors at the particle surface were visually observed and recorded as a function of time, and subsequently transformed to particle surface temperature versus time relationships. The analytical solution to the heat conduction problem for a sphere with uniform initial temperature, heated by a medium of constant temperature, with convective boundary conditions given by (66) was used together with the experimentally obtained particle surface temperatures to determine h_p. The effects of fluid viscosity, density, and flow rate, as well as particle size, were investigated.

For the experimental ranges studied, that is, $700 < Re < 22000$, $5 < Pr < 100$, and $0.2 < D_p/D_t < 0.3$, the following correlation equation was developed

$$Nu = 2.0 + 1.51 \, Re^{0.54} \, Pr^{0.24} \, (D_p/D_t)^{1.09}$$

with a correlation coefficient between predicted and experimental values of $R^2 = 0.88$.

Although the described methodology seems adequate in determining heat transfer coefficients at the liquid-particle interface for particles carried through a flowing medium, experimentation with actual food products is considered essential before equations of the above form could be used with aseptic processing.

PARTICLE RESIDENCE TIME DISTRIBUTION

In general, residence time of an element (*e.g.*, a fluid element, a particle, etc.) in a system (*e.g.*, a pipe, a tank, etc.) can be defined as the time elapsed from the element entering and leaving the system, or in other words, the time the element spends in the system. Presumably, for the cases where different elements travel through the system with different velocities, there is a distribution of the residence times. For homogeneous products and for the ideal cases where the velocity profiles are known, the residence time distribution can be predicted based on product and system characteristics, for example, for fully developed laminar flow of a Newtonian or a power-law fluid in a circular pipe (67). However, this is not the case for heterogeneous products. Currently, the residence time distribution of particulate foods processed in an aseptic system must be determined experimentally.

Considering the various components of the aseptic system, it is conceivable that particle residence time distribution experiments must be performed for each component (*e.g.*, holding tube, heater). Several investigators have studied particle residence time distribution in holding tubes, (28), (31)-(34), (39)-(41), or scraped surface heat exchangers (27), (33), (35)-(38), (41). Most of the above studies, with the exception of (27) and (41), were conducted at atmospheric pressure. Furthermore, residence times were mostly determined by monitoring (visually or by videotaping) colored particles as they were passing through transparent sections of the system. An alternative methodology for residence time measurements, suitable for opaque foods, has been developed using electro-magnetic induction (34). This method, with minor variations, has been used under commercial production conditions (41). A summary of this work, (41), is presented next.

The methodology is based on the induced electrical current as a result of the motion of a magnet towards or away from a circuit. Small magnetic strips were embedded in food particles (potato, carrots, or chicken alginate, 0.127 cm, cubes) and the voltage drop across coils, wrapped around the system pipes at selected positions was monitored as a function of time. Voltage readings above or below a baseline indicated the times that the tracer particles were passing through the coils. Residence time distribution data were collected for a range of experimental variables in a commercial aseptic system consisted of horizontal scraped surface heaters and coolers and a holding tube. The product was diced potatoes (1.27 cm cubes) in a starch slurry. Starch concentration was varied between 2 and 6%. The volume fraction of the potatoes was 12 to 25%. Product flowrate was 0.19 to 0.57 l/s. The scraped surface heat exchanger mutator speed was varied between 150 and 250 rpm. Product temperature at the exit at the last heater was controlled to 120 to 132 °C.

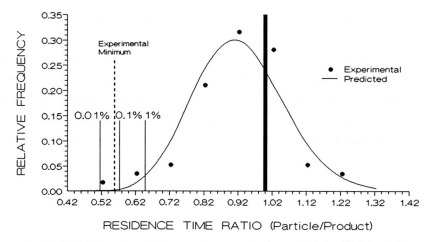

Figure 1. Relative residence time ratio frequency for the holding tube.

Figure 1 shows a typical relative frequency histogram of the residence time ratios (particle residence time over mean -based on the flow rate- product residence time) for the holding tube. Note that the majority of the particles were moving faster than the mean product velocity. In designing aseptic processes both data for the fastest moving particle and the distribution of residence times are needed: the former to ensure commercial sterility for the particle receiving the least heat treatment, while the latter to optimize processing conditions. In traditional in-container processing, thermal process design is based on the experimentally determined slowest heating container. For aseptic processing, process design can be based either on the experimentally determined, following the traditional approach, or on the statistically predicted, based on the residence time distribution data, fastest moving particle. However, several factors have to be considered before any statistical interpretation of the experimental data. Figure 1 shows a gamma distribution fitted to the experimental data together with selected critical residence time ratios below which only some small percentage of the data falls. The specific level upon which the critical residence time ratio will be based is still to be decided by the thermal processing authorities. If the obtained distribution cannot be described mathematically, then distribution free tolerance limits must be set based on the observed minimum residence time and the number of observations.

During this study, two distinct sets of experiments were performed. One in which multiple tracer particles were introduced at the same time, and another in which the tracer particles were introduced one at a time. For the experimental conditions studied, minimum particle to mean product residence time ratios greater than 0.5 (the laminar flow situation) were obtained for all the components of the aseptic system, except for two cases (one for the heater and one for the cooler) for the multiple particle introduction tests where values of 0.40 and 0.46, for the heater and the cooler, respectively, were found. This was attributed to the conservative way of analyzing the data for the multiple particle experiments; the possibility that the last particle entering could be the first one exiting the system had to be considered. However, this can lead to conservative estimations of minimum residence times. The importance of introducing tracer particles one at a time must be emphasized.

MATHEMATICAL MODELING

Several mathematical models applicable to aseptic processing of particulate foods have been proposed in the literature. Early models assumed an infinite liquid-particle film heat transfer coefficient (43), (44). A number of researchers, in order to decouple the fluid and particle temperatures for the solution of the governing equations, assumed a predescribed function for the fluid temperature (usually of a linear or exponential nature) for at least one of the components (e.g., heater) of the aseptic system (23), (43), (44), (55), (56). Several investigators have solved for fluid and particle temperatures simultaneously, using finite difference methods, (49) and (52), finite element methods, (47), or analytical procedures (45), (48), (57). Contrary to the numerical methods, the analytical solutions mentioned above were restricted to spherical particles. In addition, the concept of residence time distribution has been incorporated in the mathematical models by several investigations (44), (47), (52). The solution presented by (57) was used by (58) to study the effects of various parameters on process optimization. This work (58) is summarized below.

The differential equations governing the heat transfer problem under consideration are given by (refer to the nomenclature for symbol definitions)
Overall energy balance:

$$\varepsilon V \rho_f \frac{dT_f}{dt} = \frac{3 h_p (1-\varepsilon) V}{R_p} (T_p|_{r=R_p} - T_f) + H(T_m - T_f)$$

$$T_f(0) = T_{fi}$$

Heat conduction to spherical particles:

$$\frac{\partial^2 (r T_p)}{\partial r^2} = \frac{1}{\alpha_p} \frac{\partial (r T_p)}{\partial t}$$

$$-k_p \frac{\partial T_p}{\partial r}\Big|_{r-R_p} = h_p (T_p|_{r-R_p} - T_f)$$

$$T_p(0,t) = finite$$

$$T_p(r,0) = T_{pi}(r)$$

Basic assumptions that characterize the governing equations and their solution include: steady state conditions, spherical particles of uniform radius, constant thermal and physical properties for both particles and fluid, constant overall and liquid-particle heat transfer coefficients within each section, uniform fluid temperature in the radial direction, constant external medium temperature in each section, and plug flow, that is, particles and fluid travel through each section at the same velocity. Note, that h_p and the parameter H, defined as $H=U_oA$ can be different at each section (heater, holding tube, cooler). Furthermore, T_{fi} and T_{pi}, the initial fluid and particle temperatures, respectively, at the entrance of each section, are given by the corresponding temperatures at the exit of the previous section.

Using the solutions to the above equations presented by (57) and values for the heat transfer coefficients obtained through literature correlations, (26), (68) and (69), the effect of various parameters, including particle diameter, percent particles, fluid viscosity, target F_o value, heating medium temperature, and heating time, on microbial destruction and thiamine retention were studied. Microbial destruction was characterized by the center point F_o value given by

$$F_o = \int_0^t 10^{(T_p(r,\tau)-T_{ref})/z} d\tau$$

for r=0, T_{ref}=121.1 °C and z=10 °C.

Mass average thiamine retention in the particles was calculated by appropriate weighing averaging thiamine concentrations calculated at specific positions inside the particle, (70), through the following formula (2)

$$F^{27.8} = D_{T_{ref}}(\log a - \log b)$$

for D_{Tref}=130 min, and $F^{27.8}$ calculated by a similar equation as for F_o for z=27.8 °C and the appropriate $T_p(r,t)$.

The effect of particle size on optimum processing temperature based on thiamine retention on the particles, is shown in Figure 2. Smaller diameter particles retained more thiamine after processing. For larger particles, higher steam temperatures were required for

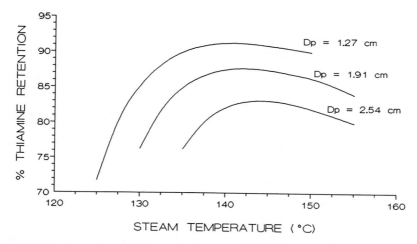

Figure 2. Effect of particle size on optimum steam temperature based on thiamine retention.

optimum processing and the optimum steam temperature range narrowed. Summarizing some of the results of the simulation, thiamine retention increased and optimum steam temperature decreased with decreasing fluid viscosity. In addition, higher steam temperatures were required when reducing the heating time or increasing the percent particles. Both these factors, however, seem to not significantly affect thiamine retention.

FUTURE WORK

To improve our understanding of aseptic processing of particulate foods, determinations of the liquid-particle film heat transfer coefficient and the particle residence time distribution using actual food products, under commercial conditions, must be performed. Studies with model food systems are considered necessary as starting point, in order to eliminate inherent variability of food characteristics. However, the results from model systems should not be extrapolated to food systems without precaution.

Finally, the effect of particle residence time distribution on the fluid and particle temperature profiles has not been fully explored and it is suggested as a possible topic for further research.

NOMENCLATURE

A	wall heat transfer area, m²
a	initial concentration of a heat labile substance, number of microorganisms/ml, g/ml, or any other appropriate unit
b	final concentration of a heat labile substance, number of microorganisms/ml, g/ml, or any other appropriate unit
C_{pf}	specific heat of fluid, J/kgK
C_{pp}	specific heat of particle, J/kgK
D_p	particle diameter, m
D_t	holding tube inside diameter, m
D_{Tref}	time at a constant reference temperature, T_{ref} required to achieve a decimal reduction of the initial concentration of a heat labile substance, s
F	time at a reference temperature, T_{ref}, required to destroy a given percentage of a heat labile substance whose thermal resistance is characterized by z, s
F_o	the F value for T_{ref} = 121.1 °C and z = 10 °C
$F^{27.8}$	the F value for T_{ref} = 121.1 °C and z = 27.8 °C
H	heat transfer parameter, between the external medium and the internal fluid, $H = U_o A$, W/K
h_p	liquid-particle film heat transfer coefficient, W/m²K
k_f	thermal conductivity of fluid, W/mK
k_p	thermal conductivity of particle, W/mK
Nu	Nusselt number, $Nu = h_p D_p / k_f$, dimensionless
Pr	Prandtl number, $Pr = \mu_f C_{pf} / k_f$, dimensionless
Re	Reynolds number, $Re = \rho_f V_f D_t / \mu_f$, dimensionless
R_p	particle radius, m
r	particle radial distance, m
$T_f(t)$	fluid temperature, °C
T_{fi}	initial fluid temperature, °C
$T_m(t)$	external medium temperature, °C
$T_p(r,t)$	particle temperature, °C
$T_{pi}(r)$	initial particle temperature, °C
T_{ref}	reference temperature, °C
t	heating time, $t = x/V_{avg}$, s
U_o	overall heat transfer coefficient, heating medium/wall/internal fluid, W/m²K

V	system volume, m^3
V_{avg}	average product velocity, m/s
V_f	average fluid velocity, m/s
x	longitudinal distance, m
z	temperature interval required for the time required to destroy a certain percentage of a heat labile substance to traverse a logarithmic cycle, °C
α_p	thermal diffusivity of particle, $\alpha_p = k_p/\rho_p C_{pp}$, m^2/s
ε	volume fraction of fluid, dimensionless
μ_f	fluid viscosity, Pa s
ρ_f	fluid density, kg/m^3
ρ_p	particle density, kg/m^3

REFERENCES

1 C.O. Ball and F.C.W. Olson, Sterilization in Food Technology. Theory, Practice, and Calculations, McGraw-Hill Book Co., New York, 1957.
2 C.R. Stumbo, Thermobacteriology in Food Processing. Academic Press, New York, 1973.
3 C.O. Ball, Food Res., 3 (1938) 13-55.
4 D.B. Lund, Food Technol., 31 (1977) 71-78.
5 D. Rose, D. Dairy Industries International, 51 (1986) 25-26, 29.
6 R.L. Merson and T.K. Wolcott, in: M. LeMaguer and P. Jelen (Eds), Food Engineering and Process Applications. Vol. 1: Transport Phenomena, Elsevier Science Publishing Co., New York, 1986, pp. 501-520.
7 E.L. Mitchell, in: C.O. Chichester, E.M. Mrak, and B.S. Schweigert (Eds), Advances in Food Research, Vol. 32, Academic Press, New York, 1987, pp. 1-37.
8 R.T. Toledo and S.Y. Chang, Food Technol., 44 (1990) 72-76.
9 N.G. Stoforos and R.L. Merson, in: W.E.L. Spiess and H. Schubert (Eds), Engineering and Food. Vol. 2: Preservation Processes and Related Techniques, Elsevier Applied Science Publishers LTD., Essex, England, 1990, pp. 50-59.
10 D.R. Heldman, Food Technol., 43 (1989) 122-123, 131.
11 D.M. Dignan, M.R. Berry, I.J. Pflug, and T.D. Gardine, Food Technol., 43 (1989) 118-121, 131.
12 I.J. Pflug, M.R. Berry, and D.M. Dignan, J. Food Protection, 53 (1990) 312-321.
13 D.I. Chandarana, presented at the Conference of Food Engineering, Food Engineering: Advances and Technologies, Chicago, IL, March 10-12, 1991.
14 G.M. Hunter, Food Technol. in Australia, 4 (1972) 158-165.
15 N.J. Heppell, presented at the Fourth International Congress on Engineering and Food, Edmonton, Alberta, Canada, July 7-10, 1985.
16 C.A. Zuritz, S. McCoy, and S.K. Sastry, ASAE Paper No. 87-6538, American Society of Agricultural Engineers, St. Joseph, MI, 1987.
17 S.K. Sastry, B.F. Heskitt, and J.L. Blaisdell, Food Technol., 43 (1989) 132-136, 143.

18 S.K. Sastry, M. Lima, J. Brim, T. Brunn, and B.F. Heskitt, J. Food Proc. Eng., 13 (1990) 239-253.
19 K.V. Chau and G.V. Snyder, Trans. ASAE, 31 (1988) 608-612.
20 D.I. Chandarana, A. Gavin III, and F.W. Wheaton, Food Technol., 43 (1989) 137-143.
21 D.I. Chandarana, A. Gavin III, and F.W. Wheaton, J. Food Proc. Eng., 13 (1990) 191-206.
22 D.I. Chandarana, A. Gavin III, and D.R. Heldman, in: W.E.L. Spiess and H. Schubert (Eds), Engineering and Food. Vol. 2: Preservation Processes and Related Techniques, Elsevier Applied Science Publishers LTD., Essex, England, 1990, pp. 31-49.
23 S.Y. Chang and R.T. Toledo, J. Food Sci., 54 (1989) 1017-1023, 1030.
24 S.Y. Chang and R.T. Toledo, J. Food Sci., 55 (1990) 199-205.
25 N.G. Stoforos and R.L. Merson, paper 47g, AIChE Annual Meeting, Washington, D.C., November 27 - December 2, 1988.
26 N.G. Stoforos, K.H. Park, and R.L. Merson, paper 545, IFT Annual Meeting, Chicago, IL, June 25-29, 1989.
27 D. Taeymans, E. Roelans, and J. Lenges, presented at the Fourth International Congress on Engineering and Food, Edmonton, Alberta, Canada, July 7-10, 1985.
28 S.C. McCoy, C.A. Zuritz, and S.K. Sastry, ASAE Paper No. 87-6536, American Society of Agricultural Engineers, St. Joseph, MI, 1987.
29 S.K. Sastry and C.A. Zuritz, J. Food Proc. Eng., 10 (1987) 27-52.
30 S.K. Sastry and C.A. Zuritz, ASAE Paper No. 87-6537, American Society of Agricultural Engineers, St. Joseph, MI, 1987.
31 B. Dutta and S.K. Sastry, J. Food Sci., 55 (1990) 1448-1453.
32 B. Dutta and S.K. Sastry, J. Food Sci., 55 (1990) 1703-1710.
33 L. Alkskog, L. Mejvik, and E. Karlsson, presented at the National Food Processors Association Annual Convention, Anaheim, CA, January 26 - February 1, 1989.
34 W.P. Segner, T.P. Ragusa, C.L. Marcus, and E.A. Soutter, J. Food Proc. Pres., 13 (1989) 257-274.
35 J.H. Lee and R.K. Singh, ASAE Paper 90-6522. American Society of Agricultural Engineers, St. Joseph, MI, 1990.
36 J.H. Lee and R.K. Singh, (J. Food Proc. Eng.), in press.
37 J.H. Lee and R.K. Singh, (J. Food Sci.), in press.
38 J.H. Lee and R.K. Singh, (J. Food Eng.), submitted for publication.
39 C.W. Hong, B. Sun Pan, R.T. Toledo, and K.M. Chiou, J. Food Sci., 56 (1991) 255-256, 259.
40 M.R. Berry, in: J.V. Chambers (Ed.), Innovations in Aseptic Processing. Proceedings of the First International Congress on Aseptic Processing Technologies, Indianapolis, IN, March 19-21, 1989, pp. 6-17.
41 D.I. Chandarana, J.A. Unverferth, N.G. Stoforos, A. Gavin III, and K.A. Koshute, paper 534, IFT Annual Meeting, Dallas, TX, June 1-5, 1991.
42 R.J. Hampton, in: Proceedings on Aseptodynamics, The Food Processors Institute, Washington, D.C., 1972, pp. 43-47.
43 P.W. de Ruyter and R. Brunet, Food Technol., 27 (1973) 44-51.
44 J.E. Manson and J.F. Cullen, J. Food Sci., 39 (1974) 1084-1089.
45 J.W. Hemmings and J. Kern, Int. J. Heat Mass Transfer., 22 (1979) 99-109.
46 R. Dail, J. Food Sci., 50 (1985) 1703-1706.
47 S.K. Sastry, J. Food Sci., 51 (1986) 1323-1328, 1332.
48 H. Sawada and R.L. Merson, in: M. LeMaguer and P. Jelen (Eds), Food Engineering and Process Applications. Vol. 1: Transport Phenomena, Elsevier Science Publishing Co., New York, 1986, pp. 569-581.

49 A. Aström, T. Ohlsson, C. Skjöldebrand, and C. Falk, presented at the International Symposium on Progress in Food Preservation Processes, CERIA, Brussels, Belgium, April 12-15, 1988.
50 J.W. Larkin, Food Technol., 43 (1989) 124-131.
51 T. Ohlsson, in: J.V. Chambers (Ed.), Innovations in Aseptic Processing. Proceedings of the First International Congress on Aseptic Processing Technologies, Indianapolis, IN, March 19-21, 1989, pp. 46-55.
52 D.I. Chandarana and A. Gavin III, J.Food Sci., 54 (1989) 198-204.
53 J.H. Lee, R.K. Singh, and D.I. Chandarana, J. Food Proc. Eng., 12 (1990) 295-321.
54 J.H. Lee and R.K. Singh, Chem. Eng. Comm., 87 (1990) 21-51.
55 J.H. Lee and R.K. Singh, J. Food Eng., 11 (1990) 67-92.
56 P.M. Armenante and M.A. Leskowicz, Biotechnol. Prog., 6 (1990) 292-306.
57 R.L. Merson and H. Sawada, presented at the Conference of Food Engineering, Food Engineering: Advances and Technologies, Chicago, IL, March 10-12, 1991.
58 N.G. Stoforos, H. Sawada, and R.L. Merson, paper 172, IFT Annual Meeting, Anaheim, CA, June 16-20, 1990.
59 W.E. Ranz and W.R. Marshall, Chem. Eng. Prog., 48 (1952) 173-180.
60 S. Whitaker, AIChE J., 18 (1972) 361-371.
61 M.F. Berry, presented at the 7th World Congress of Food Science and Technology, Singapore, 1987 (abstract).
62 M.F. Berry, in: J.V. Chambers (Ed.), Innovations in Aseptic Processing. Proceedings of the First International Congress on Aseptic Processing Technologies, Indianapolis, IN, March 19-21, 1989, pp. 128-156.
63 G. Cerny, A. Fink, and A. Pecher, in: J.V. Chambers (Ed.), Innovations in Aseptic Processing. Proceedings of the First International Congress on Aseptic Processing Technologies, Indianapolis, IN, March 19-21, 1989, pp. 112-123.
64 N.G. Stoforos and R.L. Merson, (Biotechnol. Prog.), in press.
65 N.G. Stoforos and R.L. Merson, (J. Food Sci.), submitted for publication.
66 H.S. Carslaw and J.C. Jaeger, Conduction of Heat in Solids, 2nd ed. Clarendon Press, Oxford, England, 1959.
67 M.A. Rao and M. Loncin, Lebensm. -Wiss. u. Technol., 7 (1974) 5-13.
68 A.M. Trommelen, W.J. Beek, and H.C. van de Westelaken, Chem. Eng. Sci., 26 (1971) 1987-2001.
69 C.C. Monrad and J.F. Pelton, (1942), cited by D.R. Heldman and R.P. Singh, Food Process Engineering, 2nd ed. AVI Publishing Co. Inc., Westport, CT, 1981.
70 K. Hayakawa, Can. Inst. Food Technol. J., 4 (1971) 133-134.

G. Charalambous (Ed.), Food Science and Human Nutrition
© 1992 Elsevier Science Publishers B.V. All rights reserved.

DIABETES: FOOD, NUTRITION, DIET AND WEIGHT CONTROL

A. A. KHAN

Applied Research, Inc; P. O. Box 1486, Hawthorne, California 90250 (U.S.A.)

SUMMARY

Diabetes is on the increase in every country. In the United States there are more than 12 million known diabetics, and it is the third ranking cause of death. It has been shown that diet low in fat and rich in complex carbohydrates can reverse the diabetic condition or decrease the severity. Increasing fiber in the diet can lower cholesterol in the blood, and it can also control or cure diabetes. Moreover, it has been demonstrated that a diet low in fat and as high as 70% beans can reduce blood pressure, cancer and heart disease. Though there is no cure for diabetes, it can be controlled by diet, exercise, hypoglycemic drugs and insulin therapy.

HISTORY OF DIABETES

The disease known as diabetes has been recognized from antiquity. Over two thousand years ago Hippocrates described it. The word diabetes is of Greek origin and means "going through." Celsus, a Roman medical writer, gave it the name diabetes mellitus. This comes from the Greek and Latin: diabetes (to pass through) and mellitus (honey). It was applied to conditions in which too much water "went through" the body, as when excessive thirst is associated with an abnormally increased urinary output. In the days when no clinical laboratories existed, an important diagnostic test was the taste of urine, in addition to its smell and appearance. It was found that in some cases of diabetes, the urine tasted sweet, and so they called this condition diabetes mellitus, the "honey sweet going through." In other cases, the urine was clear and neither sweet nor salty, it tasted just like water. The diagnostics of the fourteenth century called this disorder diabetes insipidus, the "tasteless going through." These two designations are still in common use, though it is now known that diabetes mellitus has nothing to do with diabetes insipidus. Here we are only concerned with diabetes mellitus, the passage of sugar in the urine, also known as glycosuria.

It was not, however, until the year 1922 that any major breakthrough occurred related to the treatment of diabetes. At that time, two Canadians, Dr. Frederick Banting and Charles Best, who worked in the University of Toronto, discovered insulin, and revolutionized the treatment of diabetes.[1] Simply stated, diabetes mellitus is an "energy crisis" in the body. It is a state in which the body does not use glucose properly to produce energy. The major reason for this condition is inadequate production or use of insulin by the body. Insulin, a hormone produced by the pancreas, is necessary in order for the body to efficiently use sugar for energy.

Though accurate statistics are not available, it is known that diabetes has increased markedly during the past 10 years. It is estimated that there are more than 12 million known diabetics in the United States.

Diabetes may develop at any age, but most of the cases appear after middle life. There is a higher incidence of diabetes among urban rather than rural populations. The exact cause of diabetes is not known definitely. Observations show that an overweight condition and overeating, especially of sugars and starches together with a lack of exercise, are all contributing factors. Diabetes occurs in all races and nationalities. Statistics show that diabetes is most likely to occur in persons who have diabetic relatives, hence, heredity is a factor.

Recent studies on genetic and environmental factors influencing the development of diabetes have led to considerable advancement in the understanding of the disease, but the cause (causes?) of it remain a mystery. Diabetes is the third ranking cause of death in the United States, and remains one of the most crippling of all diseases because of its chronicity and complications (i.e. arteriosclerotic heart disease, hypertension, renal failure and blindness).

Detection of diabetes in its earliest stages is absolutely essential to the future health of the person who suffers from this condition. Although diabetes cannot be cured by current available treatments, it can be controlled by hypoglycemic drugs and insulin therapy. As a result, large numbers of diabetics are able to lead normal, productive and fulfilling lives.

Over the centuries diet has been considered as a possible cure for many medical problems: thus it is not surprising that early Physicians considered diet a way to control diabetes. One of the first pioneers in this field was Dr. John Rollo, who in

1796, suggested a diet regimen low in carbohydrates and high in protein to treat diabetic patients.[2] An Italian Physician, Dr. Arnold Cantani, who practiced in the second half of the 19th century, introduced alternate fast days to his patients in addition to lean meats and fat diet. The really pace-setting doctrine for diabetics, introduced by Dr. Frederick Allen of the Rockefeller Institute for Medical Research called for systematic undernutrition. In a typical case, treatment began with a seven-day fast during which the patient was daily allowed four bran muffins and some fluids, none of which provided any calories. Since the diet emphasized total restriction of calories, various foods were recommended which offered bulk without nutrition. One of these foods was bran, a major part of the bulk in the Allen Diet.[3] During the 1940s and 1950s, Walter Kemper in the United States treated hundreds of diabetics and cardiovascular patients with a diet consisting of rice, fruits and low sodium vegetables.[4]

Although the importance of dietary restrictions has been demonstrated objectively, a report indicates that only three out of four diabetics are given diets, and only about one-half of those patients appear to understand their purpose. The American Diabetes Association estimates that roughly only 15 percent of patients follow prescribed diets. Therefore, motivation in patients is essential if control of diabetes is to be successful.

PANCREAS

The pancreas is a soft, fleshy, pinkish gland lying on the posterior wall of the abdomen in the curve of the duodenum.

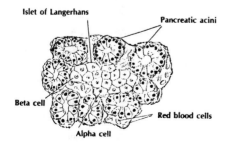

Figure I. Physiologic Anatomy of the Pancreas.

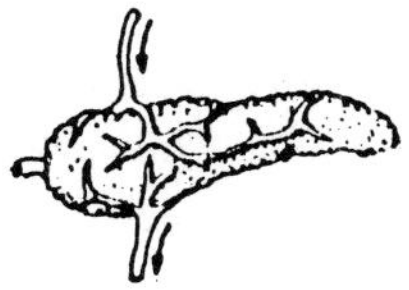

Figure II. A Human Pancreas Islets of Langerhans secrete insulin which reduces blood glucose level.

Its main function is the production of digestive enzymes, which enter the duodenum through the pancreatic duct. It also contains numerous Islets of Langerhans, which are clumps of specialized cells producing hormones (insulin and glucagon). Fig. 1

The normal functioning of all the cells in the body depends upon an adequate supply of glucose in the blood which reaches them, and the amount present (the blood sugar level) varies from 4.0 to 6.0 mml/l (70 to 120 mg per 100 ml) in the fasting state. The blood sugar level is controlled partly by the dietary intake and mainly by the hormones of the pancreas (insulin and glucagon), pituitary and suprarenal glands. Insulin is secreted in response to a rise in blood sugar level above its normal value. It stops the breakdown of liver glycogen into glucose and increases the tissue utilization and storage of glucose; it therefore helps to reduce the level of blood sugar. The hormone glucagon raises the blood sugar level when it descends too far by stimulating the breakdown of glycogen into glucose in the liver. A rise in blood sugar level increases the secretion of insulin and reduces that of glucagon.

In diabetes mellitus, the blood sugar level is abnormally high, and there is little or no secretion of insulin in response to a carbohydrate meal. The high blood sugar level leads to the excretion of much sugar in the urine, together with large quantities of water because of the osmotic pressure effect of sugar in solution.

Langerhans first described small nests of the islets as highly vascularized cells which are independent of the duct system of the pancreas.[5] These islets maintain their functional integrity following legation of the pancreatic ducts, whereas the acinar tissue becomes atrophic. The total volume of islet tissue makes up about 1% to 3% of the entire pancreas. Three cell types have been shown to be present in the Islets of Langerhans, and they have been differentiated on the basis of their solubility and affinity to certain stains. The alpha cells contain fine granules that are soluble in alcohol and which stain bright red with Mallory or Mason staining methods. They are relatively few in numbers and are a source of glucagon. The beta cells contain small alcohol soluble granules which stain orange-brown with the above methods. They are the source of insulin and make up about 75% of the islet tissue. The delta cells do not contain granules and their functional significance is unknown, but they act as mother cells to the alpha and beta cells.

Insulin is synthesized in the beta cells of the pancreas and is stored in the cell in the form of packets of granules. Zinc is essential for the formation and storage of insulin granules. When the blood glucose level rises, the granules in the beta cells move toward the cell membrane and fuse with it, thereby releasing their contents. Insulin then enters the circulatory system through the portal vein.

The normal functioning of all the cells in the body depends upon an adequate supply of glucose in the blood which reaches them. The blood sugar level is controlled partly by the dietary intake but mainly by the hormones of the pancreas (insulin and glucagon), pituitary, and suprarenal glands. Insulin is secreted in response to a rise in the blood sugar level above its normal value. The hormone glucagon raises the blood sugar level when it descends too far by stimulating the breakdown of glycogen into glucose in the liver. A rise in the blood sugar level increases the secretion of insulin and reduces that of glucagon.

The normal concentration of sugar in the blood under fasting conditions is usually from 80mg to 115mg per 100ml. This may vary due to your state of health or age. Following a meal containing carbohydrates, there is an elevation of the blood sugar to a concentration of 130mg to 140mg per 100ml of blood. This may also vary with the increase of age. This concentration of sugar is soon reduced to the normal level, partly by the conversion of glucose to glycogen and the storage of the latter (in the liver), and partly by the oxidation of glucose to carbon dioxide and water. Continuous hyperglycemia, or elevation of the blood sugar level above normal, is an abnormal condition. If under fasting conditions, the circulating level of the blood sugar is found to be in excess of 120mg per 100ml, there is some bodily dysfunction. The condition in which there is an insufficient production or inefficient use of insulin by the body is known as diabetic mellitus. In this disease there is a failure to store and burn glucose. It is characterized by an increased blood sugar and by glycosuria. The high blood sugar leads to the secretion of much sugar in the urine, together with large quantities of water because of the osmotic pressure effect of sugar in solution.

THE FOOD YOU EAT

What a person eats for breakfast depends greatly on who he is. A man who works all day in his office should not eat the same breakfast as a soldier who is on the march all day. You do not have the same breakfast as that of a two-year-old child. A person's needs at breakfast, and during the rest of the day, depend on that person's age, occupation, state of health, sex, or the season. These factors do not entirely cover the case, for habit and custom have much to do with what one eats. For example, oranges are habitually used for breakfast in American homes. When a large number of people have the same habit, it is called a custom. Evidence of the effect of the customs on what people eat is found by comparing the typical American, English and Mexican menus. The division of the day's food into meals is largely a matter of custom and varies in different parts of the world.

The word breakfast means exactly what it says. We break our fast. For twelve hours or more we have eaten nothing. For at least eight hours of that time we have been relaxed in sleep, or should have been. To start our bodies out for the day with no breakfast would be like trying to ride a train without buying a ticket.

Breakfast varies less than perhaps any other meal. Any breakfast menu will contain some of these foods: fruits, cereals, beverages, breads, eggs, bacon, or perhaps a meat. A breakfast consisting of all these items is termed a heavy breakfast. A breakfast consisting of a good number of these items, but not all, is considered a medium breakfast. A breakfast consisting of only two or three is considered a light or very light breakfast. You should eat a medium breakfast, and should include the following: oat bran cereal or oats and oat bran both, milk, two eggs, orange juice, and whole wheat toast. As a dietary supplement, you must take one 20mg to 25mg zinc tablet and a tablespoonful of brewer's yeast powder during breakfast.

Three meals each day is the first step to good nutrition. Growing boys and girls need proportionately more food than adults because they are building their bodies. Three meals a day are not sufficient for young children, and at times even older children need more than three meals daily.

People under twenty years of age are more often underweight than overweight. This means if they omit breakfast they miss one of the three chances to get building materials and fuel supplies. The person who goes without breakfast runs a great risk of being undernourished, a condition which may cause susceptibility to disease, bad teeth, nervousness, early old age, or other disorders.

Your lunch and dinner should consist of the following: lean meat, beans (legumes), vegetables, fruits, and whole wheat bread. You may make little changes in the menu by adding salad instead of bread, fruit, or vegetables. However, you should eat a bean of your choice with lunch and dinner. In addition, you should eat oysters and seafood twice a week.

After two or three weeks, depending on how you feel, you may discontinue the zinc tablets after breakfast. At bedtime, you may have a fruit, juice or a cup of milk.

All fruits or juices should be unsweetened. Unsweetened means that no sugar has been added to what is present naturally. Pastries, sweet rolls, doughnuts, desserts, pies, cakes, chocolates, cookies, and white bread should be avoided.

You may eat the above-mentioned diet of about 1400 cal. to 1600 cal. a day, in which 60% to 70% of the calories come from the complex carbohydrates of beans (legumes), 5% to 12% from fat, and the remaining from protein. Your diet is rich in fiber so you should not add any extra fiber to what you eat.

Under the direction of Leo Paul Krall of the Juslin Clinic in Boston, a ten-year study was conducted on diabetic airline pilots. In order to keep their jobs, the pilots were asked to control their diabetes by diet alone. They were given a diet of 1540 cal. a day that was high in nutrients. Krall found that the pilots reduced their weight and stayed in excellent physical condition.[6] A diet of 1540 cal. was not a starvation diet.

Research has shown that increasing fiber in the diet may reduce the needs of diabetics for insulin or hypoglycemic drugs. Until recently, traditional diabetic diet, recommended by physicians or dietitians, contained 40% of the total calories as carbohydrates.[7] No recommendation was made to include a specific level of dietary fiber among the carbohydrate sources. Recently, high-fiber diets comprised of complex carbohydrates have allowed reductions or even withdrawals of insulin in diabetics.

A group in the United States headed by James W. Anderson has treated diabetics on a diet consisting of seventy-five percent complex carbohydrate calories, nine percent fat calories and high fiber.[8,9] David J. A. Jenkins has given patients a high fiber and high carbohydrate diet. The diet consisted of 22% to 61% complex carbohydrate. The patients showed 64% reduction in diabetes.[10] Some patients recovered completely.

Other investigators have also found considerable improvement or total recovery in the diabetic condition using leguminous or high-fiber diets.[11] J. M. Whitaker has also recommended a diet high in complex carbohydrates, low in fat, and a natural approach to the diabetes problem.[12]

A vast majority of the people in India are lactovegetarian. Physicians have treated diabetics there by giving them a diet in which up to 70% of the calories come from legumes and grains. In Asian countries, people generally consume diets high in complex carbohydrates and have a very low incidence of diabetes.

Jenkins has found that beans are as effective as oats in lowering cholesterol levels. Jenkins has further shown that many people can lower their cholesterol 13% to 14% by eating two servings of beans each day.[13] Anderson has demonstrated that a diet of oat bran as a source of fiber reduces high blood cholesterol. Anderson's studies indicate that increased fiber intake not only lowers blood cholesterol but also provides other health benefits. Five major health problems in the United States are heart disease, cancer, high blood pressure, obesity, and diabetes. According to Anderson, fiber reduces the risk of developing these problems and also acts therapeutically to reverse most of these conditions (except cancer) after they develop.[14]

We know from research studies that fiber in the diet helps diabetics and patients suffering from heart diseases. There are several kinds of fibers present in plants, vegetables and fruits. Each kind of fiber has its own specific function in your digestive system. To simplify the fibers, they may be classified into two broad categories. One is insoluble fiber (found in bran) that does not dissolve in water. Cellulose, hemicellulose, and lignin are known to ease constipation since they speed the food through the digestive tract. Water insoluble fiber or roughage does not influence blood sugar or decrease the blood cholesterol level, but has beneficial effects on the digestive tract since it acts as nature's laxative.

The soluble fibers, pectin and gums, do help in diabetes, and they lower blood cholesterol, which can lower your chances of heart attack. Water soluble fibers are found abundantly in beans, legumes, fruits and vegetables.

Lowering of cholesterol and fat in the blood also results in better control of the blood sugar level in the diabetic. Oat bran, dried beans (legumes), and broccoli are an excellent source of soluble fiber; moreover, they are also a good source of zinc, manganese, chromium, and other trace metals in our diet.

In general, you should focus your diet on wholesome, fresh fruits, vegetables, lean meat, whole wheat bread, and unrefined grains. They will provide not only more health-promoting fiber, but also vitamins and minerals. The more "whole" and unprocessed a food is, the better it tends to be for you.

Remember, your mood, vitality, and ability to cope all depend on maintaining a normal blood-sugar level.

THE IMPORTANCE OF NUTRITION

Health is a combination of many factors, of which nutrition is one of the most important. Good nutrition means better health and happier lives to all of us. Good nutrition means eating right. It means an adequate diet. Good nutrition helps to promote strong and healthy bodies, better appearance, active and keen minds, greater resistance to disease, and longer life.

Poor nutrition means wrong eating habits. It means an inadequate diet. Poor nutrition may contribute to weak and undernourished bodies, bad teeth, poor mental development, nervousness, lowered resistance to disease, and a lack of endurance. Deficiencies of specific food essentials do not occur very often today in our country. However, certain pronounced deficiencies in the diets of some people do exist, and their effects have been known for a long time. For example, it is known that scurvy is caused by a lack of vitamin C, and rickets by a lack of vitamin D. Partial deficiencies in the diet, however, are much more common than pronounced deficiencies. Such ailments as night blindness caused by a partial lack of vitamin A and bleeding gums arising from insufficient vitamin C are examples of the effect of partial deficiencies.

You and every other human being are made up of approximately 17 different elements. Each of these 17 elements must be supplied to our body through food or drinking water. These elements are not present in the body as free elements but are combined in hundreds of ways to make the various chemical compounds which add up to being the human body.

According to a report by former U.S. Surgeon General, C. Everett Koop, there is a link between food, diabetes, cancer, high blood pressure and heart disease. Everyone needs a nutritious diet to maintain a healthy body whether they have diabetes or not. Let us look at the nutrients that make up a well balanced diet.

NUTRIENTS

Protein

The proteins are the chief nitrogen containing components of food and of the human body. They have large complex molecules built of simple amino acids in various proportions. There are twenty-three different amino acids in the human body and they can combine to form millions of different protein molecules. Thirteen amino acids can be synthesized in the body but the other ten either cannot be produced at all or not in sufficient quantities. They are, therefore, indispensable in a diet adequate for growth and are called essential amino acids. Animal proteins, which are most expensive, contain the essential amino acids in adequate quantities. Vegetable proteins contain much less essential amino acids, but even so, beans and nuts are better sources of protein than grains. Foods that are good sources of proteins are meat, eggs, milk and cheese.

Fat

Fats are used for energy and to carry fat-soluble vitamins within the body. Many types of fats cannot be made in the body. Therefore, we need to include some fat-containing foods in our diet every day. Good sources of fat are butter, margarine, oil, and salad dressings.

Carbohydrate

Carbohydrate is the scientific name for sugars and starches and is the major source of energy for the body. If too little carbohydrate and fat are eaten, the body must use protein to supply the energy needed. Carbohydrates may be divided into two categories: simple and complex. For example, table sugar, honey, and candy are simple carbohydrates; and bread, potatoes and rice are complex carbohydrates.

Foods rich in simple carbohydrates are very easily digested or broken down into sugar (glucose) which enters the bloodstream and raises the blood sugar level quickly. Starches or complex carbohydrates are more complicated in their structure than sugars and are digested more slowly. The sugar that comes from their digestion enters the bloodstream more slowly.

Vitamins and Minerals

Vitamins and minerals are also needed for good health as they are used for many purposes in the body such as good vision, strong bones and teeth, and healthy skin. These nutrients are found in varying amounts in all foods. If a well-balanced diet is eaten daily, which includes food from all of the exchange lists, the necessary amount of vitamins and minerals good health should be obtained. It should be remembered that all foods will be partly turned into a sugar called "glucose" in the body. Glucose is the fuel a person's body uses for energy.

```
        58% of Protein  . . . . . . . . . . . Glucose
        10% of Fat  . . . . . . . . . . . . . Glucose
       100% of Carbohydrate  . . . . . . . . . Glucose
```

This is the reason that all foods, including fat and protein, must be calculated in the diabetic diet, not just the carbohydrate.

There are no known advantages to consuming excess amounts of any nutrients. You may rarely need to take vitamins and minerals if you eat a wide variety of foods. There are a few important exceptions to this general statement. Women in their childbearing years may need to take iron supplements to replace the iron they lose with menstrual bleeding. Women who are no longer menstruating should not take iron supplements routinely. Women who are pregnant or who are breast feeding need more of many nutrients, especially iron, folic acid, vitamin A, calcium, and sources of energy (calories from carbohydrates, proteins, and fats).

In general, you should try to focus your diet on wholesome, fiber-rich foods such as fresh fruits and vegetables, whole wheat breads and unrefined grains. They will contribute not only more health promoting fiber, but also vitamins and minerals. The more "whole" and unprocessed a food is, the better it tends to be for you.

WEIGHT CONTROL

The first and most important function of food for the body is to supply energy. The body needs energy for metabolic purposes to support physical activities, growth, and to maintain body temperature. Food is the fuel for all metabolic purposes and its energy value is measured in calories.

Calories:

A calorie is a measure of the heat the body uses for energy. Almost every food contains some calories. Protein and carbohydrate provide four calories per gram while each gram of fat provides nine calories.

The normal adult requires sufficient calories to balance the total loss from his body. It is obvious that the manual laborer needs more calories than the individual who is engaged in light work. The caloric demands are also influenced by external temperature and, hence, by climate. When more calories are given off by an individual than are taken in the form of food, he is no longer in a state of caloric equilibrium. Calories are produced under these circumstances, at the expense of the tissues, and there is a loss of weight. It is important to bear in mind that the growing child should be provided with more food than is sufficient for the maintenance of the energy balance. The normal state for the growing child is a condition of positive caloric balance.

It is very important to the control of diabetes that you be the ideal weight for your height. Eighty percent of adults who are discovered to be diabetic are overweight at the time they are diagnosed. An individual who is 20% over their ideal weight is obese. Ideal weight is the weight at which an individual functions well and feels best.

HEIGHT AND WEIGHT TABLE

DESIRABLE WEIGHTS FOR MEN AND WOMEN
ACCORDING TO HEIGHT AND FRAME, AGES 25 AND OVER

Height (in Shoes, 1-Inch Heels)		MEN Weight in Pounds (in Indoor Clothing)			Height (in Shoes, 2-Inch Heels)		WOMEN Weight in Pounds (in Indoor Clothing)		
Feet	Inches	Small Frame	Medium Frame	Large Frame	Feet	Inches	Small Frame	Medium Frame	Large Frame
5	2	112-120	118-129	126-141	4	10	92-98	96-107	104-119
5	3	115-123	121-133	129-144	4	11	94-101	98-110	106-122
5	4	118-126	124-136	132-148	5	0	96-104	101-113	109-125
5	5	121-129	127-139	135-152	5	1	99-107	104-116	112-128
5	6	124-133	130-143	138-156	5	2	102-110	107-119	115-131
5	7	128-137	134-147	142-161	5	3	105-113	110-122	118-134
5	8	132-141	138-152	147-166	5	4	108-116	113-126	121-138
5	9	136-145	142-156	151-170	5	5	111-119	116-130	125-142
5	10	140-150	146-160	155-174	5	6	114-123	120-135	129-146
5	11	144-154	150-165	159-179	5	7	118-127	124-139	133-150
6	0	148-158	154-170	164-184	5	8	122-131	128-143	137-154
6	1	152-162	158-175	168-189	5	9	126-135	132-147	141-158
6	2	156-167	162-180	173-194	5	10	130-140	136-151	145-163
6	3	160-171	167-185	178-199	5	11	134-144	140-155	149-168
6	4	164-175	172-190	182-204	6	0	138-148	144-159	153-173

Weight control is a matter of energy balance. That is, balancing your food intake with your energy output per day. A calorie is a means of measuring energy. Food is usually measured in calories. For example:

Food Input (calories)	Body Weight	Energy Output (calories)
1800 cal.	Maintain Weight	1800 cal.
2000 cal. (+ 200 cal.)	Gain Weight	1800 cal.
1600 cal. (- 200 cal.)	Lose Weight	1800 cal.

The Food and Nutrition Board of the National Research Council has made recommendations for the number of calories required by men of different ages, engaged in moderate activity and weighing 154 pounds. Similar recommendations have been made for women weighing 128 pounds. These recommendations, however, are not for diabetics. For those who do not wish to keep a daily record of their activities and wish to make a quick estimate of calories required each day, the following allowances may be used. For men: for moderate activity, 20 calories per pound of weight; for heavy work, 24 calories; and for sedentary work, 14 calories. For women: per pound of weight for moderate activity, 13 calories; for heavy work, 18 calories; and for sedentary activity, 11 calories. Multiply total calories per pound for 24 hours by your weight in pounds to obtain your total caloric requirement for one day. If your actual weight falls outside of the desirable range in weight suggested for your height, it is preferable to multiply by your desirable weight (see Table 4, height and weight table).

If you are very much overweight, it may be desirable to arbitrarily set the caloric requirement to 1200 or 1400 calories per day. It is almost impossible to obtain from foods all the mineral elements and vitamins needed each day if the food intake is less than 1200 calories. If the food supplies 1400 calories daily, the loss of weight may be a little slower but the diet may be more adequate. A good reducing diet is one which is low in calories and high in other essential nutrients: proteins, mineral elements, and vitamins. Increasing the exercise and decreasing the calories simultaneously is an effective procedure for reducing weight.

There is no magic formula or food that will cause weight loss. It is strictly a matter of burning more calories than are eaten. A diet for weight loss should still be well balanced and should consist of three meals and a snack following your regular meal schedule.

When you accumulate 3500 calories more than you use up, you gain one pound. On the other hand, if you use up 3500 calories more than you eat, you will then lose one pound of stored body fat. Anyone who wants to lose weight must eat fewer calories than the body needs to maintain normal weight. A person must decrease food intake by 3500 calories to lose one pound of fat. To make up for the decrease in food intake, your body will burn the stored fat for energy and weight will be lost.

If you are underweight, the calories required should be increased by several hundred calories daily. The food selected for gaining weight should also provide liberal contributions of all essential nutrients as well as extra calories. Decreasing the exercise and increasing the calories simultaneously is an effective procedure for gaining weight.

Regular exercise or physical activity is as important as insulin and diet in treating diabetes. It may lower blood cholesterol levels, help maintain a normal cholesterol level, and, by increasing circulation, help the blood vessels to perform more effectively. When combined with a nutritious diet, exercise can help you lose weight or maintain your ideal weight by burning excess calories and helping to control your appetite. Proper exercise may also give you more energy, help you sleep better, improve your appearance, and contribute to good mental health.

In short, your goals are to lose excess weight and maintain optimum weight, maintain proper nutrition and control diabetes as weight changes. Also, look for imbalances in carbohydrate, protein, and fat distribution in your diet.

REFERENCES

1 Banting, F. G. and Best, C.H., J. Lab. Clin. Med. 1922, 7, 251.

2 Rollo, J., Cases of the Diabetes Mellitus with the Results of the Trial of Certain Acids, and Other Substances in the Cure of the Lens Venera, 1798, 2nd Edition, C. Dilly, London

3 Allen, F. M., J. Amer. Med. Assn. 1914, 63, 359

4 Kemper, W., Peschel, R. L., and Schlayer, C., Postgrad. Med. 1958, 24, 359

5 Langerhans, P., Zur Mikroskopischem Anatomie der Bauchspeicheldruse, 1869, Inaugural Dissertation, Berlin

6 Krall, L. P., Goals of Treatment and Why They Are Not Achieved, in Internat. Diabetes Foundation, VII Congress, 1973, Brussels, P. 645

7 Simpson, H. C. R., Lousley, S., Greehie, M., Maun, J. I., Simpson, R. W., Carter, R. D., Hockaday, T. D. R., Lancet, 1981, 3, 1

8 Anderson, J. W., and Ward, K., Diabetes Care, 1, 1977

9 Anderson, J. and Seiling, B., Geriatrics, 1981, 36, 64

10 Jenkins, D. J. A.; Wolever, T. M. S.; Bacon, S.; Nineham, R.; Leeds, R.; Love, M.; and Hockaday, T. D. R., Amer. Jrnl. Clin. Nutr., 1980, 33, 1729

11 Simpson, R. W.; Mann, J. I.; Eaton, J.; Moore, R. A.; Carter, R. D.; and Hockaday, T. D. R., British Med. Jrnl. 1982, 284, 1608

12   Whitaker, J. M., Let Us Live, Nov. 1985, p. 8

13   Hall, T., Beans, Old or New, Win Fans Among Chefs and Nutritionists, The New York Times, Jan. 25, 1989, p. C6

14   Anderson, J. W., A Diet That Can Save Your Life, The Saturday Evening Post, Sept. 1988, p. 90

CURRENT APPROACHES TO THE STUDY OF MEAT FLAVOR QUALITY.

A. M. Spanier

Food Flavor Quality - Meat Program, USDA, ARS, SRRC, 1100 Robert E. Lee Blvd., New Orleans, LA 70124

SUMMARY

The long-term goals of food technologists and biotechnologists are to design muscle foods based upon a desired function such as enriched/enhanced flavor quality. This very ambitious, yet obtainable, goal requires a complete understanding of the factors involved in the development and deterioration of flavor in muscle foods. This, of course, involves a thorough understanding of the rules governing muscle/meat structure and function and the basis for any given reaction mechanism in the muscle food. While we are still a long way from completely unlocking the puzzling relationships between meat structure and flavor, some of the technical achievements over the last few decades have provided the basic machinery to study the complex nature of the problem of food quality in general and muscle food quality in particular. Factors such as lipid oxidation, cooking temperature, storage time, Maillard product formation and activity, muscle proteins and enzymes, all play an important role in the generation and deterioration of the flavor of a muscle food. This chapter outlines some of the more recent work dealing with meat flavor.

1. **MEAT FLAVOR QUALITY:**

The flavor quality of a muscle food is dependent upon several key pre- and postmortem factors. These factors include, but are not limited to, the animal's age, breed, sex, and nutritional status as well as all of the postmortem handling and cooking protocols. While both of the pre- and postmortem factors are involved in the development of the food's final flavor and texture, the most important factors are those which develop during the postmortem aging period (1) and during postmortem handling, cooking, and storage (2-6).

As meat ages and as it is cooked or stored...during the postmortem period...it shows a significant alteration in the level of numerous endogenous chemical components such as sugars, organic acids, peptides and free amino acids, and products of adenine nucleotide metabolism, e.g., adenosine triphosphate (ATP). Many of these changes are due to enhanced hydrolytic activity (7). No matter what the history of the meat, as it is stored and heated, both desirable and undesirable flavors develop from the proteolysis, thermal degradation and interaction of sugars, amino acids, and nucleotides. Lipid oxidation is also a major producer of undesirable flavor components. These chemical modifications to the muscle food serve as a pool of reactive flavor compounds and flavor intermediates which later interact to form additional flavor notes during cooking such as the Maillard reaction products formed during the heating of sugars and amino acids (8, 9). It becomes immediately apparent, therefore, that the development of flavor in a muscle food is an extremely complicated process which occurs continuously from the moment of slaughter, continues through cooking and storage and ends when the food is eaten and the flavor perceived. The final flavor quality of the muscle food, therefore, involves several external and internal factors which will be the object of the remainder of this chapter.

2. WHAT FACTORS AFFECT MEAT FLAVOR QUALITY?

The advent of more American households needing both spouses to be an active part of the workforce has led to a decrease in the amount of time available for the couple or family to prepare food at home. A direct outgrowth of this phenomenon is the proliferation in the sales and development of more prepackaged and precooked foods and fast food outlets. A major deterrent to the purchase of these muscle food items is the rapid development of warmed-over flavor. Warmed-over flavor (WOF) was first recognized by Tims and Watts (10) who defined it as the rapid onset of rancidity in cooked meats during refrigerated storage. Oxidized flavors are readily detectable after 48 hours in cooked meats as opposed to the more slowly developing rancidity encountered in raw meats or fatty tissues which becomes evident only after prolonged freezer storage (11, 12). WOF can also develop rapidly in raw meat that has been ground and exposed to air (13, 14). It is now generally accepted that any process that involves disruption of the muscle structure (e.g. cooking, grinding or restructuring) enhances the development of WOF.

The acronym WOF is misleading in that it suggests that it is a flavor. Actually, WOF has been shown to be a dynamic process of flavor deterioration (4-7, 15, 16). Because of the dynamic nature of the change in flavor, MFD, representing meat flavor deterioration, has been proposed as a more appropriate acronym for describing the processes which occur in meat accompanying storage (7, 16). During MFD the undesirable flavors increase in intensity while the desirable meaty flavors decline.

The National Live Stock and Meat Board (NLSMB) report titled "Warmed-over flavor (WOF) in meat" (1988) indicated that consumers are aware of meat flavor deterioration, MFD, as...

> "evidenced by their dissatisfaction with 'warmed-over' roasts, chops, steaks and other meat 'leftovers.' The increasing demand for more precooked, ready-to-eat meat entrees in the marketplace, as well as their use by airlines, fast food service franchises, and specialty service restaurants, provides an ever expanding potential for consumer exposure to WOF. Thus, it is important that meat processors involved in adding value or convenience to meat products, particularly those involved in partial or complete cooking, need to understand available knowledge of WOF, and keep informed of new scientific developments with regard to meat processing, preparation, distribution and merchandising technology." The National Livestock and Meat Board report concludes that the development of meat flavor deterioration, MFD, "is a major deterrent to the introduction of such products (pre-cooked) in the market place. Only when [MFD] is eliminated or at least minimized in precooked meat products, will their market potential be realized." This report also made recommendations indicating "...a very real need for basic research on the mechanism of [MFD] and muscle foods...".

Subsequent portions of this chapter will address current research designed to address the problem of MFD.

2.1   Lipid oxidation

Of the compounds identified in meat many are products of lipid oxidation. These lipids and the products of their oxidation play an important role in the development of the distinctive flavor character of the meat, e.g., they make beef taste like beef, pork like pork, lamb like lamb, etc.. As the meat lipids oxidize, they produce many secondary reaction products, such as alcohols, hydrocarbons, ketones, fatty acids, and aldehydes, each capable of supplying a different aroma, and collectively, several different aromas. For example, increased concentrations of butanal, pentanal, hexanal, hept-2-enal, oct-2-enal and 2,4-decadienal in the lipids fraction of lambs fed a high linoleic acid diet could be responsible for the oily flavor characteristic in the cooked lamb that was similar to that found in pork (17). Watanabe and Sato (18) reported that the beef-fat flavor in heated beef could be ascribed to a specific combination of aldehydes, ketones and sulfur containing compounds. Hornstein and Crowe (19) and others (20-22) suggested that while the fat portion of muscle foods contributed to the unique flavor that characterizes the meat from these species, the lean portion of meat contributed to the basic meaty flavor which they postulated to be identical in beef, pork, and lamb. The major differences between pork and lamb are accounted for by a number of short chain unsaturated fatty acids, which are not present in beef. Bailey, Dupuy, and Legendre (23) and Hedrick et al. (24) reported higher concentration of hexanal and 2,4-decadienals (both products of linoleic acid oxidation, 25) in fat of grass-fed beef compared to grain-fed cattle. Nevertheless, even though over 600 volatile compounds have been identified from cooked beef, there has not been one single compound identified to date that can be attributed to the aroma of "cooked beef".

Meat flavor deterioration (MFD) is a process in which the desirable meaty flavor characteristics decrease with a simultaneous increase in undesirable or off-flavor notes. Yonathan and Watts (26) showed that the polyunsaturated fatty acids of cellular lipids (the phospholipids) were involved in flavor deterioration in cooked meat. Later, Igene and Pearson (27) found that phospholipids oxidize faster than triglycerides in MFD samples. Using capillary gas chromatography, Dupuy et al. (28) demonstrated that subcutaneous fat produced about fifty volatile compounds during MFD development, whereas intramuscular fat produced more than 200 volatile compounds. There is no question that oxidation of phospholipids seems to be the primary source of off-flavor notes produced during the MFD process. However, where these lipids lie in situ, which ones are the most susceptible to oxidation, and the mechanism of their catalysis is unanswered.

Since Robinson (29) first described that iron porphyrins could oxidize polyunsaturated fatty acids, there have been many theories postulated to explain the role of iron or iron containing compounds as the primary catalyst of lipid oxidation in muscle tissue. Several, but certainly not all, are reported herein. For example, Tappel (30) attributed lipid oxidation to heme catalysts, such as hemoglobin, myoglobin, and cytochromes. Sato and Hegarty (14) reported that nonheme iron, rather than myoglobin, was the active catalyst responsible for the rapid oxidation of cooked meat. Liu (31) and Liu and Watts (32) reported that both heme and nonheme iron could function as pro-oxidants in meats. Love (33) showed that metmyoglobin did not influence thiobarbituric acid (TBA) values in cooked meat, thereby, supporting the findings of Sato and Hegarty (14). Igene et al. (34) also reported that nonheme iron plays an important role in lipid oxidation in lipid tissues. McDonald, Gray and Gibbins (35) showed that myoglobin and hemoglobin were important pro-oxidants, they were not the major cause of lipid oxidation in pork muscle. Microsomal fractions from muscle were implicated in lipid oxidation (36-38). Hultin (39) reported that microsomes treated with phospholipase A showed an increased lipid oxidation based on TBA measurement. Kanner and Kinsella (40) suggested that phagocytic cells may initiate lipid oxidation in muscle tissue from contamination with microorganisms during the slaughter process. Kanner and Harel (41) suggested that hydrogen peroxide interacts with metmyoglobin to produce a species that catalyzes lipid oxidation in muscle sarcosomes. In all of the above reports, the general consensus seems to be that lipid oxidation in muscle foods involves some form of iron ions, either bound or free.

2.2   Cooking temperature

Cooking method and final internal temperature have an important effect on the formation and stability of the volatile compounds in meats (4, 7, 42 43) as well as some of the non-volatile compounds such as the proteins, peptides and amino acids (see Proteins and Enzymes section below; 7). The formation of the Maillard reaction products (see Maillard Reactions section below for more detail) is enhanced at the higher cooking temperatures. Several of these Maillard reaction products, such as reductones, have antioxidative characteristics (44). These compounds, whether formed during cooking (4, 45) or added back to the meat products (8, and references cited within), inhibit the rate of lipid autoxidation and deterioration of meat flavor. The rate of lipid autoxidation is also enhanced in meats cooked to a higher internal temperature. The enhanced myoglobin degradation (7) and subsequent release of free iron (46, 47) further augment the rate of lipid autoxidation. This causes disruption of the muscle membrane and further exposes the membrane lipids to oxygen and catalysts (48). The loss of myoglobin levels, in addition to enhancing lipid oxidation via the release of free iron, leads to an enhanced tissue proteolysis by specific thiol dependent proteinases (7, 49) thereby leading to a further decline in meat flavor. Major chemical changes, which include changes in enzyme activity and protein and amino acid composition, begin to occur between 60°C and 77°C (7). As temperature increases up to this range, lipid autoxidation also increases; beyond this range lipid autoxidation decreases. The decrease in the rate of lipid autoxidation is attributed to the formation of Maillard reaction products with antioxidative characteristics at the elevated temperatures (see below; 5, 45, 48).

The formation of the sulfur-containing compounds, benzaldehyde, and phenyl-acetaldehyde appears to be more directly influenced by temperature than are lipid degradation (16). Ground beef patties cooked to higher temperatures have a higher content of amino acids and peptides (4, 7) and sulfur containing compounds than the patties cooked to lower temperatures (16). From this it can be assumed that the content of the reductones and other Maillard reaction products with antioxidative properties is also elevated. On the other hand, there was no difference in the content of lipid degradation compounds in patties cooked to different temperatures (16). It seems plausible that the additional Maillard reaction products formed at higher internal cooking temperature may not have been sufficient to slow the rate of lipid autoxidation, thereby, resulting in no effect on the content of lipid degradation compounds. On the other hand, the free iron content may have been elevated in the patties cooked to the higher temperature, and, therefore, these two opposing effects nullified each other. The opposing effects of the role of temperature on the stability of reactive components and volatile compounds in cooked beef patties needs to be addressed in future studies that encompass a wider range of temperatures than that included in the Drumm and Spanier study (16).

2.3 Storage time

Lipid autoxidation in meats is initiated during the cooking process and continues throughout the storage period (50). The content of aldehydes, alcohols, ketones, and other lipid autoxidation products identified in cooked beef patties increases during refrigerated storage with significant ($P < 0.05$) variability as a function of storage time (5, 6, 16). Hexanal, a major lipid autoxidation product in the beef patties, is most frequently quantified as a measure of lipid autoxidation in foods (51). This compound is formed at rates significantly higher than other major lipid autoxidation products (6, 16).

The relationships between content and storage time were consistent for 28 selected compounds detected by FID (flame ionization detector; 16). Linoleic, oleic, and arachidonic acids are the primary reactants for the formation of volatile compounds during lipid autoxidation in meats (52). The decomposition of the fatty acid hydroperoxides formed during lipid autoxidation involves a complex set of reactions resulting in the formation of numerous volatile compounds (53, 54). These factors, in addition to variability in the presence of catalysts, chelators, antioxidants, and other components, affect the rate of lipid autoxidation and complicate the determination of kinetic parameters (55). In a recent study (16) the formation of lipid autoxidation compounds is shown to favor zero-order kinetics in a 4 day storage study although some compounds do favor first-order kinetics. The overriding dominance of lipid degradation compounds with tendencies to follow zero-order kinetics indicates that the content of these compounds are increasing at a linear rate throughout the storage period. A high degree of variability is seen when a comparison of the slope and intercept value for the autoxidation compounds is made. Hexanal, a major product of lipid oxidation, has a slope and intercept which is at least 5-times greater than that of many of the other volatile products of lipid oxidation. Comparison of the other major lipid autoxidation compounds reveals that the initial content of a compound (intercept) is not necessarily an indication of the rate of formation of the compound (slope) during storage and the formation of lipid degradation compounds is not proportional. The rate of formation of these compounds is independent of the initial concentration; thus, the total volatile content and distribution of volatiles change continuously during the 4-day storage time.

The compounds formed during lipid autoxidation do not contribute to desirable meaty flavor but, rather, impart green, rancid, fatty, pungent, and other off-flavor characteristics to the beef (56). The actual flavor characteristics and threshold values of these lipid autoxidation compounds are unique and several references are included for those interested (53, 57-61). Generally, the carbonyl compounds have the greatest impact on flavor due to their low flavor threshold in comparison to the hydrocarbons, substituted furans, and alcohols (53, 58). For each of these classes of compounds, flavor thresholds decrease with an increase in chain length (see references in two preceding sentences).

The aldehydes are the major contributors to the loss of desirable flavor in meats because of their high rate of formation during lipid autoxidation and low flavor threshold (60). Hexanal is the major autoxidation product of linoleic acid (60, 62). Some of these lipid oxidation products equal or exceed their flavor threshold even in freshly cooked meat (16) thereby, making an immediate negative impact on the flavor quality of meat. The alcohols contribute measurably less to the undesirable flavor quality of meat than the aldehydes due to their relatively high flavor thresholds. Among the ketones produced during the storage of precooked meat, 2,3-octanedione is unique in that the content of this compound is negligible at day 0, but is produced rapidly with storage (16). Ketones are products of lipid oxidation and have previously been identified in the off-flavors of animal and vegetable fats; the mechanism for the formation of these compounds is less clear (53, 59). It is clear that several complex, thermal and storage-dependent reactions occur in meat. Study of this process is difficult at best and should include thorough examination of all food components within the same samples and under different treatments.

2.4 Maillard Reactions

There have been suggestions that the oxidation of sulfhydryl groups on aldolase could be the initial event in the degradation of proteins to amino acids (63). It is the reaction of sugars with these amino acids that has become known as Maillard reaction products or MRPs (64). These MRPs are considered to have a vital role in the production of flavor in meat (65). A significant proportion of the organic compounds which are known to produce meaty-like flavors contain sulfur. A significant number of these organic sulfur compounds are aldehydes. The specific aldehydes produced during the Maillard reaction are controlled mainly by the specific amino acid used in the reaction (64), whereas the amount of a specific aldehyde produced is determined mostly by the type of sugar used in the reaction (64). With this information in hand, it is reasonable to expect that through control of reactants and reaction conditions, the MRPs can be controlled; furthermore, through the use of heuristic models, the MRPs can be predicted. The literature contains a notable amount of information relating to synthetic Maillard Reaction Products. There is an ever growing list of MRPs found in synthetic mixtures and in meat but we were unable to find published quantitative correlations between the levels of MRPs and the sensory response of these compounds in meat. Although much is known about the formation of MRPs *in vitro*, little is known of their formation and influence on the overall sensory perception and flavor of meat *in vivo*. Thus, the mechanism of MRP formation, the specific content of MRPs in meat, and the influence of MRPs on sensory perception need to be a major research area in food science.

Most Maillard reaction products even though generally present in the low parts per million to the parts per billion range, have a high impact potential on flavor because of their extremely low flavor threshold. Sulfur-containing compounds which have been shown to be important contributors to desirable meaty flavor (56) comprise a major group within the Maillard reaction products. However even though these compounds can be measured with great success, the instability of the sulfur-containing compounds (66) indicates the difficulty in accurately measuring these compounds in some food systems. Recent analysis of the sulfur compounds found in cooked ground beef has indicated that several of the heterocyclic compounds such as 4-methylthiazole, 2-acetylthiazole, benzothiazole, and 2-furylmethanethiol are fairly stable (16). These latter compounds were identified in ground beef patties which had undergone a fairly strenuous 4 hour steam distillation-extraction protocol. On the other hand, use of milder methods indicated that precooked ground beef does not contain any thiazoles (Fig. 1) at least at the level below 2.5 parts per billion (ppb). The milder extraction method included homogenization of the ground beef patties in 50 mL of methylene chloride followed by extraction at 50°C for 24 hours in a Soxhlet thimble. The extract was transferred to a Kadurna-Dannish apparatus for concentration and the solvent concentrated to a volume of 2.0 mL. An appropriate amount of internal standard (benzothiazole) was added and the sample injected onto a GC/MS and HPLC. Spiked samples (Fig. 2; Table 1), containing known amounts of thiazoles of interest at the 5 μg/mL, were also prepared and analyzed to determine the efficiency of recovery of thiazoles added to ground beef using this method. With the exception of 4-methyl-5-ethanol thiazole (32%), 2-acetylthiazole (88%) and 4-methyl-5-ethanol thiazole acetate (88%), all other thiazoles were recovered at above 94% (Table 1). Since muscle structure is so complex and compartmentalized, i.e., soluble, myofibrillar (structural), and organellar, it is important to perform such experiments using both gentle and more vigorous extraction protocols. These experiments will provide a means of more accurately defining the flavor characteristics of a muscle food by more precisely examining each facet of the microenvironments of meat within which the flavor is generated.

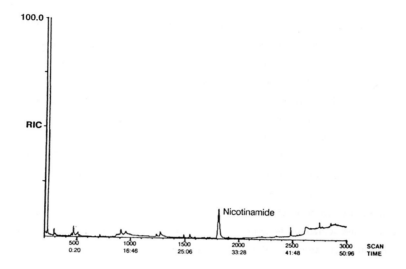

Fig. 1. Reconstructed ion chromatogram (RIC) of 1 Kg cooked meat. Sample not spiked with thiazole standards.

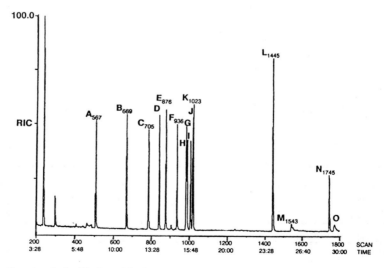

Fig. 2. RIC of meat spiked with 5 μg thiazole standard. **A.** 4-methylthiazole. **B.** 2,4-dimethylthiazole. **C.** 4,5-dimethylthiazole. **D.** 2-ethoxythiazole. **E.** 2-ethyl-4-methylthiazole. **F.** 2,4,5-trimethylthiazole. **G.** 2-isopropyl-4-methylthiazole. **H.** 2-acetylthiazole. **I.** 4-methyl-5-vinylthiazole. **J.** 2-(1-Methylp;ropyl)thiazole. **K.** 2-isobutylthiazole. **L.** Benzothiazole (Internal Standard). **M.** 4-methyl-5-ethanol thiazole. **N.** 4-methyl-5-ethanol thiazole acetate. **O.** Nicotinamide.

Other sulfur compounds found in meat are formed by Strecker degradation of cysteine, methionine and alanine and from hydrogen sulfide. Hydrogen sulfide is produced via several mechanisms including free-radical reactions (67). Hydrogen sulfide which has been shown to be a product of the degradation of dimethyl trisulfide (67) can also react with several components of meat to give ethanedithiol, (methylthio)ethanethiol, and dimethyltrithiolane. These latter compounds have been shown to increase in meat during storage (16). Hydrogen sulfide generation itself has been shown to be temperature dependent (68, in preparation).

Further research is needed to determine the effect of storage time and cooking temperature on the content and composition of the volatile compounds...both lipid and heterocyclic...that contribute to desirable and undesirable meat flavors. Generally, the heterocyclic compounds have been identified as contributors to desirable meat flavor (59, 66, 69). The content of the heterocyclic compounds quantified in several studies (16, 70) did not change significantly during storage. On the other hand, the content of lipid autoxidation products and aliphatic and cyclic sulfur compounds did increase during the storage period. The change in the level of these two groups of compounds as well as the change in the content of muscle protein and peptides (see below) has been attributed to action of similar free-radical mechanisms which account for the formation of undesirable flavors in meats during storage.

Table 1. Thiazole standards and their recoveries on GC/MS.

STANDARD	% Recovery	Quantitation M/E	Relative Response Factor	Relative Retention Time	Aldrich[§] Identification
Benzothiazole (Internal Standard)	N/A	135	1.000	1.000	
4-methylthiazole	110	99	0.409	0.351	W37160-2
2,4-dimethylthiazole	110	113	0.425	0.462	W50340-9
4,5-dimethylthiazole	110	113	0.467	0.543	W32740-9
2-ethoxythiazole	104	101	0.527	0.582	W33400-6
2-ethyl-4-methylthiazole	98	126	0.387	0.606	W36800-8
2,4,5-trimethylthiazole	104	127	0.390	0.647	W33251-8
2-isopropyl-4-methylthiazole	94	126	0.669	0.681	W35551-8
2-acetylthiazole	88	127	0.331	0.685	W33280-1
4-methyl-5-vinylthiazole	94	125	0.466	0.697	W33130-9
2-(1-methylpropyl)thiazole	98	112	0.454	0.705	W33721-8
2-isobutylthiazole	110	99	0.682	0.708	W31340-8
4-methyl-5-ethanol thiazole	32	112	0.364	1.071	W32040-4
4-methyl-5-ethanol thiazole acetate	88	125	0.666	1.211	W32050-1

[§]Aldrich Chemical Company, Inc, Milwaukee, Wisconsin

2.5 Proteins and Enzymes

The nutritional contribution of meat proteins is well established, and significant research efforts have been directed towards understanding the effect of proteinases on meat texture and tenderization (1, 2, 7, 71). However, the contribution of meat proteinases and peptides to meat "tenderness", meat "flavor" and overall meat "quality" is perhaps one of the least examined areas in meat science. The postmortem process of meat tenderization is complex and is not fully understood. Indeed, improvement in tenderness and the exact mechanisms involved in the conditioning process are still unknown. It has been emphasized that the key target of all the morphological and biochemical changes occurring in meat during the postmortem conditioning period reside with the myofibrillar matrix (2, 72-75). Many of the alterations seen in muscle ultrastructure during the postmortem period have been ascribed to the action of lysosomal enzymes, especially cathepsin B and L (7, 74, 76) and these enzymes have been implicated in the process of postmortem tenderization. However, the changes which occur during the aging/conditioning process can only be ascribed to a synergistic action of lysosomal and calcium-dependent proteinases (71).

While lipids and Maillard reaction products (MRPs; see above) contribute significantly to meat flavor and have been the area of the most intensive flavor quality research, one finds little evidence in the literature regarding research efforts given to the understanding the role of meat proteinases, proteins and peptides to overall flavor impression. Because proteins comprise the major chemical components of beef it would seem to be the ideal class of compounds to examine for their relationship to flavor quality. Increased amounts and kinds of proteinaceous components such as peptides and amino acids have been shown to occur both during postmortem aging (7, 77) and at different end-point cooking temperatures ranging from 125°F to 170°F (4). For example, two major classes of peptides are found in beef roasts during cooking (4). One of these classes, the 1800 M.W. class, is composed of two subclasses as determined by reverse phase (RP) high pressure liquid chromatography (HPLC), i.e. one enriched with hydrophilic residues and another enriched with hydrophobic residues (Fig. 3). Hydrophilic residues are associated with desirable flavor while hydrophobic residues are associated with undesirable or off-flavors. Both residues are produced during cooking and there is little evidence that their final tissue level is due to the end-point cooking temperature; it is more likely that these flavor peptides have been generated during the postmortem conditioning stage by proteolytic activity (4, 7). As precooked meat is stored in the refrigerator, there is a decline in the presence of the hydrophilic residue with no major effect on the hydrophobic residue (Fig. 3, lower). It is thought that the loss in the hydrophilic residue with storage is a function of fragmentation of the parent hydrophilic residue by free-radical mechanisms. This loss in hydrophilic peptide residue is closely related to changes observed in the flavor of the stored meat sample where one generally sees an increase in the bitter and sour notes and a decline in the cooked beef/brothy notes during storage (78).

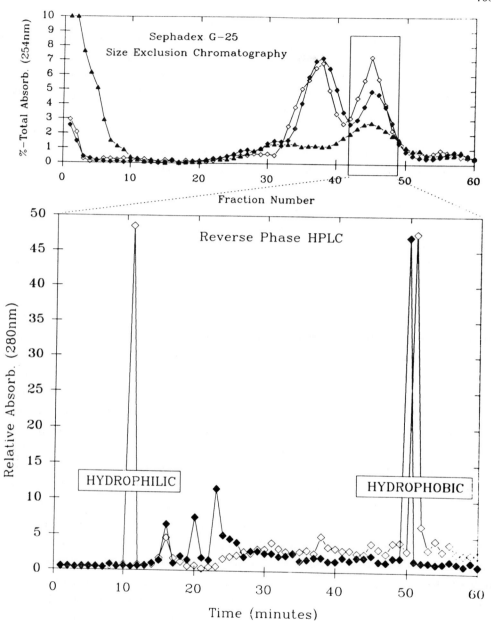

Fig. 3. **UPPER**. Size exclusion chromatography (SEC) using Sephadex G-25 of aqueous extracts from fresh uncooked meat (▲), fresh cooked meat (◊), and cooked meat stored in a refrigerator for 2 days (♦). Two major peaks are present between fractions 30 & 50. The first is approximately 2,500 M.W. while the second is approximately 1,800 M.W. **LOWER**. Reverse phase high performance liquid chromatography (HPLC) of pooled 1,800 M.W. peaks from SEC run using a gradient (5 to 95% water to acetonitrile. Fresh cooked meat is represented by ◊ and the cooked meat stored in at 4°C for 2 days is represented by ♦.

A delicious-tasting, meaty-flavored, linear, octapeptide was reported by Yamasaki and Maekawa (79) in papain digests of beef. The potential impact of peptides in general and this octapeptide in particular to beef flavor has been demonstrated by Kato et al. (3) who reported that enzymatic cleavage of the two amino-terminal residues from the "delicious meaty peptide" yielded a hexapeptide residue imparting a "bitter" taste. This is similar to our observation in precooked/stored meat in which there is a loss in the level of a hydrophilic / desirable flavored peptide and cooked beef/brothy flavor notes along with a concomitant increase in the off-flavor notes, bitter and sour (Fig. 3; 78). This octapeptide proved valuable in serving as an experimental model for examining the behavior and role of peptides in meat flavor quality as described below.

2.6 Lipid Oxidation and Meat Proteins

Since it is difficult to clearly define the mechanism(s) and targets responsible for the change in beef flavor in whole meat systems, and since lipid oxidation (see sections above) is directly involved in the alteration in beef flavor, an *in vitro* model was developed which permitted the study this process. The model used endogenous meat lipids to prepare artificial membranes called "**liposomes.**" Various meat proteins were encapsulated ore entrapped into these liposomes. Lipid oxidation and free-radical production in this model system was accomplished by addition of a solution of chemicals (80) to which the acronym, FROG, for free radical oxidation generator, was assigned. Lipid oxidation was assessed by the measurement of thiobarbituric acid reactive substances (TBARS) and by gas chromatography. The level of TBARS in the experimental samples increased as a function of increased incubation time while the controls containing an antioxidant and a chelator showed no change in initial TBARS levels; this indicated that the FROG system was capable of inducing lipid oxidation. Changes in proteins were monitored electrophoretically and indicated that exposure of the beef proteins to free radical induced via oxidation led to a decrease in the levels of several proteins and the development of some new electrophoretically identifiable protein fractions (Fig. 4).

A electrophoretic peak appearing between 5.0 and 5.3 minutes was particularly intriguing since it had the same initial shape and migration-time as a synthetically-prepared delicious-octapeptide which itself was unaffected directly by lipid oxidation. Semiquantitative analysis of integrated peak areas, indicated that there was approximately a 16% reduction in peak area due to incubation in the presence of the FROG system suggesting that the composition of this protein peak had been altered. Further semiquantitative analysis of these integrated peaks revealed the following: The area under the peak of the unincubated beef extract (Fig. 4 upper) represents 44.9% of the area of the standard or approximately 2.69 µg of octapeptide. This represents a sample containing an equivalent of 1.59 mM of octapeptide which is greater than the 1.41 mM perception-threshold reported by Dr. Okai and his colleagues for this peptide (81). Carrying this mathematical exercise a step further, an observed 16.6% reduction in the presumptive octapeptide peak area due to FROG treatment, i.e., incubation for 1 hour at 37°C, yields a 1.32 mM concentration which is just below the threshold level for its sensory perception. These data demonstrated clearly that major alterations occurred in several meat proteins following lipid oxidation. More importantly, it follows, that these altered proteins and peptides have the ability to effect significant affects on meat flavor.

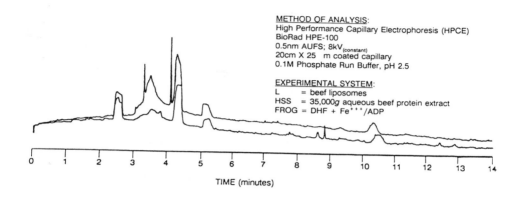

Fig. 4. Electrophoretogram (EG) of proteins separated via capillary electrophoresis. Upper pattern represents the EG obtained from HSS incubated for 0 minutes at 37°C in the presence of the FROG (free radical oxidation generating) system. The lower pattern represents the EG obtained from the same HSS incubated for 60 minutes at 37°C in the presence of the FROG system.

3. CONCLUSIONS.

Several factors contributing to the final flavor perception of muscle foods have been presented. The preceding chapter has demonstrated hopefully that meat flavor development and deterioration is a complex process involving many contributory mechanisms affecting the chemical composition...and thus flavor...of meat. A full comprehension of meat flavor and meat quality will necessarily involve the combination of several disciplines with analysis and intercorrelation of the structure/activity relationship of all contributing factors by statistical techniques such as multivariate principal components analysis (78). As of today, we know the words which constitute flavor quality, but we do not fully understand the syntax of the words which comprise the complete flavor sentences. We have to learn not just what these words are, but how they work together.

REFERENCES

1 M. Koohmaraie, A.S. Babiker, A.L. Schroeder, R.A. Merkel and T.R. Dutson, J. Food Sci., 53(1988):1638-1641.
2 D.J. Etherington, M.A.J. Taylor, and E. Dansfield, Meat Sci., 20(1987):1-18
3 H. Kato, and T. Nishimura, in: Umami: A Basic Taste. Kawamura, Y. and M.R. Kare (Eds), New York, Marcel Dekker, Inc., 1987, pp. 289-306.
4 A.M. Spanier, J.V. Edwards and H.P. Dupuy, Food Tech., 42(1988):110-118.

5   A.J. St. Angelo, J.R. Vercellotti, M.G. Legendre, C.H. Vinnett, J.W. Kuan, C. James, and H.P Dupuy, J. Food Sci., 52(1987):1163-1168.
6   A.J. St. Angelo, J.R. Vercellotti, H.P. Dupuy, and A.M. Spanier, Food Technol., 42(1988):133-138.
7   A.M. Spanier, K.W. McMillin and J.A. Miller, J. Food Sci., 55(1990):318-326.
8   M.E. Bailey, Food Technol., 42(1988):123-126.
9   M.E. Bailey, S.Y. Shin-Lee, H.P. Dupuy, A.J. St. Angelo, and J.R. Vercellotti, in: Warmed-over flavor of meat, eds. St. Angelo, A.J. and M.E. Bailey (Eds), Orlando, Florida: Academic Press, 1987 pp. 237-266.
10   M.J. Tims, and B.M. Watts, Food Technol., 12(1958):240-243.
11   A.M. Pearson, and J.I. Gray, in: The Maillard Reaction in Foods and Nutrition. Amer. Chem. Soc. Symp. Ser. 215, G.R. Waller and M.S. Feather (Eds.), Washington, D.C., American Chemical Society, 1983, pp. 287-300.
12   A.M. Pearson, J.D. Love and F.B. Shorland, in: Advances in Food Research. Vol. 23. C.O. Chichester, E.M. Mrak and G.F. Stewart (Eds), New York, Academic Press, 1977, pp. 1-74.
13   B.E. Greene, J. Food Sci., 34(1969):110-113.
14   K. Sato and G.R. Hegarty, J. Food Sci., 36(1971):1098-1102.
15   P.B. Johnsen and G.V. Civille, J. Sensory Studies, 1(1986):99-104.
16   T.D. Drumm and A.M. Spanier, J. Agric. Food Chem., 39(1991):336-343.
17   R.J. Park, A.J. Ford, and D. Ratcliff, J. Food Sci., 40(1975):1217-1221.
18   K. Watanabe and Y. Sato, Agric. Biol. Chem., 35(1971):756-763.
19   I. Hornstein and P.F. Crowe, J. Agric. Food Chem. 8(1960):494-498.
20   J.D. Sink, J. Food Sci., 44(1979):1-5.
21   A.E. Wasserman, J. Food Sci., 44(1979):6-11.
22   A.E. Wasserman and F. Talley, J. Food Sci., 33(1968):219-223.
23   M.E. Bailey, H.P. Dupuy, and M.G. Legendre, in: The Analysis and Control of Less Desirable Flavors in Foods and Beverages. G. Charalambous (Ed.), New York: Academic Press, 1980, pp. 31-52.
24   H.B. Hedrick, M.E. Bailey, H.P. Dupuy and M.G. Legendre, Proc. 26th European Meeting Meat Res. Workers, U. S. A. 1980:Abstract F.15.
25   A.J. St. Angelo, M.G. Legendre and H.P. Dupuy, Lipids, 15(1980):45-49.
26   M.T. Younathan and B.M. Watts, Food Res., 25(1960):538-543.
27   J.O. Igene and A.M. Pearson, J. Food Sci., 44(1979):1285-1290.
28   H.P. Dupuy, M.E. Bailey, A.J. St. Angelo, J.R. Vercellotti, and M.G. Legendre, in: Warmed-Over Flavor of Meats, A.J. St. Angelo and M.E. Bailey (Eds), p. 165. Orlando, Florida: Academic Press, 1987, pp. 165-191.
29   M.E. Robinson, Biochem. J., 18(1924):255-264.
30   A.L. Tappel, Food Res., 17(1952):550-559.
31   H.P. Liu, J. Food Sci., 35(1970):590-595.
32   H.P. Liu and B.M. Watts, J. Food Sci., 35(1970):596-598.
33   J.D. Love, Ph.D. Dissertation, Michigan State University, East Lansing, Michigan, 1972
34   J.O. Igene, J.A. King, A.M. Pearson and J.I. Gray, J. Agric. Food Chem. 27(1979):838-842.
35   B. MacDonald, J.I. Gray and L.N. Gibbins, J. Food Sci., 45(1980):893-897.
36   T.S. Lin and H.O. Hultin, J. Food Sci., 41(1976):1488-1489.
37   K.S. Rhee, T.R. Dutson, T.R., and Smith, G.C., J. Food Sci., 49(1984):675-679.
38   B.M. Slabyj and H.O. Hultin, J. Food Sci., 47(1982):1395-1398.
39   H.O. Hultin, in: Autoxidation in Food and Biological Systems. M.G. Simic and M. Karelп (Eds.), 1979, pp. 505-527.
40   J. Kanner and J.E. Kinsella, J. Agric. Food Chem., 31(1983):370-378.
41   J. Kanner and S. Harel, Arch. Biochem. Biophys., 237(1985):314-321.
42   G. MacLeod and B.M. Coppock, J. Agric. Food Chem., 25(1977):113-117.
43   G. MacLeod and J.M. Ames, Flavour Fragrance J., 1(1986):91-104.
44   H.E. Nursten, Food Chem., 6(1981):263-277.
45   W.J. Huang and B.E. Greene, J. Food Sci. 43(1978):1201-1209.
46   D.S. Mottram, J. Sci. Food Agric., 36(1985):517-522.

47 U. Tanchotiku., J.S. Godber, G.A. Arganosa, K.W. McMillin, and K.P. Shao, J. Food Sci. 54(1989):280-283.
48 D.A. Lillard, in: Warmed-over Flavor of Meat., St. Angelo, A.J. and M.E. Bailey (Eds.), pp. 41. Orlando, Florida: Academic Press, 1987, pp. 41-67.
49 A.M. Spanier and J.W.C. Bird, Muscle & Nerve, 5(1982):313-320.
50 D.A. Baines and J.A. Mlotkiewicz, in: recent Advances in the Chemistry of Meat, ed. Bailey, A.J.(Ed.), London: The Royal Society of Chemistry, 1984, pp. 119-164.
51 S.L. Melton, Food Technol., 37(1983):105-111.
52 D. Ladikos and V. Lougovois, Food Chem., 35(1990):295-314.
53 D.A. Forss, Prog. Chem. Fats OtherLipids, 13(1972):181-258.
54 E.N. Frankel, in: recent Advances in the Chemistry of Meat, A.J. Bailey (Ed), London, The Royal Society of Chemistry. 1984, pp. 87-118.
55 T.P. Labuza, CRC Crit. Rev. Food Technol. 2(1971):355-405.
56 S.S. Chang and R.J. Peterson, J. Food Sci., 42(1977):298-305.
57 P.W. Meijboom and G.A. Jongenotter, J. Am. Oil Chem. Soc., 58(1981):680-682.
58 M.D. Dixon and E.G. Hammond, J. Am. Oil Chem. Soc., 61(1984):1452-1456.
59 F. Shahidi, L.J. Rubin and L.A. D'Souza, CRC Crit. Rev. Food Sci. Nutr., 24(1986):141-243.
60 F. Ullrich, and W. Grosch, Z. Lebensm. Unters. Forsch., 184(1987):277-282.
61 U. Gasser and W. Grosch, Z. Lebensm. Unters. Forsch., 86(1988):489-494.
62 H.T. Badings, in: Food Flavours, I.D. Morton, and A.J. MacLeod (Eds), New York, Elsevier Scientific Publishing, 1970, pp. 325-398.
63 M.J. McKay and J.S. Bond, in: Intracellular protein catabolism. Progress in Clinical and Biological Research, Vol. 180. E.A. Khairallah, J.S. Bond and J.W.C. Bird (Eds), New York, Alan R. Liss, Inc., 1985, pp. 351-361.
64 J.P. Danehy, in: Advances in Food Research, C.O. Chichester, E.M. Mrak and B.S. Schweigert (Eds.), New York, Academic Press, 1986
65 B.K. Dwivedi, CRC Critical Reviews in Food Technology, 5(1975):487-535.
66 R.V. Golovnja and M. Rothe, Nahrung, 24(1980):141-154.
67 L. Schutte, CRC Crit. Rev. Food Technol., 4(1974):457-505.
68 A.M. Spanier and T.D. Boyleston, J. Agric. Food Chem., 1992 In preparation.
69 M.E. Bailey, in: The Maillard Reaction in Foods and Nutrition, ACS Symposium Series 215, G.R. Waller and M.S. Feather (Eds.), Washington, D.C., American Chemical Society, 1983, pp. 169-183.
70 J.R. Vercellotti, J. Kuan, A.M. Spanier, and A.J. St. Angelo, in: Thermal Generation of Aromas. ACS Symposium Series 409, T.H. Parliment, R.J. McGorrin, and C.T. Ho (Eds.), Washington, D.C., American Chemical Society, 1989, pp. 452-459.
71 A. Ouali, 1990, J. Muscle Foods, 1(1990):129-165.
72 A. Ouali, N. Garrel, A. Obled, C. Deval, C. Valin, and I.F. Penny, Meat Sci., 19(1987):83-100.
73 D.E. Goll, Y. Otsuka, P.A. Nagainis, J.D. Shannon, and S.K. Sathe, J. Food Biochem., 7(1983):137-177.
74 I.F. Penny, D.J. Etherington, J.L. Reeves, and M.A.J. Taylor, in: Proc. 30th Eur. Meet. Meat Res. Work., Bristol, 1984, pp. 133-134.
75 M. Mikami, A.H. Whiting, M.A.J. Taylor, R.A. Maciewicz, and D.J. Etherington, Meat Sci., 21(1987):81-97.
76 J.W.C. Bird, W.N. Schwartz and A.M. Spanier, Acta biol. med. germ., 36(1977):1587-1604.
77 A.W.J. Savage, P.D. Warriss and P.D. Jolley, Meat Science, 27(1990):289-303.
78 A.M. Spanier, J.R. Vercellotti and C. James, Jr. , J. Food Sci., 56(1991):IN PRESS.
79 Y. Yamasaki and K. Maekawa, Agric. Biol. Chem.. 42(1978):1761-1765.
80 I.T. Mak, H.P. Misra and W.B. Weglicki, J. Biol. Chem., 258(1983):13733-13737.
81 M. Tamura, T. Nakatsuka, M. Tada, Y. Kawasaki, E. Kikuchi and H. Okai, Agric. Biol. Chem., 53(1989):319-325.

G. Charalambous (Ed.), Food Science and Human Nutrition
1992 Elsevier Science Publishers B.V.

PREPARATION AND USE OF FOOD GRADE N-CARBOXYMETHYLCHITOSAN TO PREVENT MEAT FLAVOR DETERIORATION

A.J. ST.ANGELO AND J.R. VERCELLOTTI

Southern Regional Research Center, U.S. Department of Agriculture, New Orleans, Louisiana 70124

SUMMARY

The research described herein discusses the findings on crab chitosan, although similar modifications of shrimp and crawfish chitosan have been made in our laboratory. The effectiveness of NCMC to inhibit lipid oxidation reactions that are catalyzed by metals and the preservation of the desireable cooked beef brothy flavor have been demonstrated. In particular, NCMC as a chelating polysaccharide has been shown to possess a high activity to control those peculiar reactions in meat. The chemical and descriptive sensory analysis for the ground beef to which NCMC was added showed that the oxidative chemistry was controlled and that the flavor aromatics were preserved for the valuable beef flavor. In other words, the data showed that the patties that contained the NCMC did not develop flavor deterioration. For future research we would encourage polysaccharide synthetic and natural product chemists to be aware of this flavor stabilizing effect of chelating polysaccharides and to search for new possibilities to enhance such free radical control activity. In addition, due to health concerns such as cholesterol, markets are being lost that can only be solved by risking changes in meat flavor. We have concentrated on beef in our research but our explorations are applicable to many other meat and seafood types. Our findings should also be useful for the development of new edible products and better utilization of the surpluses presently on hand.

1. INTRODUCTION

The meat industry represents sales of more than $50 billion dollars per year in the United States. Many pre-cooked meat products such as frozen entrees for home use, institutional foods, and fast food outlets are affected by off-flavors that develop during storage. In 1958, Tims and Watts (1) described one such off-flavor as warmed-over flavor, or WOF, and defined it as the result of lipid oxidation during refrigerated storage. Since then, that definition has been altered to include raw and uncooked meat (2-5) and the process in which meat develops WOF has been called "meat flavor deterioration", or MFD (6). In addition to off-flavors, markets are being lost due to health concerns such as cholesterol, which can primarily be solved by risking changes in meat flavor. Our research has concentrated on beef but our explorations are applicable to many other meats and seafoods. Our findings are also probably useful for the development of new dairy products and better utilization of the surpluses presently on hand.

The generally accepted cause of the development of the off-flavor known as WOF is that of lipid oxdiation of the membrane bound polyunsaturated fatty acids, catalyzed by metals or metalloproteins (7). That mechanism explains why scientists began to use chelating agents, such as sodium tripolyphosphate (STP), as antioxidants in meat formulations to prevent lipid oxidation (1-3, 7). However, St. Angelo et al, (8) have shown that STP at concentrations of 500 to 1000 ppm can reduce the desirable meaty sensory note, cooked beef brothy, and increase undesirable sensory notes, cardboardy and painty. Also, there may be a question as to the heat stability of phosphate salts, since it was reported that STP injected into raw beef, cooked and stored 3 days, was ineffective in preventing warmed-over flavor in meat as judged by sensory means (9).

The purpose of this research was to find an efficient water soluble chelating polysaccharide that would be compatible with meat muscle protein and would effectively reduce free radical catalyzed lipid oxidation, which is one of the primary causes of off-flavors in meat. Because of the desire to use food additives, such as antioxidants, that are not synthetic, it would also be advantageous to isolate the compound from a natural source. Another key requirement would be that the additive not only maintain high quality meat flavor but also that no detrimental tastes be introduced by its presence.

2. PREPARATION OF FOOD GRADE N-CARBOXYMETHYLCHITOSAN (NCMC)

Although more than fifty polysaccharides as food hydrocolloids were tried in these meat flavor applications, N-carboxymethyl-chitosan was found to be the only effective compound to prevent meat flavor deterioration on storage. We, therefore, proceeded to prepare NCMC, similarly to the method of Muzzarelli (10), but with a few modifications that made the synthesis easier to manage and produce a functional food grade hydrocolloid chelator.

2.1 Starting Material

The starting material used in this research was chitosan purchased from Protan Labs (Redmond, WA). Protan made chitosan from the crab shell chitin, which is the (1-->4-linked) 2-acetamido-2-deoxy-B-D-glucan. Chitin and chitosan have a long history in carbohydrate chemistry going back more than 100 years to the

Ledderhose account (11). Chitin can also be made from the natural structural component of shellfish other than crab, such as lobster, shrimp, and crawfish. Chitin, the most plentiful natural polymer next to cellulose, is biodegradable and non-toxic. Chitosan, an unbranched (1-->4-linked) 2-amino-2-deoxy-B-D-glucan, is prepared by the chemical N-deacetylation of chitin. Similarly to chitin, chitosan is also biodegradable and nontoxic (12). Throughout the present work, it should be noted that the working limit of solution viscosity for the unmodified chitosan solutions is about 1 to 2 percent.

2.2 N-Carboxymethylchitosan (NCMC)

N-Carboxymethylchitosan, more recent in its origins than chitin or chitosan, was first well characterized by Muzzarelli in 1982 (10). Muzzarelli's product was a very interesting compound because of its action as a chelating polysaccharide that is soluble at all pH ranges, but which forms insoluble coordination compounds with transition metals and precipitates out of solution. A large number of O- and N-carboxymethylchitosan preparations were recently reviewed by Muzzarelli (13). Others who have developed methods of preparation were Hall and Yalpani (14, 15), who used monochloroacetic acid to produce predominantly O-carboxymethylation, Hayes (16), whose procedure produced both the N- and O-carboxymethylation, and Muzzarelli et al (13,17,18), whose work led to a highly substituted O- and N-carboxymethylchitosan combining O-alkylation methods with his previous N-alkylation by imine reduction.

In the procedure described in Fig. 1, we were able to: 1) synthesize N-carboxymethylchitosan by a simple method that did not introduce toxic substances to the food grade material, 2) purify the product by separation into the products of greater or less degree of substitution by preparative centrifugation, and 3) remove salts and lower molecular weight fractions by colloidal filtration, ultrafiltration and dialysis to provide a uniform product for testing in meat flavor experiments. Thus, a product was obtained that could be tested as an additive in cooked meat to determine its effectiveness in preventing meat flavor deterioration. This method also allowed us to make a chelating polysaccharide that unambiguously reflected the point of substitution on chitosan. No other chelating polysaccharides were available with quite the ease of preparation as the NCMC method of Muzzarelli (10,13,17). However, in making a food grade material, the sodium borohydride was substituted for cyanoborohydride, which we felt should not be used in the synthesis

```
                CHITOSAN (80 GRAMS, 0.5 MOLES)
                              |
              DISSOLVE IN pH 4 ACETIC ACID (8 L)
                              |
        STIR MECHANICALLY AND ADD 44 GRAMS GLYOXYLIC ACID
                              |
              ADJUST pH FROM 3.5 TO 5 AFTER 1 HOUR
              BY SLOWLY DISPERSING 25 ML. OF 10 N NaOH
                              |
              OVER 1 HOUR ADD WITH CAUTION 250 ML OF SODIUM
                       BOROHYDRIDE (46 G/250 ML)
                              |
                STIR OVERNIGHT AFTER FOAMING SUBSIDES
                              |
                         ADJUST pH to 7
                              |
                           CENTRIFUGE
                              |
           TWO FRACTIONS: SUPERNATANT IS SOLUBLE N-CARBOXYMETHYL
                CHITOSAN (NCMC) AND THE PELLET IS NCMC GEL
                              |
DIALYZE THE SOLUBLE NCMC WITH        GEL FRACTION: USE AS IS OR
ULTRAFILTRATION MEMBRANES            PRECIPITATE AND DRY.
             |                         (FRACTION 2: 80 - 85%)
PRECIPITATE WITH ALCOHOL AND DRY
  (FRACTION 1, SOLUBLE NCMC: 15 - 20%)
```

Fig. 1. The flow chart for synthesis of N-carboxymethylchitosan.

of a food grade product. Several other changes in the procedure of Muzzarelli were made. Formation of the imino intermediate at acid pH was critical to the driving force of the reaction. Manipulating pH and mode of addition permitted use of the less toxic sodium borohydride. The NCMC was centrifuged to separate by degree of substitution and possibly molecular weight two solubility classes.

Further purification of the soluble portion to obtain a food grade material was achieved through various ultrafiltration steps (19) that included utilizing colloidal cross flow filtration, ultrafiltration, diafiltration, and reverse osmosis membranes to make preparative runs on garbage can scale. A hollow fiber colloidal filter was used for filtration of suspended particulate matter. The unit used was an Enka cross flow polypropylene, 0.6 micron unit that had a molecular weight (MW) cutoff of 1 million. A Rhone-Poulenc RPC6 polyacrylonitrile plate and frame ultrafilter with 20,000 MW cutoff was followed by a cellulose hollow fiber dialyzer (Cordis Dow, C-DAK). The dialyzer has a cutoff of about 1200 MW. In this way as salts were concentrated, they could be removed so that the osmotic pressure did not build up too quickly and inhibit membrane permeability (19). A plate and frame cellulose acetate membrane was used as a concentrator for water soluble polymers such as oligosaccharides. Glucose will pass but maltose is retained. A concentrated sodium sulfate solution was used as the osmotic medium to remove water molecules from the polysaccharide solution. Reverse osmosis uses very small pore size membranes that permit water molecules to pass but retain salts and small organic molecules. Thus, a solution of 50 liters of polysaccharide preparation can be concentrated in a few hours using the reverse osmosis system described herein. The unit that was used was made by Filmtec, Minneapolis, MN, and is used for water purification (19). Running the solution of polysaccharide or oligosaccharide solution on the outside of the reverse osmosis membrane instead of water with a pump at 120 psig permitted rapid concentrations. A celluose hollow fiber dialyzer was used simultaneously with the reverse osmosis unit to keep the osmotic pressure low as salts concentrate. Usually the volume can be reduced enough with this reverse osmosis unit to permit precipitation of N-carboxymethylchitosan directly with alcohol.

3. COMPOSITION AND PROPERTIES OF NCMC

The NCMC that was produced by the above membrane methods is virtually ash free, low in borate formed on hydration of borohydride, and without residual volatiles after vacuum drying over phosphorus pentoxide at 50°C. The structure of the soluble NCMC, Fig. 1, fraction 1, and the gel, fraction 2, were identified by ^{13}C NMR spectroscopy, see Fig. 2A and B. Functional group ratios were estimated by integrals compared to reference peaks in Fig. 2A and B and are listed in Table 1 for the soluble fraction and in Table 2 for the gel fraction. Chemical shifts for the NMR of N-carboxymethyl-chitosans in this work compared well with those reported by Muzzarelli (20). The distribution of substituents and the general structure in the soluble and gel fractions are listed in Fig. 3, and were also determined from NMR data in Tables 1 and 2.

The molecular weight distributions of the chitosan derivatives were determined by gel permeation chromatography on Ultragel ACA 34 using 0.2 N sodium sulfate. Standards of polylysine were used to calibrate the column. Peaks were quantitated using the Lowry phenol-biuret copper method (21). It was found that the soluble fraction of NCMC has a molecular weight of about 150 to 250 kDaltons, comparable to molecular weight ranges in earlier reports (18, 20). Chelation properties of the soluble NCMC were also determined. Experiments demonstrated that the compound chelates the typical transition metals, copper, nickel, iron and cobalt (see Tables 3 and 4), also as had been observed previously for N-carboxymethylchitosan (13, 20).

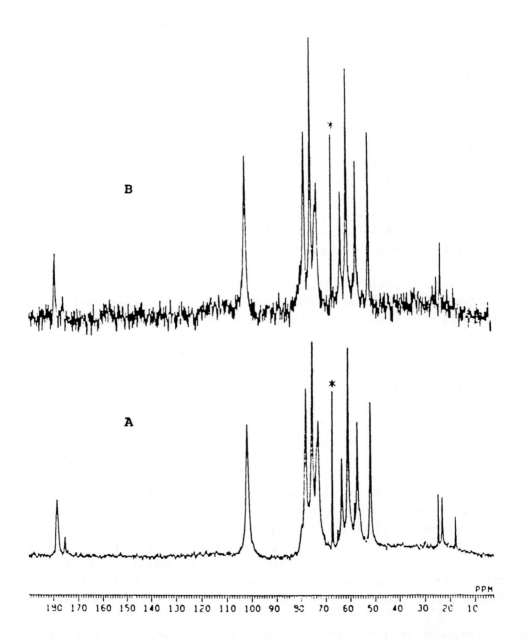

Fig. 2. Carbon-13 NMR spectrum of the soluble fraction of NCMC. *p-Dioxane as internal standard in deuterium oxide. Spectrum provided by Dr. P. E. Pfeffer, USDA-ARS, ERRC, Philadelphia, PA.

TABLE 1
N-Carboxymethylchitosan--higher degree of substitution.
^{13}C chemical shift ratios from integrals.

Functional Group	C-5	CH$_3$(NAc)	N-CH$_2$	C-1
C=O	0.216	0.364	0.331	0.388
C-1	0.556	0.938	0.851	1.000
C-4	0.719	1.212	1.101	1.293
C-5	1.000	1.686	1.531	1.799
C-3	0.570	0.961	0.873	1.025
C-2'	0.400	0.675	0.613	0.719
C-6	0.903	1.523	1.383	1.624
C-2	0.565	0.953	0.865	1.016
N-CH$_2$	0.653	1.101	1.000	1.174
CH$_3$(NAc)	0.593	1.000	0.908	1.067

TABLE 2
N-Carboxymethylchitosan--lower degree of substitiution.
^{13}C chemical shift ratios from integrals.

Functional Group	C-5	CH$_3$(NAc)	N-CH$_2$	C-1
C=O	0.374	1.545	0.581	0.476
C-1	0.785	3.244	1.219	1.000
C-4	0.672	2.777	1.043	0.856
C-5	1.000	4.132	1.553	1.274
C-3	0.862	3.562	1.339	1.098
C-2'	0.463	1.913	0.719	0.590
C-6	0.893	3.690	1.387	1.138
C-2	0.551	2.277	0.856	0.702
N-CH$_2$	0.644	2.661	1.000	0.820
CH$_3$(NAc)	0.242	1.000	0.376	0.308

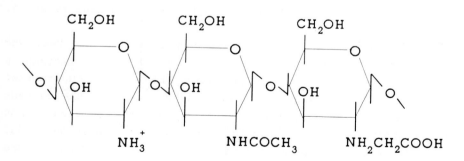

```
       GEL: 66% FREE AMINO    16% N-ACETYL    18% N-CARBOXYMETHYL
   SOLUBLE: 41% FREE AMINO    16% N-ACETYL    43% N-CARBOXYMETHYL
 COMPOSITE: 61% FREE AMINO    16% N-ACETYL    23% N-CARBOXYMETHYL
```

Fig. 3. NCMC Structure and Distribution of Substituents in the Soluble and Gel Fractions as Determined by NMR Spectroscopy.

TABLE 3
NCMC Chelation Properties.

Metal	Ratio of metal to NCMC for 80-98% Precipitation
Copper	45 mg Cu/gm NCMC
Nickel	47 mg Ni/gm NCMC
Cobalt	59 mg Co/gm NCMC

TABLE 4
Column Capacity of NCMC on Silica.

Metal	Ratio of Metal Removed to NCMC
Copper	98 mg Cu/gm NCMC
Nickel	60 mg Ni/gm NCMC
Cobalt	59 mg Co/gm NCMC

4. NCMC AS AN ANTIOXIDANT

Meat flavor deterioration is caused by the oxidation of fats, which are catalyzed my iron present in the meat. When these reactions take place, the compounds that produce the good beefy flavors are lost, and the compounds that cause off-flavors will develop. The net effect is that meat no longer will taste like meat. Eventually, the meat will become rancid. NCMC has been reported to chelate transition metal ions, such as iron (13), so that they cannot catalytically activate oxygen in free radical attack on fats in foods. With this in mind, NCMC was added to ground meat, which was then made into patties for evaluation by chemical and sensory means.

4.1 Sample Preparation

For this study, NCMC (0.5%) was added to raw ground beef and stored at 4°C as reported previously (4). Top round (<u>semimembranosus</u> and <u>adductor</u> muscles) roasts were purchased from a local supermarket on the morning of sample preparation. After removing the carcass fat, the lean meat was ground twice and separated into several 850 g portions. Total fat content ranged from 4-5%. From these portions, 85 g patties were made and cooked on a grill (7 minutes/side). One half of the patties were placed in Petri plates and stored in a refrigerator (4°C) for 2 days to develop MFD. The other 5 patties were stored in a freezer for 2 days to be thawed and used as controls. To another 850 g portion of the ground beef, 0.5% NCMC was added and thoroughly mixed for 2 minutes, made into patties, cooked similarly to the previous patties, and stored for 2 days in the refrigerator. After storage, all patties were removed and rewarmed immediately prior to presentation to a trained sensory panel, followed by analyses by two different chemical methods.

4.2. Sensory Studies

Sensory studies of experimental and control meat samples were conducted with a highly trained and skillful panel, which used a descriptive method of analysis. This method, including panel training, was described previously (8,22,23). Routinely, additives that have not been previously tested for toxicity, or are not on the "Generally Regarded as Safe" (GRAS) list, are not presented to panelists without their consent. In other words, for the sensory evaluation of non-GRAS additives, such as NCMC, panelists do so with their consent. In the case of chitosan and NCMC, a considerable amount of animal toxicity literature has been reviewed by Muzzarelli (13) demonstrating that NCMC is non-toxic and non-allergenic. He also reported that NCMC can be used in emulsion-type cosmetic creams (owing to its moisture-maintaining capacity), and in tooth paste (due to its bacteriostatic properties). Chitosan has been used as an ingredient for domestic animal feeds (24). Others have shown that the product is non-toxic and have used it in foods abroad (refs. 25-28). Included in these studies were the removal of cholesterol by chitosan.

Sensory effects of NCMC on meat flavor after 2 days storage at 4°C was demonstrated in Fig. 4. The values shown were reported as relative intensities calculated from the actual flavor scores, similarly as reported previously (8). Results showed that the desirable flavor note, cooked beef brothy (CBB), was well preserved with NCMC. After 2 days of storage the sample treated with NCMC still had its CBB intensity rated by the special panel at 5.8, only slightly below (9%) that of the zero day control (6.4), whereas the 2 day storage control had a CBB of 3.6 (or 46% below), which is indicative of MFD. The off-flavor character notes, cardboardy (CBD) and painty (PTY), were also quite low in the NCMC 2 day storage sample (0.3 CBD and 0.2 PTY) as compared to 1.8 CBD and 2.1 PTY in the 2-day storage untreated MFD control. The values of the NCMC treated sample represented a decrease of 83% for CBD and 94% for PTY. The mouth feel of the meat treated with NCMC was quite normal. Most importantly, the panel reported that NCMC made no additional off-flavors or tastes.

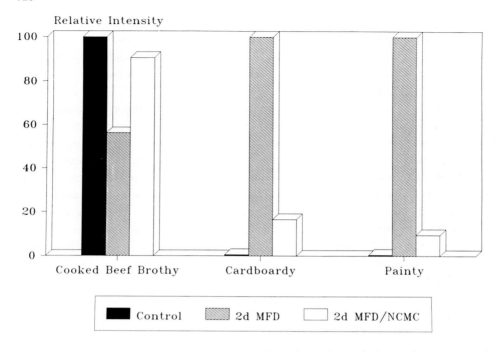

Fig. 4. Effect of 0.5% N-Carboxymethychitosan on beef flavor.

4.3 Quality Assessment by Chemical Means

Chitosan itself, at 10,000 ppm, was not very effective at inhibiting MFD in this system as measured by malonaldehyde and hexanal contents (4), which are chemical markers of lipid oxidation. Malonaldehyde was measured by the thiobarbituric acid (TBARS) assay of Tarladgis (29). Hexanal content was determined by the direct gas chromatographic method previously reported (30-32). Chitosan may be ineffective since it had to be dissolved in pH 5 acetic acid to mix it into the meat, which may lead to poor dispersal. NCMC, however, was quite effective in inhibiting the oxidative processes that form malonaldehyde and hexanal; Even at lower doses, NCMC maintained its effectiveness. For example, at a high concentration of 5000 ppm, NCMC was about 93% effective, while at 600 ppm, NCMC was still 60% effective in reducing oxidative damage. The dose response effects were proven by verification of the inhibition of lipid oxidation by the chemical means of TBARS assay and hexanal, as shown in Fig. 5.

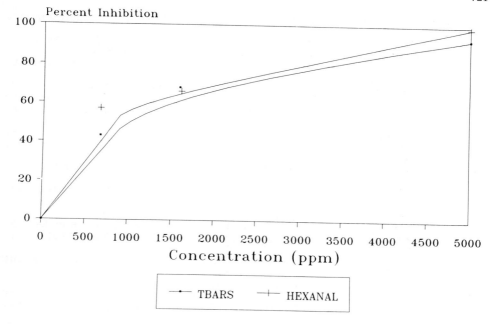

Fig. 5. Dose response of NCMC in beef patties.

REFERENCES

1. M.J. Tims and B.M. Watts, Food Technol. 12(5) (1958) 240-243.
2. B.E. Greene, J. Food Sci. 34 (1969) 110-113.
3. K. Sato and G.R. Hegarty, J. Food Sci. 36 (1972) 1098-1102.
4. A.J. St. Angelo, J.R. Vercellotti, H.P. Dupuy, and A.M. Spanier, Food Technol. 42(6) (1988) 133-138.
5. A.M. Spanier, J.V. Edwards, and H.P. Dupuy, Food Technol. 42(6) (1988) 110-118.
6. A.M. Spanier, K.W. McMillin and J.A. Miller, J. Food Sci. 55 (1990) 318-322.
7. A.M. Pearson and J.I. Gray, in: G.R. Waller and M.F. Feather (Eds.) The Maillard Reaction in Foods and Nutrition. ACS Symposium Series No. 215, American Chemical Society, Washington, DC, 1983, pp. 287-300.
8. A.J. St. Angelo, K.L. Crippen, H.P. Dupuy and C. James, Jr., J. Food Sci. 55 (1990) 1501-1505.
9. L.A. Smith, S.L. Simmons, F.K. McKeith, P.J. Bechtel, and P.L. Brady, J. Food Sci. 49 (1984) 1636-1637.
10. R.A.A. Muzzarelli, F. Tanfani, M. Emanuelli, and S. Moriotti, Carbohydrate Research, 107 (1982) 199-214.
11. G. Ledderhose, Berichte, 9, (1876) 1200-1201.
12. K. Arai, T. Kinumaki, T. Fujita, Bull. Tokai Reg. Fish. Res. Lab. 56 (1968) 89-95.
13. R.A.A. Muzzarelli, Carbohydrate Polymers, 8 (1988) 1-21.
14. L.D. Hall and M. Yalpani, Macromolecules, 17 (1984) 272-281.

15 L.D. Hall and M. Yalpani, U.S. Patent 4,424,346, Issued January 3, 1984.
16 E.R. Hayes, U.S. Patent 4,619,995, Issued October 28, 1986.
17 R.A.A. Muzzarelli, U.S. Patent 4,835,265, Issued May 30, 1989.
18 R.A.A. Muzzarelli, C. Lough, and M. Emanuelli, Carbohydrate Research, 164 (1987) 433-442.
19 J.R. Vercellotti, S.V. Vercellotti, and E. Klein, in: V. Crescenzi, I.C.M. Dea, and S.S. Stivala (Eds.) New Developments in Industrial Polysaccharides, Gordon and Breach, New York, 1985, pp. 125-136.
20 R.A.A. Muzzarelli, in: V. Crescenzi, I.C.M. Dea, and S.S. Stivala (Eds.) New Developments in Industrial Polysaccharides, Gordon and Breach, New York, 1985, pp. 207-222.
21 O.H. Lowry, N.J. Rosebrough, A.L. Farr, and R.J. Randall, J. Biol. Chem. 193 (1951) 265-275.
22 P B. Johnsen and G. V. Civille, J. Sensory Studies 1 (1986) 99-104.
23 J. Love, Food Technol. 42(6) (1988) 140-143.
24 S. Hirano, C. Itakura, H. Seino, Y. Akiyama, I. Nonaka, N. Kanbara, and T. Kawakami, J. Agric. Food Chem. 38 (1990) 1214-1217.
25 P.A. Austin, J.P. Zikakis, and C.J. Brine, U.S. Patent 4,320,150, Issued March 16, 1982.
26 D. Knorr, Food Technol., 45, (1991) 114-122.
27 I. Furda, in: I. Furda (Ed.) Unconventional Sources of Dietary Fiber. ACS Symposium Series No. 214, American Chemical Society, Washington, DC, 1983, pp. 105-122.
28 C.D. Jennings, K. Boleyn, S.R. Bridges, P.J. Wood, and J.W. Anderson, Proc. Soc. Exptl. Biol. Med. 189 (1988) 13-20.
29 B. G. Tarladgis, B. M. Watts, M. T. Younathan, and L. R. Dugan, J. Am. Oil Chem. Soc., 37 (1960) 44-48.
30 H. P. Dupuy, M. L. Brown, M. G. Legendre, Wadsworth, J. I., and E. T. Rayner, in: M.K. Supran (Ed), Lipids as a Source of Flavor. ACS Symposium Series No. 75, American Chemical Society, Washington, DC, 1978, pp. 60-67.
31 A. J. St. Angelo, J.R. Vercellotti, M.G. Legendre, C.H. Vinnett, J.W. Kuan, C. James, Jr., and H.P. Dupuy, J. Food Sci. 52 (1987) 1163-1168.
32 H.P. Dupuy, M.E. Bailey, A.J. St.Angelo, J.R. Vercellotti, and M.G. Legendre, in: A.J. St.Angelo and M.E. Bailey (Eds.) Warmed-Over Flavor of Meat. Academic Press, Orlando, FL, 1987 pp. 165-191.

CONSUMER ACCEPTABILITY OF ALGIN RESTRUCTURED BEEF

J.A. MAGA[1], L. DWYER[1] and G.R. SCHMIDT[2]

[1]Department of Food Science and Human Nutrition, Colorado State University, Fort Collins, Colorado 80523 (United States)

[2]Department of Animal Sciences, Colorado State University, Fort Collins, Colorado 80523 (United States)

SUMMARY

A questionnaire, using a 7-point intensity scale, was administered to measure consumer response among 281 individuals to 7 meat sensory attributes, along with overall acceptability, of several menu items prepared with algin restructured beef. Responses to the algin restructured beef were found to be positive in that for all measurements, mean ratings were significantly higher than the neutral response. Certain menu items were preferred more than others.

INTRODUCTION

Since 1973, the demand for red meat in the United States has decreased (1,2). Consequently, the meat industry has expended much time, effort and money to isolate reasons for the decline and to plan a successful market strategy to increase demand. One of the top priority goals identified by the beef industry is to develop and expand acceptance of intermediate value meat products such as restructured beef (1,3).

Traditionally, the cohesion among meat pieces (restructuring) is accomplished by extracting muscle proteins with salt and phosphates, and mechanically processing to form a heat-set gel matrix which binds the meat upon subsequent cooking (4). The resulting product must be marketed in the frozen or precooked form to maintain structural integrity. However, consumers prefer to buy meat in the raw refrigerated state from the retail case (5).

During the last decade, a nonthermal restructuring system based on alginate, a hydrocolloid derived from kelp, in combination with calcium carbonate and lactic acid has become available (5). The process offers several advantages over the traditional salt/thermal technique including the facts that salt is not required, meat cuts of a desired shape can be formed from pieces of the carcass that are palatable but of inadequate size, and the resulting product has the color and nonsalt flavor of raw beef. In addition, the product can be prepared in a variety of ways including open flame grilling, frying, stewing, roasting and retorting.

As with any new processed form of product, consumer acceptability is a key factor in determining the economic success of the process. Relatively few sensory studies (6-10) have been reported with restructured beef.

Therefore, the objective of this study was to utilize algin restructured beef in a variety of common beef-based menu items and to determine consumer attitudes towards specific meat properties as well as overall acceptability.

MATERIALS AND METHODS
Product Preparation

Fresh beef ball tips were procured from a local beef packer (Monfort of Colorado, Inc., Greeley, CO). The average composition was determined to be 61.5% moisture, 21.2% protein and 14.3% fat in the raw form.

The meat was ground: 80% through a kidney plate for a coarse grind and 20% through a 3/16-inch plate for a finer grind. The non-meat ingredients were sifted into the ground meat in the following sequence and percentages: sodium alginate at 0.60% (Kelco Division of Merck, San Diego, CA); calcium carbonate at 0.10% (Georgia Marble Co., Tate, GA); and encapsulated lactic acid/calcium lactate at 0.15% (Balchem Corp., Slate Hill, NY). After mixing in a paddle-type mixer, the product was extruded through a rib-eye shaped stuffing horn to form logs ranging from 8-18 Kg. The logs were wrapped and frozen and were removed to thaw approximately 48 hours before menu items were prepared.

Menu Items

Prior to formal testing, a number of traditional dishes normally incorporating beef were prepared and screened to determined suitable menu item presentations. From this preliminary study, the following six items were prepared with algin restructured beef: roast beef that was sliced and served cold, charbroiled steak, Philly cheese steak sandwich, French dip sandwich, roast beef and gravy, and beef stroganoff.

Consumer Panels

In order to obtain a wide cross-section of participants, three types of food presentation situations were utilized. These involved local banquet settings, "special of the day" at the University restaurant, and local commercial restaurants. The number of individuals evaluating each menu item is summarized in Table 1.

Questionnaire Design

A questionnaire-type survey was administered. A seven point intensity scale was chosen as the measuring instrument in the questionnaire because of its simplicity and usability in statistical analysis. Eight sensory characteristics frequently used in evaluating meat products were selected to be evaluated. These attributes were presented on the questionnaire in the following order:

appearance, aroma, juiciness, tenderness, texture uniformity, amount of fat and/or gristle, flavor and overall acceptability. A food action question was included as the final question to determine if the consumer would recommend the menu item evaluated. A sample of the questionnaire used is shown in Table 2.

TABLE 1

Menu Items and Number of Individuals Evaluating Each	
Item	Number
Sliced cold roast beef	115
Charbroiled steak	44
Philly cheese steak	40
French dip	29
Roast beef and gravy	36
Stroganoff	17
Total	281

TABLE 2

Questionnaire Used to Evaluate Consumer Acceptability of Algin Restructured Beef Menu Items
Please visually evaluate the <u>beef portion</u> of the dish and check the appropriate box on the following scale: 　　Extremely appealing [] [] [] [] [] [] [] Extremely unappealing
Before tasting the dish, please evaluate the <u>beef portion</u> by smelling and checking the appropriate box on the following scale: 　　Extremely pleasant aroma [] [] [] [] [] [] [] Extremely unpleasant aroma
Then taste the dish and evaluate the <u>beef portion</u> on the following scales by checking the appropriate box: 　　Extremely juicy　　　　　[] [] [] [] [] [] []　Extremely dry 　　Extremely tender　　　　 [] [] [] [] [] [] []　Extremely tough 　　Extremely uniform　　　　[] [] [] [] [] [] []　Extremely nonuniform in 　　　in texture　　　　　　　　　　　　　　　　　　　　texture 　　Large amounts of fat　 [] [] [] [] [] [] []　No detectable fat and/or 　　　and/or gristle　　　　　　　　　　　　　　　　　 gristle 　　Extremely desirable　　 [] [] [] [] [] [] []　Extremely undesirable 　　　flavor　　　　　　　　　　　　　　　　　　　　　 flavor
This beef product, overall is: 　　Extremely acceptable　 [] [] [] [] [] [] []　Extremely unacceptable
After evaluating this beef product, I would: 　　Highly recommend　　　 [] [] [] [] [] [] []　Highly disclaim 　　　this product　　　　　　　　　　　　　　　　　　 this product

Data Analysis

For statistical analysis, numbers were assigned to each category on the scale: one was assigned to the minimum intensity on each scale and the numbers increased to seven, the maximum on this scale. For all the attributes, seven would be the optimal response. The amount of fat and/or gristle question was stated inversely; therefore, scores were reversed for comparison so that a seven would represent the optimal (no visible fat and/or gristle).

Preliminary analysis consisted of overall frequency counts, means, and standard deviations for each measured attribute. Mean scores of each attribute were compared to the neutral midpoint on the scale, four, in a one sample T-test to conclude if the algin restructured menu items were perceived as better than the average response.

Analysis of variance was executed via SPSS (Statistical Package for Social Sciences) to determine if attribute ratings were significantly different among the dishes.

RESULTS AND DISCUSSION

Frequency distribution data for the six algin restructured beef dishes as a group are summarized in Table 3.

TABLE 3

Frequency Distribution of Various Algin Restructured Beef Dish Attributes (N = 281)								
Attribute	Scale							
	0*	1	2	3	4	5	6	7
Appearance	1.9	0.9	2.5	6.5	17.4	39.3	25.2	6.3
Aroma	6.5	0.0	1.6	5.9	23.1	33.0	24.3	6.6
Juiciness	1.9	0.3	3.1	9.3	25.9	38.3	16.2	5.0
Tenderness	1.6	0.3	0.3	2.8	12.1	33.6	35.8	18.5
Texture uniformity	1.2	0.6	0.6	5.3	16.8	29.9	34.0	11.6
Fat and/or gristle	0.0	1.8	5.2	9.7	9.7	19.5	33.3	20.8
Flavor	1.9	0.9	2.5	5.0	14.0	37.7	28.3	9.7
Acceptability	1.2	0.6	1.2	4.0	14.0	30.2	38.6	10.2
Recommendation	0.0	1.1	4.2	6.4	13.5	31.1	33.0	10.9
* Zero rating indicates no response								

For appearance, the majority of the people (70.8%) rated the algin restructured beef dishes a five or greater on the seven-point intensity scale.

The overall mean appearance rating was 4.87. These results indicate that the products were viewed as moderately appealing in appearance.

With respect to aroma, 63.9% of the responses were in the five to seven rating range. The overall mean score was 4.67, which was among the lowest mean scores obtained for all attributes evaluated. However, this was still above the critical score of 4.0.

The mean juiciness rating was 4.61 (moderately juicy). Again, the majority of the scores (51.1%) were in the five to seven range.

Ratings on tenderness were primarily in the five to seven point range (87.9%) with a 5.34 mean rating. Thus, algin restructured beef was perceived as being a tender product.

The algin restructured beef achieved a mean score of 5.17 when evaluated for uniformity. Approximately 75% of the consumers placed this property in the five to seven range, thus indicating that the product was moderately uniform in texture.

The mean score for fat and/or gristle was 4.68, with 71.8% of the respondents rating this property between a five and seven. Thus, to the vast majority, the presence of fat and/or gristle was not a significant defect.

The algin restructured beef products evoked a desirable flavor response, with a mean flavor rating of 5.03. Slightly over 75% of those questioned rated flavor in the five to seven range.

Overall acceptability scores were highly skewed to the positive end of the scale. The greater part (79%) rated algin restructured beef between five and seven. The mean score was 5.22, which fell into the moderately to very acceptable range.

The response to the food action question (Would you recommend this product?) was extremely favorable, with 75% of the consumers responding favorably. The mean rating for this important attribute was 5.12.

One sample T-tests executed between the mean scores of each attribute and the beef was significantly superior than the neutral response for each attribute.

Analysis of variance on attribute data generated from evaluations of the six dishes revealed significant differences relative to appearance, amount of fat and/or gristle, and acceptability (Table 4).

With respect to appearance, the roast beef and gravy and beef stroganoff dishes (4.14 and 4.17 respectively) were statistically less appealing than the French dip, Philly cheese steak and charbroiled steak presentations (5.17, 5.03 and 5.11 respectively).

When assessing the amount of fat and/or gristle, cold algin restructured beef slices (3.71) were considered to possess the most amount of fat/gristle, but not significantly more then beef stroganoff and charbroiled steaks (4.24 and 4.27

TABLE 4

Mean Attribute Ratings Among Various Algin Restructured Beef Dishes

Dish	Attribute						
	Appearance	Aroma	Juiciness	Tenderness	Uniformity	Fat/Gristle	Flavor	Acceptability
Cold slices	4.77[ab]	4.41	4.72	5.11	5.18	3.71[c]	4.99	5.27[a]
Charbroiled steak	5.11[a]	5.25	4.20	5.11	4.89	4.27[bc]	5.30	5.50[a]
Philly cheese steak	5.03[a]	5.53	4.65	5.55	5.43	5.60[a]	5.03	5.08[a]
Roast and gravy	4.14[b]	4.22	4.86	5.36	5.39	4.69[b]	4.93	4.58[b]
French dip	5.17[a]	4.83	4.45	5.38	5.38	5.90[a]	5.21	5.34[a]
Stroganoff	4.17[b]	5.06	4.88	5.06	5.00	4.24[bc]	5.24	5.29[a]
Grand mean	4.87	4.67	4.61	5.34	5.17	4.68	5.03	5.22
Standard deviation	1.33	1.28	1.22	1.30	1.75	1.36	1.28	1.35

Subscripts denote significant differences among attribute rating at $p<.05$.

respectively). Roast beef and gravy was judged to statistically have less fat/gristle (4.69) than the aforementioned dishes. French dip and Philly cheese steak dishes evoked the most positive responses with respect to fat/gristle with mean scores of 5.90 and 5.60 respectively.

When evaluating overall acceptability, the dishes were rated similarly (5.08-5.50), except for roast beef and gravy, which received a statistically lower mean acceptability score of 4.58.

Therefore, this study demonstrated that algin restructured beef can be used with good consumer acceptability in various beef-based dishes that are prepared using a wide range of cooking techniques.

REFERENCES

1. P.J. Luby, Nat. Provisioner, 2 (1985) 13-20.
2. J.T. Yankelovich, The consumer climate for red meat. Executive Summary, National Live Stock and Meat Board, Chicago, IL, 1985.
3. B.C. Breidenstein, Intermediate value beef products. Prepared for the National Live Stock and Meat Board, Chicago, IL 1982.
4. G.R. Schmidt and G.R. Trout, Meat Science and Technology International Symposium Proceedings, Lincoln, NE, National Live Stock and Meat Board, Chicago, IL, 1982.
5. G.R. Schmidt and J.N. Sofos, Trends in Modern Meat Technology 2. Proceedings of the International Symposium, Den Dolder, Netherlands, 1987.
6. A.D. Clarke, J.N. Sofos and G.R. Schmidt, J. Food Sci., 53 (1988) 711-713.
7. A.D. Clarke, J.N. Sofos and G.R. Schmidt, J. Food Sci., 53 (1988) 1266-1277.
8. H.R. Cross and M.S. Stanfield, J. Food Sci., 41 (1976) 1257-1258.
9. P.R. Durland, S.C. Seideman, W.J. Costello and N.M. Quenzer, J. Food Protect. 45 (1987) 127-131.
10. W.J. Means, A.D. Clarke, J.N. Sofos and G.R. Schmidt, J. Food Sci. 52 (1987) 252-256.

FORMATION OF DIALKYLTHIOPHENES IN MAILLARD REACTIONS INVOLVING CYSTEINE

G. P. RIZZI, A. R. STEIMLE and D. R. PATTON
Procter & Gamble Company, Miami Valley Laboratories
Cincinnati, Ohio 45239-8707 (U.S.A.)

SUMMARY

Thiazolidinecarboxylic acids (1) derived from cysteine and common food aldehydes decompose into volatile products at roasting temperatures. Examples of (1) were synthesized, pyrolyzed and resultant products were analyzed by GC/MS. Prominent reaction products were 2,4-dialkylthiophenes with identical substituents. A mechanism for dialkylthiophene formation is proposed in which all thiophene carbons are derived from carbonyl precursors of (1) and only the sulfur is contributed by cysteine.

1. INTRODUCTION

Cooked meat and deep fried foods contain many heteroaromatic flavor compounds with long sidechains i.e. 2-n-butyl, pentyl and hexylpyridines, pyrazines, thiazoles and thiophenes etc. which have been postulated to originate via joint reactions of proteins, carbohydrates and lipids (ref. 1). Model studies have further suggested that some of these alkylheterocycles are formed in reactions of lipids with amino acids or ammonia; for example, the formation of 2-n-pentylpyridine from linoleate (ref. 2). Also, Maillard reaction intermediates like aldehydes and dihydropyrazines undergo aldol condensation to form chain elongated products such as methylpentylpyrazines (ref. 3).

Formation of long chain thiazole and thiophene derivatives is less clearly understood. Recently, model reactions with cysteine and 2,4-decadienal generated alkylthiazoles and thiophenes similar to those observed in cooked meat (ref. 4). Cysteine has long been considered a precursor of meat flavor compounds, but pathways linking it to long chain thiazoles or thiophenes have not been described.

Cysteine reacts readily with aldehydes or ketones to form

derivatives of 4-thiazolidinecarboxylic acid (1) (ref. 5).
Compounds (1) are stable at room temperature, but decompose at
their melting points to form complex mixtures of volatile
products. Recently, similar thiazolidines derived from arabinose
and glucose (2, n=3,4) were patented for use as meat flavor
precursors (ref. 6). 4-Thiazolidinecarboxylic acid (1, R_1=H)
occurs in food (ref. 7) and its decomposition at 200°C was
shown to produce thiazolidine, a thiazoline and cyclic sulfur
compounds containing three sulfur atoms (ref. 8).

The foregoing evidence suggested that food aldehydes derived
from Strecker degradation of amino acids or from lipid oxidation
could react with cysteine during cooking/frying to form
thiazolidines (1, R_1=alkyl) which could later decompose to form
structurally related thiazoles. The objective of this work was
to test this hypothesis by heating authentic thiazolidines (1,
R_1=alkyl) to their decomposition points to see which, if any,
heterocyclic compounds might be formed. In principle,
thiazolidines (1) are naturally occurring, efficient precursors
of flavor significant long chain derived heteroaromatics.

2. EXPERIMENTAL
  2.1 Materials and Synthetic Procedures
    4-Thiazolidinecarboxylic acids (1a-g) were prepared by
reacting ethanal, propanal, n-butanal, 2-methylpropanal,
3-methylbutanal, n-hexanal or 2-phenylethanal with L-cysteine
according to literature procedures (ref. 5). Structures were
confirmed by proton and carbon NMR and by mass spectrometry
(Table 1). 2-n-Butyl-2-octenal was obtained by base-catalyzed
aldol condensation/dehydration of n-hexanal.

Pyrolyses of (1) were done either in flame-sealed 1 mL glass
ampules (0.1-0.3 mmol scale) or in glass flasks attached to
atmosphere-vented reflux condensors (5-40 mmol scale). Heat was
provided by a stirred, thermostated oil bath. Smaller scale

reaction mixtures were dissolved in methylene chloride and analyzed directly by GC/MS. Preparative scale reaction mixtures were stirred with hexane or pentane to extract relatively non-polar products. The hydrocarbon extracts were column chromatographed on 70-230 mesh silica gel [Merck Kieselgel 60] using hexane or pentane as eluant and fractions were analyzed by thin-layer chromatography (TLC) on 0.25 mm silica gel G plates [hexane or 75-25 v/v hexane-benzene solvent with I_2 vapor spot visualization]. Early fractions containing at most two of the least polar reaction products were pooled for GC/MS analysis. To simplify spectral interpretation, mixtures containing dihydrothiophenes were also dehydrogenated with chloranil (2,3,5,6-tetrachlorobenzoquinone) to form thiophenes (ref. 9).

2.1.1 <u>Pyrolysis of (1c)</u> Thiazolidine (1c), 5.91 g. (34 mmol) was heated at 190-195°C for 2 hrs during which time the compound melted, turned dark and evolved a considerable amount of gaseous products. The cooled mixture was stirred with pentane (150 mL). The concentrated pentane solution was chromatographed over 50 g. of silica gel. Pentane fractions (60 mL) were analyzed by TLC and those containing the two components with highest R_f value were combined, concentrated to yield 0.071 g. of pale yellow oil and analyzed by GC/MS (Table 2). The oil, consisting mainly of (3c) and (4c), was treated with 0.080 g. of chloranil in benzene (2 mL) and heated at reflux for 1.5 hrs. Benzene was carefully evaporated under partial vacuum and the pentane soluble portion of the reaction residue was chromatographed over 15 g. of silica gel. Early fractions containing a single component were combined and evaporated to yield 0.015 g. of 2,4-diethylthiophene (4c) as a colorless oil with a strong sulfurous, onioney aroma and UV max at 235 nm (log e = 3.78). Proton NMR data agreed well with literature values (ref. 10).

2.1.2 <u>Pyrolysis of (1g)</u> Thiazolidine (1g) 1.18 g. (5.3 mmol) was heated at 190°C for 2 hrs., cooled and extracted with benzene. The benzene solubles (0.65 g.) were chromatographed over 20 g. silica gel using benzene and early fractions were pooled to yield 0.0926 g. of yellow oil. No attempt was made to isolate a dihydrothiophene. The oil was treated directly with 0.098 g. of chloranil in benzene (3 mL) and heated at reflux for

1.5 hrs. Benzene was evaporated and hexane soluble products were chromatographed over silica gel (10 g.) using hexane. Initial fractions eluted 0.016 g. of 3-phenylthiophene (6, R_2= phenyl), a colorless solid; UV max 225 nm (log e = 4.08), 257 nm (log e = 4.04) (ref. 11); IR showed characteristic bands at 625, 675, 740, 790, 860 and 900 cm^{-1} (ref. 12); MS (probe sample) m/z (rel. int.) 160(100) M^+, 115(47), 161(14), 116(13) and 89(12). Further elution with 95-5 v/v hexane-benzene gave 0.016 g. of 2,4-diphenylthiophene (4g), a colorless solid; UV max 255 nm (log e = 4.35), inflection at 294 nm (log e = 3.75) (ref. 11); MS data are given in Table 2.

2.2 Analytical Methods

GC/MS was done with a Finnegan Model 800 (ion trap detector) mass spectrometer interfaced to a Hewlett-Packard 5880A GC. A 30 m x 0.25 mm fused silica column containing RTX-5 (0.5 u) [Restek Corp.] was programmed for zero hold time at 50°C and 4°C/min. to 130°C.

Mass spectra were obtained in the electron ionization (EI) mode (70eV) at a scan acquisition of 26-200 amu/spectrum/sec. GC without MS was done on a 30 m x 0.32 mm fused silica column containing DB-5 (1 u) [J&W Scientific Co.] programmed as follows: 7 min. hold at 37°C; 3°C/min. to 80°C; 1°C/min. to 90°C; 3°C/min. to 190°C and 5°C/min. to 250°C. Thiophene (4a) was quantitated via an external reference standard.

NMR data were obtained on a General Electric Co. QE-300 (300 MHz) spectrometer using $CDCl_3$ solvent. Spectrum calibration was provided by deuterium lock signals at 7.26 ppm (proton spectra) and 77.0 ppm (carbon spectra).

UV spectra were obtained in hexane solution on a Beckman DU-50 spectrophotometer.

IR spectra were obtained on samples dispersed in KBr pellets with a Perkin-Elmer Model 298 instrument.

Melting points were determined in open capillaries on a Mel-Temp apparatus and are uncorrected.

Mass spectra other than GC/MS were 70eV EI data acquired on a Hewlett-Packard Model 5985B instrument using a source temperature of 200°C and with a probe temperature programmed to rise ballistically from ambient to 325°C.

3. RESULTS AND DISCUSSION

Thiazolidine formation with cysteine is a special case of the Maillard reaction (ref. 13). With cysteine the initially formed Schiff's base does not undergo normal Amadori rearrangement, but instead cyclization occurs with nearby sulfhydryl groups to form a thiazolidine ring. Like Amadori compounds thiazolidines (1) and (2) decompose on heating to form complex mixtures of volatile products.

Thiazolidines (1a-g) were synthesized by reacting common food aldehydes with cysteine according to published procedures (Table 1). Compounds (1a-g) are colorless, odorless crystalline solids which all melted with complete decomposition at ca.

TABLE 1

4-Thiazolidinecarboxylic acids (1).

Compd	R_1	yield %	m.p. °C	mass spectral data m/z (relative intensity)
1a	CH_3	59	158-164	147[M^+](19), 75(100), 102(55), 86(54), 85(47) 132(43)
1b	C_2H_5	75	161-162	161[M^+](12), 132(100), 86(63), 69(15), 70(15), 114(13)
1c	$n-C_3H_7$	48	166-167	175[M^+](8), 132(100), 86(46), 59(11), 82(10) 87(9)
1d	$i-C_3H_7$	21	173-174	175[M^+](3), 132(100), 86(50), 87(9), 59(8), 133(7)
1e	$i-C_4H_9$	40	164-166	189[M^+](6), 132(100), 86(46), 100(12), 69(10), 59(10)
1f	$n-C_5H_{11}$	54	160-162	203[M^+](2), 132(100), 86(35), 100(9), 69(9), 68(8)
1g	$PhCH_2$	55	172-174	132[M^+](100), 86(64), 91(27), 59(10), 65(9), 77(9)

150-180°C to form sulfurous odors resembling roasted meat. GC/sniff-port analysis of decomposition products typically indicated 100-200 compounds of which some had potent aromas. Initially, compound (1f) was studied in greater detail to learn more about it's decomposition mechanism.

Thiazolidine (1f) decomposed rapidly at 190°C to form six major products tentatively identified by GC/MS as: hexanal; an n-butylthiophene; 2-n-pentyl-2-thiazoline; 2-butyl-2-octenal; a di-n-butylthiophene and a di-n-butyldihydrothiophene. Column chromatography on silica gel separated the dialkylthiophene fraction from the rest of a complex reaction mixture. The least polar fraction was analyzed by GC/MS and shown to be mainly a mixture of di-n-butylthiophene (4f) and the corresponding dihydrothiophene (3f) (Table 2). The mass spectrum of (4f) was similar to the published spectrum of 2,5-di-n-butylthiophene (ref. 14) and was characterized by facile loss of 3-C units resulting from McLafferty-type rearrangement (ref. 15). The mass spectrum of the dihydrothiophene (3f) differed significantly from the fully aromatic compound (4f). Compound (3f) exhibited a prominent molecular ion at m/z 198 and showed evidence for loss of an intact sidechain (4-C), m/z 141 (34% of base peak). Similar fragmentation has been reported for 2-methyldihydrothiophene (ref. 16).

(or C=C isomer)

3   4

To simplify the thiophene structure proof mixtures of (3f/4f) were treated with chloranil (2,3,5,6-tetrachlorobenzoquinone) to convert (3f) into more (4f). Complete reaction was evidenced by GC analysis which showed loss of (3f) and enhancement of (4f). Repeated column chromatography on silica gel afforded pure (4f) for spectral characterization.

The gross chemical structure of (4f) was confirmed by proton NMR. Ring substitution was obviously unsymmetrical as evidenced by unique ring methylene signals (triplets) at 2.58 and 2.81 ppm; i.e. evidence for a 2,4- or a 2,3-disubstituted thiophene. The ^{13}C NMR spectrum contained signals for four ring carbons consistent with an unsymmetically substituted dialkylthiophene (Table 3). The two peaks at greater chemical shifts had relatively smaller areas indicative of ring substitution at these points. The relative position of alkyl groups was established as 2,4 by proton-proton coupling constant data (Table 3). The small J value observed (0.5-1.0 Hz) for ring hydrogens is more indicative of 2,4-dialkylthiophenes than the 4.8 Hz expected for

TABLE 2

Pyrolysis products of 4-thiazolidinecarboxylic acids (1).

Precursor/Product	R_2	R_t min.	Yield[a] %	Product mass spectral data[b] m/z (relative intensity)
1a/4a	H	(5.3)[c]	0.16	not determined
1b/3b	CH_3	10.1	---	114[M$^+$](35), 99(100), 39(57) 45(45), 65(39), 41(32)
1b/4b	CH_3	9.4	1.5	112[M$^+$](70), 111(100), 97(64) 45(51), 39(45), 39(45)
1c/3c	C_2H_5	15.5	---	142[M$^+$](6), 125(100), 85(90) 113(73), 27(61), 45(57)
1c/4c	C_2H_5	13.0	6.5	140[M$^+$](26), 125(100) 45(26), 27(18), 39(17) 111(13)
1e/3e	i-C_3H_7	19.3	---	170[M$^+$](31), 41(100), 85(97) 153(87), 43(78), 39(78)
1e/4e	i-C_3H_7	17.0	18	168[M$^+$](22), 153(100) 111(31) 39(27), 41(24), 27(22)
1f/3f	n-C_4H_9	28.7	---	198[M$^+$](28), 41(100), 39(68) 155(55), 154(54), 111(45)
1f/4f	n-C_4H_9	26.9	11	196[M$^+$](16), 154(100) 111(82), 112(59), 27(44) 39(31)
1g/4g	Phenyl	---	15	236[M$^+$](100), 237(21) 234(15), 121(13), 202(13) 189(12)

[a] Percent of theoretical based on wt. of crude 3+4 mixture from column chromatography.
[b] Molecular ion plus five most intense peaks in spectrum.
[c] GC/MS conditions, except (5.3) = GC without MS.

TABLE 3

Thiophene NMR data[a].

Compd	ring carbons				ring protons	
	C-2	C-3	C-4	C-5	H-3, J	H-5, J
4c	147.2	116.4	144.3	124.5	6.66, 0.6	6.71, 1.2
4e	153.0	115.0	149.2	122.0	6.75, 0.9	6.76, 0.8
4f	145.5	117.0	142.8	125.4	6.66, 0.5	6.72, 1.0
4g	144.5	119.2	142.6	121.8	---	---

[a] Chemical shifts in ppm, J in Hz.

vicinal substitution (ref. 17).

Similar results were obtained by pyrolyzing thiazolidines (1b), (1c) and (1e) (Tables 2 and 3). In all cases the major products isolated by column chromatography were 2,4-dialkylthiophenes (plus dihydro derivatives) with identical ring substituents each having one fewer carbon atom than the sidechain originally present in respective thiazolidines (1). In addition to mass and NMR data the thiophenes (4c), (4e) and (4f) showed characteristic UV absorption maxima at 232-235 nm (log e = 3.50 to 3.78). Pyrolysis of thiazolidines (1a) and (1b) gave mixtures that we could not separate by column chromatography, however thiophene (4a) and 2,4-dimethylthiophene (4b) were tentatively identified by GC and GC/MS respectively.

The pyrolysis of thiazolidine (1g) derived from 2-phenylethanal produced somewhat different results in that 3-phenylthiophene (6, R_2=phenyl) was isolated in addition to the expected product, 2,4-diphenylthiophene (4g) (see EXPERIMENTAL). The presence of the 3-substituted thiophene suggested that the n-butylthiophene observed as a pyrolysis product of (1f) may actually have been 3-butylthiophene (6, R_2= n-butyl).

The odors of dialkylthiophenes (4b-4f) ranged from sulfurous/onioney for (4b) and (4c) to sulfurous/estery for (4e) and camphoraceous/aromatic for (4f). Phenylthiophenes had no odor at room temperature.

3.1 Reaction Mechanism

A possible mechanism for the pyrolysis of 4-thiazolidinecarboxylic acids is presented in Figure 1. Initial thermal decomposition is envisioned as a fragmentation process that produces three primary products: thioaldehydes (5); vinylamine and/or its tautomer iminoacetaldehyde and carbon dioxide. The absence of 2-pentylthiazolidine among the pyrolysis products of (1f) suggested that simple decarboxylation is not a major reaction pathway. Thioaldehydes are extremely unstable and predictably undergo further reactions (ref. 18). Aldol condensation of (5) followed by loss of hydrogen sulfide can lead to a dimeric alpha, beta-unsaturated thioaldehyde. Such a thioaldehyde can undergo hydrolysis with further loss of hydrogen sulfide to form a related sulfur-free aldehyde i.e. our observation of n-butyl-2-octenal by GC/MS analysis of (1f)

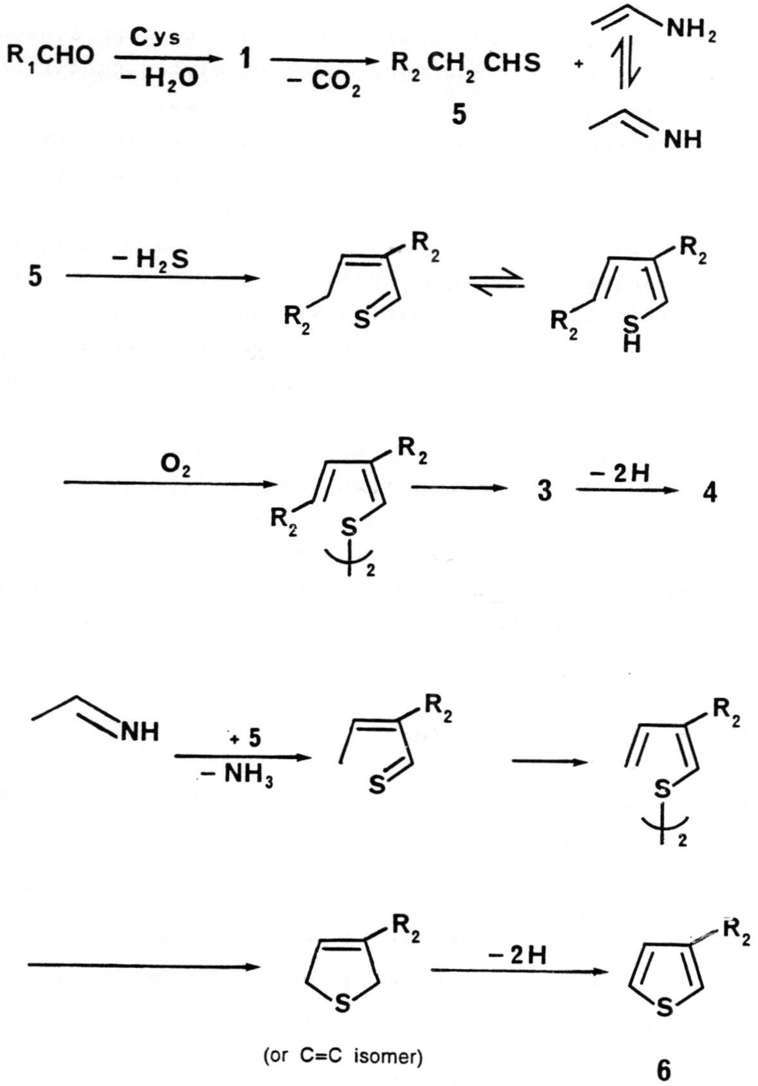

Fig. 1. Mechanism of alkylthiophene formation.

pyrolysate. The thioaldehyde dimer may also react (in its tautomeric dienemercaptan form) with oxygen to form a predicably more stable disulfide. However, under pyrolytic conditions such disulfides can undergo homolytic S-S bond cleavage, cyclization and chain transfer protonation to form dihydrothiophenes (3). Further oxidation or disproportionation of (3) finally leads to thiophenes (4).

Aldol condensation of initially formed thioaldehydes with co-produced iminoacetaldehyde followed by loss of ammonia leads to another thioaldehyde containing a single R_2 substituent. Further reactions like those already described can lead to 3-substituted thiophenes (6) as evidenced by our observation of (6), (R_2= phenyl, n-butyl).

Thioaldehydes are intriguing intermediates since they are also reasonable precursors of food important poly-sulfur heterocycles like: s-trithianes; 1,2,4-trithiolanes; 1,3,5-dithiazines and 1,3,5-oxadithianes (ref. 15). The thioaldehydes have not been reported in food per se, but as S-oxides they comprise a pungent component of onions (ref. 19).

REFERENCES

1   L.J. Farmer, D.S. Mottram and F.B. Whitfield, J. Sci. Food Agric., 49 (1989) 347-368.
2   S.K. Henderson and W.W. Nawar, J. Am. Oil Chem. Soc., 58 (1981) 632-635.
3   E.-M. Chiu, M.-C. Kuo, L.J. Bruechert and C.-T. Ho, J. Agric. Food Chem., 38 (1990) 58-61.
4   Y. Zhang and C.-T. Ho, J. Agric. Food Chem., 37 (1989) 1016-1020.
5   R. Riemschneider and G.-A. Hoyer, Z. Naturforsch., 17b (1962) 765-768.
6   Anon. Res. Discl., 179 (1979) 113-114; Chem. Abst., 90 (1979) 520.
7   Y. Kurashima, M. Tsuda and T. Sugimura, J. Agric. Food Chem., 38 (1990) 1945-1949.
8   F. Ledl, Z. Lebensm. Unters.-Forsch., 161 (1976) 125-129.
9   J.M. McIntosh and H. Khalil, Can. J. Chem., 53 (1975) 209-211.
10 L.I. Belen'kii and A.P. Yakubov, Tetrahedron, 42 (1986) 759-762.
11 H. Wynberg, H. van Driel, R.M. Kellogg and J. Buter, J. Am. Chem. Soc., 89 (1967) 3487-3494.
12 H. Rosatzin, Spectrochim. Acta, 19 (1963) 1107-1118.
13 R. Bognar, L. Somogyi and Z. Gyorgydeak, Justus Liebigs Ann. Chem., 738 (1970) 68-78.
14 A. Cornu and R. Massot, Compilation of Mass Spectral Data, Heyden & Son Ltd. (1966).

15   G. Vernin, Chemistry of Heterocyclic Compounds in Flavours and Aromas, John Wiley & Sons, New York (1982).
16   R.G. Arnold, L.M. Libbey and R.C. Lindsay, J. Agric. Food Chem., 17 (1969) 390-392.
17   E. Pretsch, J. Seibl, W. Simon and T. Clerc, Tables of Spectral Data for Structure Determination of Organic Compounds, Springer - Verlag, New York (1983) H265.
18   J. March, Advanced Organic Chemistry, 3rd Edition, John Wiley & Sons, New York (1985) 793.
19   M.H. Brodnitz and J.V. Pascale, J. Agric. Food Chem., 19 (1971) 269-272.

Listeria monocytogenes AND ITS FATE IN MEAT PRODUCTS

J.N. SOFOS

Departments of Animal Sciences and Food Science and Human Nutrition, Colorado State University, Fort Collins, CO 80523, U.S.A.

SUMMARY

Listeria monocytogenes is a well recognized human and animal pathogen which has been involved in several foodborne outbreaks of listeriosis in the past ten years. Listeriosis is exceptionally severe when it afflicts immunocompromised individuals, including pregnant women and their fetuses, where it is more than 20-30% fatal. The pathogen is commonly found in nature from where it contaminates plants, animals, water and foods. This emphasizes the need to increase our knowledge on this pathogenic bacterium in order to develop procedures for assurance of food product safety. Work in our laboratory has examined the potential of *L. monocytogenes* to survive and proliferate in meat plant environments, meat products, meat processing additives, and during thermal processing of various formulations of beef and pork. In general, the organism appears to be more resistant to adverse environments and processes than other nonspore-forming bacterial pathogens. Good hygiene and appropriate sanitation during product processing and handling, however, should reduce levels of contamination, which should permit traditional preservation procedures to control the pathogen.

1. GENERAL

1.1 The Disease

The disease caused by the facultative intracellular bacterium of *L. monocytogenes* is called listeriosis (1,2), and was first recognized as an animal infection in the early 1920s, while the first reported incidence of human listeriosis was in 1929 (3,4). Presently, it is known that more than 50 species of wild and domesticated animals are susceptible to the pathogen, and that it is the cause of infant and adult septicemia, meningitis and encephalitis (4). Other clinical manifestations produced by *L. monocytogenes* are flu-like illness, abortion, stillbirth, cerebritis, bacteremia, endocarditis, conjuctivitis, endophthalmitis, peritonitis, septic arthritis, osteomyelitis, cholecystitis, hepatitis, and brain and splenic abscesses (5). The primary manifestations in foodborne infections, however, have been meningitis, abortion and perinatal septicemia. In the absence of medical treatment death usually results from listeric meningitis. Abortion is usual in the last half of pregnancy, resulting in stillbirth or acutely ill infants, which die soon after delivery or develop meningitis, leading to death or mental deficiencies.

The incidence of the disease is generally sporadic, but in the past decade some major foodborne outbreaks were documented, indicating that the gastrointestinal tract may be the primary infection site through consumption of contaminated food (6). It is apparent from the above manifestations, however, that the pathogen affects tissues other than the gastrointestinal tract (7). Although the mechanisms by which *L. monocytogenes* causes listeriosis are not well defined, the pathogen is known to produce toxins, including hemolysins, lipolytic toxins, an extracellular hemorrhagic toxin, a pyrogenic fraction, and others. In addition, substances found in the cell wall of the organism may also contribute to its pathogenicity (6,7).

Although not defined for humans, cell numbers needed to infect susceptible individuals may be low, and the severity and symptoms of the disease are variable and depend on the susceptibility of the infected individual. In healthy adults, the infection is usually symptomless or takes the form of a mild, flu-like illness. The infection, however, is of pronounced severity in sensitive segments of the population. These include immuno-compromised or-deficient individuals such as infants, pregnant women, elderly, and people with hematological malignancy receiving immunosuppressive therapy (5). In general, the ingestion of *L. monocytogenes* should not result in disease in the absence of underlying risk factors. When it does strike sensitive segments of the population, however, it results in mortality rates of 20-35%.

1.2 Food-borne Outbreaks

In the past decade, *L. monocytogenes* has been implicated in some major food-borne documented outbreaks of listeriosis through consumption of raw vegetables, coleslaw, milk, and soft cheeses (8-12). In general, however, most cases of listeriosis are sporadic (13). In 1986, when listeriosis became a reportable disease in the United States, a total of 229 cases were identified (14,15). Current estimates project an annual incidence of 1600-1860 cases per year in the United States with approximately one-third resulting in death or stillbirths (13,15,16). Total annual estimated costs due to listeriosis amount to $480 million (16). It is also estimated that at least 1% of the humans may be asymptomatic carriers of the pathogen (12).

1.3 The Organism

The genus *Listeria* includes the species *L. monocytogenes*, *L. innocua*, *L. welshimeri*, *L. seeligeri* and *L. ivanovii* (17). Other species of *Listeria*, which have now been transferred to the genus *Jonesia*, are the previously known as *L. denitrificans*, *L. grayi* and *L. murrayi* (18,19). There are 16 distinguishable serovars associated with the five most common species of *Listeria* (20). Serovars associated with *L. monocytogenes* are 1/2a, 1/2b, 1/2c, 3a, 3b, 3c, 4a, 4ab, 4b, 4c, 4d, 4e and 7. Presently, *Listeria* is classified under Section 14 of Bergey's

Manual, "Regular, Nonsporing, Gram-positive Rods," which is comprised of seven very different genera (17). Previously, *L. monocytogenes* was placed in the family of *Corynebacteriaceae*.

Listeria spp. organisms are small regular rods or coccobacilli of 0.4-0.5 µm by 0.2-2.0 µm with rounded ends. Young cultures are Gram-positive, while old cultures may stain irregularly. They are asporogenous, not acid-fast and do not form capsules. They are motile, especially at 20-25°C by a few peritrichous, flagella (20). The organisms are aerobic and facultatively anaerobic, oxidase-negative, catalase-positive, methyl red-positive, Voges-Proskauer-positive, indole-negative, and urea-negative. They utilize glucose and esculin producing acid without gas, while only *L. murrayi* reduces nitrate. All species, with the exception of *L. grayi* and *L. murrayi*, hydrolyze sodium hippurate. Certain species utilize xylose and mannitol. *Listeria monocytogenes* is differentiated based on ß-hemolysis on blood agar and the CAMP-test, mouse pathogenicity, lack of utilization of mannitol and xylose, utilization of rhamnose, and tumbling motility in wet mount at 20-25°C (19,20). When grown on nutrient agar, the organisms form round colonies 0.5-1.5 mm in diameter, dew-drop in appearance, low convex with a fine texture and complete margin. On exposure to 45 degree incident transmitted white light, the colonies appear bluish, while under magnification and oblique lighting they have the appearance of bluish crushed glass (20).

1.4 Occurrence

Listeria monocytogenes is found in the environment worldwide, but its ecological niche is difficult to be established (3,21). The organism is found in the soil, water, sewage, feces, leaves, silage, plants, and animals (22). These sources contaminate plant and animal food products and humans (23). In general, *L. monocytogenes* has been found to be widely distributed in the environment contaminating in excess of 40 mammalian species and 17 avian species including chicken and turkey, as well as amphibians, fish, and insects (22,24,25).

More specifically, *L. monocytogenes* has been isolated from effluents of sewage treatment plants (26), and meat animal slaughter and processing environments (27), among other food processing operations. Sites in food processing plants found contaminated with the pathogen include cool and wet areas, legs of equipment, drains, refrigeration units, air handling systems, conveyors, unchlorinated water, and damaged or rusted stainless steel or other metal surfaces (3,28). These sources of the pathogen contaminate food products. Foods, however, may also be contaminated before they reach the plants. For example, infection of lactating cows can result in contaminated raw milk (29).

1.5 Factors Affecting Growth

Growth of *L. monocytogenes* in foods is influenced by many factors including the type and amount of nutrients, the pH, water activity, inhibitors, temperature, and packaging conditions (30). In general, however, the organism is able to grow over a wide range of temperatures, pH values and water activities (21), which makes it widely distributed in the environment, and of great concern in food products (31). The pathogen is capable of growing at refrigeration temperatures, and it can persist for long periods of time under adverse environmental conditions such as frozen storage and in dried materials. The temperature range allowing growth of *L. monocytogenes* is 1-45°C with an optimum at 30-37°C (17,25,32). The generation time in broth and foods such as milk decreases with increasing storage temperature (33,34). The pH range supporting growth of *L. monocytogenes* is 6-9 (17), although growth has been reported at pH values as low as 4.4-5.0 depending on substrate, acid, strains and storage temperature (34-41). In general, the pH range allowing growth of *L. monocytogenes* is wide enough that it includes most foods as well as fermented milk and meat products (30).

Listeria monocytogenes can tolerate low water activities, and is able to grow at sodium chloride concentrations as high as 10%, and to survive for long periods of time at higher levels (42). Survival of the organism in high amounts of sodium chloride depended on storage temperature. In 25.5% salt it could survive for five days at 37°C, 32 days at 22°C, and more than 132 days at 4°C (43). Although aerobic conditions allow growth of *L. monocytogenes* (17,44), proliferation is enhanced in anaerobic environments (39,45-47). Absence of oxygen also improved recovery of heated *L. monocytogenes* (48).

2. **BEHAVIOR OF** *Listeria* **IN FOODS**

The behavior of the organism in various foods depends on individual products and conditions (31,44). The organism was able to grow in raw shredded cabbage stored at 5°C (49), and during refrigerated (4°C) storage of liquid eggs (50). In Cheddar cheese made with inoculated milk the pathogen survived for more than 400 days (51), while in Camembert cheese, which is soft and of high pH, the organism was able to multiply during ripening (52). *Listeria monocytogenes* also survives frozen storage (53,54) and has been isolated from a variety of frozen foods, including meat, dairy and seafood products. The pathogen also survived spray drying of skim milk, and persisted for at least 12 weeks in the dried product (55). In dry cured fermented salami, *L. monocytogenes* also survived for 12 weeks at 5°C (56). In general, the organism has been shown to survive during the manufacture of fermented meat and dairy products, and it can be present in products of reduced pH during storage at refrigeration temperatures (31).

Several antimicrobial compounds, in addition to acid, have been shown to be inhibitory against *L. monocytogenes*. The inhibitory activity of sodium benzoate, potassium sorbate and sodium propionate against *L. monocytogenes* in tryptose both increased as the pH and storage temperature decreased (57-60). Lysozyme in combination with a chelating agent was inhibitory against the pathogen (61,62), while hydrogen peroxide may selectively enrich for *L. monocytogenes* in raw milk (63). Other inhibitors of *L. monocytogenes* include phenolic antioxidants, liquid smoke and sodium lactate (64-66).

In addition to surviving in high concentrations of sodium chloride (43), *L. monocytogenes* could proliferate, at pH 7.4 and in the absence of sodium chloride, in sodium nitrite concentrations as high as 1% at 4°C (67,68). Nitrite levels (0.02%) used in meats, however, were effective in inhibiting the organism in broth when combined with at least 3% sodium chloride, pH of 5.5, and storage at 4°C. In general, the bacteriostatic activity of sodium nitrite should be enhanced by low pH, low temperature, high sodium chloride concentration, and anaerobic environment (45).

As indicated by Donnelly (69), the scientific literature includes conflicting results relative to the heat resistance of *L. monocytogenes*. In general, it appears that *L. monocytogenes* is appreciably more resistant than *Salmonella* serotypes, but less resistant than *Salmonella seftenberg* 775W (70). Current milk pasteurization practices, however, are expected to inactivate the pathogen (71,72). Several studies have indicated that *L. monocytogenes* can survive cooking of red meat and poultry products to temperatures as high as 82°C (73-77). Heating of frankfurters for 70 minutes to 71.1°C should inactivate 10^3 cells/g (78). Heating sausage mixtures in beakers inoculated with 7×10^4 *L. monocytogenes* per gram to 51.7°C for eight hours or 57.2°C for four hours reduced the counts by >2 log CFU/g, while heating to 62.8°C inactivated the pathogen to undetectable levels (79). Heating pepperoni at 31.7°C for four hours, after fermentation but before drying, destroyed most *L. monocytogenes*, but the organism was occasionally detected in samples during drying. Heating after drying eliminated the pathogen completely.

Thermal resistance of *L. monocytogenes* in meat increases with addition of fat and curing salts (80-83). Sensitivity to heat may increase or remain the same for various strains when grown in media containing sodium chloride (84). Thermal resistance, however, may increase upon exposure of *L. monocytogenes* cells to heat shocking conditions (85,86). The heat shock condition of 48°C for 10 minutes increased the D-value at 55°C by 2.3-fold in nonselective and 1.6-fold in selective plating agar (87). D-values at 62.8°C in milk for *L. monocytogenes* heat-shocked at 43°C and plated anaerobically were 6-fold higher than those for cells held at 37°C and plated aerobically (48). Sokolovic and Goebel (88) found that heat shocking of *L. monocytogenes* at 48°C for 30 minutes resulted in detection of 12-14 proteins varying from 20 to 120 kilodaltons in molecular weight. The major heat shock protein detected was listeriosin, which may help the cell to lyse the phagosomal membrane. Increased heat resistance was also observed when cells of *L. monocytogenes* had formed microcolonies adherent to glass or stainless steel (89,90).

Cells of *L. monocytogenes* subjected to sublethal stress may be injured, as indicated by failure to grow in media containing selective agents which permit growth of noninjured cells (49,53,84,91-94). Injured cells do not grow in presence of selective agents such as acriflavin, polymyxin, sodium chloride, phenylethanol and tellurite. In addition to heat, *L. monocytogenes* may be injured by acid and freeze-thaw treatments, while addition of sugars, salts or polyols to the heating medium protect the cells from heat injury. Fructose and ammonium chloride, however, enhanced thermal destruction.

Although selective media are necessary for the isolation of *L. monocytogenes* in mixed cultures, they do not permit detection of injured organisms, and thus, they may be underestimating the extent of contamination with the pathogen. Smith and Archer (91) indicated that addition of pyruvate did not enhance recovery of *L. monocytogenes*, but Farber et al. (95) found that decreasing the temperature of resuscitation and increasing the incubation time in combination with added pyruvate enhanced recovery of heat injured cells. Lovett (96,97) reported that 25°C was the optimum temperature for repair of sublethally heat injured *L. monocytogenes*, while there is preliminary evidence that repair may be very slow or nonexistent at low temperatures (98).

3.   LISTERIOSIS FROM MEAT

Evidence of involvement of meat and meat products in food-borne human listeriosis is limited , and was reviewed by Johnson et al. (19). Almost forty years ago, sheep were infected experimentally with *L. monocytogenes*, which indicated that meat products could thus be contaminated and infect humans (99). Also mice were infected when fed meat contaminated with the pathogen (100). It has been indicated that four neighbors in Sweden were infected probably due to consumption of meat from the same source (101). Consumption of meat from a stillborn calf was also presumed to have resulted in listeriosis (102).

In recent years, the Centers for Disease Control conducted an epidemiologic case-control study to determine risk factors for occurrence of sporadic listeriosis in the United States (103). It was concluded that case-patients were significantly more likely than controls to have consumed undercooked chicken or uncooked hot dogs, with odds-ratio of 20.5 and 12.3, respectively. This conclusion, however, has been considered controversial because it is based only on epidemiological evidence and without established cause-and-effect association (19).

There are at least two cases of documented listeriosis from consumption of poultry products. One of these involved consumption of commercial cooked and chilled chicken which resulted in materno-fetal infection (104). The second incidence involved consumption of contaminated turkey frankfurters by an immunocompromised cancer patient (105). This infection occurred in April 1989 in Oklahoma and it was confirmed by finding a L. monocytogenes serotype 1/2a strain with identical isoenzyme types in the patient, an opened package of turkey frankfurters in her refrigerator, and in two of five unopened packages of the same brand purchased in local stores. Subsequent to this incidence, a study (106) evaluated the facility that produced these turkey frankfurters, and found the pathogen in 2/41 environmental samples from the plant and from 12/14 (86%) samples from the frankfurter peeler-conveyor.

4. CONTAMINATION OF MEAT AND POULTRY PRODUCTS

As indicated above, the environment and food processing plants are possible sources of contamination of animals and their products with L. monocytogenes. Several studies have examined contamination of meat and poultry plant environments and products with the pathogen (19,107). In addition to L. monocytogenes meat may be contaminated with other Listeria species. These include the nonpathogenic L. innocua, whose incidence may be higher than that of L. monocytogenes, and L. seeligeri and L. welshimeri. Furthermore, L. grayi, L. murrayi, L. denitrificans and atypical Listeria organisms have been isolated from meats, while the other pathogen, L. ivanovii, is found in sheep, but rarely in meat (19,108).

A study reported by the American Meat Institute (109) examined environmental samples from 41 meat processing plants and found that 20% of the food contact surfaces were contaminated with L. monocytogenes. Sources of contamination also include animal feces, hides and pelts (108,110,111). Thus, L. monocytogenes may be present in meat through contamination and infection of various tissues of the animal antemortem. Cells of the pathogen inoculated intravenously into cattle were found in muscles two days after inoculation (112). Thus, in some instances presence of L. monocytogenes in meat may not indicate post-slaughter contamination. Johnson et al. (113) examined interior muscle cores from 50 beef, 50 pork and 10 lamb roasts, and found that three beef and three pork roasts were contaminated with L. monocytogenes, presumably through antemortem exposure of the animal to the pathogen.

In general, studies from throughout the world have found that 0-90% of meat and poultry product samples examined were contaminated with *L. monocytogenes* (103,108,111,114-127). Several reports have presented evidence of contamination of fresh or frozen beef and pork with *L. monocytogenes*. In ground beef, *L. monocytogenes* was found in 29/50 (122) samples (48%), and 20/41 (118) samples (49%). In Denmark, *L. monocytogenes* was found in 19% of ground pork (111) and in 68% of ground beef samples (108). In Taiwan, the pathogen was present in 38.8% of pork samples and 24% of beef steaks (128).

An increasing number of studies has also isolated *L. monocytogenes* from poultry (108,119). Such studies have involved examination of chicken (129) and turkey (130) samples with 13-15% of the samples being positive, as well as environmental samples from poultry processing plants. Pini and Gilbert (121) in the United Kingdom found that 70/160 chicken samples (44%) were contaminated. Bailey et al. (115) in the Southeastern United States found that 21/90 (23%) of broiler carcasses were contaminated with *L. monocytogenes* and 34/190 (38%) with *Listeria* spp. In Australia, Varabioff (131) isolated *L. monocytogenes* from 2.1% (1/48) of fresh and 15% (12/80) of frozen chicken carcasses, while *L. innocua* was present in 10% and 17.5% of fresh and of frozen chicken carcasses, respectively. In Taiwan, Wong et al. (128) found *L. monocytogenes* in 50% of chicken carcasses and 38% of turkey parts, while in Canada, Farber et al. (126) showed that 56.3% of chicken legs were contaminated with the pathogen. *Listeria monocytogenes* was also isolated from 27/102 (26.5%) of precooked, ready-to-eat chicken samples (124).

Processed meat products have also been found contaminated with *L. monocytogenes*. Farber et al. (125) reported that 6/30 (20%) of fermented sausages examined were positive, while others have reported positive fermented sausage samples in the range 5-33% (116,117). Other processed meats found contaminated with *L. monocytogenes* include wieners (21%), luncheon meats (13%) and sliced meats (14%) (132,133); pork sausage (32%) (118); and processed, ready-to-eat meat products (22%) (134). The American Meat Institute (135) reported that in its 1987 survey 11.5% of the samples of ready-to-eat meat products examined were positive, while the incidence was 13% for 1988. In 1988, 38% of the frankfurter, 7% of the luncheon meat and 7% of the ham samples examined were positive for *L. monocytogenes* (135).

The Food Safety and Inspection Service of the United States Department of Agriculture has been involved in a national monitoring program for the incidence of *L. monocytogenes* in meat products (107). The program was initiated for raw meats in January 1987, for cooked products in September 1987, and for canned-cured meat in January 1988. Results indicated incidence in raw beef of 6.23% (41/658) for *L. monocytogenes*, 1.67% (36/2151) for *Salmonella* and 0% (0/906) for

Escherichia coli 0157:H7. *Listeria monocytogenes* incidence in canned-cured meats was 0% (0/140) and 2.2% (3/136) in Prosciutto ham (107). Incidence in cooked beef through October 1990 was 2.78% (44/1580), while in ready-to-eat meat and poultry products in the period of October-December, 1990, there were 48 positive samples identified (136).

It can be concluded that *L. monocytogenes* is a frequent contaminant and that it is virtually impossible to completely avoid its presence in meat and poultry products. Thus, it must be assumed that the pathogen will be present in the raw material and processing environment, and procedures must be designed to eliminate it or to avoid its proliferation, especially when introduced after product processing.

5. BEHAVIOR OF *Listeria* IN MEAT AND POULTRY PRODUCTS

A few studies have examined the fate of *L. monocytogenes* in raw meat and poultry products. It appears that cell numbers at refrigeration temperatures either remain constant or increase with storage time. Constant cell numbers have been reported for lamb meat at 0°C for 24 days (50); beef at 4°C for 14 days (56); and for ground meat or liver at 4°C for 30 days (137). The number of cells in inoculated sterile ground beef decreased initially, but then remained constant at 8°C (138). Another study with vacuum packaged strip loins found increased cell numbers with storage (139). The increase was more rapid at 5.3°C than at 0°C and at pH 6.0 than 5.6. Another interesting observation was that cell numbers were higher in fat than lean tissue or weep. Other studies found a decrease in cell numbers in lamb meat at 0°C and no change at 8°C (140). Problems associated with studies examining the fate of *L. monocytogenes* in meat are that they used only a limited number of strains and that the cultures used were propagated at temperatures (30-35°C) optimum for growth, while such cultures may behave differently when stored at colder temperatures.

It was reported that reduced numbers of the pathogen could survive fermentation, drying and refrigerated storage of hard salami and pepperoni (56,79). Since there was no growth in these products, the lactic acid cultures used in the fermentation reduced cell numbers and controlled growth. The fate of the pathogen in various cooked meat products appeared to be related to product type and pH (141). Growth was generally more pronounced in products of pH 6.0 or higher, and inhibited in products of pH 5.0 or lower. Storage of cooked chicken meat at 10°C allowed increases of *L. monocytogenes* cell numbers within 3-10 days (74-76). The pathogen also proliferated in previously sterilized chicken loaves stored under modified atmospheres (142). In general, the fate of *L. monocytogenes* in meat should depend on product pH, temperature of storage, amount of fat and lean tissue, strain of the pathogen, other contaminants present, and chemical additives.

6. EXPERIMENTAL
6.1 Objectives

Continuing studies in our laboratory are examining the potential of *L. monocytogenes* strains to survive and proliferate in meat plant environments, and in meat products with or without meat processing additives (82,83,143-146). More specifically we have examined the potential of the pathogen to survive and proliferate in waste fluids present in slaughterhouses and in meat processing facilities; its survival in meat curing brine solutions; and its thermal destruction in beef and pork without or with added nonmeat ingredients.

6.2 Procedures

Waste fluids tested to examine their potential to support growth of *L. monocytogenes* strain Scott A included: a lamb carcass rinsing fluid (after removal of pelt and offal); a floor waste fluid (containing a composite of all waste during the slaughtering operation); a floor drain fluid (drawn from the drain after slaughter and cleanup were complete); a meat grinder rinsing fluid (after washing); a sanitizer rinsing fluid (collected during meat grinder sanitation with 25 ppm titratable iodine); and a floor drain fluid sample (collected after cleaning and sanitation of the meat grinder was complete (143,144). Examination of the fate of the pathogen in curing brine solutions involved inoculation of aqueous solutions of sodium chloride (0-20%) and other curing agents with *L. monocytogenes* strain Scott A and incubation at 5°C (146). Examination of thermal destruction of *L. monocytogenes* (83,145) involved heating of strain Scott A inoculated in a ground beef slurry (20% ground beef/80% water); and in ground beef; or heating of a 9-strain composite inoculum in pork with or without nonmeat ingredients such as sodium chloride (0-3%), dextrose (0 or 1%), sodium phosphate (0 or 0.4%), sodium erythorbate (0 or 0.055%) and sodium nitrite (0 or 0.0156%). Detection of surviving cells of *L. monocytogenes* involved plating of serial dilutions in selective agar media such as modified Doyle-Schoeni Selective Agar (144), its modification (Mannitol-Phenol red-Esculin-Ferric ammonium citrate; MPEF) agar, Lithium chloride-Phenylethanol-Moxalactam (LPM) agar, and Lithium chloride-Phenylethanol-Moxalactam-Tellurite (LPMT) agar. When no colonies were detected by direct plating, the samples were enriched according to USDA procedures (147) for detection of injured cells.

6.3 Results and Discussion

In our studies (143,144) the pathogen, *L. monocytogenes*, was able to multiply within 24 hours at 8°C and 35°C in the waste fluids collected from a slaughterhouse and from cleaning of a meat grinder (Table 1). Proliferation varied with type of waste fluid and incubation temperature. Growth, however was present even at 8°C, while at 35°C was more rapid. The only fluid not supporting growth of the pathogen was the sanitizer solution collected as the washed and rinsed meat grinder was being sanitized. The pH of this solution was 3.50, while the other fluids had pH values in the range 6.60-7.40. This indicates that proper and frequent cleaning and sanitation is essential for reduction of the potential of contaminating meat with pathogenic *L. monocytogenes*.

Other studies (146) have indicated that *L. monocytogenes* is resistant to destruction by ingredients present in meat curing aqueous solutions (brines), especially, when meat residues are present in the solution. The pathogen may survive for long periods of time, during storage of brines, especially at lower temperatures (5°C). Brine ingredients not affecting survival of *L. monocytogens* included sodium chloride (up to 20%), dextrose, sodium phosphates, sodium lactate and sodium nitrite. Inactivation of the pathogen was recorded in brines containing acidic phosphates (sodium acid pyrophosphate and sodium hexametaphosphate) due to reduced brine pH. Also, in the absence of meat residue, sodium erythorbate (0.18%) resulted in inactivation of cells.

TABLE 1

Generation times (hours) of *L. monocytogenes* Scott A in waste fluids from meat plant environments.

Waste fluid	Generation time	
	8°C	35°C
Lamb carcass rinsing	25.5 ± 20.0	2.9 ± 0.4
Slaughterhouse floor waste	35.1 ± 31.0	2.1 ± 0.3
Slaughterhouse floor drain	12.3 ± 8.0	6.4 ± 2.4
Meat grinder rinsing	10.1 ± 0.4	8.9 ± 0.7
Meat grinder sanitizing	---[a]	---
Meat grinder floor drain	2.3 ± 0.1	2.2 ± 0.3

[a] No growth; pH 3.50.

Studies on thermal destruction (145) of *L. monocytogenes* in ground beef (80% lean, 20% fat) indicated that when an initial inoculum of 7-8 log colony forming units (CFU)/g was present, cells of the pathogen survived heating even to 70°C (Table 2). Thus, the safety of a meat product will depend on minimizing initial contamination and proper cooking to destroy cells of the pathogen that may be present.

TABLE 2

Thermal destruction of *L. monocytogens* strain Scott A in 80% lean ground beef heated in sealed tubes submerged in a 75°C water bath.

Final internal product temperature (°C)	Time of heating (min)	Reduction in *L. monocytogenes* (log CFU/g)
50	6.2	0.2-0.9
60	8.4	1.6-3.4
65	10.6	4.4-6.1
70	13.6	*

*Eight out of nine samples (8.08 log CFU/g initial inoculum) were positive for *L. monocytogenes* after enrichment.

In ground pork (pH 6.36-6.60) of 15% fat, destruction (83) of a composite of nine strains of *L. monocytogenes* by heat (83) was more difficult in cured than in uncured products (Tables 3 and 4).

TABLE 3

Effect of sodium chloride on thermal destruction of *L. monocytogenes* in ground pork cooked to 60°C.

Sodium chloride (%)	Reduction in *L. monocytogenes* (log CFU/g)
0	7.1
0.5	6.8
1.0	6.4
2.0	5.0
3.0	4.1

TABLE 4

Effect of curing ingredients on thermal destruction of *L. monocytogenes* in ground pork cooked to 60°C.

Curing ingredients	Reduction in *L. monocytogenes* (log CFU/g)
None	7.1
Sodium chloride (2%)	5.0
Dextrose (1%)	4.9
Sodium phosphates (0.4%)	6.4
Sodium erythorbate (0.055%)	6.8
Sodium nitrite (0.0156%)	6.9
All of the above	3.3

Curing ingredients protecting cells of *L. monocytogenes* from thermal destruction in ground pork included sodium chloride, dextrose and sodium phosphates (a mixture of sodium tripolyphosphate and sodium hexametaphosphate), while sodium erythorbate and sodium nitrite had no influence on extent of thermal destruction. Death of *L. monocytogenes* cells by heat was reduced with increasing concentration of sodium chloride, and when all curing ingredients were used as a complete cure. Other nonmeat ingredients which did not influence extent of thermal destruction included sodium lactate, kappa-carrageenan and the algin-calcium meat binder (83).

Additional studies in our laboratory have indicated that when cooked to a constant internal temperature, products with more fat (17-34%) required more cooking time, but the extent of thermal destruction of *L. monocytogenes* was similar to products with lower fat (5-8%) (82). Products with added water (25%) also showed similar extent of destruction of *L. monocytogenes* by heat when cooked to the same internal temperature, as products with no added water.

In general, animal slaughterhouse and meat processing facilities are potential sources of *L. monocytogenes* hazards because the organism can proliferate in waste fluids even at 8°C. Thus, sanitation programs should be based on the assumption that the pathogen is present and should react accordingly. Frequent cleaning and proper application of effective sanitizers are essential for control of *Listeria*. Improper cooking of meat may result in a is a potential *L. monocytogenes* hazard because high initial cell numbers of the pathogen can survive refrigerated storage and cooking of ground beef even to 70°C. Our studies have also indicated that *L. monocytogenes* is difficult to inactivate, especially in cured meat, since several curing ingredients protect it from thermal destruction. Thus, it is important for meat processors to reinforce meat plant sanitation guidelines so that raw material contamination is minimal, especially in cured meat products, where destruction is less efficient.

7. REFERENCES

1. S. Kathariou and L. Pine, in: A.J. Miller, J.L. Smith and G.A. Somkuti (Eds), Laboratory studies of virulence of *Listeria monocytogenes*. *Foodborne Listeriosis*, Elsevier, Amsterdam, 1990, pp. 55-60.
2. W.F. Schlech, III, in: A.J. Miller, J.L. Smith and G.A. Somkuti (Eds), *Listeria*, animals and man: aspects of virulence. *Foodborne Listeriosis*. Elsevier, Amsterdam, 1990, pp. 51-54.
3. S.A. McCarthy, in: A.J. Miller, J.L. Smith and G.A. Somkuti (Eds), *Listeria* in the environment. *Foodborne Listeriosis*, Elsevier, Amsterdam, 1990, pp. 25-29.
4. H.P.R. Seeliger, in: A.J. Miller, J.L. Smith and G.A. Somkuti (Eds), Listeriosis-avoidable risk? *Foodborne Listeriosis*, Elsevier, Amsterdam, 1990, pp. 1-3.
5. B. Lorber, in: A.J. Miller, J.L. Smith and G.A. Somkuti (Eds), Clinical listeriosis--implications for pathogenesis. *Foodborne Listeriosis*, Elsevier, Amsterdam, 1990, pp. 41-49.
6. W.F. Schlech, III, Food Technol. 41, 4 (1988) 176-178.

7   E.H. Marth, Food Technol., 41, 4 (1988) 165-168.
8   Anonymous, Bull l'Office Fed. Sante. Publ., 3 (1988) 28-29.
9   D.W. Fleming, S.L. Cochi, K.L. MacDonald, J. Brondum, P.S. Hayes, B.D. Plikaytis, M.B. Holmes, A. Audurier, C.V. Broome and A.L. Reingold, N. Engl. J. Med., 312 (1985) 404-407.
10 J.L. Ho, K.N. Shands, G. Friedland, P. Ecking and D.W. Fraser, Arch. Intern. Med., 146 (1986) 520-524.
11 M.J. Linnan, L. Maxcola, X.D. Lou, V. Goulet, S. May, C. Salminen, D.W. Hird, L. Yonekura, P. Hayes, R. Weaver, A. Audurier, B.D. Plikaytis, S.L. Fannin, A. Kleks and C.V. Broome, N. Engl. J. Med., 319 (1988) 823-828.
12 W.F. Schlech, III, P.M. Lavigne, R.A. Bortolussi, A.C. Allen, E.V. Haldane, A.J. Wort, A.W. Hightower, S.E. Johnson, S.H. King, E.S. Nicholls and C.V. Broome, N. Engl. J. Med., 308 (1983) 203-206.
13 B. Schwartz, R.W. Pinner and C.V. Broome, in: A.J. Miller, J.L. Smith and G.A. Somkuti (Eds), Dietary risk factors for sporadic listeriosis: association with consumption of uncooked hot dogs and undercooked chicken. *Foodborne Listeriosis*. Elsevier, Amsterdam, 1990, pp. 67-70.
14 J. Bille, in: A.J. Miller, J.L. Smith, G.A. Somkuti (Eds), Epidemiology of human listeriosis in Europe, with special reference to the Swiss outbreak. *Foodborne Listeriosis*, Elsevier, Amsterdam, 1990, pp. 71-74.
15 C.V. Broome, B. Gellin and B. Schwartz, in: A.J. Miller, J.L. Smith and G.A. Somkuti (Eds), Epidemiology of listeriosis in the United States. *Foodborne Listeriosis*, Elsevier, Amsterdam, 1990, pp. 61-65.
16 T. Roberts and R. Pinner, in: A.J. Miller, J.L. Smith and G.A. Somkuti (Eds), Economic impact of disease caused by *Listeria monocytogenes*. *Foodborne Listeriosis*, Elsevier, Amsterdam, 1990, pp. 137-149.
17 H.P.R. Seeliger and D. Jones, in: Sneath, Mari, Sharpe and Holt (Eds), Genus *Listeria* Pirie, 1940, 383. *Bergey's Manual of Systemic Bacteriology*, Vol. 2, Williams and Wilkins, Baltimore, MD, 1986.
18 J. Rocourt and H.P.R. Seeliger, Zbl. Bakteriol. Hyg. A, 259 (1985) 317-330.
19 J.L. Johnson, M.P. Doyle and R.G. Cassens, J. Food Prot., 53 (1990) 81-91.
20 J. Lovett, in: A.J. Miller, J.L. Smith and G.A. Somkuti (Eds), Taxonomy and general characteristics of *Listeria* spp. *Foodborne Listeriosis*. Elsevier, Amsterdam, 1990, pp. 9-12.
21 D.L. Archer, in: A.J. Miller, J.L. Smith and G.A. Somkuti (Eds). *Listeria monocytogenes*: what is its ecological niche? *Foodborne Listeriosis*, Elsevier, Amsterdam, 1990, pp. 5-8.
22 M.L. Gray, and A.H. Killinger, Bacteriol. Rev., 30 (1966) 309-382.
23 L.R. Beuchat, M.E. Berrang and R.E. Brackett, in: A.J. Miller, J.L. Smith and G.A. Somkuti (Eds), Presence and public health implications of *Listeria monocytogenes* on vegetables. *Foodborne Listeriosis*. Elsevier, Amsterdam, 1990, pp. 175-181.
24 J. Weis and H.P.R. Seeliger, Appl. Microbiol., 30 (1975) 29-32.
25 R.E. Brackett, Food Technol., 42, 4 (1988) 162-164, 178.
26 M.R. Al-Ghazali and S.K. Al-Azawi, J. Appl. Bacteriol., 60 (1986) 251-254.
27 J. Watkins and K.P. Sleath, J. Appl. Bacteriol., 50 (1981) 1-9.
28 M.T. Knight, J.F. Black and D.W. Wood, J. Assoc. Off. Anal. Chem., 71 (1988) 682-683.
29 E.H. Marth and E.T. Ryser, in: A.J. Miller, J.L. Smith and G.A. Somkuti (Eds), Occurrence of *Listeria in foods: milk and dairy foods*. *Foodborne Listeriosis*, Elsevier, Amsterdam, 1990, pp. 151-164.
30 J. Lovett, D.W. Francis and J.G. Bradshaw, in: A.J. Miller, J.L. Smith and G.A. Somkuti (Eds), Outgrowth of *Listeria monocytogenes* in foods. *Foodborne Listeriosis*. Elsevier, Amsterdam, 1990a, pp. 183-187.
31 A.M. Lammerding and M.P. Doyle, in: A.J. Miller, J.L. Smith, G.A. Somkuti (Eds), Stability of *Listeria monocytogenes* to non-thermal processing conditions. *Foodborne Listeriosis*, Elsevier, Amsterdam, 1990, pp. 195-202.

32 J.R. Junttila, S.I. Niemela and J. Hirn, J. Appl. Bacteriol., 65 (1988) 321-327.
33 R.L. Petran and E.A. Zottola, J. Food Sci., 54 (1989) 458-460.
34 E.M. Rosenow and E.H. Marth, J. Food Prot., 50 (1987) 452-459.
35 N. Ahamad and E.H. Marth, J. Food Prot., 52 (1989) 688-695.
36 N. Ahamad and E.H. Marth, J. Food Prot., 53 (1990) 26-29.
37 K.M. Sorrells, D.C. Enigl and J.R. Hatfield, J. Food Prot., 52 (1989) 571-573.
38 M.E. Parish and D.P. Higgins, J. Food Prot., 52 (1989) 144-147.
39 R.L. Buchanan and J.C. Phillips, J. Food Prot., 53 (1990) 370-376, 381.
40 D.E. Conner, R.E. Brackett and L.R. Beuchat, Appl. Environ. Microbiol., 52 (1986) 59-63.
41 S.M. George, B.M. Lund and T.F. Brocklehurst, Lett. Appl. Microbiol., 6 (1988) 153-156.
42 H.P.R. Seeliger, Listeriosis, Hafner Publishing Co., New York, 1961.
43 M. Shahamat, A. Seaman and M. Woodbine, Zb. Bakteriol. Hyg., I. Abt. Orig. A, 246 (1980a) 506-511.
44 M.P. Doyle, Food Technol., 42, 4 (1988) 169-171.
45 R.L. Buchanan, H.G. Stahl and R.C. Whiting, J. Food Prot., 52 (1989) 844-851.
46 R.L. Buchanan and L.A. Klawitter, J. Food Sci., 55 (1990) 1754-1756.
47 L. Wimpfheimer, N.S. Altman and J.H. Hotchkiss, Int. J. Food Microbiol., 11 (1990) 205-214.
48 S.J. Knabel, H.W. Walker, P.A. Hartman and A.F. Mendonca, Appl. Environ. Microbiol., 56 (1990) 370-376.
49 L.R. Beuchat, R.E. Brackett, D.Y.-Y. Hao and D.E. Conner, Can. J. Microbiol., 32 (1986) 791-795.
50 M.A. Khan, I.A. Newton, A. Seaman and M. Woodbine, in: M. Woodbine (Ed), The survival of *Listeria monocytogenes* inside and outside its host. Problems of Listeriosis, Leicester University Press, Leicester, England, 1975.
51 E.T. Ryser and E.H. Marth, J. Food Prot., 50 (1987a) 7-13.
52 E.T. Ryser and E.H. Marth, J. Food Prot., 50 (1987b) 372-378.
53 D.A. Golden, L.R. Beuchat and R.E. Brackett, Appl. Environ. Microbiol., 54 (1988a) 1451-1456.
54 D.A. Golden, L.R. Beuchat and R.E. Brackett, Food Microbiol., 5 (1988b) 17-23.
55 M.P. Doyle, L.M. Meske and E.H. Marth, J. Food Prot., 48 (1985) 740-742.
56 J.L. Johnson, M.P. Doyle and R.G. Cassens, Int. J. Food Microbiol., 6 (1988) 243-247.
57 M.A. El-Shenawy and E.H. Marth, J. Food Prot., 51 (1988a) 525-530.
58 M.A. El-Shenawy and E.H. Marth, J. Food Prot., 51 (1988b) 842-847.
59 M.A. El-Shenawy and E.H. Marth, Int. J. Food Microbiol., 8 (1989) 85-94.
60 E.T. Ryser and E.H. Marth, J. Food Prot., 51 (1988) 615-621.
61 V.L. Hughey and E.A. Johnson, Appl. Environ. Microbiol., 53 (1987) 2165-2170.
62 V.L. Hughey, P.A. Wilger and E.A. Johnson, Appl. Environ. Microbiol., March, 1989, 836-888.
63 L. Dominguez, J.F.F. Garayazabal, E.R. Ferri, J.A. Vazquez, E. Gomez-Lucia, C. Ambrosio and G. Suarez, J. Food Prot., 50 (1987) 636-639.
64 K.D. Payne, E. Rico-Munoz and P.M. Davidson, J. Food Prot., 52 (1989) 151-153.
65 M.C. Messina, H.A. Ahmad, J.A. Marchello, C.P. Gerba and M.W. Paquette, J. Food Prot., 51 (1988) 629-631.
66 E. Harmayani, J.N. Sofos and G.R. Schmidt, Behavior of *Listeria monocytogenes* in raw and cooked ground beef with meat processing additives, Proceedings of the 51st Ann. Meeting Inst. Food Technol., Dallas, Texas, 1 June - 5 June 1991, Abstract No. 404.

67 M. Shahamat, A. Seaman and M. Woodbine, in: G.W. Gould and J.E.L. Corry (Eds), Influence of sodium chloride, pH and temperature on the inhibitory activity of sodium nitrite on *Listeria monocytogenes*. *Microbial growth and survival in extremes of environment*, Academic Press Inc., New York, 1980b, pp. 227-237.
68 J. Junttila, J. Hirn, P. Hill and E. Nurmi, J. Food Prot., 52 (1989) 158-161.
69 C.W. Donnelly, in: A.J. Miller, J.L. Smith and G.A. Somkuti (Eds), Resistance of *Listeria monocytogenes* to heat. *Foodborne Listeriosis*, Elsevier, Amsterdam, 1990, pp. 189-193.
70 B.M. Mackey and N. Bratchell, Lett. Appl. Microbiol., 9 (1989) 89-94.
71 J. Lovett, I.V. Wesley, M.J. Vandermaaten, J.G. Bradshaw, D.W. Francis, R.G. Crawford, C.W. Donnelly and J.W. Messer, J. Food Prot., 53 (1990b) 734-738.
72 J.G. Bradshaw, J.T. Peeler and R.M. Twedt, J. Food Prot., 54 (1991) 12-14.
73 P.G. Karaioannoglou and G.C. Xenos, Medecine Veterinaire Hellenique, 23 (1980) 111-118.
74 M.A. Harrison and S.L. Carpenter, J. Food Prot., 52 (1989a) 376-378.
75 M.A. Harrison and S.L. Carpenter, Food Microbiol., 6 (1989b) 153-157.
76 S.L. Carpenter and M.A. Harrison, J. Food Sci., 54 (1989) 556-557.
77 J.E. Gaze, G.D. Brown, D.E. Gaskell and J.G. Banks, Food Microbiol., 6 (1989) 251-259.
78 L.L. Zaika, S.A. Palumbo, J.L. Smith, F. Del Corral, S. Bhaduri, C.O. Jones and A.H. Kim, J. Food Prot., 53 (1990) 18-21.
79 K.A. Glass and M.P. Doyle, J. Food Prot., 52 (1989) 226-231, 235.
80 J.M. Farber, Int. J. Food Microbiol., 8 (1989) 285-291.
81 B.M. Mackey, C. Pritchet, A. Norris and G.C. Mead, Lett. Appl. Microbiol., 10 (1990) 251-255.
82 N. Boonmasiri, J.N. Sofos and G.R. Schmidt, Thermal destruction of *Listeria monocytogenes* in ground pork with different levels of fat, Presented at the Ann. Meet. Inst. Food Technol.,16 June - 20 June 1990, Anaheim, CA, Abstract No. 387.
83 L. Yen, J.N. Sofos and G.R. Schmidt, Effect of sodium chloride on thermal destruction of *Listeria monocytogens* in ground pork. Presented at the Ann. Meet. Inst. Food Technol., Anaheim, CA, 16 June - 20 June 1990, Abstract No. 385.
84 A.W. Dallmier and S.E. Martin, Appl. Environ. Microbiol., 54 (1988) 581-582.
85 W.M. Fedio and H. Jackson, Lett. Appl. Microbiol., 9 (1989) 157-160.
86 J.M. Farber and B.E. Brown, Appl. Environ. Microbiol., 56 (1990) 1584-1587.
87 R.H. Linton, M.D. Pierson and J.B. Bishop, J. Food Prot., 53 (1990) 924-927.
88 Z. Sokolovic and W. Goebel, Infect. Immun., 57 (1989) 295-298.
89 S.-H. Lee and J.F. Frank, J. Food Safety, 11 (1991) 65-71.
90 J.F. Frank and R.A. Koffi, J. Food Prot., 53 (1990) 550-554.
91 J.L. Smith and D.L. Archer, J. Ind. Microbiol., 3 (1988) 105-110.
92 J.T. Smith and S.E. Hunter, Lebensm.-Wissench. und Technol., 21 (1988) 307-311.
93 J.L. Smith, in: A.J. Miller, J.L. Smith and G.A. Somkuti (Eds), Stress-induced injury in *Listeria monocytogenes*. *Foodborne Listeriosis*. Elsevier, Amsterdam, 1990, pp. 203-209.
94 J.L. Smith and B.S. Marmer, J. Food Safety, 11 (1991) 73-80.
95 J.M. Farber, G.W. Sanders and J.I. Speirs, J. Assoc. Off. Anal. Chem., 71 (1988) 675-678.
96 J. Lovett, J. Assoc. Off. Anal. Chem., 71 (1988a) 658-660.
97 J. Lovett, Food Technol., 42, 4 (1988b) 172-175.
98 R.G. Crawford, C.M. Beliveau, J.T. Peeler, C.W. Donnelly and V.K. Bunning, Appl. Environ. Microbiol., 55 (1989) 1490-1494.

99   J.W. Osebold and T. Inouye, J. Infect. Dis., 95 (1954) 67-78.
100 K. Temper, Archiv fur Lebensmittelhyg., 12 (1961) 1-4.
101 L. Olding and L. Philipson, Acta Pathol. Microbiol. Scand., 48 (1960) 24-30.
102 E.H. Kampelmacher, in: M.L. Gray (Ed), Animal products as a source of listeric infection in man. In Second Symposium on *Listeria* Infection, Montana State College, Bozeman, MT, 1962, pp. 146-156.
103 B. Schwartz, C.A. Ciesielski, C.V. Broome, S. Gaventa, G.R. Brown, B.G. Gellin, A. W. Hightower, L. Mascola and the Listeriosis Study Group, Lancet, 11, 8614 (1988) 779-782.
104 K.G. Kerr, S.F. Dealler and R.W. Lacey, Lancet, ii (1988) 1133.
105 Anonymous, Morbid. Mortal. Weekly Rep., 38 (1989) 267-268.
106 J.D. Wenger, B. Swaminathan, P.S. Hayes, S.S. Green, M. Pratt, R.P. Pinner, A. Schuchat and C.V. Broome, J. Food Prot., 53 (1990) 1015-1019.
107 J.M. Carosella, in: A.J. Miller, J.L. Smith and G.A. Somkuti (Eds), Occurrence of *Listeria monocytogenes* in meat and poultry. *Foodborne Listeriosis*, Elsevier, Amsterdam, 1990, pp. 165-173.
108 N. Skovgaard and C.-A. Morgen, Int. J. Food Microbiol., 6 (1988) 229-242.
109 Anonymous, Microbial control during production of ready-to-eat meat products. Controlling the incident of *Listeria monocytogenes*. American Meat Institute, Washington, DC 20007, 1987.
110 P.D. Lowry and I. Tiong. The incidence of *Listeria monocytogenes* in meat and meat products factors affecting distribution. Proc. 34th Int. Congress Meat Sci. Technol., part. B, 1988, pp. 528-530.
111 N. Skovgaard and B. Norrung, Int. J. Food Microbiol., 8 (1989) 59-63.
112 J.L. Johnson, M.P. Doyle, R.G. Cassens and J.L. Schoeni, Appl. Environ. Microbiol., 54 (1988) 497-501.
113 J.L. Johnson, M.P. Doyle and R.G. Cassens, J. Food Sci., 55 (1990) 572, 574.
114 C. Breer and G. Breer, The isolation of *Listeria* spp. in meat and meat products, Proc. 34th Int. Congress Meat Sci. Technol., part B, 1988, pp. 520-521.
115 J.S. Bailey, D.L. Fletcher and N.A. Cox, J. Food Prot., 52 (1989) 148-150.
116 V.J. Breuer and O. Prandl, Archiv. Lebensmittelhyg., 39 (1988) 25-56.
117 World Health Organization, Report of the informal working group on foodborne listeriosis. WHO/EHE/FOS/88.5, Geneva, Switzerland, 1988, pp. 1-18.
118 D. McClain and W.H. Lee, J. Assoc. Off. Anal. Chem., 71 (1988) 660-664.
119 M. Gitter, Vet. Rec., 99 (1976) 336.
120 P.N. Pini and R.J. Gilbert, Int. J. Food Microbiol., 6 (1988) 317-326.
121 P.N. Pini and R.J. Gilbert, Int. J. Food Microbiol., 7 (1988) 331-337.
122 R.B. Truscott and W.B. McNab, J. Food Prot., 51 (1988) 626-628.
123 K.G. Kerr, S.F. Dealler and R.W. Lacey, Lancet, ii (1988) 37-38.
124 K.G. Kerr, N.A. Rotowa, P.M. Hawkey and R.W. Lacey, J. Food Prot., 53 (1990) 606-607.
125 J.M. Farber, F. Tittinger and L. Gour, Can. Inst. Food Sci. Technol. J., 21 (1988) 430-434.
126 J.M. Farber, G.W. Sanders and M.A. Johnston, J. Food Prot., 52 (1989) 456-458.
127 J.A. Nicolas, Sci. Aliments, 5 (1985) 175-180.
128 H.-C. Wong, W.-L. Chao and S.-J. Lee, Appl. Environ. Microbiol., 56 (1990) 3101-3104.
129 C.A. Genigeorgis, D. Dutulescu and J.F. Garayzabal, J. Food Prot., 52 (1989) 456-458.
130 C.A. Genigeorgis, P. Oanca and D. Dutulescu, J. Food Prot., 53 (1990) 282-288.
131 Y. Varabioff, J. Food Prot., 53 (1990) 555-557.
132 N.P. Tiwari and S.G. Aldenrath, J. Food Prot., 53 (1990) 382-385.

133 N.P. Tiwari and S.G. Aldenrath, Can. Inst. Food Sci. Technol. J., 23 (1990) 109-113.
134 J. Gledel, Vetmed-Hetic., 5 (1987) 9-20.
135 G.D. Wilson, *Listeria monocytogenes*-1988. Proceedings of the Reciprocal Meat Conference, vol. 41, National Live Stock and Meat Board, Chicago, 1988, pp. 11-13.
136 Anonymous, FSIS reports increased positives for listeria, American Meat Institute Newsletter, 1 February 1991, p. 5.
137 L.A. Shelef, J. Food Prot., 52 (1989) 379-383.
138 P. Gouet, J. Labadie and C. Serratore, Zbl. Bakteriol. Hyg. I. Abt. Orig. B, 166 (1978) 87-94.
139 F.H. Grau and P.B. Vanderlinde, J. Food Prot., 53 (1990) 739-741.
140 M.A. Khan, C.V. Palmas, A. Seaman and M. Woodbine, Acta Microbiol. Acad. Sci. Hung., 19 (1972) 357-362.
141 K.A. Glass and M.P. Doyle, Appl. Environ. Microbiol., 55 (1989) 1565-1569.
142 S.C. Ingham, J.M. Escude and P. McCown, J. Food Prot., 53 (1990) 289-291.
143 D.L. Boyle, G.R. Schmidt and J.N. Sofos, J. Food Sci., 52 (1990a) 277-278.
144 D.L. Boyle, J.N. Sofos and G.R. Schmidt, J. Food Prot., 53 (1990b) 102-104, 1118.
145 D.L. Boyle, J.N. Sofos and G.R. Schmidt, J. Food Sci. 55 (1990c) 327-329.
146 B.D. Gildemeister, J.N. Sofos and G.R. Schmidt, Survival of *Listeria monocytogenes* in aqueous solutions of meat curing ingredients, Presented at the Ann. Meet. Inst. Food Technol., 16 June - 20 June 1990, Anaheim, CA, 1990, Abstract No. 384.
147 D. McClain and W.H. Lee, FSIS method for the isolation and identification of *Listeria monocytogenes* in meat and poultry products. Laboratory Communication No. 57. U.S. Department of Agriculture - FSIS, Microbiology Division, Beltsville, MD.

EXTRUSION COOKING OF CHICKEN MEAT WITH VARIOUS NONMEAT INGREDIENTS

A.S. BA-JABER[3], J.N. SOFOS[1]*, G.R. SCHMIDT[1] and J.A. MAGA[2]

[1]Departments of Animal Sciences and Food Science and Human Nutrition, Colorado State University, Fort Collins, CO 80523, U.S.A.

[2]Department of Food Science and Human Nutrition, Colorado State University, Fort Collins, CO 80523, U.S.A.

[3]Department of Food Science, King Saud University, Riyadh (Saudi Arabia)

SUMMARY

Although extrusion-cooking of raw meat of high moisture and fat content is generally difficult, several studies have attempted to accomplish meat texturization by extrusion of precooked or dried meat, or by extrusion after mixing with plant materials, including corn starch, soy proteins, wheat flour, potato products and gums. Problems encountered during extrusion cooking of raw meat include material gushing from the extruder die and backflowing of the raw material from the extruder inlet. Studies in our laboratory have examined extrusion-cooking of chicken meat in combination with corn starch, oat fiber, whey protein concentrate and soy protein products. Other variables evaluated included level of nonmeat ingredient (10-20%), screw speed (60-100 rpm) and extrusion temperature (75-125°C). Extruder screw speed had no influence on the properties of any of the extruded products. Of all six nonmeat ingredients tested soy proteins resulted in extrusion-cooked chicken meat products with better binding than other ingredients. The highest binding scores of all products were achieved with soy protein isolate. Certain treatments received binding scores above 5, with 6 being the maximum and corresponding with binding of commercial frankfurters.

1. **INTRODUCTION**

Results of several published and unpublished studies have demonstrated that formation of extrusion-cooked products from meat is possible, and that the process can be useful in upgrading animal products and byproducts (1-4). Extrusion cooking of animal tissues either alone or in combination with plant materials and other ingredients is also widely reported in the patent literature (5-9).

One underutilized, economical source of animal protein, mechanically deboned meat, was restructured with a twin screw extruder in the presence of gelling and binding agents such as soy protein isolates, wheat flour, corn starch, egg white concentrate, carrageenan, sodium chloride, sodium phosphate, sodium alginate and calcium chloride (10). Another study on restructuring mechanically deboned chicken meat with a twin-screw extruder found that soy protein isolate and wheat gluten were less effective than starch for increasing apparent tensile stress and Warner-Bratzler shear stress of extruded products. These parameters also increased as a function of temperature up to 104°C (11).

Other researchers have also attempted to develop meat-containing products including low-fat snacks, processed by extrusion cooking, with nonmeat ingredients such as corn products (12,13), modified potato starch and hydrolyzed vegetable proteins (14), gums, maltodextrins and soybean proteins (15). Meats tested included beef, pork and mechanically deboned turkey meat, with nonmeat ingredient levels as high as 50-60% (12) and meat up to 10% in the dehydrated state (14). Other studies have used similar principles to develop extrusion cooked products based on raw materials from fish (16-18). Texturized blends of meat proteins and corn starch were formed with a twin screw extruder at various feeding rates, temperatures, shear rates and pH values (19). The results indicated that lower extrusion temperatures and higher pH values produced extrudates of better quality. Ground meat with 20-40% moisture was extrusion processed to form an expanded meat product (20).

Extrusion cooking of raw meat of high moisture and fat is generally difficult. Major problems observed in this process include product gushing out of the die in small individual granules or backflowing of the raw material from the extruder inlet (10,21). These problems are due to lubrication provided by fat and moisture in the extruder barrel which results in product slippage or blockage of the die outlet. In these instances, the material exiting the extruder die is of limited cohesion, crumbly and friable. These technical problems are avoided by drying the meat; defatting it; and/or mixing it with nonmeat binders and gelling agents. Potentially effective nonmeat ingredients include corn starch, soy proteins, wheat flour, potato products and gums. Addition of these ingredients to the meat may not only eliminate the above technical problems, but it may also improve binding and texture of the extruded material. In addition, the extruded products should be of low fat (<10%) and high protein (>20%) contents, which are desirable to consumers.

Extrusion of meat mixed with plant materials can be used to produce meat-based snacks, chunks or powders for soups or stews, and pasta products fortified with meat. It should be mentioned again that these products are based on lower value raw meat, are of low fat, no added sodium chloride, and high protein contents, and if they can be made shelf-stable they should be very useful in development of value-added items which should increase overall consumption of meat by providing consumers with nutritious, safe, and reasonably priced food items.

The objective of studies in our laboratory was to compare the ability of six nonmeat ingredients to bind meat particles, and hold water and fat during extrusion cooking of chicken meat. In designing the study, the extrusion temperature, the screw speed and the level of the nonmeat ingredients were considered to be the most important factors in determining the properties of the extruded products.

2. MATERIALS AND METHODS

2.1 Experimental Design

Four extrusion variables, namely screw speed, temperature, and type and level of nonmeat ingredients were tested in an experiment of fractional factorial design (Table 1). The fractional factorial design (22) consisted of one-sixth of the total factorial combinations. The results of the evaluation of the extruded products were statistically analyzed by analysis of variance and by response surface methodology with the SPSS-X Release 2 Package (SPSS-X, inc., Chicago, IL).

2.2 Raw Material Preparation and Extrusion Processing

The hand-deboned chicken meat used was derived from broilers purchased from a supermarket. The chicken meat was skinned, deboned and cut. Then it was ground through a plate with 0.3 cm diameter holes in a Univex grinder (#PB2, Univex Co., Somerville, NC) and mixed at low speed for one minute in a laboratory mixer (Model K45 SS, Hobart Mfg. Co., St. Joseph, MO). Next, the nonmeat ingredients were slowly added during low-speed mixing to avoid spattering. The mixing of the meat and nonmeat ingredients was continued at low speed for 5 min, after which the mixing process was stopped. All of the nonmeat ingredients on the sides of the bowl were pushed down with a plastic spatula. Mixing was then resumed for another 8-10 min until the ingredients became uniform and no lumps appeared in the dough. The dough was then removed from the mixer bowl and divided into two portions of 200 g each. Each portion was placed in a plastic bag, labeled A and B, and refrigerated (4°C) until it was extruded later on the same day.

Extrusion was performed in a Brabender plasticoder extruder, Model PL-V500 (C. W. Brabender Instruments, Inc., South Hackensack, NJ). The diameter of the barrel of the extruder was 19.00 mm, with a 20:1 length-to-diameter ratio and eight 0.79 x 3.18 mm longitudinal grooves. A screw configuration of 1:1 compression ratio was used, and the die plate used was 5.10 cm long with a 0.87 cm diameter opening. The two zones of the extruder were electrically heated and compressed air-cooled collars controlled by thermostats were used to control the temperature of the barrel. Two thermocouples were placed through the barrel wall and indicated the temperature of the dough in the extruder (23,24). The extruder was equipped with a variable speed D-C drive unit, a tachometer, and a balanced-type torque meter (Model 7540, Eaton Corporation, Troy, MI).

TABLE 1

Fractional factorial experimental design used to study extrusion-cooked products consisting of chicken meat and nonmeat ingredients at different screw speeds and extrusion temperatures.

A	B	C	D	A	B	C	D	A	B	C	D
0	0	0	0	0	0	2	4	0	0	4	2
0	2	0	4	0	2	2	2	0	2	4	0
0	4	0	2	0	4	2	0	0	4	4	4
1	0	0	4	1	0	2	2	1	0	4	0
1	2	0	2	1	2	2	0	1	2	4	4
1	4	0	0	1	4	2	4	1	4	4	2
2	0	0	2	2	0	2	0	2	0	4	4
2	2	0	0	2	2	2	4	2	2	4	2
2	4	0	4	2	4	2	2	2	4	4	0
0	0	1	1	0	0	3	5	0	0	5	3
0	2	1	5	0	2	3	3	0	2	5	1
0	4	1	3	0	4	3	1	0	4	5	5
2	0	1	3	2	0	3	1	2	0	5	5
2	2	1	1	2	2	3	5	2	2	5	3
2	4	1	5	2	4	3	3	2	4	5	1
1	0	1	5	1	0	3	3	1	0	5	1
1	2	1	3	1	2	3	1	1	2	5	3
1	4	1	1	1	4	3	5	1	4	5	5
0	1	0	1	0	1	2	5	0	1	4	3
0	3	0	5	0	3	2	3	0	3	4	1
0	5	0	3	0	5	2	1	0	5	4	5
1	1	0	5	1	1	2	3	1	1	4	1
1	3	0	3	1	3	2	1	1	3	4	5
1	5	0	1	1	5	2	5	1	5	4	3
2	1	0	3	2	1	2	1	2	1	4	5
2	3	0	1	2	3	2	5	2	3	4	3
2	5	0	5	2	5	2	3	2	5	4	1
0	1	1	0	0	1	3	4	0	1	5	2
0	3	1	4	0	3	3	2	0	3	5	0
0	5	1	2	0	5	3	0	0	5	5	4
1	1	1	4	1	1	3	2	1	1	5	0
1	3	1	2	1	3	3	0	1	3	5	4
1	5	1	0	1	5	3	4	1	5	5	2
2	1	1	2	2	1	3	0	2	1	5	4
2	3	1	0	2	3	3	4	2	3	5	2
2	5	1	4	2	5	3	2	2	5	5	0

A = Screw speed (0 = 60 rpm; 1 = 80 rpm; 2 = 100 rpm).
B = Extrusion temperature (0 = 75°C; 1 = 85°C; 2 = 95°C; 3 = 105°C; 4 = 115°C; 5 = 125°C.
C = Nonmeat ingredients (0 = Oat fiber - Mira oat fiber, Canadian Harvest, Ontario, Canada; 1 = Corn starch - Mira-gel 463, Staley, Decatur, IL; 2 = Whey protein concentrate - Lo-Lac 360, Foremost Whey Products, Baraboo, WI; 3 = Soy flour - Nuvupan, Lucas Meyer, Decatur, IL; 4 = Soy protein concentrate - Promosoy Plus, Central Soya, Fort Wayne, IN; 5 = Soy protein isolate - Mira-Pro 121, Staley, Decatur, IL).
D = Nonmeat ingredient level (0 = 10%; 1 = 12%; 2 = 14%; 3 = 16%; 4 = 18%; 5 = 20%).

Ground, moistened corn grits were choke-fed into the extruder until a steady state of operation was achieved. Samples of the mixtures from Bag A were then fed manually and continuously into the extruder. Ground, moistened corn was fed between treatments. After the A samples were extruded, the B samples were extruded in the same manner. Each sample was collected from the die outlet in a plastic cup and transferred to a plastic bag. The extruded samples were allowed to cool for approximately 30 minutes and were stored for one day in the refrigerator (4°C) for subsequent evaluation. Observations on the behavior of the products during extrusion were recorded.

Since the total number of treatments was large (108 treatments), they were divided into five groups, and each group was extruded on a given day (a total of 5 days). After each group of treatments was extruded and packaged, the products were refrigerated at 4°C. On the sixth day, after all five groups had been extruded, the products underwent sensory evaluation.

2.3 Product Evaluation

Sensory evaluation of product texture involved rating samples for binding, hardness and gumminess. Samples of common commercial products were assigned scores for hardness, binding and gumminess (Table 2), and were used as anchor points in the evaluation process (25). Hardness was evaluated on a 6-point scale against six foods assigned scores from 1 to 6: 1 was the hardness of cream cheese and 6 was the hardness of peanuts. For gumminess, a 6-point scale was also used (40 percent flour paste was point 1 and 65% flour paste was point 6). For evaluation of product binding the anchor points were a score of 6 for commercial frankfurters, and a score of 1 for commercial ground turkey meat (26).

TABLE 2

Sensory panel scores and products used as anchor points for the evaluation of extrusion-cooked chicken meat with nonmeat ingredients.

Panel scores	Gumminess	Hardness	Binding
1	40[a]	Cream cheese (Kraft Inc., Glenview IL)	Ground turkey
2	45	Hard-boiled egg whites	-----
3	50	Frankfurters (Bar-S Foods, Phoenix AZ)	-----
4	55	American cheese (Kraft Inc., Glenview IL)	-----
5	60	Ripe black olives (Food Club, Top Co Assn., Inc., Skokie, IL)	-----
6	65	Peanuts (Gold Crest, Inter-American Food, Inc., Cincinnati, OH)	Frankfurters

[a] Percent flour in paste.

A 4-member sensory panel consisting of three males and one female with ages ranging from 30 to 45 years, was individually trained to score the extruded products for the textural responses of hardness, gumminess and binding. They were trained on how to press food samples to test for hardness, and then were given samples of the extruded products to press in order to become familiar with the range of the differences in hardness (26). For binding, they were trained to pull apart a 1 cm slice of frankfurter, which was given a score of 6 on the binding scale, and to pull apart a similar amount of ground turkey meat, which was given the binding score of 1 on the 6-point scale. The panelists were trained to evaluate gumminess by pressing and pulling different flour paste samples to compare their gumminess with that of the extruded products. Upon completion of the training (training time depended on the individual; the average time was 20 minutes), each panelist was allowed to ask questions and make comments before evaluating the products. The same panel members did the sensory evaluation on all of the products.

The extruded samples were removed from the refrigerator on the day of sensory evaluation and allowed to reach room temperature (1.5-2 h). The 16 to 20 samples, 20 to 30 g each, were presented during each session to each panelist on a white, waxy sheet of paper that was divided into 20 boxes. The anchor samples were placed in a 6-muffin baking tin form next to the extruded samples with the evaluation sheet for reference.

3. RESULTS AND DISCUSSION

3.1 The Effect of Whey Protein

When whey protein concentrate (WPC) was used as the nonmeat ingredient, none of the variables examined (WPC level, screw speed and extrusion temperature) had any significant effect ($P>0.05$) on the binding of the extruded products (Table 3). On the other hand, the level of WPC had a significant effect ($P<0.05$) on the gumminess and hardness of the final product. Variation in screw speed did not contribute to the regression coefficients of product binding, gumminess or hardness. The interaction between the level of WPC and the extrusion temperature had a positive, but not significant, effect on the three properties (Table 3).

At low extrusion temperatures (75°C), increasing the WPC level from 10% to 20% reduced product binding, but not significantly (Fig. 1). Extrusion at higher temperatures (125°C), however, had no influence on binding of products with 20% WPC. Increasing the extrusion temperature from 75°C to 125°C in products with 10% WPC had only a minor positive effect on binding. Figure 1 also shows that the maximum binding score (4.80) was recorded at the extrusion temperature of 125°C, and a WPC level of 10%. However, at this high temperature, product gushing from the die and fluid separation during extrusion were significant, and thus resulted in drier and harder products.

TABLE 3

Regression coefficients for binding, gumminess and hardness of extrusion-cooked chicken meat with different levels of whey protein concentrate (10-20%). Screw speed varied in the range of 60-100 rpm at extrusion temperatures of 75-125°C.

Extrusion variables	Binding		Gumminess		Hardness	
	Regression coefficients	Significance	Regression coefficients	Significance	Regression coefficients	Significance
Constant	3.77	0.0000	4.98	0.0000	4.21	0.0000
Level of WPC	-0.50	N.S.	-0.82	0.0342	-0.43	0.0068
Temperature	0.38	N.S.	0.21	N.S.	0.27	N.S.
(Level of WPC)^2	-0.01	N.S.	0.11	N.S.	-0.06	0.0225
(Temperature)^2	-0.04	N.S.	-0.04	N.S.	-0.04	N.S.
Temperature x WPC level	0.06	N.S.	0.06	N.S.	0.02	N.S.

WPC = Whey protein concentrate.
N.S. = Not significant.

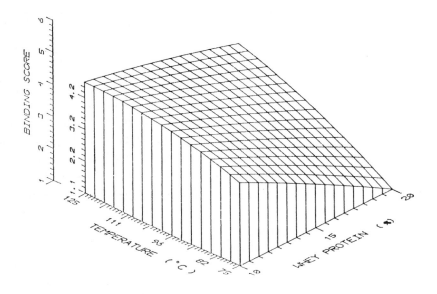

Figure 1. A response surface diagram for predicted binding of extrusion-cooked chicken meat with different levels of whey protein concentrate (10-20%) at different extrusion temperatures (75-125°C) (the screw speed was 60-100 rpm).

As the extrusion temperature increased from 75 up to 125°C, product gumminess increased, especially at WPC levels above 12% (Table 4). At 75°C, however, as the WPC level increased above 10%, product gumminess decreased. The lowest predicted gumminess (3.40) was recorded at 18% WPC and the extrusion temperature of 75°C.

TABLE 4

Predicted gumminess and hardness scores of extrusion-cooked chicken meat with different levels of whey protein concentrate at different extrusion temperatures (the screw speed was 60-100 rpm).

Extrusion temperature (°C)	Level of whey protein concentrate (%)					
	10	12	14	16	18	20
	Predicted gumminess					
75	4.98	4.25	3.74	3.46	3.40	3.57
85	5.15	4.51	4.10	3.91	3.94	4.19
95	5.26	4.71	4.38	4.28	4.40	4.74
105	5.29	4.83	4.60	4.58	4.79	5.22
115	5.25	4.88	4.73	4.81	5.11	5.63
125	5.14	4.86	4.80	4.97	5.36	5.97
	Predicted hardness					
75	4.21	3.84	3.58	3.44	3.41	3.50
85	4.44	4.09	3.85	3.73	3.72	3.83
95	4.59	4.26	4.04	3.93	3.94	4.07
105	4.66	4.34	4.14	4.06	4.09	4.23
115	4.65	4.35	4.17	4.10	4.15	4.32
125	4.55	4.27	4.11	4.06	4.13	4.32

The predicted hardness of the extruded products was affected only slightly by extrusion temperature and WPC level (Table 4). The lowest hardness scores were observed at WPC levels above 16% and at 75°C. Maximum hardness was at temperatures above 95°C and 10-20% WPC. This may be related to increased moisture retention at higher WPC and low temperature, and greater moisture losses at higher temperatures.

3.2 The Effect of Corn Starch

The results showed no influence of the screw speed on the regression coefficients for binding, gumminess and hardness of extruded products in the presence of starch. Neither the extrusion temperature nor the level of starch or their interaction had significant ($P>0.05$) effects on the three properties of the final products (Table 5). In general, binding of products extruded with corn starch was poor (Fig. 2). Increasing the extrusion temperature from 75°C to 125°C, however, caused a slight increase in the binding of the extruded chicken products. This increase was more pronounced at the low level of starch (10%), but the improvement in bind was only minor. Increasing the level of starch from 10 to 20% did not cause any major change in the binding of the products, which ranged from a score of 0.94 to 2.56. In general, binding of extruded chicken meat in the presence of 10-20% corn starch was very weak, especially at the lower extrusion temperature (75°C). However, the lower the starch level (10%) and the higher the extrusion temperature (125°C), the stronger the binding (Fig. 2).

TABLE 5

Regression coefficients for binding, gumminess, and hardness of extrusion-cooked chicken meat with different levels of corn starch (10-20%). Screw speed varied in the range of 60-100 rpm at extrusion temperatures of 75-125°C.

Extrusion variables	Binding		Gumminess		Hardness	
	Regression coefficients	Significance	Regression coefficients	Significance	Regression coefficients	Significance
Constant	1.10	0.0189	1.98	0.0011	2.06	0.0037
Level of starch	0.003	N.S.	0.01	N.S.	0.06	N.S.
Temperature	0.32	N.S.	0.15	N.S.	0.28	N.S.
(Level of starch)^2	-0.0005	N.S.	0.01	N.S.	0.06	N.S.
(Temperature)^2	-0.005	N.S.	0.08	N.S.	0.03	N.S.
Temperature x starch level	-0.07	N.S.	-0.08	N.S.	-0.07	N.S.

N.S. = Not significant.

The predicted gumminess of the extruded chicken meat product with corn starch was the highest at the high extrusion temperature of 125°C and in the presence of 10% starch (Table 6). At 10% starch, the predicted gumminess was increased from a score of 1.98 at 75°C to 4.75 at 125°C. In general, increasing the extrusion temperature caused an increase in the gumminess of the products, probably by increasing gelation of starch, which also caused an increase in binding. At a given level of starch, as the temperature increased, hardness scores increased (Table 6). The higher hardness at increased temperatures should be due to more gelatinization and evaporation of water during extrusion cooking and cooling. A higher temperature alone can cause more evaporation and more hardness of the product. The higher temperatures, together with the mixing motion of the screw inside the barrel, should have caused more breakdown of starch granules, which may result in more water release from the granules and from the dough.

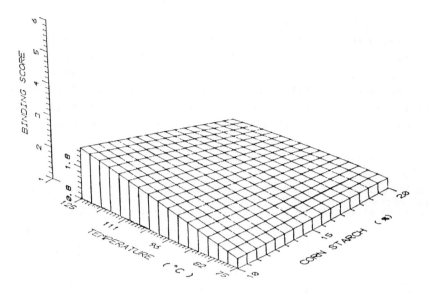

Figure 2. A response surface diagram for predicted binding of extrusion-cooked chicken meat with different levels of corn starch (10-20%) at different extrusion temperatures (75-125°C) (the screw speed was 60-100 rpm).

TABLE 6

Predicted gumminess and hardness scores of extrusion-cooked chicken meat with different levels of corn starch at different extrusion temperatures (the screw speed was 60-100 rpm).

Extrusion temperature (°C)	Level of corn starch (%)					
	10	12	14	16	18	20
	Predicted gumminess					
75	1.98	2.00	2.04	2.58	2.19	2.29
85	2.21	2.15	2.12	2.10	2.10	2.13
95	2.60	2.46	2.35	2.26	2.19	2.14
105	3.15	2.94	2.75	2.03	2.43	2.30
115	3.87	3.58	3.31	3.07	2.84	2.63
125	4.75	4.38	4.04	3.71	3.41	3.12
	Predicted hardness					
75	2.06	1.76	1.57	1.50	1.54	1.71
85	2.37	2.00	1.74	1.60	1.58	1.68
95	2.73	2.29	1.97	1.76	1.68	1.71
105	3.15	2.64	2.25	1.98	1.82	1.79
115	3.62	3.04	2.59	2.25	2.03	1.92
125	4.14	3.50	2.98	2.57	2.28	2.11

3.3 The Effect of Oat Fiber

The results showed that neither the level of oat fiber nor the extrusion temperature had any significant effect on the gumminess or hardness of the extruded products (Table 7). The screw speed did not contribute to the regression coefficients for predicted binding, gumminess and hardness. However, Figure 3 does show that as the oat fiber level increased, binding decreased, at least at the lower extrusion temperatures. Increasing the extrusion temperature up to approximately 100°C inceased binding, but extrusion at higher temperatures (105-125°C) caused the binding to decrease (Fig. 3). Although at all of the extrusion temperatures this pattern held, the degree of the decrease differed from lower temperatures (75 to 95°C) to higher temperatures (105 to 125°C). At the lower temperatures, the degree of decrease in binding between the lower and higher levels was notably greater than between the higher temperatures (Fig. 3). In general, product binding with oat fiber was weak, with scores in the range 0.32-2.89.

TABLE 7

Regression coefficients for binding, gumminess and hardness of extrusion-cooked chicken meat with different levels of oat fiber (10-20%). Screw speed varied in the range of 60-100 rpm at extrusion temperatures of 75-125°C.

Extrusion variables	Binding		Gumminess		Hardness	
	Regression coefficients	Significance	Regression coefficients	Significance	Regression coefficients	Significance
Constant	1.89	0.0059	1.45	0.0000	4.94	0.000
Level of oat fiber	-0.42	N.S.	-0.26	N.S.	-0.13	N.S.
Temperature	0.81	0.0460	0.19	N.S.	0.036	N.S.
(Level of oat fiber)^2	0.02	N.S.	0.11	N.S.	-0.007	N.S.
(Temperature)^2	-0.16	0.0410	-0.07	N.S.	-0.016	N.S.
Temperature x oat fiber level	0.03	N.S.	-0.03	N.S.	0.07	N.S.

N.S. = Not significant.

At all of the levels of oat fiber, gumminess increased as the temperature increased (Table 8). In general, the gumminess of these products was very low and similar to 45-50% flour paste. This phenomenon of increasing gumminess by increasing the temperature can be related to more gelatinization of the free starch or other carbohydrates. In general, these products were harder than those with WPC, starch and soy proteins (Table 8). The reason may be a loss of more water during extrusion in products with fiber than with other ingredients.

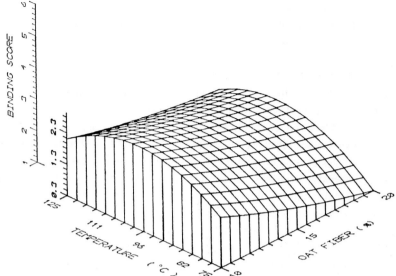

Figure 3. A response surface diagram for predicted binding of extrusion-cooked chicken meat with different levels of oat fiber (10-20%) at different extrusion temperatures (75-125°C) (the screw speed was 60-100 rpm).

TABLE 8

Predicted gumminess and hardness scores of extrusion-cooked chicken meat with different levels of oat fiber at different extrusion temperatures (the screw speed was 60-100 rpm).

Extrusion temperature (°C)	Level of oat fiber (%)					
	10	12	14	16	18	20
	Predicted gumminess					
75	1.45	1.31	1.39	1.70	2.23	3.00
85	1.63	1.45	1.50	1.88	2.28	3.02
95	1.80	1.59	1.60	1.85	2.32	3.02
105	1.95	1.71	1.69	1.91	2.35	3.02
115	2.09	1.82	1.77	1.95	2.36	3.00
125	2.22	1.91	1.83	1.98	2.36	2.97
	Predicted hardness					
75	4.94	4.80	4.64	4.47	4.29	4.10
85	4.96	4.89	4.81	4.71	4.60	4.48
95	4.95	4.95	4.94	4.92	4.88	4.83
105	4.90	4.98	5.04	5.09	5.13	5.16
115	4.83	4.98	5.12	5.24	5.35	5.44
125	4.73	4.95	5.16	5.35	5.53	5.70

Generally, as the level of fiber increased at the extrusion temperature of 75°C, hardness decreased. At 10% oat fiber, hardness did not change in the temperature range of 75-125°C. At 20% fiber and 75°C, hardness was at a minimum, while at 125°C and the same fiber level, it received its maximum score.

3.4 The Effect of Soy Protein Isolate

Table 9 shows significant effects ($P<0.05$) of both the extrusion temperature and soy protein isolate (SPI) level on the binding of the final product. The effect of temperature was greater than that of the SPI level. Neither of these two variables had a significant ($P>0.05$) effect on the gumminess or hardness of the extruded products. The screw speed had no effect on any of the three properties, binding, gumminess or hardness, of the extruded products.

TABLE 9

Regression coefficients for binding, gumminess and hardness of extrusion-cooked chicken meat with different levels of soy protein isolate (10-20%). Screw speed varied in the range of 60-100 rpm at extrusion temperatures of 75-125°C.

Extrusion variables	Binding		Gumminess		Hardness	
	Regression coefficients	Significance	Regression coefficients	Significance	Regression coefficients	Significance
Constant	2.04	0.0004	4.44	0.0000	3.11	0.000
Level of SPI	1.12	0.0015	0.27	N.S.	0.13	N.S.
Temperature	1.19	0.0009	-0.15	N.S.	0.07	N.S.
(Level of SPI)^2	-0.21	0.0016	-0.03	N.S.	-0.06	N.S.
(Temperature)^2	-0.24	0.0006	0.06	N.S.	0.01	N.S.
Temperature x SPI level	0.03	N.S.	-0.03	N.S.	-0.02	N.S.

SPI = Soy protein isolate.
N.S. = Not significant.

The results showed that SPI had some unique effects on the properties of the extruded chicken meat, which were different than the effects of the other nonmeat ingredients. At a given level of SPI (10-20%), as the extrusion temperature increased (from 75 to 105°C), the predicted binding of the extruded products increased, then it decreased again as the temperature was increased to 125°C (Fig. 4). For example, at the level of 12% SPI, as the temperature increased from 75 to 105°C, the binding score increased from 2.95 to 4.47, but when the temperature was increased to 125°C, binding decreased to 3.11. At SPI levels of 10% to 16%, binding increased, but then it was reduced as the SPI level reached 20%. At the temperature of 85°C, by increasing the SPI level from 10 up to 20%, the binding increased from 2.99 to 4.54, then decreased to 4.22 and 3.47, respectively.

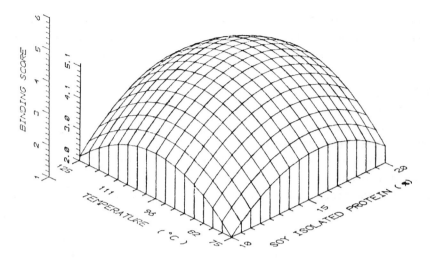

Figure 4. A response surface diagram for predicted binding of extrusion-cooked chicken meat with different levels of soy protein isolate (10-20%) at different extrusion temperatures (75-125°C) (the screw speed was 60-100 rpm).

Optimum binding of chicken meat with SPI occurred at temperatures around 100°C (Fig. 4), which coincides with results of studies indicating interactions of meat and soy proteins at temperatures of 80-100°C (27-31). At lower extrusion temperatures (75°C) there was some binding which may have been due to an interaction between the myosin and 11S soy protein, but when the extrusion temperature was above 100°C, binding started to decrease possibly because the matrix of the soy protein began to weaken and nonmatrix gelling started to form (29).

Gumminess of the extruded products showed only slight changes with variations in extrusion temperature or SPI level (Table 10). In general, at the lower levels of SPI (10-12%), as the extrusion temperature increased (from 75 to 125°C), gumminess increased. For example, at 10% SPI, product gumminess increased from a score of 4.44 to 5.10 when the extrusion temperature was increased from 75°C to 125°C. At the higher levels of SPI, such as 20%, gumminess had proportionately higher scores. These results agree with the discussion concerning gelling of SPI, which, in this study, started at a temperature of around 100°C. It is assumed, however, that higher gumminess is an indicator of higher degree of gelling. In general, the gelling behavior of the SPI in high moisture conditions (70%) inside the extruder increased by increasing the temperature; the best gelling was found to be at 180°C (32). The formation of the matrix is not necessarily involved in the gelation of the SPI at high extrusion temperatures (above 100°C).

TABLE 10

Predicted gumminess and hardness scores of extrusion-cooked chicken meat with different levels of soy protein isolate at different extrusion temperatures (the screw speed was 60-100 rpm).

Extrusion temperature (°C)	Level of soy protein isolate (%)					
	10	12	14	16	18	20
	Predicted gumminess					
75	4.44	4.68	4.86	4.98	5.04	5.05
85	4.35	4.56	4.71	4.81	4.85	4.83
95	4.37	4.55	4.68	4.75	4.77	4.72
105	4.50	4.66	4.76	4.81	4.80	4.73
115	4.75	4.88	4.96	4.98	4.94	4.85
125	5.10	5.21	5.26	5.26	5.19	5.07
	Predicted hardness					
75	3.11	3.30	3.61	4.04	4.58	5.25
85	3.20	3.36	3.65	4.05	4.57	5.22
95	3.30	3.44	3.70	4.08	4.59	5.21
105	3.42	3.54	3.78	4.14	4.62	5.22
115	3.57	3.67	3.88	4.22	4.68	5.25
125	3.74	3.81	4.01	4.32	4.75	5.31

Changes in hardness (Table 10) were similar to those found when chicken meat was extruded with ingredients other than SPI. At a given level of SPI, increasing the extrusion temperature caused hardness to increase. Also, increasing the level of SPI at the same temperature caused hardness to increase. For example, at 10% SPI, by increasing the temperature from 75 to 125°C, the hardness score increased from 3.11 to 3.74. In addition, at the extrusion temperature of 125°C increasing the level of SPI from 10 to 20%, the hardness scores increased from 3.74 to 5.31. As explained earlier with other nonmeat binders, both the increased evaporation of water at higher extrusion temperatures and the higher level of the binder, which affected the level of free moisture in the product, should have been responsible for the increased hardness.

3.5 The Effect of Soy Protein Concentrate

Table 11 shows regression coefficients and significance for binding, gumminess and hardness of extruded chicken meat products in th presence of soy protein concentrate (SPC). The extrusion temperature and the SPC level had a significant effect ($P<0.05$) on the binding of the final product with the effect of the level of SPC being greater. The extrusion temperature also affected product gumminess, but none of the extrusion variables affected the hardness of the products significantly. The screw speed was not involved in the regression coefficients.

TABLE 11

Regression coefficients for binding, gumminess and hardness of extrusion-cooked chicken meat with different levels of soy protein concentrate (10-20%). Screw speed varied in the range of 60-100 rpm at extrusion temperatures of 75-125°C.

Extrusion variables	Binding		Gumminess		Hardness	
	Regression coefficients	Significance	Regression coefficients	Significance	Regression coefficients	Significance
Constant	0.54	N.S.	4.05	0.0000	3.54	0.0000
Level of SPC	1.26	0.0007	0.38	N.S.	0.13	N.S.
Temperature	1.05	0.0026	0.50	0.0494	0.08	N.S.
(Level of SPC)^2	-0.22	0.0004	0.05	N.S.	0.03	N.S.
(Temperature)^2	-0.15	0.0076	-0.07	N.S.	0.003	N.S.
Temperature x SPC level	-0.02	N.S.	0.06	N.S.	0.02	N.S.

SPC = Soy protein concentrate.
N.S. = Not significant.

Due to differences in protein concentration between SPI (90%) and SPC (70%) and processing involved in their manufacture, binding of the extruded products in presence of these two nonmeat ingredients was somewhat different. In general, however, it followed a similar pattern. Overall, binding scores were lower with SPC than SPI. As the extrusion temperature increased, so did binding scores. When the temperature was 75°C at 10% SPC, the binding score was only 0.54, but by increasing the temperature to 125°C, the binding score rose to 2.09 (Fig. 5).

The need for the higher extrusion temperature for maximum binding with SPC compared to SPI may be due to the higher amount of carbohydrate in the SPC. In addition, the method of manufacturing SPC may have influenced the temperature for maximum binding. Further, presence of more carbohydrate in the SPC may have caused binding to become weaker compared to SPI.

The highest gumminess scores with SPC occurred at the levels of 14 to 16% and at 95 to 110°C (Table 12). In general, as the temperature or the level of SPC was increased, gumminess increased. These changes were similar to those with SPI, with one exception, that the increase in gumminess with SPC started at 75°C rather than 95°C. Maximum gumminess (5.07) was recorded at 95°C and 105°C. At the highest level of SPC (20%), the highest gumminess scores (4.7) was at the lower temperature (75°C).

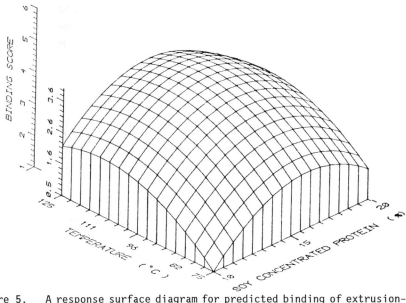

Figure 5. A response surface diagram for predicted binding of extrusion-cooked chicken meat with different levels of soy protein concentrate (10-20%) at different extrusion temperatures (75-125°C) (the screw speed was 60-100 rpm).

TABLE 12

Predicted gumminess and hardness scores of extrusion-cooked chicken meat with different levels of soy protein concentrate (SPC) at different extrusion temperatures (the screw speed was 60-100 rpm).

Extrusion temperature (°C)	Level of soy protein concentrate (%)					
	10	12	14	16	18	20
	Predicted gumminess					
75	4.05	4.38	4.61	4.73	4.75	4.67
85	4.48	4.75	4.91	4.98	4.94	4.79
95	4.75	4.96	5.07	5.07	4.97	4.76
105	4.88	5.03	5.07	5.02	4.85	4.59
115	4.86	4.95	4.93	4.81	4.59	4.26
125	4.69	4.72	4.64	4.46	4.18	3.79
	Predicted hardness					
75	3.54	3.58	3.67	3.81	4.01	4.25
85	3.63	3.69	3.80	3.96	4.18	4.45
95	3.71	3.80	3.93	4.12	4.36	4.65
105	3.81	3.91	4.07	4.28	4.54	4.86
115	3.91	4.04	4.22	4.45	4.74	5.07
125	4.02	4.17	4.37	4.63	4.93	5.29

Hardness of the final products was affected by extrusion temperature, level of SPC and their interaction. As the extrusion temperature increased, hardness of the product also increased (Table 12). As an example, at the SPC level of 10%, increasing the temperature from 75 to 125°C increased hardness scores from 3.54 to 4.02. At 85°C, hardness increased from a score of 3.63 to 4.45 by increasing the SPC level from 10 to 20%. Hardness also increased at higher temperatures (125°C) when the SPC level was raised from 10 to 20%. The higher extrusion temperature and the higher level of SPC should have resulted in products with a lower free moisture content, which should have resulted in increased product hardness.

3.6 The Effect of Soy Flour

Various levels of soy flour (41% protein), had a significant effect ($P<0.05$) on the binding of the extruded products, but the extrusion temperature showed a stronger effect on binding than the level of soy flour (Table 13). The level of soy flour and the other extrusion variables used in this study had no significant effect ($P>0.05$) on the gumminess or hardness of the extruded products. The screw speed had no influence on the regression coefficients for product binding, gumminess or hardness.

TABLE 13

Regression coefficients for binding, gumminess and hardness of extrusion-cooked chicken meat with different levels of soy flour (10-20%). Screw speed varied in the range of 60-100 rpm at extrusion temperatures of 75-125°C.

Extrusion variables	Binding		Gumminess		Hardness	
	Regression coefficients	Significance	Regression coefficients	Significance	Regression coefficients	Significance
Constant	0.87	0.0274	4.45	0.0000	3.18	0.0000
Level of soy flour	0.68	0.0097	-0.12	N.S.	-0.02	N.S.
Temperature	1.10	0.0003	0.02	N.S.	-0.20	N.S.
(Level of soy flour)^2	-0.13	0.0096	0.01	N.S.	0.05	N.S.
(Temperature)^2	-0.12	0.0142	-0.009	N.S.	0.04	N.S.
Temperature x soy flour level	0.02	N.S.	0.03	N.S.	0.06	N.S.

N.S. = Not significant.

Binding (Fig. 6) was improved by changing either the temperature or the level of soy flour, in a manner similar to that caused by SPI and SPC (Fig. 4 and 5). At a given level of soy flour (from 10 to 20%), as the extrusion temperature increased, binding increased. For example when the level was 10%, binding increased gradually from 0.87 to 3.33, and at 16% soy flour, binding increased from 1.75 to 4.55, when the extrusion temperature was increased from 75°C to 125°C, respectively (Fig. 6). In general, maximum binding occurred at temperatures approaching 125°C and at soy flour levels between 14 and 17%.

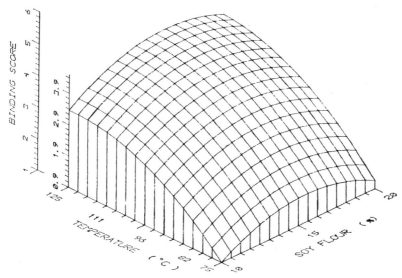

Figure 6. A response surface diagram for predicted binding of extrusion-cooked chicken meat with different levels of soy flour (10-20%) at different extrusion temperatures (75-125°C) (the screw speed was 60-100 rpm).

Both, extrusion temperature and soy flour level changes, had no notable effect on the gumminess of the products (Table 14). Overall changes in gumminess, however, were only minor. At a given temperature (from 75 to 125°C), hardness increased as the level of soy flour was increased (Table 14). For example, at 105°C and 125°C, an increase of the level from 10 to 20% increased the hardness from 2.95 to 5.01 and from 3.23 to 5.86, respectively. Hardness, in general, followed the same pattern as discussed before: as the soy level increased, the moisture of the product would be lower, and at a higher extrusion temperature, more water would evaporate from the product. Both, low moisture content and higher evaporation should have produced harder products.

Upon gelation around 100°C, soy protein can function as a matrix to hold fat and water (33,34), which should result in optimum binding. Other factors affecting binding in presence of soy products, however, should be the concentration of carbohydrate and lecithin in the product. These ingredients may have enhanced gelatinization and binding at higher temperatures (120-125°C). In general, the soy flour gave better binding than either SPI or SPC at a high extrusion temperature (125°C), with scores of 4.07 for soy flour (Fig. 6), 3.15 for SPI (Fig. 4) and 2.36 for SPC (Fig. 5).

TABLE 14

Predicted gumminess and hardness scores of extrusion-cooked chicken meat with different levels of soy flour at different extrusion temperatures (the screw speed was 60-100 rpm).

Extrusion temperature (°C)	Level of soy flour (%)					
	10	12	14	16	18	20
	Predicted gumminess					
75	4.45	4.34	4.26	4.21	4.19	4.19
85	4.46	4.39	4.35	4.33	4.34	4.37
95	4.46	4.42	4.41	4.43	4.47	4.54
105	4.44	4.44	4.46	4.51	4.58	4.69
115	4.40	4.43	4.49	4.57	4.68	4.82
125	4.35	4.41	4.50	4.62	4.76	4.93
	Predicted hardness					
75	3.18	3.21	3.35	3.59	3.93	4.38
85	3.02	3.11	3.30	3.60	4.00	4.50
95	2.95	3.09	3.34	3.70	4.15	4.71
105	2.95	3.16	3.47	3.88	4.39	5.01
115	3.05	3.31	3.68	4.14	4.72	5.39
125	3.23	3.55	3.97	4.50	5.13	5.86

4. **CONCLUSIONS**

Of all six nonmeat ingredients tested, soy proteins resulted in extrusion-cooked chicken meat products with higher binding scores. Certain products with whey protein concentrate also exceeded the binding score of 4, while products formulated with corn starch and oat fiber had binding scores of less than 3. Products with scores approaching 6 (binding of frankfurters) should be of optimum binding, while a binding score of 1 (ground meat) is completely unacceptable.

In addition to better binding, the soy flour and soy proteins, in general, produced smoother and better texturized products than the other nonmeat ingredients. Although at low soy levels the products displayed some fluid separation, the appearance of the final products was more acceptable than that of products prepared with nonsoy binders.

The highest binding scores of all products, were achieved with soy protein isolate (SPI) in the formulation. At 16% SPI, the binding scores of products extruded at 95°C and 105°C were 5.11 and 5.21, respectively. Thus, future studies should examine the potential for developing extrusion-cooked chicken meat products formulated with soy protein, and especially soy protein isolate products. Utilization of mechanically deboned poultry meat in such products should also be examined.

5. REFERENCES

1. R.A. Lawrie and D.A. Ledward, in: D.A. Ledward, A.J. Taylor and R.A. Lawrie (Eds), Texturization of recovered proteins. *Upgrading Waste for Feeds and Food*, Butterworths, London, 1983, pp. 163-182.
2. P. Mittal and R.A. Lawrie, Meat Sci., 10 (1984) 101-116.
3. J.A.G. Areas and R.A. Lawrie, Meat Sci., 11 (1984) 275-299.
4. K.H. Kristensen, P. Gry and F. Holm, in: P. Zeuthen, J.C. Cheftel, C. Eriksson, M. Jul, H. Leniger, P. Linko, G. Varela and G. Vos (Eds), Extruded protein-rich animal by-products with improved texture. *Thermal Processing and Quality of Foods*, Elsevier Appl. Science Publish., London, 1984, pp. 113-121.
5. K. Buckley, Gelatinized animal food product. U.S. patent 4,143,171 (1979).
6. G.B. Stupec, Reconstituted fried puffed pork skins, U.S. Patent 4,119,742 (1978).
7. T.J. Ernst. Process for the production of a formed high-moisture pet food product, U.S. Patent 4,011,346 (1977).
8. R.H. Meyer, Composition containing animal parts for production of a fried snack food and method for production thereof, U.S. Patent 4,262,028 (1981).
9. A. Feldbrugge, Process for preparing meat-like fibers, U.S. Patent 3,886,299 (1975).
10. D. Megard, N. Kitabatake and J.C. Cheftel, J. Food Sci., 50 (1985) 1364-1369.
11. V.B. Alvarez, D.M. Smith, R.G. Morgan and A.M. Booren, J. Food Sci., 55 (1990) 942-946.
12. A.D. Clarke, F. Hsieh and S. Mulvaney, Processing of mechanically deboned turkey and corn flour mixtures by twin screw extrusion. Presented at the Ann. Meet. Inst. Food Technol., Chicago, IL, 25 June - 29 June 1989, Abstract 127.
13. R. Tarte, R.A. Molins and M. Kazemzadeh, Development of a beef/corn extruded snack model product. Presented at the Ann. Meet. Inst. Food Technol., Chicago, IL, 25 June - 29 June 1989, Abstract 284.
14. L. Thomas, P. Bechtel and R. Villota, Effects of composition and process parameters on twin-screw extrusion of expanded meat-based products. Presented at the Ann. Meet. Inst. Food Technol., Chicago, IL, 25 June - 29 June 1989, Abstract 118.
15. S. Chung, P. Bechtel, and R. Villota, Production of meat-based intermediate moisture snack foods by twin-screw extruder. Presented at the Ann. Meet. Inst. Food Technol., Chicago, IL, 25 June - 29 June 1989, Abstract 258.
16. H. Suzuki, B.S. Chung, S. Isobe, S. Hayakawa and S. Wada, J. Food Sci., 53 (1988) 1659-1661.
17. Y. Sasamoto, Y. Kammuri, K. Sawa, M. Araki, S. Morimoto, F. Mitsui and N. Miyazaki. Process for processing and treating raw materials of marine products, U.S. Patent 4,816,278 (1989).
18. S. Bhattacharya, H. Das, and A.N. Bose, Food Chem., 28 (1988) 225-231.
19. K.C. Chakraborty, S. Richardson, and R. Villota, Twin-screw extrusion performance of meat proteins and interactions with starch. Presented at

Ann. Meet. Inst. Food Technol., Las Vegas, Nevada, 16 June - 19 June 1987, Abstract 18.
20 D. Hale, Expanded meat product, Canad. Patent 842,723 (1970).
21 A.S. Ba-Jaber, Restructuring poultry meat with nonmeat ingredients by extrusion cooking. Ph.D. Dissertation, Colorado State University, Fort Collins, Colorado (1990).
22 O. Kempthorne, *Design and Analysis of Experiments*. Huntington, New York: Robert E. Krieger Publishing Company (1973).
23 T.A. Likimani, J.N. Sofos, J.A. Maga, and J.M. Harper, J. Food Sci., 55 (1990) 1388-1393.
24 T.A. Likimani, J.N. Sofos, J.A. Maga, and J.M. Harper, J. Food Sci., 56 (1991) 99-105, 108.
25 A.S. Szczesniak, M.A. Brandt, and H.H. Friedman, J. Food Sci., 28 (1963) 397-403.
26 A.D. Clarke, J.N. Sofos, and G.R. Schmidt, J. Food Sci., 53 (1988) 1266-1277.
27 N.L. King, J. Agric. Food Chem., 25 (1977) 166-171.
28 I.C. Peng, W.R. Dayton, D.W. Quass and C.E. Allen, J. Food Sci., 47 (1982a) 1976-1983.
29 I.C. Peng, W.R. Dayton, D.W. Quass, and C.E. Allen, J. Food Sci., 47 (1982b) 1984-1994.
30 I.C. Peng, and S.S. Nielsen, J. Food Sci., 51 (1986) 588-590.
31 K. Shiga, Y. Nakamura, and Y. Taki, Jpn. J. Zoo. Sci., 56 (1985) 897-904.
32 J.E. Kinsella, CRC Crit. Rev. Food Sci. Nutr., 11, 11, (1978) 147-207.
33 A.M. Hermansson, Amer. Oil Chem. Soc. J., 63 (1986) 658-666.
34 R. Schmidt, and H. Morris, Food Technol., 38, 5 (1984) 85-96.

G. Charalambous (Ed.), Food Science and Human Nutrition
© 1992 Elsevier Science Publishers B.V. All rights reserved.

A METHOD FOR DETERMINING BINDING OF HEXANAL BY MYOSIN AND ACTIN USING EQUILIBRIUM HEADSPACE SAMPLING GAS CHROMATOGRAPHY

RICHARD A. GUTHEIL and MILTON E. BAILEY

University of Missouri, Department of Food Science & Human Nutrition, 21 Agriculture Building, Columbia, MO 65211

SUMMARY

An equilibrium headspace sampling method was developed and used to investigate the binding of hexanal to muscle myofibrillar proteins in aqueous solution. Utilizing a diphasic system (lipid/water), headspace concentrations were measured by headspace sampling gas chromatography over a range of ligand concentrations and binding constants calculated. Coefficient of variation between duplicate headspace measurements averaged 4% and less than 10% between replications; however, calculated Klotz constants varied significantly. In an attempt to reduce Klotz plot variation, linear regression was applied to headspace measurements prior to the calculation of BOUND verses FREE variables used to plot Klotz plots. Headspace data modification of hexanal standard curves (with and without added protein) did not reduce variation in calculated Klotz constants N, the number of binding sites (number of molecules of hexanal per protein molecule) or in the Klotz constant (K). In a second attempt to reduce Klotz plot variation, two calculation methods were compared. A nonlinear calculation method should be used on nonlinear Klotz plots while the traditional linear calculation method should be used on linear Klotz plots to calculate binding constants. There were significant ($P < 0.05$) differences in binding of hexanal due to protein concentration, pH, temperature, and salt concentration.

1. INTRODUCTION

Proteins have little flavor, but they can modify flavors by selective binding of flavorants (1). Knowledge of the binding behavior of flavor compounds to food components is of great practical importance in the flavoring of foods (2). The binding of flavors to food components and their rates of partitioning between different phases is important in the flavoring of foods, in determining the relative retention of flavors, and in the release of flavors during processing, storage, and mastication. The selective binding of one component of a flavor blend to food components or packaging material can markedly alter the overall flavor impact (2).

A better understanding of the nature of flavor-protein interactions may be useful in minimizing the interaction between flavor compounds and protein to prevent the generation of unwanted compounds and improve the stability of desirable flavors in foods (3).

An excellent review on the advantages and disadvantages of several methods used to study flavor protein interactions has been published by Wilson (4). Methods that have been used to investigate interactions between flavor compounds and proteins include: equilibrium dialysis, equilibrium gel filtration, liquid-liquid partition equilibrium, and headspace sampling after an equilibrium has been established. These methods have been used in attempts to determine the amount of bound and free ligand under equilibrium conditions. It is important that equilibrium conditions are observed so that binding calculations (which are based on measurement under equilibrium conditions) can be made. Aqueous protein solutions insure that the protein is homogeneously available to the ligand.

Equilibrium dialysis methods (5, 6,7) used a semipermeable membrane in a diffusion cell to separate the aqueous protein solution from the flavor (ligand) solution (4). The protein solution is placed into one sample chamber and ligand solution is placed into a second chamber separated from the first chamber by a semipermeable membrane. Ligand molecules can diffuse throughout the cell, but protein molecules are retained in the first chamber. After the protein becomes saturated with ligand, the system comes to equilibrium.

Wilson (4) listed a number of disadvantages to the equilibrium dialysis method that included potential problems with (A) flavor binding to the membrane, (B) protein coating of the membrane which would slow or prevent equilibrium from being reached, (C) leakage around the membrane, (D) headspace areas in the dialysis cell where ligand can volatilize and be lost from measurement (E) permeation of the membrane by protein, while (F) the flavor (ligand) does not always permeate the membrane easily, and (G) incomplete extraction of the ligand from the aqueous solution can occur.

Equilibrium Gel Filtration involves the use of size exclusion to separate free ligand from ligand bound to a larger protein molecule (8). The column support material is equilibrated with ligand and added to a column. As a dilute solution of protein travels down the column, ligand is bound by the protein and is carried down the column with the protein. The amount of ligand bound by the protein is measured by various methods such as absorbance, radioactive counts (radioactively labeled ligand), and fluorescence specific to the ligand. Problems with this method include: (A) the difficulty of setting up a column at equilibrium, (B) volatility of the ligand, and (C) the difficulty of preparing identical control columns to measure the concentration of ligand in the column.

Liquid-Liquid Partition Equilibrium involves a biphasic system with the ligand in an organic solvent layered over an aqueous solution of the protein (9). After equilibration, the amount of ligand in the organic solvent is measured and compared to a similar setup without the protein being present. Unfortunately, there are problems with this method (4) which include: (A) denaturing of the protein at the liquid/liquid interfaces, (B) removal of weakly bound flavor compounds from the protein due to solvent extraction problems, and (C) the formation of surface foams and emulsions which increase measurement error. Denaturation can change the number of binding sites available and remove weakly bound flavor compounds from the protein which can decrease the flavor binding observed (4).

Equilibrium Headspace Sampling has the advantage that no additional extractions are used which could alter the protein binding or increase error by the procedure (4). However, disadvantages of the headspace sampling procedure include: (A) the flavor compound must be volatile in sufficient concentration to be measured, and (B) that only low flavor concentration ranges can be used to avoid saturating the headspace with ligand (4).

Equilibrium Headspace Sampling is the method of choice for studying the interaction of flavor components with protein. There are less problems than with other methods, and if a semi-automatic or automatic headspace sampler is used, quantitative results can be obtained. With headspace sampling, sample preparation is minimal because it is not necessary to extract the flavor compound. Volatiles characteristic of aroma are sampled directly from the headspace.

Equilibrium Headspace Sampling Gas Chromatography has been used effectively to measure the binding of hexanal to the soy protein glycinin and beta-conglycinin (10). In the present study, equilibrium headspace sampling gas chromatography was used to measure the binding of hexanal to the myofibrillar proteins myosin and actin. The methodology is described in detail as a guide to future studies.

2. MATERIALS AND METHODS

2.1 Prerigor Beef Muscle

An 18 month old Angus steer raised on the University of Missouri Beef Farm was slaughtered at the University of Missouri abattoir and the Longissimus dorsi muscle was removed prerigor and immediately chilled by immersion into ice. Time was kept short to minimize actomyosin formation. Myofibrillar protein myosin was extracted immediately after grinding using a salt extraction procedure by Margossian and Lowey (11). The procedure by Pardee and Spudich (12) was used to extract actin from the muscle residue remaining after myosin was extracted. All myosin solutions were stored at $4°C$ with 0.05% sodium azide to inhibit microbial growth. Freezing or drying denatures myosin; therefore, refrigeration was the only option for the storage of myosin. Actin was extracted with water from frozen acetone powder (12) as needed.

2.2 Determination of Molar Protein Concentration

For binding calculations, the number of moles of protein must be known. The microKjeldahl method (13) was used to determine the amount of nitrogen in the relatively pure protein samples. The amount of nitrogen determined was converted to protein on a weight basis with conversion factors calculated from the amino acid composition of the protein (14). The calculated conversion factors used were 6.05 for myosin and 6.29 for actin. The amount of purified protein measured in aqueous solutions of myofibrillar protein was then calculated on a molar basis.

2.3 SDS-PAGE Electrophoresis

Sodium dodecyl sulfate polyacrylamide gel electrophoresis (SDS-PAGE) was used to estimate the purity of the protein preparations (14). Tubes were filled with 7% polyacrylamide gel (15 ml gel buffer, 9.5 ml stock acrylamide-Bis solution, 4.0 ml distilled water, 1.5 ml Ammonium persulfide (10 mg/ml), and 0.045 ml TEMED). Gel buffer was prepared by adding 6.7 g sodium phosphate, monobasic (anhydride), 20.45 g sodium phosphate, dibasic (anhydride), plus 2.0 g sodium dodecyl sulfate to a 1 liter volumetric flask and diluting to volume with distilled water. The stock acrylamide-methylene bisacrylamide solution contained 22.2% acrylamide and 0.6% methylene bisacrylamide. TEMED (N,N,N',N'-Tetramethylethylenediamine) was purchased as a liquid (Sigma Chemical Co., St. Louis, MO) and served as a catalyst for the polymerization of the polyacrylamide gel. The protein (approximately 4 mg/ml) was diluted 1:1 with denaturing solution (0.02 M Sodium phosphate, monobasic, pH 7.0, 2% Sodium dodecyl sulfate (w/v), 2% Beta-mercaptoethanol (v/v), and 8 M urea and heated at 80-90°C for 15 min. The denatured protein was diluted 1:1 with tracking dye to yield a concentration of approximately 1 mg/ml. Fifteen or thirty microliters of the protein/tracking dye mixture was added to the gel. Current was applied at 3 mAmps/tube for 30 min followed by 8 mAmps/tube until the tracking dye was 2-3 cm from the bottom of the gel tubes using a Bio-Rad model 500 Power Supply (Bio-Rad Laboratories, Richmond, CA). Each gel was fixed with 10% (w/v) trichloroacetic acid (TCA) for 18 hr. For staining, the fixer was drained and Commassie Blue staining solution (2.5%) was added for 2-3 hr followed by destaining. Destaining solution was prepared by adding 60 ml 95% ethanol, 100 ml methanol, and 150 ml glacial acetic acid to a 2 liter volumetric flask and diluting to volume with distilled water.

2.4 Gel Scans of SDS-PAGE Gels

Gel scans (absorbance scans) of the SDS-PAGE gels were prepared using a Gel Scan Assessory attached to a Beckman DU-64 Spectrophotometer (Beckman Instruments, Inc., Fullerton, CA). Seven percent polyacrylamide gels were scanned spectrophotometrically from 0 to 100 mm at a wavelength of 560 nm to produce integration area counts representing protein bands (14). Approximate purity was estimated by dividing the area count of each band by the total area count of all bands scanned. The purity of the myosin preparations were estimated to be approximately 95% and the actin purity was approximately 98%.

2.5 Headspace Sampling Gas Chromatography

Headspace Sampling Gas Chromatography (HSGC) was carried out using a Perkin-Elmer semi-automatic headspace sampler (model HS-6) attached to a Perkin-Elmer model 8500 Gas Chromatograph (Perkin-Elmer Corporation, Norwalk, CT). Integration of peaks were performed on a Perkin-Elmer LCI-100 integrator. Perkin-Elmer headspace vials (borosilicate glass) had a volume of 9.2 cc and were cleaned in dilute Micro cleaning solution (Micro Liquid Laboratory Cleaner, Cole-Parmer Instrument Co., Chicago, IL) prior to use. Teflon-coated silicone headspace septa (19 mm) were obtained from Alltech Associates, Inc., Applied Science Labs (Deerfield, IL) and star springs were obtained from Perkin-Elmer. Aluminum seals (also called crimp caps) were used to seal the vials (Alltech Associates, Inc., Applied Science Labs, Deerfield, IL).

All vials contained 1.0 ml of buffer or protein solution. Using a 1.0 microliter plunger-in-needle syringe (Scientific Glass Engineering Pty. Ltd., 7 Argent Place, Ringwood, Australia), microliter amounts of hexanal were added to each vial. The volatile lipid was deposited on the glass just above the liquid level to avoid liquid contamination of the syringe. One microliter (1 mg) solute added to 1.0 ml of sample was equivalent to 1000 PPM. Larger amounts were added using a 5.0 microliter syringe. Immediately after adding the volatile, the headspace vial was assembled and sealed to minimize volatile loss. Septa could not be punctured by sample addition without destruction of the Teflon lining on the septa; therefore, headspace septa were purchased new and used once with the Teflon coating facing down into the sample vial. Headspace vials were submerged in a water bath (25°C or 35°C) to insure that the entire vial was at a uniform temperature and incubated for 18 hours to insure equilibrium between the air/water phase. Operating headspace sampler parameters, gas chromatograph parameters, and integration parameters are listed as follows:

```
GAS CHROMATOGRAPH CONTROL
    Isothermal oven temperature            190°C
    Injector temperature                   250°C
    FID Detector temperature               275°C
    Headspace Sampler temperature          25°C or 35°C
    FID sensitivity                        high
    Gas Chromatograph equilibration time   1.0 min
    Headspace Sampler pressure             35 PSIG
    Carrier gas                            Helium
    Detector zero                          on
    Carrier gas flow                       46 ml/min
    Headspace Sampler apparatus purge      5.0 ml/min
    Hydrogen pressure (zero grade)         18 PSIG
    Air pressure (grade D)                 22 PSIG
    Helium pressure (zero grade)           35 PSIG
```

HEADSPACE SAMPLER CONTROL--TIMED EVENTS
Hold (pressurization)	-0.50 min
Relay 0 on	-0.01 min
Relay 1 on	0.00 min
Relay 1 off (sampling)	0.20 min
Relay 0 off	0.21 min

PERKIN-ELMER LCI-100 INTEGRATION CONTROL
Area sensitivity	100
Base sensitivity	4
Skim sensitivity	2
Type of integration	base to base integration
Response factor	1.00
Area/Height rejection	0.00

A packed 10' x 1/8" stainless steel column containing 8% Poly MPE on Tenax GC 60/80 mesh was used.

2.6 Calculation of Binding Constants

The Free ligand concentration was the amount of ligand (not bound by the protein) measured. A duplicate vial containing the same ligand concentration, but no protein was measured to represent the Total ligand concentration. By subtraction (Total - Free = Bound), the amount of ligand bound in the aqueous phase was calculated. A standard curve (Total concentration values) was used to convert bound peak areas to the concentration bound in parts per million (PPM). The Bound/Free ligand concentrations were recalculated to BOUND/FREE thermokinetic values using a SAS program (15) and plotted as double reciprocal plots (Klotz Plot). For nonlinear Klotz plots, a nonlinear regression program was used to calculate N, the number of molecules of lipid bound per molecule of protein (also called the number of binding sites), and K, the Klotz binding constant. The Klotz constant was used to calculate Gibbs free energy and a modification of the Arrhenius equation was used to calculate enthalopy from Klotz variables determined at two temperatures.

2.7 SAS Program

Statistical Abstracts Service (SAS) release 5.16 (SAS Institute Inc., Cary, NC, copyright 1984, 1986) was the software used on the University of Missouri mainframe computer to run the SAS Program. A SAS program (15) was used to calculate FREE ligand concentrations (moles/liter) and the amount BOUND (moles ligand bound/mole protein). The program is listed as follows:

In the following program, the data file is called HEXANAL and the SAS program is called TEST. The molecular weight of hexanal was entered as 100.16, density as 0.8139, moles of actin as 1.060×10^{-7}, and moles of myosin as 7.690×10^{-9}.

DATA HEXANAL; CMS FILEDEF TEST 1 DISK HEXANAL DATA A; INFILE TEST 1; INPUT PPM BUFF MYO ACT; MOLEACT = (1.0600E-07); MOLEMYO = (7.6900E-09); L = PPM*10**-9; MOLWT = 100.16; DENS = 0.8139; MOLES = ((DENS/MOLWT)*1000)*L; BB7 = ((BUFF - MYO)/BUFF)*MOLES; BB11 = ((BUFF - ACT)/BUFF)*MOLES; BNDMYO = BB7; BNDACT = BB11; B7 = BNDMYO/MOLEMYO; B11 = BNDACT/MOLEACT; F7 = (MOLES-BNDMYO)/1000; F11 = (MOLES BNDACT)/1000; IB11 = 1/B11; IF11 = 1/F11; IF11SQ = IF11**2; IF7 = 1/F7; IF7SQ = IF7**2; IB7 = 1/B7; FB7 = F7/B7; FB11 = F11/B11; BF7 = B7/F7; BF11 = B11/F11; CARDS;

PROC PRINT; PROC PLOT; PLOT B7*F7; TITLE 'SATURATION PLOT FOR MYOSIN'; PROC GLM; MODEL B7 = F7/P; OUTPUT OUT = NEW P = YSAT7 R = RESAT7; PROC PLOT; PLOT RESAT7*F7; TITLE 'RESIDUAL PLOT FOR MYOSIN SATURATION'; PROC PLOT; PLOT IB7*IF7; TITLE 'KLOTZ PLOT FOR MYOSIN'; PROC GLM; MODEL IB7 = IF7/P; OUTPUT OUT = NEW P = YHATK7 R = RESIDK7; PROC PLOT; PLOT RESIDK7*IF7; TITLE 'RESIDUAL PLOT FOR MYOSIN KLOTZ'; PROC PLOT; PLOT IB7*IF7SQ; TITLE 'MODIFIED KLOTZ PLOT FOR MYOSIN'; PROC GLM; MODEL IB7 = IF7SQ/P; OUTPUT OUT = NEW P = YHATM7 R = RESIDM7; PROC PLOT; PLOT RESIDM7*IF7SQ; TITLE 'RESIDUAL PLOT FOR MYOSIN MODIFIED KLOTZ'; PROC PLOT; PLOT B11*F11; TITLE 'SATURATION PLOT FOR ACTIN'; PROC GLM; MODEL B11 = F11; OUTPUT OUT = NEW P = YSAT1 R = RESAT1; PROC PLOT; PLOT RESAT1*F11; PROC PLOT; PLOT IB11*IF11; TITLE 'KLOTZ PLOT FOR ACTIN'; PROC GLM; MODEL IB11 = IF11/P; OUTPUT OUT = NEW P = YHATK11 R = RESIDK11; PROC PLOT; PLOT RESIDK11*IF11; TITLE 'RESIDUAL PLOT FOR ACTIN KLOTZ'; PROC PLOT; PLOT IB11*IF11SQ; TITLE 'MODIFIED KLOTZ PLOT FOR ACTIN'; PROC GLM; MODEL IB11 = IF11SQ/P; OUTPUT OUT = NEW P = YHATM11 R = RESIDM11; PROC PLOT; PLOT RESIDM11*IF11SQ; TITLE 'RESIDUAL PLOT FOR ACTIN MODIFIED KLOTZ'; PROC PLOT; PLOT FB7*F7; TITLE 'Y RECIPROCAL PLOT FOR MYOSIN'; PROC GLM; MODEL FB7 = F7/P; OUTPUT OUT = NEW P = YY7 R = RY7; PROC PLOT; PLOT RY7*F7; TITLE 'RESIDUAL PLOT FOR Y RECIPROCAL FOR MYOSIN'; PROC PLOT; PLOT FB11*F11; TITLE 'Y RECIPROCAL PLOT FOR ACTIN'; PROC GLM; MODEL FB11 = F11/P; OUTPUT OUT = NEW P = YY1 R = RY1; PROC PLOT; PLOT RY1*F7; TITLE 'RESIDUAL PLOT FOR Y = RECIPROCAL FOR ACTIN'; PROC PLOT; PLOT BF7*B7; TITLE 'X RECIPROCAL PLOT FOR MYOSIN'; PROC GLM; MODEL BF7 = B7/P; OUTPUT OUT = NEW P = YX7 R = RX7; PROC PLOT; PLOT RX7*F7; TITLE 'RESIDUAL PLOT FOR X-RECIPROCAL FOR MYOSIN'; PROC PLOT; PLOT BF11*B11; TITLE 'X RECIPROCAL PLOT FOR ACTIN'; PROC GLM; MODEL FB11 = F11/P; OUTPUT OUT = NEW P = YX11 R = RX11; PROC PLOT; PLOT RX11*F7; TITLE 'RESIDUAL PLOT FOR X-RECIPROCAL FOR ACTIN'; RUN;

The term FREE was used to indicate the concentration in moles/liter not bound. The term BOUND was used to indicate the amount bound per protein molecule (moles ligand bound/mole protein). Note that FREE refers to concentration and that BOUND refers to an amount. The terms FREE and BOUND are capitalized in order to distinguish them from the Free and Bound raw data (peak areas). BOUND verses FREE was plotted directly to produce a saturation plot and the reciprocals were plotted (1/BOUND verses 1/FREE) to produce a Klotz Plot.

2.8 Nonlinear Regression Program (16)

A nonlinear regression program was written by Dr. Pat Murphy, Professor of Food Technology, Iowa State University (16) in Applesoft basic based on Wilkinson's curve fitting technique (17). Murphy's program was rewritten in basica by Richard Gutheil to run the program on an IBM or IBM compatible computer. In addition to calculating N and K, the program also calculates the Standard Error (S.E.) associated with the values. FREE data must be entered as moles/liter and BOUND data as moles of ligand bound/mole protein. The nonlinear regression program is listed as follows:

150 REM WILKINSON PLOT, 155 CLS, 160 PRINT "   WILKINSON STATISTICAL ESTIMATIONS", 165 PRINT "   OF V-MAX AND KM": PRINT, 170 PRINT "BY DR. PATRICIA MURPHY, 171 PRINT "DEPARTMENT OF FOOD TECHNOLOGY", 172 PRINT "IOWA STATE UNIVERSITY', 180 PRINT : PRINT, 200 DIM S(10,10),V(10,10), 210 PRINT "ENTER NUMBER OF S,V PAIRS", 220 INPUT N1, 230 FOR I1 = 1 TO 10, 240 Q1 = I1, 250 FOR J1 TO 10, 260 R1 = R1 + 1, 270 PRINT "ENTER S", 280 INPUT S, 290 S(I1,J1) = S, 300 PRINT "ENTER V", 310 INPUT V, 320 V(I1,J1) = V, 330 X = (V * V), 340 Y = X / S, 350 A = A + (V * X), 360 B = B + (X * X), 370 C = C + (V * Y), 380 D = D + (X * Y), 390 E = E + (Y * Y), 400 IF R1 = N1 GOTO 430, 410 NEXT J1, 420 NEXT I1, 430 D1 = (A * E) - (C * D), 440 KM = ((B * C) - (A * D)) / D1, 450 VO = ((B * E) - (D * D)) / D1, 460 K5 = INT (KM * 10 ^ 4) / 10 ^ 4, 470 V5 = INT (VO * 10 ^ 4) / 10 ^ 4, 480 PRINT "K-PRO="K5"   V-PRO="V5, 485 PRINT : PRINT, 490 PRINT "ENTER 'GO' WHEN READY", 510 INPUT T$, 515 R1 = 0, 520 FOR I1 = 1 TO 10, 530 Q1 = I1, 540 FOR J1 TO 10, 550 R1 = R1 + 1, 560 S = S(I1,J1) 570 V = V(I1,J1), 580 U = S + KM, 590 F = (VO * S) / U, 600 G = - (VO * S) / (U * U), 610 FG = (F * G), 620 VG = (V * G), 630 VF = (V * F), 640 G2 = (G * G), 650 F2 = (F * F), 660 H = H + F2, 670 H2 = H2 + FG, 680 H3 = H3 + VF, 690 K = K + G2, 700 L = L + VG, 701 X = (V * V), 702 X1 = X1 + X, 710 IF R1 = N1 GOTO 740, 720 NEXT J1, 730 NEXT I1,740 M = (H * K) - (H2 * H2), 750 N = ((K * H3) - (H2 * L)) / M, 760 O = ((H * L) - (H2 * H3)) / M, 770 V1 = (N * VO), 780 K1 = KM + O / N, 790 S2 = (X1 - (N * H3) - (O * L)) / (N1 - 2), 792 S3 = SQR (S2), 795 S4 = (S3) * (SQR (H / M)) / N, 797 S5 = (VO * S3) * (SQR (K / M)), 800 V9 = INT (V1 * 10 ^ 4) / 10 ^ 4, 805 S7 = INT (S4 * 10 ^ 4) / 10 ^ 4, 810 K9 = INT (K1 * 10 ^ 4) / 10 ^ 4, 820 S8 = INT (S5 * 10 ^ 4) / 10 ^ 4, 830 PRINT "VM="V9" S.E.="S8, 840 PRINT "KM="K9" S.E.="S7, 850 END

Each instruction is preceded by a line number. Commas are used to separate instructions and are not part of the program. V-MAX or V_m = N, the number of binding sites; K_m = K, the Klotz binding constant; S = substrate concentration (for binding plots, this is the FREE concentration in moles/liter); V = velocity of the reaction (for binding plots, this is the BOUND value (moles ligand bound/mole protein).

The IBM basica program was originally designed to compute enzyme kinetic data; therefore, the values V_m and K_m are the same as enzyme kinetics. The program is similar for binding calculations except that K_m becomes K, the Klotz binding constant and V_m becomes N, the number of binding sites.

2.9 Step by Step Instructions for Calculating Binding Data:

1. Using the headspace peak area data for all concentrations, calculate % CV among and between replications to determine experimental precision.

2. Check that the standard curve is linear over a range of concentrations.

3. Enter headspace peak areas (standards and protein samples) along with corresponding concentration in PPM into SAS data files. Enter molarity of protein solution, molecular weight of ligand and density of ligand into the SAS program in order to calculate number of moles and FREE/BOUND values.

4. Plot BOUND verses FREE for a Saturation plot and 1/BOUND verses 1/FREE for a Klotz plot. Compute regression values (y-intercept and slope) from linear Klotz plots.

5. Subjectively examine the Klotz Plot to determine if the plot is linear or nonlinear. If the plot looks like a scattergram, then there is too much variation in the data and/or little or no binding. If the Klotz plot is linear, compute N and K thermokinetic values from the linear regression equation. If the Kotz plot is predominantly linear, use the linear portion of the plot to determine the y-intercept and the slope of the line.

6. If the Klotz Plot is nonlinear, enter SAS calculated values for FREE and BOUND for each concentration into the nonlinear regression program to calculate N and K. FREE data must be entered as moles/liter and BOUND data as moles ligand bound/mole protein.

7. Calculate the Gibb's free energy of interaction (ΔG).

    $\Delta G = -RT \ln K$ where R = 1.987 cal/deg mol

8. Using two temperatures for binding, calculate ΔH, enthalpy change.

    $\Delta H = (-\ln K_2/K_1) / 1/T_2 - 1/T_1$ where

    K_1 = Klotz constant K at one temperature
    K_2 = Klotz constant K at second temperature
    T_1 = Temperature first Klotz constant measured
    T_2 = Temperature second Klotz constant measured

9. Calculate ΔS, entropy (randomness change).

    $\Delta S = (\Delta H - \Delta G)/T$

3. STEP BY STEP CALCULATION EXAMPLE

The following is an example of the methodology used to calculate binding of hexanal by myosin and actin. Representative data has been used in these calculations.

3.1 <u>Step 1</u>. Calculate the precision of the raw data. Data points that have a percent coefficient of variation of 5.0% or less are highly precise.

Example 1. Percent coefficient of variation (% CV) of headspace peak areas between duplicate measurements over a range of concentrations.

Concentration (PPM)	Hexanal peak area[a]	%CV	Hexanal plus Myosin peak area[a]	%CV	Hexanal plus Actin peak area[a]	%CV
1600	6418.51	0.5	3573.64	0.9	4739.50	3.9
1600	6372.72		3529.16		5011.79	
1400	5819.47	0.3	3266.77	1.3	4349.75	2.0
1400	5792.51		3205.95		4230.16	
1200	4965.04	1.6	2669.32	4.2	3825.32	0.9
1200	4855.08		2516.38		3874.13	
1000	4354.66	3.8	1780.31	2.1	2972.27	3.0
1000	4595.21		1728.00		3099.89	
900	3887.87	3.7	1498.72	2.9	2811.34	2.3
900	4095.36		1437.72		2723.12	
800	3304.16	4.0	1183.49	0.6	2440.78	0.3
800	3497.59		1194.07		2452.24	
700	2934.79	2.1	813.91	0.8	2160.94	1.5
700	3022.32		805.14		2114.17	
600	2539.83	0.8	358.00	3.9	1835.75	1.7
600	2567.43		378.27		1879.31	
500	2098.40	0.1	8.13	1.4	1582.44	2.6
500	2101.55		8.29		1525.28	
400	1660.16	0.7	.		1214.38	3.4
400	1677.29				1273.77	
300	1247.84	1.1	.		911.77	2.9
300	1228.87				875.27	
200	805.32	1.9	.		618.54	3.1
200	826.81				591.88	
100	368.47	5.6	.		262.06	4.4
100	398.59				278.98	

[a] Peak areas have been multiplied by 10^{-4}. Hexanal plus 0.44% Myosin or 0.44% Actin, 0.6 M KCl, pH 7.0, 25°C, 18 hr equilibration time.

3.2 **Step 2.** Check the hexanal standard curve for linearity using linear regression.

Example 2. Headspace peak areas modified by linear regression plus regression output.

Hexanal Concentration (PPM)	Original Headspace data (peak area)	Modified[a] Headspace data (peak area)
1600	6418.51	6622.52
1600	6372.72	6657.22
1400	5819.47	5799.31
1400	5792.51	5837.17
1200	4965.04	4976.10
1200	4855.08	5017.13
1000	4354.66	4152.89
900	4595.21	4197.08
900	3887.87	3741.28
900	4095.36	3787.06
800	3304.16	3329.67
800	3497.59	3377.04
700	2934.79	2918.07
700	3022.32	2967.02
600	2539.83	2506.46
600	2567.43	2556.99
500	2098.40	2094.86
500	2101.55	2146.97
400	1660.16	1683.25
400	1677.29	1736.95
300	1247.84	1271.64
300	1228.87	1326.93
200	805.32	860.04
200	826.81	916.90
100	368.47	448.43
100	398.59	506.88
0		36.82
0		96.86

REGRESSION OUTPUT

y-intercept	36.82
	96.86
Standard error of y-intercept	103.09
	194.36
R Squared	0.9973
	0.9905
Number of Observations	13
	13
Degrees of Freedom	11
	11
Slope	4.1161
	4.1002
Standard error of Slope	0.06
	0.12

[a] Linear regression applied to headspace data.

3.3 Step 3. Calculate FREE and BOUND Hexanal. Enter headspace peak areas with corresponding concentration in PPM into a SAS data file. Modify the SAS program to include the name of the SAS data file, enter molarity of protein solution, molecular weight of ligand, and density of ligand.

Example 3. FREE and BOUND hexanal calculated using SAS from headspace peak areas for each concentration.

Hexanal Concentration (PPM)	Myosin[a]		Actin[a]	
	FREE (M)[c]	BOUND[b]	FREE (M)[c]	BOUND[b]
1600	7239	749.4	9601	32.1
1600	7200	754.4	10225	26.2
1400	6386	648.9	8503	27.1
1400	6296	660.6	8308	28.9
1200	5242	586.3	7513	21.1
1200	5054	610.8	7781	18.6
1000	3322	624.7	5546	24.3
900	3056	659.3	5482	24.9
900	2819	584.4	5288	19.1
800	2567	617.2	4863	23.1
800	2328	542.6	4802	16.0
800	2219	556.8	4558	18.3
700	1578	534.5	4188	14.1
700	1515	542.6	3979	16.1
600	687	544.6	3524	12.8
600	718	540.6	3569	12.3
500			3064	9.4
500			2949	10.5
400			2378	8.2
400			2468	7.4
300			1781	6.2
300			1736	6.6
200			1248	3.6
200			1163	4.4
100			578	2.2
			569	2.3

[a] Hexanal plus 0.40% Myosin or 0.44% Actin, 0.6 M KCl, pH 7.0, 25°C, 18 hr equilibration time.
[b] BOUND is moles hexanal bound/mole protein.
[c] (M) = moles/liter

3.4 <u>Step 4</u>. Plot Saturation plots (FREE vs BOUND) and Klotz plots (1/FREE vs 1/BOUND). Calculate the linear regression equation for each Klotz plot.

Example 4. Saturation plots and Klotz plots were made from the data given in Example 3 (See Figure 1 for myosin and Figure 2 for actin).

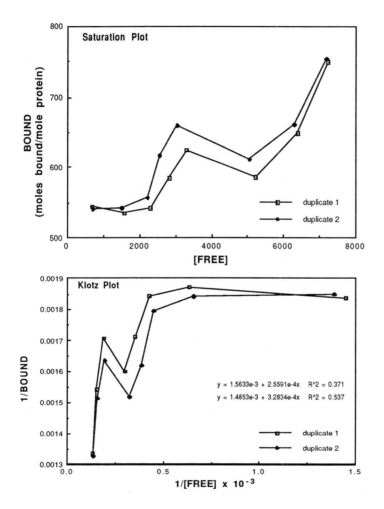

Figure 1. Saturation and Klotz plots for hexanal plus 0.44% myosin, 0.6 M KCl, pH 7.0, 25°C, 18 hours, 12 second sampling. Linear regression equations for duplicate Klotz plots are given.

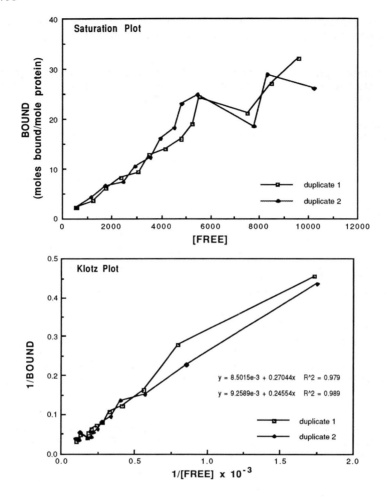

Figure 2. Saturation and Klotz plots for hexanal plus 0.44% actin, 0.6 M KCl, pH 7.0, 25°C, 18 hours, 12 second sampling. Linear regression equations for duplicate Klotz plots are given.

Eliminate data points that can be attributed to error and replot the graphs. A single data point that causes a sharp spike (due to a relatively low BOUND value) in a plot is most likely in error. Also points that are greatly different from similar points in a duplicate plot may be due to experimental error.

3.5 **Step 5**. Calculate N and K from Klotz plots. Subjectively determine linearity of Klotz plots. Use nonlinear regression on nonlinear Klotz plots and linear regression on linear Klotz plots.

Example 5. Nonlinear regression was applied to BOUND and FREE values used to construct Klotz plots and N and K calculated. Linear regression was used on Klotz plots (1/BOUND vs 1/FREE) to obtain y-intercept and slope used to calculate N and K.

Linear regression calculation method		Nonlinear regression calculation method				Klotz Plot subjective appearance
N[a]	K	N[a]	S.E.[b]	K	S.E.[b]	
Myosin 25°C						
639.7	6108.8	660.7	40.0	230.0	140.7	Nonlinear
673.3	4523.4	694.6	37.8	289.6	132.1	Nonlinear
Actin 25°C						
117.6	31.4	189.6	87.4	46180.0	19507.5	Linear
108.0	37.7	58.7	14.3	10432.9	3347.9	Linear

[a]N is a dimensionless number. N = the number of binding sites. N is also the number of hexanal molecules on each molecule of protein. [b]S.E. = Standard error

Notice in the above example that nonlinear regression should be used on nonlinear Klotz plots and that linear regression should be used on linear Klotz plots to get reasonable values of N and K. When calculations involving large numbers required more memory than available, the nonlinear regression program aborted. Negative intercept refers to Klotz plots in which the linear regression line intersects the y-axis at a negative value. N and K values can not be calculated from negative y-intercepts.

3.6 **Step 6**. Calculate Gibb's free energy of interaction for each temperature used. Using two temperatures for binding, calculate ΔH, enthalpy change. Calculate ΔS, entropy (randomness change) when ΔG and ΔH are known.

Example 6. Binding constants for the binding of hexanal to myosin and actin. Nonlinear regression used on nonlinear Klotz plots and linear regression used on linear Klotz plots for the calculation of Klotz constant K. Additional measurements at 35°C enabled the following calculations since calculation of ΔH requires that the Klotz constant K be measured at two temperatures.

	duplicate	ΔH (kcal/mole)	ΔG (kcal/mole)		ΔS (cal/mole°K)	
			25°C	35°C	25°C	35°C
Myosin						
Hexanal	1	3.42	-3.22	-3.10	22.3	21.2
Hexanal	2	2.75	-3.36	-3.65	20.5	20.8
Actin						
Hexanal	1	2.24	-2.04	-1.96	14.4	13.6
Hexanal	2	3.43	-2.15	-2.45	18.7	19.1

3.7 Standard Error of N

The following calculation was used to estimate the standard error of N derived from linear Klotz plots (14):

$$S.E.(N) = \frac{1 \; (S.E. \; of \; \mu)}{\mu^2}$$

where μ represents the y-intercept.

3.8 Standard Error of K

The following calculation was used to estimate the standard error the the Klotz constant (K) from linear Klotz plots (14).

$$S.E.(K) = Var(K)^{-1/2}$$

where K represents the Klotz constant K.

3.9 Analysis of Variance

Two way Analysis of Variance (ANOVA), described by Snedecor and Cochran (19) was used to determine if variation associated with the Klotz constant or N could be significantly reduced by modification of the headspace peak areas prior to calculation of FREE/BOUND values used to plot Klotz plots.

ANOVA's were calculated using the Statistical Abstract Service (SAS) general linear model using least significant differences (LSD) and Duncan's new multilple range test as means separation techniques to determine if significant differences existed between means (SAS Institute Inc., Cary, NC). Negative values of N (due to a negative intercept on the y-axis), negative values of K (due to negative slopes and/or negative values of N), and values that were inconsistent with the trend (or with its duplicate determination) in the data were deleted.

4. RESULTS AND DISCUSSION

4.1 Selection of Hexanal as Model Compound

Hexanal was chosen as the model compound since it has been used as an indicator compound for warmed-over flavor in meats (20, 21, 22). The concentration of hexanal was directly related to lipid oxidation.

4.2 Reproducibility of Headspace Peak Areas

Variation was determined by calculating the percent coefficient of variation (% CV) which is also referred to as the coefficient of relative variation or as the relative standard deviation (23). The advantage of using the coefficient of variation instead of the standard deviation is that the coefficient of variation expresses variation relative to the size of the observations summarized (24). Therefore, it is useful to compute % CV when one compares variability between different sets of data (24). The average % CV for duplicate measurements of headspace standards (hexanal standard curve) was 3.4% over the entire range of concentrations (Figure 3). The % CV improved slightly when measurements were made in the presence of myosin (3.1%) or actin (2.2%).

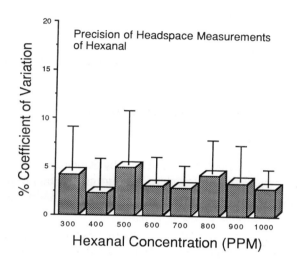

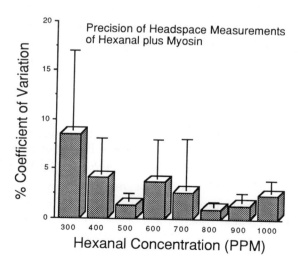

Figure 3 (continued next page)

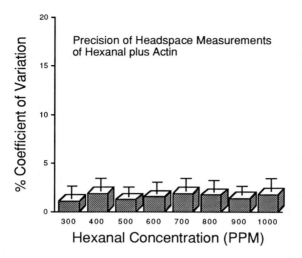

Figure 3. Precision of headspace measurements. Percent coefficient of variation (%CV) over a range of hexanal concentrations with and without added protein. Each concentration represented the mean of nine determinations.

Protein concentration (0.22%, 0.44% myosin; 0.19%-0.44% actin) did not affect variation among headspace measurements. In general, % CV less than 4% between duplicate headspace sampling determinations was achieved. This excellent precision was a result of good technique in the addition of ligand to individual headspace vials, good technique in operating the Perkin-Elmer Headspace Sampler (model HS-6), and good technique in operating the Perkin-Elmer 8500 gas chromatograph (selection of optimal measurement conditions). The use of a semiautomatic headspace sampler was critical to attaining excellent precision for the external standard curves.

It is difficult to attain this level of precision using gas syringes to manually collect and inject gases into a gas chromatograph. Manual gas syringe injection problems include, column back pressure, inaccurate sampling at varying temperatures (syringe should be same temperature as gas), temperature changes due to handling syringes with warm hands, loss of volatiles at the needle valve used to split injections (needle valves can not be completely closed off), and pressure changes within the gas chromatograph. In accordance with the ideal gas law $PV = nRT$, pressure (P), volume (V), and temperature (T) must be kept constant if n, the amount injected is to be quantitatively measured. R is the ideal gas constant and T is the absolute temperature..

Hexanal concentration (300-1000 PPM) did not affect the precision of duplicate measurements (% CV); however, at lower concentrations (<300 PPM), precision suffered. This was in part due to the difficulty in quantitatively adding small amounts of hexanal to headspace vials prior to sealing the vials. Since septa could not be punctured to add ligand, ligand was deposited on the inside wall of the vial followed by immediate crimping of the vial. At low concentrations, all the ligand may be bound by the protein which leaves nothing to measure in the headspace. Samples with high concentrations (generally greater than 900 PPM) of ligand suffered from poor reproducibility due to saturation of the headspace. It was necessary to keep ligand concentrations in the headspace below saturation for the standard curve to be linear. High % CV's often occurred in protein-containing samples when almost all of the ligand in the headspace had been bound by the protein. These data points were not used since they did not conform to the linearity of the standard curve.

For valid Klotz plots, the protein must be saturated with an excess of ligand in the aqueous phase. When most of the ligand was bound to the protein in the aqueous phase, it was likely that the protein in the aqueous phase was not saturated with ligand. There are two saturation conditions that must be met in the equilibrium headspace sampling method for diphasic systems (lipid/water). First, the headspace must be below saturation levels and second, the aqueous phase must always be saturated with ligand.

Therefore, there were upper and lower limits of ligand concentration that could be studied in binding experiments. If the ligand concentration was too low, all of the headspace volatiles were bound and there was no ligand left in the headspace to measure. In general, for single ligand binding experiments a range of 300 to 900 PPM could be measured precisely (duplicate determinations). The most important requirement for a Headspace Sampling-Gas Chromatography system is to achieve a high degree of reproducibility of analytical conditions (25).

4.3 Percent of Hexanal Bound to Protein

The amount of hexanal bound to myosin was affected by protein concentration. Increased protein concentration resulted in disproportionately more binding at similar ligand concentrations. A concentration of 0.11% myosin was found to be too low for binding experiments since most of the binding amounted to less than 10% of hexanal was bound to the protein. It is recommended that 0.22% protein content or greater be used in binding experiments with myosin when using equilibrium headspace sampling.

The binding of hexanal with actin was not affected by protein concentration to the same extent as myosin. Regardless of the protein concentration, the percent bound was approximately the same at similar ligand concentrations. An average of 25-30% of the added hexanal was bound to actin over a concentration range of 200-

1000 PPM hexanal. These results indicated that the protein concentration was important when binding hexanal to myosin, but of less importance when binding hexanal to actin. If a relatively large percentage of the ligand concentration was bound to the protein (such as greater than 95%), the headspace data were not used to calculate BOUND/FREE values which are used to construct Klotz plots (x and y-axis variables).

4.4 Variation in Headspace Measurements over a Range of Concentrations

When protein was incorporated into vials containing a series of hexanal standards, the resulting plot (headspace peak area verses Hexanal concentration) was generally linear. The correlation R squared statistic (R^2) for standard curves was generally greater than 0.98.

The linearity of standard curves was affected when the ligand headspace concentration approached saturation levels. Standard curves were checked for linearity at ligand headspace concentrations in excess of 1000 PPM by comparing the linear regression modified standards to the nonmodified standards. If the standards were not linear at high ligand concentrations, the peak areas for the linearized standards were substantially higher. In general, hexanal standard curves equal to or less than 1000 PPM were linear for all ligand concentrations selected and therefore valid to use. Different compounds have different volatilities and therefore become saturated at different concentrations.

If the headspace was saturated with ligand the standard curve results were erratic. Droplets of lipid formed on the inside of the glass vial which resulted in a decrease in the headspace concentration. Conversely, if a droplet of lipid was drawn into the headspace sampler, a large error occurred. In general, if the headspace was saturated with ligand, the amount of standard measured was erroneously less than the actual amount in the vial.

The slopes of standard curves with or without protein resulted in some variation, but this variation generally was less than 20% coefficient of variation (% CV). However, after the long equilibrium time period, there was a large amount of variation associated with the y-intercept of hexanal external standard curves (155% CV). Standard curves of samples containing protein had less variation; however, the variation associated with the y-intercept was still high (myosin, 74% CV; actin, 81% CV). This lack of precision was not important, however, since standard curves were plotted for each individual experiment and Free and Bound ligand concentrations calculated from these data as described in section 2.6.

The best approach was to calculate the amount bound by measuring the Total amount of hexanal in the headspace (hexanal standard only) and subtracting the Free amount of unbound hexanal (hexanal standard plus protein) for each ligand concentration. By using a pair of samples to measure Total and Free headspace concentrations of hexanal (with and without protein), the amount bound was calculated at individual concentrations for each sample.

4.5 Calculation of BOUND/FREE Values

Binding data is unique in that there are many variables associated with obtaining reproducible data and in calculating BOUND/FREE values. Without the original data, it is not easy or practical to calculate backwards from a thermokinetic plot to the original data and clearly not possible to determine the precision of the original chromatographic data. BOUND values represent moles of ligand bound to protein by each mole of protein and were calculated as amounts bound to a specific amount of protein. Conversely, FREE values were calculated as molar concentrations of measured ligand. Calculation of FREE and BOUND values involves separate calculations using the same headspace peak area measurements.

4.6 Saturation and Klotz Plots

The BOUND/FREE data were directly plotted (BOUND verses FREE) to produce Saturation plots. These plots are similar to Michaelis-Menten plots, except in Saturation plots, the protein is saturated with ligand and in Michaelis-Menten plots the ligand is in equilibrium with the protein (enzyme).

Some proteins bind irreversibly with ligand. Saturation plot and Klotz plot data take this into account by assuming the protein is saturated with ligand and not necessarily in reversible equilibrium with it. Since all proteins are not enzymes, it is invalid to assume that the protein-ligand interaction will be completely reversible. In actuality, most proteins will irreversibly bind to many ligands. It is often not possible to strip all bound flavor components from a protein without destroying protein functionality (26).

Considering, the variation associated with the y-intercept and the slope of external headspace standard curves, it was logical that this variation would cause problems in binding plots constructed from headspace data. Therefore, variation in binding values calculated from Klotz plots were most likely due to variations associated with the y-intercept and to the slope.

This was found to be true in the case of Klotz plots where the y-intercept and the slope were used to calculate binding values N and K. N, the number of binding sites, was calculated by taking the reciprocal of the y-intercept (1/y-intercept). The Klotz constant K was calculated by taking the reciprocal of N multiplied by the slope.

Saturation plots are useful because they graphically show upper limits of the amount of ligand that can be bound to protein. If at increasingly higher FREE ligand concentrations, there was no corresponding increase in BOUND values, then the plot levels out to a maximum BOUND value for the protein. However, if there are no upper limits to the amount that the protein binds, then the slope of the plot will continue to increase. In order to calculate binding values from Saturation plots, it is necessary to reach a maximum amount bound that is not affect by increased FREE ligand concentration (27). Klotz plots do not have this limitation.

Klotz plots (1/BOUND verses 1/FREE) are double reciprocal plots of Saturation plots (BOUND verses FREE), and do not require the protein to reach a maximum BOUND for calculation of binding constants. The maximum BOUND value (N) can be calculated based on the intersection of the curve with the y-axis.

A small amount of variation on Saturation plots at higher ligand concentrations translated to a large amount of variation on Klotz plots in the area where the plot intersected the y-axis. This was due to the effect reciprocal calculations have on data. Evenly spaced ligand concentrations (100, 200, 300, and higher) when converted to reciprocals, become increasingly more packed as the curve approaches the y-axis intercept.

Linear regression was applied to Klotz plots and subsequent linear regression equations were calculated for each Klotz plot. The linear regression equation yielded the value of the y-intercept and the slope which was used to calculate binding values from the plot (by a linear calculation method).

4.7 Headspace Data Modifications to Improve Reproducibility

Modified headspace measurements prior to calculating BOUND/FREE values (used to construct Klotz plots) were used in an effort to reduce variation associated with binding constants calculated from Klotz plots. In theory, linear regression eliminates variation among data points.

Headspace data were calculated into three categories, unmodified data, standards modified, and both standards and protein modified. Standards modified referred to the headspace measurements of nonprotein containing standards used to construct standard curves for converting peak areas into the amount BOUND at particular FREE ligand concentrations. Protein plus standards referred to the inclusion of protein into vials containing known ligand concentrations. All headspace sampling determinations involved two identical vials containing exactly the same ligand concentration, except one vial also contained protein. Binding of ligand in the aqueous phase resulted in a reduction in the headspace concentration for that ligand.

Analysis of variance (ANOVA) was used to determine if headspace data modification significantly affected the calculation of binding values using data from a variety of experiments (Table 1). Treatments included varying salt concentration (0.3 M KCl, 0.6 M KCl, 0.9 M KCl), pH (4,5,6,7,8), protein concentration (0.22% and 0.44% myosin; 0.19% and 0.41% actin), azide addition, and whether the use of a stir bar affected results. Treatment effects will be discussed in more detail in following sections.

Table 1. Analysis of Variance (ANOVA) on the Calculation of Binding Constants N and K and their Associated Standard Errors SE(N) and SE(K) from Klotz plots using the Linear Regression Calculation Method.

experiment	Linear N					Linear K				
	trt	Data mod	trt x mod	R^2	% CV	trt	Data mod	trt x mod	R^2	% CV
Salt concentration	S	N	N	0.82	20.7	N	N	N	0.57	529.9a
pH	S	N	N	0.94	35.5	N	N	N	0.93	34.8
Actin concentration	N	N	N	0.42	97.0	S	S	S	0.99	16.0
Myosin conc.	S	N	N	0.85	31.0	N	N	N	0.65	52.7
Azide plus myosin	N	N	N	0.44	53.8	N	N	N	0.59	94.1
Azide plus actin	S	S	S	0.94	50.2	S	S	S	0.99	18.5
Stir bar use	N	N	.	0.96	37.3	N	N	.	0.25	175.8
	linear SE(N)					linear SE(K)				
Salt conc.	S	N	N	0.72	67.2	S	N	N	0.66	114.7
pH	S	N	S	0.92	33.8	N	N	N	0.59	208.4
Actin conc.	N	N	N	0.37	126.8	N	N	N	0.53	70.7
Myosin conc.	N	N	N	0.45	235.8	S	N	N	0.60	124.9
Azide plus myosin	N	N	N	0.40	106.5	N	N	N	0.62	90.3
Azide plus actin	N	S	N	0.77	148.2	S	S	S	0.99	14.4
Stir bar use	N	N	N	0.51	52.4	N	N	N	0.35	165.5

trt = treatment, exp = experiment, Data mod = data modification, CV = coefficient of variation, S = significant ($P<0.05$), N = not significant.

Binding values in Table 1 were calculated from Klotz plots using the linear regression calculation method. Pearsons correlation coefficient R squared (R^2) was calculated as a measure of plot linearity of the original data (unmodified) and the percent coefficient of variation (% CV) was calculated as a measure of overall variation of the data. Since vials could be sampled only once, duplicate determinations represented individual sampling; therefore, duplicate determinations represented individual observations which made duplicate Klotz plots independent of each other.

In general, data modifications of headspace peak areas had no significant effect compared to the original data. It was assumed that applying linear regression to headspace measurements would reduce variation associated with Klotz plots because headspace measurements were linear ($R^2 > 0.98$) over a range of ligand concentrations. This did not occur. Visual inspection of plots created with raw headspace peak area data that were modified by linear regression prior to calculation of FREE/BOUND values (used to plot Klotz plots) gave the illusion that variation could be reduced by linear regression.

The only significant effect found with respect to data modification was in the azide experiment with actin. However, this result must be ignored because one of the azide concentrations tested was high enough (0.50% sodium azide) to result in a salt effect. Apparently, it is possible to attain good precision associated with the raw data (headspace data), but this does not necessarily mean that there will be good reproducibility of binding values. Data in Table 2 indicate that it is possible to have good precision with the analytical data, but have large standard errors (linear SE(N) and linear SE(K) associated with individual treatments). The reason this standard error was high was in part due to the additive nature of variation. That is, total variation was the sum of its parts. Variation associated with binding values not only included variation associated with the plot (y-intercept and slope variation), but also the increase in variation due to the calculation of standard error associated with binding values using Taylor's expansion.

Table 2. Analysis of Variance (ANOVA) of Individual Treatments on Binding constants N and K and their Associated Standard Errors SE(N) and SE(K).

experiment	Nonlinear N					Nonlinear K				
	trt	Data mod	trt x mod	R^2	% CV	trt	Data mod	trt x mod	R^2	% CV
Salt concentration	S	N	N	0.72	32.2	S	N	N	0.70	80.2
pH	S	N	N	0.98	25.1	S	N	N	0.97	18.1
Actin concentration	N	N	N	0.62	128.0	N	N	N	0.52	154.1
Myosin conc.	S	N	N	0.87	28.4				0.73	24.9
Azide plus myosin	N	N	N	0.44	156.3	N	N	N	0.41	150.9
Azide plus actin	S	N	N	0.83	35.9	S	N	N	0.84	38.9
Stir bar use	S	S	S	0.99	22.8	N	N		0.74	72.9
	Nonlinear SE(N)					Nonlinear SE(K)				
Salt concentration	N	N	N	0.43	97.9	N	N	N	0.44	98.2
pH	S	S	N	0.92	49.2	N	N	N	0.43	192.9
Actin concentration	N	N	N	0.32	363.5	N	N	N	0.53	170.5
Myosin conc.	N	N	N	0.38	98.9	S	N	N	0.54	174.4
Azide plus myosin	N	N	N	0.29	107.3	N	N	N	0.42	200.9
Azide plus actin	N	N	N	0.53	155.6	N	N	N	0.57	75.8
Stir bar use	N	N	N	0.21	121.6	N	N	N	0.32	108.8

trt = treatment, exp = experiment, Data mod = data modification of headspace data, CV = percent coefficient of variation, S = significant ($P<0.05$), N = not significant.

Similar results were found for K; data modification had no significant effect on Klotz constants (K) calculated using the linear regression calculation method. In addition, headspace data modifications (linear regression applied to headspace peak areas prior to calculation of FREE/BOUND values) did not reduce the variation associated with the Klotz constant K. The average precision among K values calculated by the linear regression calculation method was 66%. An average of individual standard errors was calculated to be 139%.

Since the calculation of N involved the y-intercept (N = 1/BOUND) of the Klotz plot, this variation influenced K since N was part of the calculation of K ((K=1/(N)(slope)). Therefore, the Klotz constant K was affected by large variations as was N. The more nonlinear the plot, the poorer the precision.

4.8 Use of Linear verses Nonlinear Regression

In an additional attempt to improve precision associated with Klotz binding values, a Nonlinear Regression method was used. The individual experimental data used to produce Table 1 were recalculated using a nonlinear regression calculation method (16) and the results tabulated in Table 2. Unfortunately, the use of nonlinear regression to calculate binding constants from Klotz plots as opposed to linear calculation was not immediately conclusive. There was no improvement in the average precision (% CV) of binding constants N or K or in their standard errors. However, the regression method affected treatment means. In Figure 4, values of N were calculated by the linear calculation method and also by the nonlinear calculation method, then plotted (linear calculation of N verses nonlinear calculation of N). If there were no differences, the points would be randomly distributed about a 45° line. Treatment means calculated by the nonlinear method were generally higher that if the linear regression method was used.

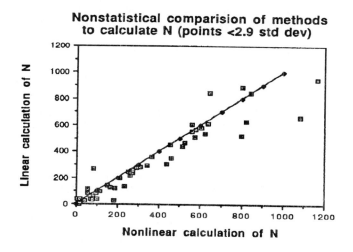

Figure 4. Nonstatistical comparison between calculation methods. Linear verses nonlinear calculation of the number of binding sites (N).

4.9 Effect of protein Concentration

There was an increase in binding with increased protein as would be expected; however, the increase in binding with increased protein was not a direct relationship. Higher protein concentrations disproportionately bound more hexanal than lower protein concentrations. The effect of protein concentration was a complex interaction. Changes in the number of binding sites due to increased concentration were not directly related. Perhaps, agglomerization of myosin at higher concentrations affected binding sites. Changes in myosin solubility due to increased protein concentration would affect binding. The same salt concentration may affect binding differently at higher protein concentrations. Protein concentration had a significant effect on the binding of hexanal to myosin ($P < 0.05$); but not with actin. Binding at protein concentrations as low as 0.10% was considered inadequate. At low protein concentrations there were more undesirable effects encountered with the Klotz plots such as negative slopes and negative intercepts. Binding at concentrations such as 0.22% and 0.44% resulted in few problems with negative Klotz plot slopes. A negative slope results in a negative Klotz constant.

The azide experiment with actin resulted in a significant difference due to concentration; however, this effect was discounted since it was observed from the Klotz constants that there was no trend in the data. The calculation of the Gibb's free energy of interaction is directly affected by the Klotz constant (Gibb's energy = -RTlnK) since it is part of the calculation. Since the conversion of the Klotz constant to the Gibb's free energy constant is a direct calculation, any variation found with K would be the same with the Gibb's constant. Therefore, energy required for binding hexanal to either myosin or actin was not significantly affected by protein concentration.

Myosin has a molecular weight of approximately 520,000 daltons, while actin has a molecular weight of 42,000 daltons. Therefore, in all binding experiments, myosin bound more than actin on a mole basis. Binding calculations are on a molar basis; therefore, the additional binding by myosin is not simply based on the number of molecules or on protein concentration, but rather is due to size. If larger molecules are more hydrophobic, then it is probable that more hydrophobic interactions are involved in the binding of hexanal to large molecules such as myosin.

4.10 Salt Concentration Effects

The salt concentration had a significant effect on the binding of myosin and actin (Table 3). Myosin is a salt-soluble protein; therefore, at high salt concentrations, myosin will salt in (become more soluble). This was reflected in an increase in N with samples having increased salt concentrations. At low salt concentration (0.15 M KCl), myosin precipitated from solution. When myosin was precipitated, less binding sites were available. This was reflected in the lower values of N, the number of binding sites on the protein. N is a dimensionless number which was calculated as the number of moles of ligand bound per mole of protein. Since N is a molar relationship, N can also be used to indicate the number of ligand molecules (hexanal molecules) that are bound to each protein molecule.

Table 3. Effect of Salt Concentration on the Binding of Hexanal to Myosin.

salt concentration (M)	linear calculation method			
	N	SE(N)	K	SE(K)
0.90	598.4[a]	100.4	333[a]	1
0.60	358.2[b]	43.6	-2834[a]	140
0.30	457.5[ab]	25.1	1199[a]	1225
0.15	256.2[c]	26.5	-1700[a]	435

salt concentration (M)	nonlinear calculation method			
	N	SE(N)	K	SE(K)
0.90	729.0[a]	155	4811[a]	1881
0.60	397.9[bc]	58	1106[bc]	572
0.30	591.1[ab]	160	2568[b]	1478
0.15	266.0[c]	46	8[d]	611

salt conc. (M)	Gibb's free energy (kcal/mole)	
	Linear calculation	Nonlinear calculation
0.90	-3.55	-5.19
0.60	4.86	-4.29
0.30	-4.34	-4.80
0.15	4.55	-1.27

Means followed by different letters are significantly different ($P < 0.05$).

Gibb's free energy values were erratic when the linear calculation method was used for calculating values of K. Results of the nonlinear calculation method indicated that myosin in 0.15 M KCl (precipitated myosin), required more energy to bind hexanal than when the myosin was soluble. It was apparent that precipitation of the protein interferes with binding.

Therefore for binding experiments, a salt concentration of 0.6 M KCl was chosen to insure solubility of myosin. Myosin isolation procedures include 0.6 M KCl for solubilizing myosin during extraction and storage (11). In the salt concentration data there were problems with negative values of N (not included in the means) and particularly with K (included in the means) with the linear calculation method. In addition, there were individual binding values that varied greatly from the trend. Values judged as erratic were not included if they differed greatly from the means of other values for the same analysis.

From the salt concentration experiment, it was concluded that salt concentration should be kept constant throughout all experiments. By keeping salt concentration constant throughout all experiments, results among different proteins could be compared. Therefore, the concentration of KCl was kept at 0.6 M KCl in all experiments with myosin and actin.

4.11 Effects due to pH

The pH had a significant effect on the binding of hexanal to myosin (Table 4). When pH was lowered from pH 8.0 to pH 4.0, the amount of hexanal bound to myosin uniformly decreased over the entire pH range. At pH 7.0, myosin was stable (11). At pH 8.0, myosin was denatured and the number of binding sites (N) increased due to unfolding of the myosin chains. Myosin is composed of two heavy chains and 4 light chains that can be separated after denaturation. In acid conditions, particularly at pH 4.0 and 5.0, the myosin was visibly precipitated. Precipitation or agglomeration of myosin resulted in decreased binding sites.

Gibb's free energy of interaction was also affected by pH (Table 4). The energy required for binding decreased in acid conditions (as compared to pH 7.0 where myosin is stable). This was probably due to precipitation of the myosin in acid conditions. In alkali (pH 8.0) some unfolding may have occurred due to denaturation. Unfolding exposed more binding sites thereby resulting in increased binding. The energy required for binding decreased with increasing pH. Since myosin was stable at pH 7.0 (11), it is recommended that binding experiments involving myosin be carried out at pH 7.0 in an effort to avoid pH effects.

4.12 Effect of Protein Concentration

The effect of protein concentration on the binding of hexanal with myosin and actin was inconclusive (Table 5). There was an increase in binding with increased protein as would be expected; however, the increase in binding with increased protein was not a direct relationship. Higher protein concentrations disproportionately bound more hexanal than lower protein concentrations. The influence of protein concentration on binding is complex. Changes in the number of binding sites due to increased protein concentration were not directly related. Perhaps, agglomerization of myosin at higher concentrations affected binding sites. Changes in myosin solubility due to increased protein concentration would affect binding. The same salt concentration may affect binding differently at higher protein concentrations. Protein concentration had a significant effect on the binding of hexanal to myosin ($P < 0.05$); but not with actin.

Table 4. Effect of pH on the Binding of Hexanal to Myosin.

pH	Linear Calculation Method			
	N	SE(N)	K	SE(K)
8	984.6[a]	70.8	342[b]	31280
7	477.9[b]	35.7	788[a]	58734
6	157.6[c]	23.9	64[b]	1102
5	62.1[cd]	12.7	-1264[d]	59
4	28.6[d]	18.1	-381[c]	13

pH	Nonlinear Calculation Method			
	N	SE(N)	K	SE(K)
8	1395.0[a]	325	6092[a]	2019
7	497.8[b]	70	724[b]	469
6	210.4[c]	77	-2126[c]	2093
5	61.0[cd]	31	-2838[c]	2733
4	18.5[d]	189	1044[b]	4148

pH	Gibb's free energy (kcal/mole)	
	Linear calculation	Nonlinear calculation
8	-3.57	-5.33
7	-4.08	-4.03
6	-2.55	4.69
5	4.37	4.86
4	3.64	-4.25

Means followed by different letters are significantly different ($P < 0.05$).

Table 5. Binding of Hexanal to Actin and Myosin at several protein concentrations.

Protein	ligand	Protein (%)	N	Linear calculation method		
				SE(N)	K	SE(K)
actin	hexanal	0.22	28.3[a]	19	1729[a]	0
		0.44	132.3[a]	64	72[b]	0
myosin	hexanal	0.11	117.3[b]	19	-2190[b]	67
		0.22	221.3[b]	89	-819[b]	139
		0.44	612.4[a]	30	5043[a]	2890
				Nonlinear calculation method		
actin	hexanal	0.22	53.9[a]	28	11347[a]	13269
		0.44	464.7[a]	6077	121986[a]	66167
myosin	hexanal	0.11	142.7[b]	34	-1151[b]	243
		0.22	213.1[b]	139	-1372[b]	2139
		0.44	634.1[a]	66	330[a]	129

Means followed by different letters within a protein group are significantly different ($P < 0.05$).

4.13 Effect of Sodium Azide Concentration

Sodium azide concentration (0.05 - 0.20%) had no effect on the binding of hexanal to myosin; however, an effect was found associated with the actin experiment (Table 6). Azide is commonly used as an antimicrobial inhibitor. Since, myosin is denatured by drying or freezing, azide was used as a preservative of myosin when it was stored in aqueous solution at 4°C. There was no significant differences between azide concentrations of 0% and 0.1%; however, there was a significant difference with the 0.5% concentration. Most likely the increase in binding to actin was actually a salt effect. Therefore, it was concluded that azide did not affect binding when used at low levels.

Table 6. Effect of Sodium Azide Concentration on the Binding of Hexanal to Myosin or Actin.

Protein	Azide (%)	Linear calculation method			
		N	SE(N)	K	SE(K)
actin	0.00	80.2^b	5	326^a	21
	0.10	130.0^b	87	19^b	0
	0.50	403.2^a	183	15^b	12
myosin	0.05	737.3^a	117	138^a	1126
	0.10	650.0^a	689	289^a	1
	0.20	583.3^a	143	549^a	2
		Nonlinear calculation method			
actin	0.00	93.2^b	18	6521^b	2091
	0.10	204.6^{ab}	37	17420^{ab}	3615
	0.50	320.3^a	175	20813^a	7930
myosin	0.05	845.3^a	911	6779^a	5528
	0.10	672.4^a	152	4166^a	2002
	0.20	495.3^a	580	2819^a	4030

Means followed by different letters within a column for each protein are significantly different ($P < 0.05$).

	Azide (%)	Gibb's free energy (kcal/mole)	
		linear calculation	nonlinear calculation
actin	0.00	-3.54	-5.38
	0.10	-1.80	-5.98
	0.50	-1.66	-6.08
myosin	0.05	-3.02	-5.40
	0.10	-3.47	-5.10
	0.20	-3.86	-4.86

4.14 Effect of Magnetic Stirring Using a Stir Bar

The use of a small stir bar inside sealed headspace vials had no effect on binding results (Table 7). The advantage of using a stir bar was to insure that the protein was homogeneously saturated with ligand. However, the use of a stir bar could disrupt the air/water equilibrium in the vial. Volatile ligands could be forced out of solution due to the stirring agitation and would enrich the headspace. This could lead to headspace saturation problems and a shift in equilibration could affect results.

Table 7. Effect of Magnetic Stirring on the Binding of Hexanal to Actin.

Stir bar used	Linear calcualtion method			
	N	SE(N)	K	SE(K)
yes	31.3^a	5	203^a	6
no	62.6^a	7	255^a	4

Means followed by different letters within a column are significantly different ($P < 0.05$).

For binding experiments, magnetic stirring was not used. The experiment to test stir bar use was carried out at room temperature since there was no practical way to simultaneously stir vials while submerged in a water bath. Also, there was no way to standardize magnetic stirrer operation to insure uniform rates of stirring.

4.15 Effect of Reusing Headspace Septa

Headspace septa became expensive to use when only one could be used per determination. Headspace septa are punctured during sampling. When reused, volatiles escaped through the first puncture hole and could be detected by smelling which represented a significant loss of headspace volatiles (Table 8). Pressurization was normally 35 pounds per square inch gas (PSIG) which resulted in leakage. The precision of headspace sampling is directly related to constant pressure control. Vials were pressurized to the same pressure that the gas chromatograph column was operating. Any reuse of headspace septa would invalidate results due to the massive loss of headspace volatiles.

5. SUGGESTED EXPERIMENTAL CONDITIONS FOR EQUILIBRIUM HEADSPACE SAMPLING

The following experimental conditions should be kept constant for all studies of binding of volatile ligands by muscle proteins: salt concentration, 0.6 M KCl; pH buffered to pH 7.0; azide concentration, 0.05%; and that protein concentration should be kept constant in experiments at approximately 0.2% to 0.44% protein. In addition, magnetic stirring is not necessary when 9-10 ml size headspace vials are used with 1.0 ml sample volumes.

Table 8. Effect of Reusing Septa on the Binding of Hexanal to Myosin or Actin.

Protein	Septa use	Linear calculation method			
		N	SE(N)	K	SE(K)
myosin	first use	917.6[a]	22	735	336
	second use	-1.8[b]	3428	-1568	0
actin	first use	129.6[a]	22	38	1115
	second use	4.8[b]	257	-157	38
		Nonlinear calculation method			
myosin	first use	749.3[a]	73	4342	583
	second use	-3428.5[b]	-268	-4465	64
actin	first use	58.8[a]	-140	1684	6981
	second use	-1.0[a]	1804	-4508	257

Percent protein for myosin was 0.22% and 0.41% for actin.

REFERENCES

1   J.E. Kinsella and S. Damodaran, in: G. Charalambous (Ed), The Analysis and Control of Less Desirable Flavors in Foods and Beverages, Academic Press Inc, New York, 1980, pp. 95-131.

2   J.E. Kinsella, Inform 1 (1990) 215-226.

3   H Kim and D.B. Min, in: D.B. Min and T.H. Smouse (Eds), Flavor Chemistry of Lipid Foods, The American Oil Chemists Society, Champaign, IL, 1989. pp. 404-421.

4   L.A. Wilson, in: M.R. Okos (Ed), Physical and Chemical Properties of Food. ASAE Publication 09-86. American Society of Agricultural Engineers, St. Joseph, MI, 1986, pp. 382-395.

5   S. Damodaran and J.E. Kinsella, J. Agric. Food Chem. 28 (1980) 567-571.

6   S. Damodaran and J.E. Kinsella, J. Agric. Food Chem. 29 (1981) 1249-1253.

7   S. Damodaran and J.E. Kinsella, J. Agric. Food Chem. 29 (1991) 1253-1257.

8   R.G. Einig, Interaction of Meat Aroma Volatiles with Soy Proteins. Ph.D. Dissertation, University of Missouri--Columbia, Missouri, 1983.

9   S.F. O'Keefe, Binding of Volatile Flavor Compounds to Purified Soy Proteins in an Aqueous Model System. Ph.D. Dissertation. Iowa State University, Ames, Iowa,1988.

10 S.F. O'Keefe, L.A. Wilson, A.P. Resurreccion and P.A. Murphy, J. Agric. Food Chem. 39 (1991) 1022-1028.

11 S.S. Margossian and S. Lowey, Methods in Enzymology 85 (1982) 55-71.

12 J.O. Pardee and J.A. Spudich, Methods in Enzymology 85 (1982) 164-181.

13 C.E. Meloan and Y. Pomeranz, in: Food Analysis Laboratory Experiments, Second Edition, The AVI Publishing Company, Inc., Westport, Connecticut, pp. 102-110, 1980.

14 R.A. Gutheil, Interaction of Warmed-Over Flavor Volatiles and Myofibrillar Proteins. Ph.D. Dissertation. University of Missouri--Columbia.

15 S.F. O'Keefe, Personal Communication, Iowa State University, Department of Food Technology, Ames, IA. September, 1987.

16 P. Murphy, Nonlinear regression program written for an Apple II computer by Pat Murphy, professor, Iowa State University, Department of Food Technology, Ames, IA. Compiled from G.N. Wilkinson (17), 1989.

17 G.N. Wilkinson, Biochem. J. 80 (1961) 324-332.

18 G.F. Krause, Personal communication. University of Missouri Agriculture Experiment Station Statistician, Columbia, MO, 1990.

19 G.W. Sedecor and W.G. Cochran, Statistical Methods, Eighth edition, Iowa State University Press, Ames, IA, 1989.

20 M.E. Bailey, H.P. Dupuy and M.G. Legendre, in: G. Charalambous (Ed), The Analyses and Control of Less Desirable Flavors in Foods and Beverages, Academic Press, New York, pp. 31-52, 1980.

21 H.P. Dupuy, M.E. Bailey, A.J. St Angelo, M.E. Legendre and J.R. Vercellotti, in: Warmed-Over Flavor of Meat, A.J. St Angelo and M.E. Bailey (Eds), Academic Press, Orlando, FL, pp. 165-191, 1987.

22 S-Y, Shin-Lee, Warmed-Over Flavor and its Prevention by Maillard Reaction Products, Ph.D. Dissertation, University of Missouri--Columbia, MO, 1988.

23 A. Coladarci and T. Coladarci, Elementary Descriptive Statistics. For Those Who Think They Can't, Wadsworth Publishing Company, Belmont, CA, pp. 50-66, 1980.

24 B.P. Korin, Introduction to Statistical Methods, Winthrop Publishers, Cambridge, MA, pp. 53-72, 1977.

25 B. Kolb, D. Boege and L.S. Ettre, Am. Lab. 20 (1988) 33-44.

26 S. Arai, in: J.R. Whitaker and M. Fujimaki (Eds), Chemical Deterioration of Proteins, ACS Symposium Series 123, American Chemical Society, Washington, D.C., pp.195-209, 1980.

27 K. A. Conners, Binding Constants. The measurement of molecular complex stability., John Wiley & Sons, Inc., New York, pp. 21-101.

SUBJECT INDEX

A

Acetaldehyde, "freshness"
in processed foods, 1
Agaricus
  bisporus, aromagrams, 252
  campestris, submerged culture, 229-238
    effect of
      different nitrogen sources, 233
      yeast extract concentrations, 236
Alcohol oxidase, enzyme systems, 2
Alcoholic
  beverage analysis, multidimentional
  GC system, 351-369
  beverages, aged, compounds in, 469-470
  fermentation, raisin extract, 475-489
Algin-restructured beef, consumer
acceptability, 723-729
Alkylthiophene, formation
mechanism, 739
Amioca, effective water
diffusivity, 333, 334, 336, 337
Anise bread, volatiles in vapor
of, 179-181
Anti-Markovnikov addition, 86
Antioxidants, alternates to
synthetic, 27-42
  tocopherols, mixed, 31
Aroma
  Chinese scented green tea, 347-350
  compounds, formation of, computer
  aided organic synthesis, 75-97
  formation, by hydrolysis of
  glycosidically bound compounds, 99-114
  production of *P. italicum*, effect
  of carbon and nitrogen sources on
  115-122
Aseptic processing, particulate
foods, 665-677

B

Baked potato aroma, influence of
variety/clone, 537-541
Beer aroma
  extract, chemical composition, 423
  extraction procedure, 406
Beers, unhopped and hopped, sensory/
analytical evaluation of, 403-426

Binding of hexanal by myosin and
actin, 783-820
Biotechnological processes
  microbially catalysed oxidation
  system, 1-14
  (4R)-(+)-Limonene, enzymatic hydration
  to (4R)-(+)-alpha Terpineol, 571-584
  interesterification of palm oil
  triacylglycerols by lipase, 585-593
Birch syrup, flavor compounds in, 133
Bombardment, fast atom, of glycosides,
103-106
Bramble dried leaf volatiles, 145-152
  influence of variety and growth
  location on, 151
Buchu leaf oil analysis, 361-363

C

Candida utilis, acetaldehyde and
ethyl acetate production, 1
Capsaicinoids, analogue composition
of commercial products, 526-529
Carbon dioxide, supercritical,
separations in soybean processing, 595-616
N-Carboxymethylchitosan, preparation
and use in meat flavor deterioration 711-722
  composition and properties, 715-718
  dose response in beef patties, 721
  effect on beef flavor, 720
  preparation, 712-715
  synthesis flow chart, 714
  use as an antioxidant, 718-720
Carotenoid composition of *Eugenia
uniflora* and *Malpighia glabra*, 643-650
Cathechins and proanthocyanidins,
in grape seeds, extractability of, 437-450
Chardonnay seeds, epicatechin and
procyanidin in, 444, 444-446
CharmAnalysis, 372
Cheese, Turkish white pickled, microbial
changes in ripening, 491-498
Cucumber pickles, processing of,
problems in, 499-513
Chicken meat, extrusion cooking
with non-meat ingredients, 761-782
Cocoa butter-like fats, biotechnological
production, 585-593

Coffee, soluble, new biotechnology, 341-346
Citrus aurantium, 347-350
Colossoma macropomum, fatty acid composition of, 633-642
  moisture and lipid contents, 637
    neutral lipids, 640
    phospholipids, 641
    total lipids, 638
Computer
  aided organic synthesis, 75-97
  simulation, chemical kinetics of flavor compounds in heated foods, 123-130
Corn starch, effect of on chicken meat extrusion cooking, 768-770
Cottonseed protein, new edible food products, 43-74
  cottonseed characteristics, 44-50
  gossypol removal, 50-55

D

Dairy products, cottonseed, 66
Dealcoholization of wines, by
  column rectification, 455-456
  flash evaporation, 454-455
Dealcoholized wines, storage stability of, 451-468
Diabetes: food, nutrition, diet and weight control, 679-694
Dialkylthiophenes, formation of, in Maillard reactions, 731-741
Diallyl sulfide, thermal degradation of, 75-97
Diels-Alder reaction, new products prediction by, 79-91
Dried distilled grains, in spaghetti products, 551-563

E

Emulsions, food, in extruded glassy materials, 651-664
Encapsulated flavors, in food glassy substances, 651-661
Ethanol to acetaldehyde, batch bioconversion, 13
Ethyl carbamate determination, in whisky, 364-366
Eugenia uniflora, carotenoid composition of, 645, 646, 648, 649

Extruded glassy material containing corn syrup and maltodextrins,
  DSC thermogram, 655
  TMA softening profile, 656
Extrusion
  cooking of chicken meat, 761-782
  corn starch/soy protein blends, 515-518

F

Fatty acid solubility isotherms in supercritical carbon dioxide, as a function of
  density, 608
  pressure, 605
Fermentation of
  cucumbers, 500, 509
  raisin extract, 477
Flavor
  compounds in
    birch syrup, 133
    heated foods, 123-130
    maple syrup, 131-140
  gas chromatography, purge and trap assembly, 207
  retention, mushrooms, in microwave-hot air drying, 249-256
  roasted peanuts, 211-227
    correlation with
      FID active chemical compounds, GC, 217-218
      FPD active chemical compounds, GC, 220
    intensity across the degrees of roast, 225-227
  stability, model salad, effect of glucose oxidase-catalase on, 617-631
  umami vs. salty, preference, 565-570
  industry, biotechnology-based, 1-14
Flavorant, added, effect on
  binding during extrusion, 519-525
  starch/protein interactions during extrusion processing, 515-518
Flavoring compounds, naturally derived, 1-14
Flavours, salty and umami, comparison 565-570
Florunner peanuts
  direct GC, 189, 190, 193, 208
  purge and trap, 194, 195, 209
  sulfur compounds in, 196, 197
  thresholds for FID compounds, 199
      - FPD compounds, 200
Food volatiles, rapid monitoring method, 141-144

Furaneol in wine, 358-360

G

GC
 olfactometry, hop varieties, 394
 MSD multifunctional system, alcoholic beverage analysis, 351-369
Glassy materials, extruded, food emulsions in, 651-664
Gliadin-water interactions, 303-311
Glucose oxidase-catalase, effects on model salad flavor stability, 617-631
Gossypol, 43, 50-55
Grape seeds, catechins and proanthocyanidins in, 437-450

H

Hallertauer Mittelfrüh hops
 hopping of beers with, 404-425
 oxygenated fractions of, 371-402
Hedonic scores, soup formulations
 Malaysian and Scottish assessors, 568
 Scottish assessors, 569
Hop oil oxygenated fractions
 chemical composition, 390-391
 sensory/analytical evaluation, 371-402
Hops and hop extracts
 chemical composition of, 375, 381
 contaminants in, 430

I

Inverse gas chromatography
 moisture sorption by wheat and soy flour, 277-286
 setup equipment, lysozyme and gliadin studies, 291
 PVC and VCM interaction, 257-276
 water vapor diffusion through plastics packaging materials, 321-327
Isomers, closely eluting, preparative separation of, 366-368

L

Lard induction time in, 33
Lecithin addition, effect of, on interesterification of palm oil mid fraction, 585-593
Light wine, 453-454

(4R)-(+)-Limonene, enzymatic hydration to (4R)-(+)-alpha-Terpineol, 571-584
Linalool in
 dried bramble leaves, 145, 147
 P. italicum isolate, 115-122
 lulo pulp, 171
Lysozyme-water interactions, 287-302
Lipid oxidation, meat flavor quality, 697-699, 706
Lipase, immobilized, interesterification of palm oil mid fraction, 585-593
Listeria
 behavior in meat and poultry products, 751-752
 fate in meat products, 743-760
 monocytogenes, effect on destruction of, sodium chloride, temperature, curing ingredients, 754
 listeriosis from meat, 748-749
Lulo, 163, 172-173
 components in, 170-171
 pulp GC profiles, 172-173

M

Maillard reactions, dialkyl thiophenes, formation in, 731-741
Maple syrup, flavor compounds in, 131-140
Malpighia glabra, carotenoid composition of, 647-649
Meat flavor
 deterioration, N-carboxymethyl chitosan in prevention of, 711-722
 quality, current approaches to the study of, 695-709
Microflora evolution, Turkish white pickled cheese, 494, 496
Microwave-assisted process, 141-144
Momordica charantia L., volatiles from seeds of, 153-161
Multi column switching GC system GERSTEL, 353-358 - applications
 closely eluting isomers, 366-368
 diastomeric ratioing, 361-363
 ethyl carbamate, in whisky, 364
 furanenol in wine, 358-360
Mushroom
 edible, growth of
  Agaricus campetris, 229-237
  Pleurotus ostreatus, 239-248
 flavor, retention in microwave-

hot air drying, 249-256
Myosin and actin, binding of
hexanal, method for determining 783-815

N

Nitrate, mass balance, in
brewing industry, 427-436
 levels in
  brewing raw materials, 434
  malt and adjuncts, 431
Non-meat ingredients, effect of,
on chicken meat extrusion cooking
 corn starch, 768-770
 oat fiber, 771-773
 soy
  flour, 778-780
  protein isolate, 773-775
  concentrate, 775-778

O

Oat fiber, effect of on chicken
meat extrusion cooking, 771-773
Odor active peaks, GC olfactometry
 beers, hopped/unhopped, 420-421
 hop varieties, 394
Off-flavor compounds, removal
from soybean flour, supercritical
carbon dioxide, 598-599, 602-603, 612
Oil droplets in water, particle
size analysis, probability area
density graphs, 659, 669
Oleic acid, extraction from
oleic acid/olive oil mixtrues, 610
Osme technique for odor activity
evaluation of GC eluates, 372, 373, 379, 388
Osmegrams and FID chromatograms, 392, 393
Oxygen, dissolved, depletion in
salad dressings, effects of
 glucose, 627
 pH, 623
 temperature, 625

P

Palm oil, mid fraction, interesterification, 585-593
Particulate foods, aseptic
processing of, 665-677

PCA graphs
 beers brewed with various hops, 415
 hop oil oxygenated fractions, 383
Peach drink, acceptability, influence
of cultivar and processing, 531-536
Peanut, roasted, flavor quality
estimated from correlation of
 butter control, volatiles profiles
 replication, 188
 GC volatiles and
 roast color, 183-209
 sensory flavor attributes, 211-227
Penicillium italicum, growth and
aroma production of, 115-122
Pichia pastoris, biological oxidation
process
 alcohol oxidase enzyme system, 2
 bioconversion of ethanol to
 acetaldehyde, 5
 catabolite inactivation of, 12, 13
 growth, correlation with alcohol
 oxidase activity, 5
 temperature effect on, 8, 9, 10
 tris buffer concentration effect on, 9, 10
Plastics packaging materials, water
vapor diffusion through, 321-327
Pleurotus ostreatus, growth/biomass
composition, 239-248
Potato starch and egg albumin, sorption
isotherms, 319
Potentiators, flavor, 565-570
Popcorn popping quality, effect of
properties, 543-549
Prerigor beef muscle, 785
Protein concentration, effect on
binding of hexanal, 808-810
Proteins, selective of flavorants, 783
Pyrazines, in baked potatoes, 540-541

R

Raisin extract, alcoholic fermentation, 475-489
Rancidity inhibitors, 37
L-Rhamnosidase, 110-113
Rosemary/ascorbic system, 91
Rosemary phenolics, 34-37, 91

S

Salad, model, flavor stability, effect
of glucose oxidase-catalase, 617-631
Sorption, moisture by wheat and soy

flour by IGC, 277-286
SOS program, 75-97
Salt concentration, effect on binding of myosin and actin, 808-809
Sampling for equilibrium headspace, experimental conditions, 813-814
SAS program, 788-789
Saturation and Klotz plots, hexanal, 795, 796, 803, 807, 808
SDS PAGE electrophoresis, 786
- gel scans, 786
Sodium azide concentration, effect on hexanal binding to myosin, 812
Soy, effect on chicken meat extrusion cooking
  fiber, 771-773
  flour, 778-780
  protein
    concentrate, 775-778
    isolate, 773-775
Soybean processing, supercritical carbon dioxide separations, 595-616
Spaghetti products containing dried distillers grains, 551-563
  attributed evaluation, 561-562
  proximate compositions, 557
Stearic acid, interesterification with palm oil triacy glycerols by immobilized lipase, 585-593

T

Tea, chinese, green, aroma of, 347-350
Alpha-Terpineol dehydratase, 571-583
Thiazole standards, recoveries, GC/MS, 703
Thiazolidine, pyrolysis, 733
Thiazolidinecarboxylic acids,
  mass spectral data, 735
  pyrolysis products, 737
Thiophene, NMR data, 737
Tocopherols, 30
Triacylglycerols, palm oil mid fraction, interesterification, 585-593
Turkey's range test, 622-625, 627, 629, 630

U

Umami flavor, 565-570

Urtica species,
  amino acid composition, 20
  fatty composition, 21
  macronutrient composition of seeds, 19
  vitamins and mineral composition, 22

V

Van Deemter curves, PVC/polymeric plasticizer, 326-327
Volatiles in
  anise white bread, 175-182
  birch syrup, 133
  bramble dried leaf, 145-148
  food, rapid monitoring method, 141-144
  glycosidically bound, in apricot and grapes, 100-102, 107
  maple syrup, 131-140
  Momorica charantia L., seeds from, 153-161
  naranjilla fruit, 163-174
  roasted peanuts, 183-227

W

Warmed-over flavor
  beef patties, 40
  chicken nuggets, 39
Water sorptional behavior
  gliadin-water interactions, 303-311
  lysozyme-water interactions, 287-302
  potato starch and eg albumin, 313-319
Wheat and soy flour
  proximate analysis, 278
  water sorption isotherma, 279-282
Whey protein as non-meat ingredient in chicken meat extrusion cooking, 766-768
Whisky, ethyl carbamate in, 364-366
Wine
  catechins and proanthocyanidins in, 440-441, 446-448
  furaneol in, 358-360
Wine-like beverages, 451-468
  analytical characteristics, light vs. original wines, 458
  microbial content, 459

Y

Yeasts, methylotrophic, 3